ANNUAL REVIEW OF PHYSIOLOGY

ANNUAL REVIEW OF PHYSIOLOGY

JULIUS H. COMROE, JR., *Editor*
University of California Medical Center, San Francisco

I. S. EDELMAN, *Associate Editor*
University of California Medical Center, San Francisco

RALPH R. SONNENSCHEIN, *Associate Editor*
University of California, Los Angeles

VOLUME 35

1973

ANNUAL REVIEWS INC.
4139 EL CAMINO WAY
PALO ALTO, CALIFORNIA 94306, USA

ANNUAL REVIEWS INC.

PALO ALTO, CALIFORNIA, USA

© 1973 BY ANNUAL REVIEWS INC.
ALL RIGHTS RESERVED

International Standard Book Number 0–8243–0335–0
Library of Congress Catalog Card Number 39–15404

Assistant Editor: Christina M. Smillie
Indexers: Victor E. Hall, Frances M. Hall,
Mary Glass, Leigh Dowling
Compositor: George Banta Co., Inc.

PRINTED AND BOUND IN THE UNITED STATES OF AMERICA
BY GEORGE BANTA COMPANY, INC.

PREFACE

Dr. Arthur Giese, who has been Associate Editor of this Review since 1947, has retired from this position. We wish to express our deep appreciation for his invaluable advice and editorial assistance throughout all these years, and wish him well.

The Editors, with Dr. Giese's successor, Dr. I. S. Edelman, look forward to continued fruitful collaboration with our Editorial Committee and ever-changing group of dedicated authors.

The most important task of the Editorial Committee is the selection of subjects to be reviewed and of authors to write the chapters. This has become more difficult over the years. One reason is the growing number and complexity of scientific papers. In 1939, when Volume 1 of the *Annual Review of Physiology* appeared, one physiologist was expected to and did review all of the advances in Respiration, another all of those in Endocrine Glands, a third all of the reports on the Digestive System, and a fourth, all of Blood (including blood cells, plasma, and blood coagulation); only the Nervous System required specialists, each reviewing one component: Brain, Spinal Cord and Reflexes, Nerve, and Autonomic Nervous System. Almost every branch of physiology in 1973 is as large and complex as the nervous system was in 1939 and now requires three or four reviewers to evaluate critically the several aspects of the field. This, in many cases, requires scheduling reviews of some organ systems over a three year period.

The job of the Editorial Committee has also become more difficult because of the increased number of other *Annual Reviews,* and the fact that some of these, with some justification, regard certain aspects of Physiology as parts of their own disciplines; the boundaries between Physiology and Medicine, Pharmacology, Biochemistry, Biophysics and Bioengineering, and Psychology are often difficult to delineate. In addition, more review journals have been started and more non-review journals have begun to publish review articles in the last decade. This trend has increased our confidence in the importance of reviews and in the necessity for thoughtful planning so that they appear at appropriate intervals and at the most advantageous times. But to achieve this, and to avoid overworking a limited number of critical, and willing, reviewers, requires knowledge of the schedules both of the reviews planned by the editors of many volumes and journals and of the reviewers who write for these publications. To help in this planning we ask the help of the Editors of other *Annual Reviews* and of *Physiological Reviews*. The result is usually imperfect even with excellent intentions, because, at times, the increasing responsibilities of scientists interfere with the completion of reviews in the year scheduled. We welcome your telling us how well we have succeeded in meeting your needs and how we might do better.

We express our sincere appreciation to the authors of our reviews, who spent a considerable amount of time reading a voluminous literature, selecting and analyzing papers, and writing these critical reviews.

We also express our appreciation to our capable Assistant Editor Christina Smillie for careful editing of manuscripts to clarify obscure or awkward phrases and to correct errors in references, spelling and grammar; we are grateful to her even when authors are not.

JHC
ISE
RRS

CONTENTS

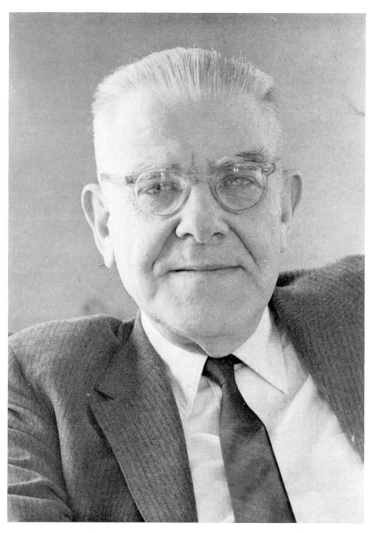

Philip Bard

Ann. Rev. Physiol. 1973. 35:1–16

THE ONTOGENESIS OF ONE PHYSIOLOGIST 1087

Philip Bard

*Professor Emeritus of Physiology, The Johns Hopkins University
School of Medicine, Baltimore, Maryland*

The circumstances that determine the choice of a career form a fascinating subject for speculation in the realm of human psychology. Few generals have duplicated George S. Patton's almost neonatally developed ambition to become a soldier (my father appointed him to West Point), and I have encountered only one physician or surgeon who cannot recall the time when he did not expect to be a doctor. During long service on committees charged with the selection of medical students, I have interviewed hundreds of young people who had decided to study medicine. After a couple of years of this duty I concluded that little was to be gained by asking the trite and obvious question: "Why do you want to be a doctor?" Many, including not a few who went on to successful careers in scientific medicine, were unable to give any very definite answer. I learned to regard this as a better omen than a flowery profession of a desire to help mankind. When I put the same question to a number of senior clinical colleagues I usually got an answer which indicated that some rather trivial incident had directed their attention to the idea of studying medicine. Thereafter some ill-defined inner urge sufficed to potentiate the original slightly supraliminal stimulus. That is surely an effective form of motivation.

Joseph Erlanger (5) has told us that the idea of medicine as an occupation came to him from an older sister "who, in my youth, had nicknamed me Doc because of my interest in lower forms of life." A noted clinical microbiologist told me that he went to medical school because of the impact of an incident related in a book for children he had read at the age of eight: the recovery of a child from a severe head injury without any specific treatment! Sometimes discouragement encountered in attempting another *metier* serves to lower the threshold for an excitatory suggestion that medicine may be a way out. Such was the case of Claude Bernard, whose literary activities during his apprenticeship to an apothecary in Lyon caused his employer to request that the young man be restored to his parents. The story has been beautifully told by Olmsted (7). Although disenchanted with the rolling of pills and preparing certain compounds—including shoe polish—Bernard had been much interested in what he saw when he delivered drugs to a nearby veteri-

1

nary school, an interest which surely adumbrated his later classical excursions in animal experimentation. During the subsequent year of unemployment he wrote a play which, when submitted to a famous Parisian critic, elicited the comment "You have done some pharmacy, study medicine. You have not the temperament of a dramatist." These were the circumstances that launched the career of the greatest physiologist of the nineteenth century. I hope it will not be out of place to relate how I became a student of the foremost American physiologist of the first half of the twentieth century. To do that properly I must present some early autobiographical information.

I was born in 1898 a mile from the then somnolent village of Hueneme on the coast of Ventura County, California. This place, once the most active town in the county, had developed in connection with a wharf that my father, Thomas R. Bard, had built in 1871 to make possible the shipping of grain and other farm products which were beginning to appear as the Hispanic pastoral use of the land gave way to an agriculture plied by Anglo-Americans. Three years later he had built a house and begun a garden of trees, flowering plants, and shrubs, which shortly became an oasis in a large treeless plain—and an acceptable residence for the eighteen year old bride he brought there in 1876. My mother was a native of San Francisco, where her father had arrived in 1850, eight years before her birth, and founded the *Evening Bulletin*. Her older sister had married my father's younger brother, Dr. Cephas L. Bard, a pioneer California physician (of whom more presently).

Shortly after the beginning of American participation in World War II my home was taken over permanently by the United States Navy and made the Pacific headquarters of the famous Seabees. There remain few traces of the erstwhile beauty, charm, and botanical distinction of its forty odd acres. The surrounding area which in my youth consisted of orchards and fields of alfalfa and sugar beets is now a maze of houses on small lots constituting the city of Port Hueneme. The newer name is the result of the building of a true harbor, a nonprofit undertaking originated and completed by my brother Richard. It was finished just in time to become a major outlet of supplies for the Pacific phase of the war. All these developments took place on land that had been a part of a Mexican grant which, along with six other *ranchos* in Ventura County, had come sight unseen into the possession of Thomas A. Scott of Philadelphia, Assistant Secretary of War during the Civil War and Vice President of the Pennsylvania Railroad. It was Scott who sent my father to California.

My father, born in Chambersburg, Pennsylvania, in 1841, graduated during his eighteenth year from the local Academy with a thorough reading knowledge of Greek and Latin and such a foundation in mathematics that fifty years later he was able with ease and clarity to tutor my older brother in calculus. A decline in the financial situation of his widowed mother led him to refuse a scholarship to Princeton College and to go to work, first as a surveyor and then as a business assistant to an uncle in Hagerstown, Maryland. With the beginning of the Civil War he managed to combine business with support of the Union cause by acting as a dispatcher of military rolling stock, as a military telegrapher, and as an occasional source of military information he obtained during excursions by horse or handcar into Confederate territory. It was these activities that attracted the attention of T. A. Scott, who at that time was seeking a personal representative to protect his interests in California and to determine the validity of certain claims—especially one made by Professor Benjamin Silliman, Jr., of Yale, that enormous deposits of petroleum lay beneath the surface of Scott's lands.

It was late in 1864 when my father arrived in California, via Panama, to begin a career that encompassed many activities and exerted no small influence on the agricultural, economic, and political development of the state. His biographer has written (4) that T. R. Bard's was "a life compounded of many stories and distinguished by that grace under pressure which marks any man who has it as worth knowing." He explored Scott's properties for oil, boring five dry wells before bringing in California's first "gusher," but the lack of a nearby market lead to the abandonment of any serious follow-up of this success. He then focused his energies on the sale of Scott's many acres, a task made difficult by the need to clear, under American law, titles based on Mexican grants. Finally, by personally making credit available at low interest rates, he was able to implement his long range view that these large tracts should be partitioned to provide farms for many buyers rather than large holdings for a few. This was the first of many acts that gained for him the trust and respect of the inhabitants of that region. Later his influence became statewide largely because he led a vigorous opposition to the control by the Southern Pacific Railroad of both the California Republican Party and the State government. This activity was the chief factor in his election by the legislature in 1900 to the United States Senate. He had been a reluctant candidate and he neither enjoyed nor admired most of what he found in Washington. A really conservative Republican who opposed every effort to bestow privilege on special interests, he did much to check the exploitation of the public domain, supported the efforts of Gifford Pinchot in conservation, and, for good physiographic and economic reasons, led the opposition to the admission of the territories of Arizona and New Mexico as a single state, thus adding one star to the flag. He made no personal effort to be re-elected and his old enemy, the Southern Pacific Railroad, saw to it that he was not. But he continued the fight that was finally won with the election of Hiram Johnson to the governorship in 1910. Earlier he had acquired some lands and an interest in the forerunners of the Union Oil Company, of which he became the first president and from which he withdrew because of his dislike of the policies of the controlling interest. It is ironic that no oil was ever produced on his property or that of his descendants. After several long illnesses he died in 1915 during my sixteenth year. Of the many tributes perhaps the best was that of a newspaper publisher who had both supported and opposed his policies: "Of all her posessions California had none more valuable than his consistent, upright, instructive life" (4).

I have devoted much space to my father's life because my thinking about myself has been directed to a considerable extent by the impact of his actions and character. Although I saw less of him than did my four older sisters and two older brothers, I discerned through the veil of his dignified reserve his fairness, kindliness, affection, and even some confidence that I might sometime do something well. My childhood at home was in a country setting with horses and dogs and much unoccupied space in which to move. When I was ten my father taught me to handle a rifle properly and encouraged straight shooting by an agreement that I would get five cents for every garden-raiding jack rabbit I hit in the head—and would forfeit twenty-five cents for each extracranial hit. A sister, the youngest of the four but ten years my senior, who could break and train any horse, taught me to ride. My brothers tutored me in the art of catching a baseball behind a plate and a batter. But these pleasant activities were mainly during vacations, for at eight I was sent to a very good school in Pasadena. It was conducted by Miss Virginia Pease (later my stepmother-in-law), a fabulous person who left her imprint on many young people. The gratifying aspects of my five years there were attenuated only by the lady in whose home I boarded; she was a Christian Scientist who spent almost as much time praying over her epileptic cat as she did doubting my veracity. Then in 1913 I entered the Thacher School in the Ojai Valley of Ventura County. Founded in 1889 by Mr. Sherman Day Thacher of New Haven and Yale College, it was small, required each student to own, care for, and ride a horse, and provided a good scholastic preparation for college. Mr. Thacher dominated the school by engendering in the boys and many of the teachers a fine blend of anxiety, respect, and admiration. His personality and his philosophy of life exerted a lifelong effect on most of them.

It was Mr. Thacher who put into my head the idea of becoming a doctor. This happened while we were returning to the school from a public memorial service for my father. He reminisced about my uncle, Dr. Cephas L. Bard, whom I knew only as a legend, for he died when I was three. Two years younger than my father, he had joined a Pennsylvania regiment, fought through Fredericksburg and Chancellorsville, and, when his enlistment was up, entered the Jefferson Medical College. He obtained his M.D. after one year of study, and re-entered the Union Army as a medical officer, to finish his military career amputating arms and legs somewhere between Five Forks and Appomattox Court House. He followed my father to California, becoming the most beloved citizen of Ventura County as well as attaining a high place in California medicine. Mr. Thacher's suggestion that I might enter my uncle's profession struck me as a new, startling, and provocative idea. Very soon I announced to my family and friends that I was going to go into medicine. My brother Dick, always sympathetic and helpful, then a senior at Princeton, sent me a copy of the then current edition of Dr. William H. Howell's *Text-book of Physiology* (3). I proceeded to read that lucid treatise with much interest and little understanding. But I vividly recall getting the gist of the chapters on digestion, especially that part which described the experiments of Walter B. Cannon on gastrointestinal motility. My wildest imaginings, however, could not include my ever becoming one of Cannon's students at Harvard, or Dr. Howell's successor, once removed, at the Johns Hopkins University School of Medicine.

My academic performance at school indicated no scholarly talent; I was better at baseball, tennis, camping, and student affairs. Many years later I learned that one of my best teachers had concluded that I was not "college material." In June, 1917, I passed only two of the last six College Board examinations I took for admission to Princeton. A possible factor in this poor showing was the fact that I had, along with the rest of the school, just spent two nights and days fighting a forest fire which descended on the Ojai Valley. At any rate the problem of getting into college was postponed by my enlistment in a Stanford University section of the United States Army Ambulance Corps. A year before, I had tried to obtain my mother's permission to join the old American Field Service whose ambulances had been evacuating French wounded since 1915, but she insisted that I wait until I was eighteen. Meanwhile the United States entered the war and that private organization was replaced by similar units of the American Army. I joined the Stanford group in Allentown, Pennsylvania, where we spent the summer and fall in close order drill, long marches with full packs, and the laborious construction of what were thought to be typical western front dugouts. Except that it put us into excellent physical condition, this training was irrelevant; we were to drive Model T Ford ambulances, and the first time any of my section did so was shortly before we arrived at the French front.

Once in France we soon saw action, first with the French and then with the American Second Division on the Marne, where we removed many hundreds of wounded marines from Belleau Wood and nearly as many infantrymen from adjacent areas. Thereafter we worked with five more American divisions, but mainly with the Seventy-Seventh—composed of draftees from the several boroughs of New York City, many of whom spoke only Yiddish or Italian. Being with this group was a valuable and eye-opening experience for a youth from an area where the only "foreigners" were Orientals (I had been taught that Hispano-Americans, with or without Indian genes, were not to be distinguished from "the rest of us"; the great influx of workers from Mexico came later). Thus we served with a division of the regular army, with several National Guard divisions, and with the Seventy-Seventh. The extraordinary discipline of the Marine and regular army units stood in contrast to the relatively disorderly procedures of some of the inexperienced National Guard regiments, but in the end all did remarkably well. We were especially impressed by the performance of our draft division, commanded at higher levels by competent West Pointers but at the battalion and company levels by young officers who had received only brief but intensive military training during or just after college. This earlier experience with a cross section of the United States military service in World War I, as well as some knowledge of its organization in World War II, causes me to look now with much concern at the current campaign to abolish the ROTC units in our colleges: it seems to me the only way to offset any militarism of the professional officer corps is to provide well educated civilian reserve officers.

After the armistice in 1918, our section spent about six months in Chateau Thierry, which we had first entered in July as the Germans were leaving. Our official duty was to transport French rations to nearby camps of German prisoners, but this left much time for other activities, and I had the good luck to be selected to aid the *archiviste* of the Department of the Aisne in his task of returning records of towns and villages evacuated in 1914. M. Broche was an historian, a graduate of the Sorbonne, and a student of the Roman occupation of the valley of the Aisne. On each excursion we were accompanied by his charming family and an elderly priest—who surveyed the damage to churches and blessed our picnic lunches with a superb vin rosé, the special product of his order. Young Jacques Broche, aged fourteen, brought along a copy of Caesar's *Commentaries* from which he translated into English those passages which concerned the Aisne Valley. During this period I again read Dr. Howell's textbook, which I had carried in my barracks bag, and was thereby stimulated to do something experimental. I did about the only thing possible: I constructed from a spring, some wire, and a pencil, an ergograph with which I was able to record on paper, jerkily moved by my right hand, the development of fatigue in the flexor muscles of my left index finger. In this way I maintained my early interest in physiology.

Shortly after returning home in June, 1919, I went to San Francisco, ostensibly to consult a physician about some curious after-effects of the influenza I had contracted in October, but actually to see a girl at Stanford who, after a half year with the Red Cross, was taking summer courses to make up for lost time. This venture turned out well, for we were married three years later, and, during the forty-two years that preceded her death, we had a wonderful life together, no small part of which was her self-sacrificing concern for my career in physiology.

The physician I had gone to consult was Dr. Walter C. Alvarez, whom I had known since my twelfth year, when my mother had asked him to examine me for any possible physiological flaws. Now, about to enter college, I told him of my ambition to study medicine. He encouraged me and spoke of his sojourn in Walter Cannon's laboratory (1913) and how that had started him on his quest for functional gradients in the gastrointestinal tract. He spoke enthusiastically of Sir William Bayliss' *Principles of General Physiology*. The second edition of this unique book had just appeared and I at once bought a copy and took it with me to Princeton.

I had discovered, much to my relief, that as a veteran I could enter the freshman class—with four conditions (corresponding to the four examinations I had failed in 1917), which could be absolved if I achieved an average standing at mid-year examinations; if I didn't I would be dropped. Thus I was forced to study harder than I had previously thought possible, and, in the process, I learned how to study. My burden was lightened and my interest stimulated by three superb courses, biology, chemistry, and English, each taught by a great scholar. By midyear I found that I stood at the top in each of these three classes and had not done badly in my other two. I was so elated by this unwonted success that I spent the short holiday in New Haven to celebrate with old Thacher friends, but they, now Yale undergraduates, explained my scholastic reversal as evidence of low Princeton standards. Nevertheless, I maintained those standards and graduated in 1923 with highest honors, the result of hard work, rather than of any modicum of brilliance.

Mine was a very satisfactory undergraduate experience. Since I was about two years older than most of my classmates, and had a definite purpose and the impetus created by my delay in getting started, I did not find extracurricular activities very enticing, but I did form some close and lasting friendships with undergraduates of similar tastes, and I came to know well several great scholars of the faculty in the humanities as well as in the sciences.

In biology I first had the stimulus of Edwin Grant Conklin, embryologist and cytologist, whose excellence as a lecturer I have praised before (1). With a wealth of knowledge of science, literature, and philosophy, with a fine sense of humor, and with a clarity that was almost unbelievable, he lectured in a manner that excited the interest and admiration of generations of Princeton students. But it was E. Newton Harvey who had the greatest influence on me. His remarkable course in general physiology, the clarity of his thought, and the ingenuity of his experiments were prime factors in my decision to proceed toward a Ph.D. in physiology. This change in plans made it necessary to withdraw my application for admission to The Johns Hopkins University School of Medicine. My letter was answered longhand by the Dean, Dr. J. Whitridge Williams, who wished me well. Thirty years later, when I became Dean of the Hopkins Medical Faculty, Dr. Williams' courtesy to an unknown applicant was a memory I still cherished, and one I hope I emulated in spirit if not in longhand. But I still do not know whether I could have gotten in as a student.

I spent one additional year at Princeton as a graduate student, took advanced courses, and carried out, with Newton Harvey's encouragement, some experiments on the effect of ultraviolet radiation on the skin. I had the idea that the erythema of sunburn might be the result of an axon reflex, but I was unable to obtain any evidence for this from the ear of the albino rabbit, thereby learning something about the difficulties in denervating a skin area. I did find, however, that egg albumin but not gelatin protected the skin of the rabbit's ear and that of my own arm from sunburn, and I managed to show that, in accord with their absorption spectra, tyrosine and tryptophane but not glycine or alanine had a protective effect. And much to my disappointment I failed to convert histidine to a vasoactive substance by ultraviolet radiation. Toward the end of that year I concluded that mammalian rather than general physiology was the field I wanted to enter and, remembering my discussions with Walter Alvarez, I applied for admission to the Division of

Medical Sciences at Harvard to work for the Ph.D. under the direction of
Dr. Cannon.

It may be that my decision was in part based on my experiments with
rabbits (I never again used them) which led me to extensive reading about
the vasomotor system. But there was another factor. In school I had not gone
beyond plane geometry and when I entered college I began a course that covered trigonometry, analytical geometry, and calculus. But I was just out of
the army and in no mood to put up with the overt inadequacy of an indifferent and arrogant instructor. So I dropped out and took Latin instead (my
best subject in school), which made me a candidate for the A.B. instead of
the B.S. degree. Consequently I became a graduate student with no knowledge of mathematics, and, although I attempted not very successful self-tutor-
ing in calculus to remedy this ridiculous situation, it became clear that I
would have difficulties in any field which required a rigorous quantitative approach. I discussed this matter with Professor Conklin who agreed that it
would be wise to gain some competency in mathematics since biological research was becoming more quantitative. But he remarked that some of the
so-called quantitative procedures then being used reminded him of the method
used in Georgia for weighing hogs: one drives the animals onto one scale of a
large weighing device, loads the other scale with rocks until the two balance,
drives off the hogs, and then guesses at the weight of the rocks.

When I went to see Dr. Cannon I was affected by his kindly interest in an
eager student who wasn't quite sure what he wanted to do. He accepted me
as a graduate student; thus began what was to become a close friendship—
and a major factor in whatever success I have had as a physiologist. At that
time it was required that a candidate for the Ph.D. in physiology take all the
courses of the first year of medicine except gross anatomy. Consequently,
during the first semester, more than half of my time was unscheduled and, at
Dr. Cannon's suggestion, another student and I devoted this to an intensive
reading of the classical literature on the circulation. We began with William
Harvey, proceeded to Richard Lower, Stephen Hales, Claude Bernard, W. H.
Gaskell, H. P. Bowditch and concluded with papers by E. H. Starling, W. M.
Bayliss, and August Krogh. Our reading was accompanied by some attempts to repeat classical experiments. It was fairly easy and great fun to
follow Harvey's experiments on amphibian and reptilian hearts, or to measure arterial and venous pressures directly and manometrically in an anesthetized dog by the technique used in the early 18th century by Stephen Hales
on unanesthetized dogs and horses, but I vividly recall a horribly messed up
Starling heart-lung preparation.

All this was splendid experience, for it gave me a background and interest
in the history of physiology. The task of the investigator is to advance knowledge, but as he works he needs caution as well as inspiration. He can get both
from the history of his discipline. For example, reading Claude Bernard's
description of his discovery of the vasomotor nerves is inspiring, but knowing

that he went to his grave convinced that their primary action is on the heat production of the innervated tissues may make the young researcher (and the old one too) wary of too expansive an interpretation of experimental results.

The rest of that first year (1924–25) I spent taking two courses. One was an excellent course in biochemistry given by Otto Folin with the the aid of Cyrus Fiske (the codiscoverer of phosphocreatine) and Harry Trimble. The other was the course in physiology. The senior staff were Dr. Cannon, Alexander Forbes (the founder of American neurophysiology), Alfred Redfield, and Cecil Drinker and the junior staff were Hallowell Davis, William B. Castle, David Brunswick, and Harold Himwich. These eight constituted a stimulating group which virtually radiated a demand for excellence. I especially recall the conferences that groups of students had each week with Dr. Cannon, where his provocative questions and comments caused even more interest than apprehension. Here he was a superb teacher, and no little part of his students' appraisal of him as such was their awareness that he was also a great investigator. Over many years of academic activities at the undergraduate, graduate, and faculty level, I have found it true that with very few exceptions the best teachers are also productive scholars. Nowadays, however, one too often hears that the teacher who is an investigator is ipso facto a poor teacher, a claim usually explained on the basis of that denigrating shibboleth "publish or perish." But a great many who publish abundantly are poor scholars as well as poor teachers. I hope it is not too exceptional that I never experienced any academic pressure to write more scientific papers than I was ready to write and never exerted any such pressure on junior colleagues.

During my second year at the Harvard Medical School I studied pharmacology and began some research. Dr. Cannon suggested that since there was some evidence of increased sympathetic activity during muscular exercise, stimulation of the motor cortex might evoke secretion of the adrenal medulla. So I spent some time learning how to denervate the cat's heart and thus have that indicator of circulating "adrenin" which he was employing at that time. I worked diligently but before long had to conclude that the task was hopeless because the only anesthesia then available which left the motor cortex excitable, namely, light etherization, caused a potent sympathetic discharge to the adrenal medulla. Both Dr. Cannon and I were disappointed by this result, but he was not as upset as was Carl Ludwig when one of his students failed to obtain a result the professor fully expected. The student was John J. Abel who, on arriving at Leipzig in 1884, had been put to work testing the professor's idea that a nerve could be stimulated by a change in temperature between two nearby points. He was given two tubes, one to convey warm water, the other cold. On touching these to a frog's sciatic nerve the gastrocnemius regularly twitched; the report of this greatly pleased the professor. But a little later Dr. Abel noticed that one tube was of iron, the other of copper. When he repeated the experiment using tubes made of the same metal there was no excitation; the report of this did not please the professor. When Dr. Abel told me this story in 1933, he concluded in his grave and deliberate manner, "That is how I learned to properly control every experiment I have ever carried out."

At the time I entered the Harvard laboratory and for some time afterwards the famous controversy between Cannon and Stewart & Rogoff was at its height. It raged over the question whether or not certain physiological and emotional states were accompanied by secretion or an increased secretion from the adrenal medulla. The issue concerned all of Dr. Cannon's students and colleagues, and many of us became fairly emotional over the arguments put forward. But outwardly Dr. Cannon remained cool and simply stated that the matter could not be settled by vocal or printed arguments but only by doing more experiments. These he carried out, with results which left little doubt about the correctness of his original position. I was privileged to witness those extraordinary studies of animals from which the sympathetic chains had been completely removed surgically. Their deficiencies on exposure to various stressful conditions gave the final proof of the emergency function of the sympathetic system. In them no trace of any adrenergic action could be induced. Later claims that after denervation there remain postganglionic fibers from "intermediary" ganglia may be true of some species (e.g., man and dog), but Cannon's supersensitive indicators of circulating catecholamines, capable of detecting a discharge through only one pair of remaining lateral ganglia, gave no sign that any such fibers were operative in his cats, and I know of no evidence to the contrary.

On arriving at the Harvard laboratory I had expressed considerable interest in endocrinology, but I was soon led elsewhere. When I had to abandon the motor cortex/adrenal medulla problem, a much more interesting one appeared. In searching for conditions that induce vigorous sympatho-adrenal medullary activity, Dr. Cannon took advantage of the observation made by both Goltz and Rademaker on dogs and by Dusser de Barenne on cats that the animal surviving decortication displays anger on very slight provocation. With Britton he had just completed a series of acute experiments in which the cerebral cortices were disconnected from the brain stem. When these cats emerged from the ether anesthesia they exhibited a remarkable group of activities which Dr. Cannon termed "sham rage." He suggested that I attempt to ascertain the locus of the central mechanisms essential for this activity which so closely resembles the behavior of the infuriated normal animal and is accompanied by widespread sympathetic discharges. This I managed to accomplish by first decorticating and then transecting the brain stem at different levels and at different planes. It turned out that the region requisite for sham rage (I have always preferred the term "quasi-rage") is situated in the caudal half of the hypothalamus. I had of course placed much emphasis on the sympathetically determined components of the activity and, since this was to be the work for my Ph.D. thesis, I was worried about any claim of originality, for between 1909 and 1927 Karplus & Kreidl had shown that electrical stimulation of the surface of the hypothalamus could induce in the anesthetized cat almost every bodily response mediated by the sympathetic system. But I came to the conclusion that the hypothalamus is not an "autonomic center," but rather a part of the brain that contains neural mechanisms requisite for complicated patterns of behavior—such as the display of emotion and defense against heat and cold—in which there are autonomic components. This investigation was the beginning of a permanent interest in the physiology of the nervous system and it led me to a long series of experiments on brain stem mechanisms which, in turn, caused me to ascend, from time to time, to studies of the cerebral cortex and even of the cerebellum.

During my last year as a graduate student and the year after I held an instructorship in physiology. It was Dr. Cannon's custom to give a junior member of the staff the responsibility of organizing the course for medical students. I found this a valuable experience, and later as a department head I adopted a similar policy. During that postgraduate year I began to do sterile intracranial operations with a view to preparing some chronically decorticate cats, and I learned the fundamentals of surgical technique from Dr. Harlan Newton, a former resident of Harvey Cushing who was spending a year in Cannon's laboratory.

It was also during that year that I collaborated for the only time with Dr. Cannon. In 1915, on the basis of the idea that the sympathetic innervation of the thyroid gland might be secretomotor, he had done some experiments with Carl Binger and Reginald Fitz in which the anterior root of the phrenic nerve was anastomosed to the cephalic portion of the cut cervical sympathetic trunk, and in due course some of their animals had developed signs which resembled those of hyperthyroidism. But World War I had interrupted this work. Now that it was possible to measure the oxygen consumption of resting cats, he proposed that I join him in an attempt to repeat the earlier experiments. This we did in a large number of animals—in most of which there developed ocular signs of abundant innervation of the superior cervical ganglion by phrenic fibers, but no detectable changes in metabolic rate. In this manner I learned more about negative results. Many years later I had occasion to repeat experiments carried out by a competent, wholly honest physiologist whom I knew well and greatly respected. My results were negative. I reread his report and with a student repeated his experiments many times over, making sure that we followed every detail of his procedures, but still we got only negative results. Convinced that we must be doing something wrong I decided to visit him to discuss the discrepancy, but as I was leaving a telegram informed me of his death. Within the following year two groups of investigators told me that they too had been unable, on repeating these experiments, to get any of the results which had been reported. None of these studies, which involved much time and effort, was ever reported. Should there not be some means of communicating carefully obtained negative results?

In 1928 I accepted an assistant professorship in the biology department at Princeton. I was to conduct the course in general physiology which Newton Harvey, now a research professor, had so long and so brilliantly taught, and I would have a laboratory and facilities for experiments in mammalian physiology. I spent three very pleasant years back at Princeton, then a really small town where we had many old friends. My quarters were in the "Vivarium," a small building which I had all to myself. I converted its janitor, an ex-carpenter, to the combined role of animal caretaker, anesthetist, and operating room assistant. I have never worked with anyone better in any of those three roles. Laboratory and operating room faced two large tanks for aquatic plants and animals. Into one of these my first chronically decorticate cat fell and demonstrated that the feline cortex is not necessary to assure adequate swimming with nose held high. At Princeton I was wholly on my own, there being no colleague able to share my interests or advise me in the details of my research activities. But the helping hand of Dr. Cannon was always present. Scarcely a week passed without a note or letter from him directing my attention to a new publication or giving me the benefit of some new thought which had occurred to him. Because of this relative isolation I was forced to improvise, to learn to do things I had never done before, and so to take stock of my capabilities. I carried out a lot of experiments with results that proved worthless when submitted to statistical analysis. I also prepared cats with one or another cortical area removed, and one wholly decorticate cat which in due time displayed rage and fear and, when in estrus, the full pattern of sexual behavior. During my third year at Princeton I found myself in strong opposition to certain administrative policies and tendered my resignation to take effect in June, 1931.

Shortly before the end of my last year on the Princeton faculty a piece of good fortune assured continuation of my work under the most favorable circumstances. Alfred Redfield had accepted a professorship in biology at Harvard and Dr. Cannon asked me to take his place as an assistant professor of physiology and tutor in normal medical sciences. The latter title involved two duties. The first was to select about eight first year medical students who would work intensively on a few somewhat elaborate laboratory projects and read the literature pertinent to them rather than take part in the extensive and somewhat diffuse laboratory part of the course in physiology. The second was to encourage these and other students to engage in some kind of research in any one of the preclinical departments. For two years I discharged these duties with pleasure and satisfaction. I was provided with ample facilities for research including an operating room suitable for intracranial procedures together with a technician and a small but adequate budget. Best of all was the collaboration of an accomplished neuroanatomist. David Rioch had just come from Hopkins to Harvard with George Wislocki, the new head of the department of anatomy. His histological studies of the brains of my animals and his wise counsel were of the utmost importance to the progress of my work. Together we studied all aspects of the behavioral capacities and deficiencies of four cats from which I had removed all cerebral cortex and different amounts of the rest of the forebrain. At the same time I explored the basic neural control of two groups of postural reactions, absent or very deficient in decorticate animals, and found that they depend on the sensori-motor cortex and, more important, that they remain unimpaired when all the rest of the cortex is removed.

In March, 1933, I received a letter from President Joseph S. Ames of the Johns Hopkins University inviting me to become professor of physiology and director of the department, a post that had become open because Dr. E. K. Marshall, Dr. Howell's successor, had switched to the department of pharmacology on Dr. Abel's retirement. I found my appointment as unexpected and strange as did many others. I was, after all, only thirty-four, and had published but five papers, of which only three were reports of original work. Later I learned that from its inception Hopkins has taken such chances; when I visited Baltimore my future colleagues, both preclinical and clinical, welcomed me as if I were a well established scholar. Transfers to pharmacology had left the department of physiology with only three staff members: Drs. C. D. Snyder, C. L. Gemmill, and Evelyn Howard. The friendly cooperation they gave me after my arrival I much appreciated. To augment the staff, I persuaded Dr. Chandler Brooks—who at Princeton had been my first PhD student and who had spent two years as a fellow of the National Research Council with Dr. Cannon—to accept an instructorship, and I was able to induce a Hopkins fourth year student—Clinton Woolsey—to give up an appointment in surgery to join the department as an assistant. At the time I estimated that both were capable of high scientific achievement and now, forty years later, there is no doubt I was correct. This kind of luck followed me in making departmental appointments over the years. For some reason I have been able to recruit several outstanding physiologists from surgery: Woolsey whom I have mentioned; Elwood Henneman, now professor of physiology at Harvard; and my successor, Vernon Mountcastle, whose superb contributions have made the department a mecca for all who would learn to explore the neurophysiological basis of perception.

I shall devote little space to the thirty-one years I served as director of the department of physiology. Although I underwent considerable growth as a teacher and investigator during that time, I believe that the end of my ontogenesis as a physiologist was attained when I arrived in Baltimore.

Dr. Cannon, discussing circumstances favorable for scholarly work (2), emphasized freedom of action. I surely had that when I was a member of his department and I have enjoyed it throughout my Hopkins career both as an investigator and as the head of a department. The organization of the medical school was quite simple and to some extent unique (it is less so now). The governing body was the Advisory Board (advisory to the trustees) composed of the heads of the twelve major departments and the director of the Johns Hopkins Hospital, with the president as chairman and the dean as secretary. Each department chairman was responsible only to the Board for the conduct of his department and had complete control of appointments to his staff and promotions within it, subject to the approval of the Board (I never witnessed a disapproval). Further, he had full control of his departmental budget once it was approved by an executive committee whose members were the president, the dean, and the director of the hospital. Thus large power was combined with equally large responsibility. The arrangement was distinctly autocratic but it worked very well and the spirit of the institution prevented tyranny. An important and delightful quality of the Board throughout my long membership was the entire absence of cliques. If differences of opinion occurred they never were based on any constant pattern. I was early impressed by the evidence of good will and the urge to agree even when circumstances made agreement difficult.

Discussing further the favorable and unfavorable conditions under which an investigator may work, Cannon (2) wrote: "Blessed is the scientist who serves under considerate and understanding administrators." I believe I have been signally blessed. Certainly at Hopkins I have never felt anything but administrative support and interest. In his office as dean for twenty-four years, Alan M. Chesney, perhaps because he had been the historian of the school and hospital, continued the traditions he knew so well. One story will illustrate his concept of the deanship: Shortly after my arrival he telephoned to say he would like to discuss a certain matter with me and I replied that I was free and would be in his nearby office in a few minutes. He replied, "No, I'll be in your office in a moment. You must understand that here the dean is the servant of the faculty, and when he wants to consult a department head he calls on him." He was a man who possessed and expressed strong opinions, but never regarded his office as one which gave him any special authority; he considered himself one member of a team whose main interest was the welfare of the medical school. Such happy, uncomplicated, and effective conditions as these cannot survive when an institution has grown beyond a certain critical mass. When that happens, administration becomes authoritative, and the faculty, becoming diffuse and divided, wastes its time trying to set up some sort of "democratic" governance, which, once established, consumes still more time of the investigator and teacher.

Of those factors unfavorable to a career of research and teaching, I experienced two. The first of these was an insidious entrapment to edit and write substantial parts of a textbook. Just after I went to Hopkins, Professor J. J. R. Macleod of Aberdeen, previously of Toronto, asked me to revise, for the seventh edition of his *Physiology in Modern Medicine* (6), the chapters on muscle, nerve, and the central nervous system. In earlier editions these had been written by Alfred Redfield and it was he who suggested that I replace him in this task. My acceptance of this invitation led me into further trouble, for Professor Macleod (whom I never met) died shortly after the seventh edition appeared (1935), and the publisher urged me to assume responsibility for the eighth (1938). I edited and contributed to three more editions before I turned over the twelfth, with great relief, to a more competent victim. The book required an inordinate amount of time which I would have preferred to devote to research. But the endeavor did have its benefits: It kept me informed about areas of physiology outside my own. When Cuthbert Bazett suddenly died, before he was able to revise his chapters on the circulation for the tenth edition, I undertook to rewrite them—thereby learning so much about the cardiovascular system that I felt for the first time qualified to lecture on this subject to our students.

Another interruption of my investigative work and my teaching was service as dean for four years (1953–1957). Well before Dr. Chesney reached retirement, a committee nominated his successor, but the distinguished individual selected took several months to decide to remain where he was. The same thing happened with a second admirable choice. Time was getting short. My colleagues and my old friend Detlev Bronk, who was about to give up the Hopkins presidency to direct the Rockefeller Institute (which he shortly converted to the Rockefeller University) insisted that I fill the gap. The situation was such that I could hardly refuse. I continued as director of the physiology department and managed that responsibility only with the help of Vernon Mountcastle, who had become the senior member of the staff. I found the duties of the deanship a curious melange of boring trivialities, unexpected problems to be solved quickly, interesting discussions of policies, too many committee meetings, and correspondence without end with everyone from fellow deans to a series of strange persons who wanted to leave their unblemished bodies to the school. Part of this I actually enjoyed, especially the close and extensive communications with my fellow department heads. And I did have wonderful help from two associate deans and a remarkable secretary who was quite capable of running the school by herself. It was, however, with pleasure and relief that I returned to full time teaching and research.

However favorable the conditions for research may be, one's performance can be limited by deficiencies in training or failure to learn or develop new methods of inquiry. In the preface of the eighth edition of the textbook I wrote, "Every worker must of necessity develop special methods of study and in so doing he becomes bound, to a greater or lesser extent, by his technique." I must confess that I became a sorry victim of such binding. I had become fairly adept at intracranial surgical procedures in cats, dogs, and monkeys, and there were so many inviting problems which seemed soluble by this approach that I neglected to learn the techniques of electrophysiology which have of course advanced our knowledge of the nervous system far beyond any other. In 1936 Woolsey and I had pushed the technique of cortical ablation as far as it could go toward determining the control of the placing and hopping reactions by the precentral and postcentral gyri of the monkey's cortex. At that time Wade Marshall introduced a cathode ray oscillograph and some amplifiers into the laboratory, and the three of us set about determining whether evoked potentials would throw further light on the cortical representation of somatic sensibility. This study resulted in the first systematic mapping of the primate postcentral gyrus by this then new technique. Woolsey went on to apply the method thoroughly and widely and many who subsequently entered the laboratory learned to use it in analyses of several central sensory systems. I encouraged this work but failed to take part in it. Instead, I retreated to the old-fashioned ablation technique.

I want to emphasize how much I have enjoyed physiology. It is said that E. H. Starling called it "the best sport in the world," and I agree. I think I have made it at least a spectator sport for many students. It is a satisfaction that not a few have gone down to the playing field and become professionals, while others have been led to the pleasures which attend any scientific inquiry into the physiological basis of clinical medicine. In this connection I am reminded of something else I wrote in the preface of the eighth edition of *Macleod's Physiology in Modern Medicine* (1938), in justification of its title: "The propriety of this lies in the assumption that the greatest service which physiology can render modern medicine is to continue to solve fundamental problems which are not necessarily of immediate practical concern, to acquaint the student in his preclinical days with the real importance of these and to imbue him with some appreciation of the nature of valid experimental evidence" (6). But I fear that recent developments in medical education place this concept of physiology in peril. Many schools have reduced the presentation of the basic medical sciences either to a minimum which may suffice for the routine practice of medicine or to a hodgepodge of correlations. This not only deprives the students of a chance to learn many important things, but keeps from them the philosophic background of scientific medicine. And there is evidence that this situation is demoralizing many teachers of physiology and of the other medical sciences. Further, some new schools seem content to make the clinical departments responsible for the teaching of the basic sciences, thus abrogating their responsibility for training those who will make the basic discoveries of the future. These developments appear to be leading to the creation of a group of trade schools; if they continue we shall soon need another Flexner report.

LITERATURE CITED

1. Bard, P. 1964. Edwin Grant Conklin, 1863–1952. The One Hundredth Anniversary of his Birth. *Proc. Am. Phil. Soc.* 108:55–56
2. Cannon, W. B. 1945. *The Way of an Investigator.* New York: Norton
3. Howell, W. H. 1905. *A Text-book of Physiology for Medical Students and Physicians.* Philadelphia: Saunders
4. Hutchinson, W. H. 1965. *Oil, Land and Politics, the California Career of Thomas Robert Bard,* 2 vols.

Norman: University of Oklahoma
5. Erlanger, J. 1964. A physiologist reminisces. *Ann. Rev. Physiol.* 26: 1–14
6. Macleod, J. J. R. 1935. *Physiology in Modern Medicine,* 1st–7th editions. (Later *Medical Physiology,* ed. P. Bard, 8th–11th Editions.) St. Louis: Mosby
7. Olmsted, J. M. D. 1939. *Claude Bernard, Physiologist.* New York and London: Harper

Ann. Rev. Physiol. 1973. 35:17–54

KIDNEY

Françoิs Morel and Christian de Rouffignac

Département de Biologie, C.E.N. Saclay, France

Introduction

About 800 papers relating to kidney physiology were published during 1971 alone. Although the volume of literature on the subject is constantly growing, the Editorial Committee suggests that reviewers cut down on length and contribute a critical analysis rather than an exhaustive survey. This meant we had to select a few topics from the vast field of kidney physiology, and the choice was extremely hard. We began by deciding to leave out sodium transport by the kidney despite its great physiological importance, because Orloff and Burg published an excellent appraisal of the question in the 1971 *Annual Review of Physiology* (108). We then narrowed our choices to four topics, dealing with sugar transport, amino acid transport, medullary concentrating mechanisms, and the physiology of the renin-angiotensin system. However, by the time most of the work was finished it was clear that even this restricted number of subjects would have to be curtailed because our manuscript was still twice the length stipulated by the editors. Therefore we have had to leave out the section on the renin-angiotensin system although no critical physiological review has been published for several years (141a). However, our present knowledge in this field is based on such inconclusive and contradictory documentation that in any case a section reviewing this question might not have been of very much use.

Even in the limited fields covered, we are painfully aware that our survey must be far from complete; we can only plead that no important contributions to the subjects discussed were left out intentionally.

Sugar Transport

The mechanisms by which functionally polarized cells—such as the intestine and proximal kidney tubule—transport sugars and amino-acids from the luminal to the serosal medium are still obscure; however, important progress has been made in the past two years, especially with regard to the intestine as a result of the widespread use of the everted intestine technique, which allows direct measurement of substrate transport rates through the apical border of the epithelial cells. Unfortunately, however, no such simple experimental approach is possible for the kidney, so that either less direct or more sophisticated methods have had to be used.

Despite these technical limitations, clear-cut differences have been observed between gut and kidney in such basic aspects of sugar transport as ionic requirements and stereospecificity. Before discussing the data recently published, it should be recalled that transepithelial sugar and amino acid net absorption is a vectorial process which generally works against a chemical concentration gradient; this implies functional polarization of the tubular cells, i.e. some differences in the way in which the substrates transported are handled at the luminal and basal borders of the epithelial cells.

In vitro studies on kidney cortex slices.—This technique generally yields complex kinetic accumulation curves, which will remain difficult to interpret as long as we have no better knowledge of the respective participations in the overall process of the different cell types, of the apical and basal membranes, of damaged or anoxic cells, and of many other factors. Nevertheless, some significant observations have been published recently, which will be discussed briefly.

The ability of renal cortical slices from newborn and young rats to accumulate α-methyl-D-glucoside, a nonmetabolizable sugar, was compared to that of adult rats by Segal et al (126). It was observed that in slices taken from newborn rats, this sugar was not accumulated against a concentration gradient; nevertheless, some transport probably occurred, since the cell-to-medium distribution ratio was found to be even lower in the absence of Na, and in the presence of either phlorizin (0.5 mM) or D-glucose (10 mM) in the incubation medium. The uptake capacity of the adult kidney was attained at the age of about 25 days. On the other hand, kidney slices from newborn rats accumulated the amino acids tested (lycine and glycine) as well as and even better than those of adult rats. These differences in transport characteristics during development suggest separate carrier systems for each of the two types of substrates. Similarly, Bailey et al (10) observed that kidney slices from newborn rats did not concentrate ^{3}H-D-galactose under conditions which, in adult tissue, allowed the establishment of three- to fivefold gradients. In contrast, a D-galactose transport mechanism was well developed in the newborn rat jejunum. In both structures, the mutarotase activity correlated well with the development of the sugar transport capacity, but such correlation does not necessarily mean that the enzyme is involved in the sugar transport mechanism.

Reciprocal inhibition of amino-acid transport by sugars and vice versa was reported on many occasions in a variety of cell types or tissues, including kidney. Since these interactions might have resulted indirectly from metabolite effects, the problem was reexamined in rat kidney cortex slices by Genel et al (43) using α-methyl-D-glucoside as the nonmetabolized transported hexose, and α-aminoisobutyric acid as the nonmetabolized transported amino acid. Active accumulation of α-(^{14}C) methyl-D-glucoside (0.2 and 1 mM) was definitely inhibited by adding 5 mM α-aminoisobutyric acid, glycine, L-valine, or L-methionine to the incubation medium. In this type of study, "active accumulation" indicates the establishment of a chemical concentration gradient. Analysis of the kinetics of uptake indicated that the inhibition was of a noncompetitive type; the interaction necessarily occurred at the influx of the transport process, since the α-(^{14}C) methyl-D-glucoside efflux from pre-loaded cells was unaffected by the addition of 20 mM glycine to the medium but was accelerated by the addition of 20 mM cold α-methyl-D-glucoside. Accumulation of the test amino acid was also inhibited by the sugar. With these results the mechanism involved remains difficult to interpret; it should be noted here (and will be stated further on) that α-methyl-D-glucoside transport in the kidneys is almost entirely Na-dependent. The influence of the incubation temperature on the accumulation of α-methyl-D-glucoside by rat kidney cortex slices was examined by McNamara et al (98); a greater cell-to-medium distribution ratio was observed at 25°C, resulting from greater inhibition of sugar efflux than influx at the lower temperature.

The steric requirements for active sugar transport by rabbit kidney slices were further analyzed by Kleinzeller (79): among a new series of monosaccharides tested, he observed active Na-dependent and phlorizin-sensitive cellular accumulation of β-methyl-D-glucoside, D-glucosamine, and D-galactosamine; 2-deoxy-D-allose and 2-deoxy-D-ribose were accumulated to a lesser extent by a Na-independent mechanism; mannitol, L--glucose, 3-deoxy-D-glucose, and D-ribose were not accumulated against their concentration gradients. Since the same author's previous work (82) established that both 2-deoxy-D-glucose and 2-deoxy-D-galactose are actively accumulated in kidney cells by a phlorizin-sensitive and Na-independent process, they suggested the following structural requirements for active sugar accumulation in kidney cells: a hemiacetal group, a hydroxyl group in position C3 (in a configuration identical to that of D-glucose) and a hydroxyl group in position C6; OH in the D-glucose configuration in position C2 is not required for active transport, but Na$^+$-dependent active transport could be related to the presence of a hydrophilic group ($^-$OH or $^-$NH$_2$) in this position. At first glance, these considerations suggest that great differences may exist between intestine and kidney in the steric requirements for sugar binding to the carrier systems, particularly as far as substituents in positions C2 and C3 are concerned; nevertheless, before accepting such a conclusion, it should be recalled that the specificity pattern defined by Crane (32a) was established for sugar transport through the apical border of the enterocytes, whereas the sugar accumulation pattern in kidney cortex slices concerns the whole structure and may well be mainly related to peritubular membrane properties rather than to those of the luminal border. The differences from sugar to sugar in Na requirements for active transport were further analyzed by Kolinska (84) and Kleinzeller (80) with almost the same results. Thus, part of the uphill transport of D-galactose does not require extracellular Na; the addition of

Na increases the maximum rate of galactose transport without affecting its apparent K_m for entry. The uphill transport of both 2-deoxy-D-galactose and 2-deoxy-D-glucose is almost completely Na-independent; active transport of α-methyl-D-glucoside is Na-dependent, the Na ions increasing the V_{max} and leaving the K_m unchanged. In addition, it was observed (84) that either 2-deoxy-D-galactose and D-galactose, or α-methyl-D-glucoside and D-galactose competitively inhibit each other's transport, suggesting that these sugars share a common carrier system, although the kinetic data indicate the existence of several pathways for active sugar transport into renal tubular cells (79). Transport of these different types of sugar was in every case reduced by removing Ca from the incubation medium (80) but was affected in very different and unpredictable ways when the pH in the medium was changed from 6.2 to 8.2 (81).

Active metabolic and Na^+-dependent accumulation of myo-inositol in kidney cortex slices was reported for the first time by Hauser (49, 50); this is an interesting observation since this compound does not contain the oxygen bridge present in the pyranose or furanose structure of actively transported sugars.

In vivo whole kidney studies.—Some of the features of sugar specificity observed in vitro on kidney slices were confirmed by in vivo whole kidney clearance experiments. Thus, Woosley & Huang (150) showed that optical natural sugar isomers such as L-glucose, as well as glucose derivatives (3-O-methyl-D-glucose) may in fact be secreted by the dog kidney through a process which is blocked by phlorizin. The same authors' subsequent observations in dogs and rats (62) showed that during steady-state perfusion of L-glucose, the clearance value of this sugar exceeded that of inulin, indicating tubular excretion of L-glucose. This excretory process was clearly enhanced when D-glucose was perfused intravenously; it was blocked by phlorizin but not by probenecid. Stop-flow experiments suggested that L-glucose secretion did take place along the proximal convoluted tubule. These observations are compatible with the hypothesis that L-glucose and D-glucose tubular transport both involve common carrier systems; the difference in the direction of the net transport might be accounted for by, among other factors, differences in relative affinities for the carriers, in ionic requirements, or in transport properties of both the luminal and basal borders. Woosley et al (151) also performed clearance experiments on dogs and rats, in which they analyzed the renal handling of 2-deoxy-D-glucose, a glucose derivative not transported in the intestine but accumulated in kidney cortex slices (82) as already mentioned. In the case of this sugar, the authors observed that the greater part of the filtered load was reabsorbed (probably in the proximal tubule) by a process which, like D-glucose transport, was blocked by perfusing phlorizin but not by perfusion of DNP at a rate of 1 mg kg^{-1} min^{-1}. The administration of D-glucose in excess of its maximum tubular transport capacity inhibited tubular reabsorption of 2-deoxy-D-glucose, suggesting that both sugars share common transport mechanisms. Thus, clearance experiments roughly confirmed the observations made on kidney slices in vitro; in addition, the observation that 2-deoxy-D-glucose is both actively reabsorbed and accumulated, whereas L-glucose and 3-O-methyl-D-glucose are not, supports the conclusion that steric requirements for acting sugar transport may be different in proximal tubule and intestine.

Interesting observations were made by Silverman et al (130, 131) in relation to possible differences in the handling of sugar by basal and apical borders of the tubular cells. Their studies made use of the "sudden-injection-multiple-indicator-dilution technique" developed by Chinard et al (29). Tracer amounts of T-1824 (as vascular indicator), of creatinine (as extracellular indicator), and of labeled sugars were injected as a pulse into the renal artery of dogs, and the concentration curves of these indicators measured both in the blood of the renal vein and in the ureteral urine. Tubular reabsorption of the sugar resulted in reduced fractional recovery in the urine as compared to creatinine; increased renal artery-to-vein mean transit time of the labelled sugars compared to that of creatinine may indicate either (a) cell penetration through or "interaction" with antiluminal membranes or (b) that transtubular reabsorption contributes to the venous curve. When (^{14}C)-L-glucose was used as a tracer, urinary and venous blood curves for creatinine and ^{14}C were virtually identical. With (^{14}C)-D-glucose, the following observations were made: intravenous infusion of low doses of phlorizin (2 mg kg^{-1} over a 30 to 40 min period) completely blocked luminal reabsorption of glucose, whereas a time-requiring interaction between the glucose and the basal surface remained evident; this interaction disappeared when the phlorizin dose was 200 mg kg^{-1}. In addition, probenecid (25 mg kg^{-1}) reversed the phlorizin inhibition of the glucose-antiluminal surface interaction but did not reverse phlorizin inhibition of D-glucose reabsorption by the luminal surface. The authors concluded that D-glucose binds to or penetrates the proximal tubule's antiluminal surface by a mechanism distinct from that located at the luminal membrane. This type of experimental approach was applied to the kinetic analysis of renal handling of 14 different labeled monosaccharides (130) and led to the following observations: among the sugars tested, D-glucose, D-mannose, 2-deoxy-D-glucose and D-galactose were reabsorbed through the luminal border of the tubules; with increased blood glucose concentrations, reabsorption of D-glucose, 2-deoxy-D-glucose, and D-galactose was reduced, whereas that of D-mannose remained unchanged. Similarly, D-mannose absorption was hardly affected by phlorizin, administered in doses which greatly inhibited that of the three other sugars. Conversely, cold mannose infusion reduced labeled mannose but not labeled glucose, fructose, and 2-deoxy-glucose reabsorption. From this the authors concluded that two sets of sites exist on the luminal membrane, one accessible to D-mannose and the other accessible to the three other sugars; since 3-O-methyl-D-glucose, 6-deoxy-D-galactose, and L-glucose were not reabsorbed, the authors concluded that interaction with the latter type of luminal sites requires D-pyranoside conformation and hydroxyl groups on carbons 3 and 6; a hydroxyl group on carbon 2 is not an essential prerequisite, since 2-deoxy-D-glucose was reabsorbed. Here again, the structural specificity for luminal sugar transport differs in kidney tubule and intestinal mucosa. In addition, this study indicates that structural requirements for interaction might be different at the luminal and basal borders; thus for example, 2-deoxy-D-glucose, although reabsorbed, did not "interact" with the basal membranes, and conversely, 3-O-methyl-D-glucose, although not reabsorbed, did "interact"; this suggests that in the D-pyranoside structure, a hydroxyl group on C2 but not on C3 may be a prerequisite for antiluminal surface-sugar interaction, but the accuracy of the conclusions concerning the basal properties is somewhat limited by the rather indirect nature of the experimental information available. It should be added that these kinetic experiments resulted in two unexpected observations: (a) there was no indication of tubular secretion of L-glucose and (b) D-xylose was not found to be reabsorbed, contradicting Shannon's early observation in the dog (128) made by clearance techniques.

Interrelationships between tubular reabsorption and metabolic conversion of organic substrates may be of physiological importance; this point was analyzed by Rasmussen (112) for galactose in clearance experiments in the cat; he observed that for small galactose plasma loads when almost all the filtered galactose was reabsorbed, the metabolic conversion rate in the kidney considerably exceeded the reabsorption rate; with high plasma loads, the metabolic rate reached maximum values of 50 to 100 μg min^{-1} g^{-1} kidney weight, and the reabsorption fraction then dropped to 60%. The author suggests that when the galactose metabolic rate exceeds the reabsorption rate, the intracellular concentration of galactose in the reabsorbing cells may stay low, which may promote diffusion into the cells and account for the high reabsorption fractions. When the reabsorption rate exceeds the metabolic rate, reabsorption may be increasingly due to carrier-facilitated transcellular backdiffusion along the chemical gradient. Thus, according to the author, there is no need to postulate active transport in order to account for galactose reabsorption. Nevertheless, the data do not exclude active transport; in addition, only overall metabolic conversion was determined, and not that taking place within the cells that reabsorb most of the filtered sugar. Coupling between substrate reabsorption and cell metabolism has also been suggested by Pellet et al (109) in the case of citric acid.

Recent studies of whole kidney glucose reabsorption in the rat have indicated that glucose reabsorption as a function of the filtered load is more complex than Shannon's and Fischer's original description suggested (128a); it has been observed in the rat that glucose reabsorption is influenced by changes in both GFR (142) and the rate of tubular reabsorption of sodium (113). The situation was therefore reexamined in the dog by two groups of authors: Keyes et al (76) measured maximum glucose reabsorption (Tm$_G$) as a function of the spontaneous changes in GFR, and of decreased GFR induced experimentally either by partial constriction of the renal artery or partial ureteral clamping. The spontaneous reductions in GFR, as well as those produced by renal artery constriction, were associated with proportional reductions in Tm_G; the Tm_G/GFR ratio remained constant. In contrast, during partial ureteral clamping, the Tm_G/GFR ratio rose. Kurtzman and associates (85) recently observed similar correlation in the dog between spontaneous changes in GFR and simultaneous tubular glucose reabsorption. In addition, these authors examined the effects of large changes in sodium excretion on glucose reabsorption; sodium reabsorption was either stimulated by partial obstruction of the thoracic inferior vena cava, or depressed by volume expansion with Ringer-lactate solution. The Tm_G of those volume-expanded dogs excreting more than 10% of the filtered Na was found to be definitely lower than the Tm_G of those caval dogs excreting less than 1% of the filtered Na, when the comparison was made within the same range of absolute GFR. In the rat, Baines (11) recently observed that extracellular volume expansion reduced glucose reabsorption from 30 nmoles min^{-1} g^{-1} kidney weight (controls) to 18.4 nM in the expanded rats.

All these studies were performed under glucose plasma loading conditions assumed to ensure saturation of the glucose tubular mechanism. The drop in Tm_G observed as a function of the decrease in GFR might have resulted from many factors such as (a) complete cessation of filtration in some glomeruli, (b) redistribution of GFR among superficial and deep glomeruli, whose proximal tubules could have different maximal glucose reabsorption capacities related to their different lengths, (c) decrease in absolute proximal Na reabsorption rate (as a result of the reduced filtered load), or (d) metabolic effects due to reduction in renal plasma flow. As pointed out by Keyes et al (76), mechanical or geometrical factors at the level of the brush border itself, such as effectiveness of the contact with the microvilli surface, could also play a part since these authors observed that reduction of GFR by ureteral clamping resulted in a much smaller drop in Tm_G than did clamping of the renal artery; in principle, the first maneuver should have kept the proximal tubules wide open, whereas the second should have led to partial collapse of the tubules. The inhibition of Tm_G associated with a reduction of proximal fractional Na reabsorption appears even more difficult to explain at the present time. It is well established that active glucose transport is a Na-dependent process; nevertheless even if glucose tubular reabsorption is necessarily coupled to corresponding Na absorption (e.g. a one to one cotransport), it remains obvious that neither the Na concentration nor the Na load can act as factors limiting glucose reabsorption in the proximal tubule. Other reasons must be found to account for a reduction in Tm_G during extracellular expansion. One of them could be increased permeability of the tubular wall to glucose backdiffusion, since in single nephron microperfusion experiments by Bank et al (13), some of the ^{14}C-glucose administered to the rats was found in the recollected perfusate in the animals made natriuretic by renal vein constriction, but not in the controls. Many other mechanisms could be suggested, but in the reviewer's opinion, it would be better to postpone this discussion until mechanisms by which extracellular expansion inhibits Na reabsorption itself are better understood.

Micropuncture and microperfusion studies.—Since the pioneering work of Walker et al (143) published in 1941, micropuncture techniques were not used for further analysis of glucose reabsorption by mammalian kidneys until 1968, when Deetjen & Boylan (35) and Rohde & Deetjen (114) reported new data obtained in the rat. Micropuncture data (114) indicate that in the normal rat most of the filtered glucose is reabsorbed along the very first part of the proximal tubule, since its concentration decreased exponentially from the glomerulus onwards and reach equilibrium at a distance of 2–3 mm; the steady state concentration (0.9 mM) in late proximal fluid reported by Rohde et al (114) was later called into question by Frohnert et al (42) who found 0.25 mM with an improved micromethod for glucose analysis. Thus, about 98% of the filtered glucose was reabsorbed in the first half of the proximal convoluted tubule, and no further net flux was detectable between the proximal segment and the end of the distal tubule accessible to micropuncture. The fact that glucose concentration does not drop to zero in the tubular fluid is explained (*a*) by the presence of passive glucose backdiffusion, as proved by single tubule microperfusion experiments (89) and (*b*) by the apparent K_m of the glucose transport system, the value of which was estimated at about 0.6 mM in a kinetic study on the rat (90). Microperfusion experiments showed that although under normal conditions net glucose reabsorption is limited to the very first portion of the proximal tubule, the entire accessible convoluted segment has a similar transport capacity. In addition, in Deetjen & Boylan's experiments (35) the glucose reabsorption rate was found to depend on the perfusion rate. The maximum glucose net reabsorption observed was 63 pmoles min^{-1} per mm tubular length. This figure may not represent maximum transport capacity, since Baines (11) recently reported values as high as 160 pmoles min^{-1} mm^{-1} (assuming 5 mm for the accessible proximal tubule) in a micropuncture study on glucose loaded rats. Although Tm$_G$ was reached in these experiments, it was not possible to observe any net glucose absorption taking place in the loop (including the pars recta) since distal micropuncture samples led to values similar to those of late convoluted proximal samples.

Here too, single nephron glucose reabsorption was correlated to the corresponding single nephron GFR, demonstrating that glomerular suppression (if present) is not sufficient to explain the decrease in Tm$_G$ associated with GFR reduction in the clearance studies reported above. Baines (11) also observed that extracellular volume expansion did not result in a statistically significant reduction of the maximal glucose reabsorption rate by the superficial punctured nephrons, although the whole kidney glucose reabsorption was depressed in the same animals, as already mentioned. This discrepancy, according to the author, could be accounted for by different responses of superficial and deep nephrons to volume expansion.

Glucose transport by isolated rabbit proximal tubules was carefully analyzed by Tune & Burg (139) by using the in vitro single tubule microperfusion technique developed by Burg et al (24). Two differently labeled D-glucose molecules (^{5}H and ^{14}C) were used as glucose tracers in the tubular perfusate and peritubular medium. The following important observations were made from steady state flux and cellular radioactivity measurements: (a) Both the pars convoluta and the pars recta of the proximal tubule have the capacity to transport glucose out of the lumen, but the maximum transport rate was found to be much larger in the former (78.5 pmoles min^{-1} mm^{-1}) than in the latter (about 6 pmoles min^{-1} mm^{-1}). (b) Glucose transport, expressed as a function of the perfused glucose load, was a saturable process, and the maximum glucose transport observed was independent of the perfusion rate (in the range of 7–50 nliter/min) at rates of glucose delivery in excess of 200 pmoles min^{-1}. (c) Steady state cell analysis demonstrated that glucose concentration in cell water (14.5 mM as a mean value) exceeded that of both the tubular perfusate and the peritubular medium (7.1 mM); the larger fraction of the cell glucose originated from the peritubular fluid, although maximum lumen to plasma net flux was achieved in these experiments. These results indicate that the glucose permeability of the basal cell surface was much greater than that of the luminal surface, and that the active transport step was localized at the luminal cell border. (d) Some backflux of glucose from peritubular medium to luminal fluid was measured, but it could not be established whether this flux entered the cells or passed along intercellular spaces.

Biochemical studies.—Great efforts have been made during the last few years to approach experimentally the first step of the transport, namely the interaction between transported substrates and postulated membrane carrier molecules. Binding of labeled substrate molecules to membrane fractions may be related to transport only if such precise criteria as similar affinity, specificity, competitive inhibitors, etc, for both binding and transport are fulfilled. A few results dealing with glucose transport by renal proximal tubules have been published. Busse et al (25) reported binding of ^{14}C-D-glucose to a brush border fraction from rabbit renal tubules. The fraction was prepared by sequential use of collagenase, EDTA, and differential centrifugation. Phlorizin (0.1 mM) and D-galactose (10 mM) inhibited ^{14}C-glucose (0.01 mM) binding to this membrane fraction, but L-glucose (10 mM) did not. In addition, the binding was Na-dependent and abolished by SH reagents, e.g. PCMB. From kinetic analysis it was concluded that two kinds of glucose binding sites, each with a very different affinity, were present in the preparation. Furthermore, Bode et al (19) studied binding of ^{3}H-phlorizin to rat brush border membrane fractions and, here again, two sets of binding sites were observed: the high affinity sites ($K_D = 3.4 \times 10^{-6}$ M) were blocked by PCMB; the low affinity sites ($K_D = 3.9 \times 10^{-4}$ M), about 100 times more numerous than the high affinity sites, were not PCMB-sensitive. The authors have suggested that the high affinity sites are located in the brush border membrane and might be related to the glucose carrier system. Since ^{3}H-phlorizin binding was observed to be a reversible process, Frasch et al (40) analyzed competition between sugars and ^{3}H-phlorizin for binding to these high affinity sites. They observed that D-glucose decreased the apparent affinity of ^{3}H-phlorizin for binding to the membrane with kinetics typical of competitive inhibition. The affinity calculated for D-glucose binding was very low (12 to 25 mM depending on the preparations). Na ions increased phlorizin binding affinity, and so did L-glucose! Although these results satisfy many of the above mentioned criteria and thus appear promising, some discrepancies (regarding D-glucose affinity for binding sites, for example) still need clarification before the observed glucose-membrane interaction can be considered conclusive evidence of binding to the molecules which act as carriers in glucose transport.

Amino Acid Transport

As already mentioned with reference to sugar transport, functional polarization of the tubule cells makes this system difficult to analyze, since transepithelial fluxes and metabolic uptake of amino acids cannot be delineated in experiments using cortex slices or isolated tubules incubated in vitro. The large number of different physiological substrates and transport systems constitutes an additional complication in the case of amino acids. On the other hand, when in whole kidney clearance experiments it is necessary to increase the plasma concentration of a given amino acid by appropriate perfusions, the concentration of other amino acids may change as a result, which sometimes makes the specificity of the variations observed in amino acid reabsorption difficult to interpret. Finally, the current methods of amino acid analysis are laborious, or do not have enough sensitivity to be used for micropuncture samples. The availability of ^{3}H and ^{14}C labeled amino acids of high specific activity has indeed improved the situation very much, but chemical determinations remain necessary as controls, owing to rapid metabolic transformations or to the incorporation of amino acids into proteins in kidney cells.

Amino acid reabsorption sites.—Those segments along the nephron in which amino acids are reabsorbed have been more precisely defined. Thus, Bergeron (14) injected tritiated leucine and lysine in vivo into the lumen of rat proximal tubules and, with autoradiographic techniques, observed the radioactivity uptake by the cells of the entire proximal tubule including the straight portion. Similar localization with maximum radioactivity over the pars recta was found by Carneiro et al (26) in mice injected with proline, leucine and tyrosine. Since the technique used by Carneiro et al permitted the diffusion of free amino acid molecules during the fixation process, it remains possible that the radioactivity accumulation observed constituted a measurement of the protein synthesis rate after peritubular uptake of the label instead of the luminal absorption rate. To avoid these difficulties, Wedeen & Thier (145) recently developed a freeze dry autoradiography technique (144) and injected two nonmetabolized amino acid analogs as tracers [(^{3}H)-α-aminoiso-butyric acid and (^{3}H)-cycloleucine]. Maximal cellular accumulation was demonstrated in the terminal portion of proximal tubules including the straight portion; in contrast, (^{3}H)-p-aminohippuric acid was shown to accumulate relatively homogeneously throughout the entire length of the proximal tubule. The amino acid reabsorption site was analyzed by Bergeron & Morel (15) using the single tubule tracer microinjection technique. When labeled amino acids were injected in vivo into a distal convolution, nearly 100% of the radioactivity injected was recovered in the ureteral urine; when similar injections were performed into a proximal tubule, even into the last convolution accessible to injection, most of the radioactivity was reabsorbed. Although direct free flow micropuncture evidence is not available, these results, when added to those obtained in earlier stop-flow experiments, suggest that amino acid reabsorption is restricted to the proximal tubule, and that the straight portion might have a greater capacity to transport amino acid than glucose, compared to the proximal convoluted portion.

Active intracellular accumulation of amino acids by the cells of different kidney structures has been analyzed by means of in vitro incubation techniques. It has been observed that slices of rat medulla and papilla concentrate amino acids (92) even in media of high Na concentration and osmolality. In a recent study, Lowenstein et al (91) stated that a maximum tissue/medium concentration ratio of (^{14}C)-α-aminoisobutyric acid was obtained with 200 meq/liter (Na concentration in the medium). The distribution ratios varied from 4 to 5 for two nonmetabolized amino acids—cycloleucine and α-amino-isobutyric acid; lysine accumulation was inhibited by arginine and ornithine but not by alanine. These results, obtained in rat papilla slices, are almost the same as those observed in cortex slices. Thus, Brown et al (22) found a distribution ratio of 4.1 for ^{14}C-α-aminoisobutyric acid and 3.3 for ^{14}C-cyclo-leucine in rat cortex slices incubated under conditions comparable to those of the above experiments in temperature, duration, and substrate concentration.

The kinetics of proline accumulation were analyzed in cortical slices, isolated tubules and isolated glomeruli. In rat kidney cortex slices, Mohyuddin and Scriver (99) obtained two-component uptake kinetics as a function of proline concentration in the medium: the high affinity component (apparent K_m: 0.1 mM) corresponded to a transport system shared by hydroxyproline; the low affinity component (apparent K_m: 5mM) had a much higher maximum transport capacity and less specificity since it was competitively inhibited by hydroxyproline, aminoisobutyric acid, glycine, and alanine. Both proline transport systems were Na-dependent and depressed by metabolic inhibitors such as cyanide or iodoacetamide (10^{-2} M). In isolated rabbit renal tubules prepared by collagenase digestion, Hillman & Rosenberg (53) also found two-limbed curves for L-proline accumulation, which indicated the presence of at least two transport systems for proline. Sodium dependency as well as inhibition by DNP (10^{-4} M), cyanide (10^{-2} M), and ouabain (5×10^{-4} M) were observed. The apparent K_m values of the two components (0.3 and

7 mM respectively) were of the same order of magnitude as those reported by Mohyuddin & Scriver (99). The low affinity proline transport system had a maximum capacity about 10 times greater than that of the high affinity system. Inhibition of L-proline uptake by either glycine or alanine was also observed by Hillman & Rosenberg (53), but their interpretation in relation to the two systems differs from that of Mohyuddin et al. Proline transport by isolated rat glomeruli was studied by Mackenzie & Scriver (93, 94) in in vitro incubation experiments. L-Proline was actively accumulated in the glomeruli up to a fivefold concentration ratio, although at a somewhat slower rate than in other cortical structures. The uptake was largely Na-dependent and was inhibited by 10^{-2} M cyanide or iodoacetamide. Here again, kinetic studies clearly showed two components, suggesting the existence of two systems for L-proline transport in glomeruli, for which the respective K_m values calculated were 0.1 and 5.3 mM. Thus, in vitro accumulation of L-proline by either isolated glomeruli, isolated tubules, or cortex slices turn out to be roughly similar; the same is true of α-aminoisobutyric acid and cycloleucine in both papilla and cortical slices. It can reasonably be assumed that neither the glomeruli (at least their vascular portion), nor the epithelial structures of the inner medulla are involved in amino acid reabsorption by the kidney; the conclusion should therefore be that the transepithelial reabsorption capacity of the proximal tubules does not greatly influence the in vitro kinetics of amino acid accumulation in kidney cortex slices and isolated tubules. Thus the similarity noted may be accounted for, if it is postulated that (a) most of the amino acid transport observed did take place at the basal border of the epithelial cells and (b) the peritubular cell membranes have similar transport properties in the different nephron segments and in glomeruli. Indeed, substrates added to the medium probably have little or no direct access to the luminal border of the cells in incubated slices or tubule fragments, since their lumen must quickly collapse in vitro and any net reabsorption therefore stop. It is hard to estimate how far the functioning of such cells is modified compared to conditions in vivo; Tune & Burg (139) reported that glucose concentration in cell water falls in nonperfused isolated rabbit proximal tubules, compared to glucose perfused tubules. Peritubular cell membrane properties may well be preserved during in vitro incubation experiments but luminal transport probably reaches a standstill.

Amino acid transport systems.—Earlier evidence obtained from in vivo and in vitro competition studies as well as from genetic defect analysis suggested the existence of at least four distinct amino acid transport systems in mammalian kidney: (a) the neutral system, chiefly involved in the transport of glycine, alanine, serine, threonine, valine, leucine, isoleucine, phenylalanine, tyrosine, glutamine, asparagine, methionine, and cysteine; (b) the basic system, involved in the transport of lysine, arginine, ornithine, and possibly cystine; (c) the acidic system, for the transport of glutamic acid and aspartic acid, and (d) the iminoglycine system, transporting proline, hydroxyproline, and glycine. In the kidney, a fifth system might possibly be responsible for transport of β-alanine, β-aminobutyric acid, and taurine. Although generally accepted, such a subdivision will probably appear oversimplified in the future. Many observations suggest that the number of systems might be much larger and that their specificity regarding substrates cannot be so simply delineated. There are indications however, that two functionally different types of transport systems may exist: high-capacity, low-affinity, and low-specificity systems which would transport a relatively large variety of amino acids, and low-capacity, high-affinity, and high-specificity systems which transport only a few closely related amino acids.

Thus, in vivo tracer microinjection experiments in rat kidney tubules showed that both L-leucine and L-isoleucine were reabsorbed by common low affinity and high capacity transport systems. On the other hand, arginine and lysine competed for a different transport system, characterized by a higher affinity and a much lower capacity (15). With the same technique, Baines et al (12) observed that aspartic and glutamic acid reabsorption was T_M limited. They also demonstrated marked mutual competition for transport between these two acidic amino acids when they were injected into the nephron simultaneously. Injected under the same conditions, a variety of neutral amino acids did not inhibit acidic amino acid transport. These data confirm glutamic and aspartic acid reabsorption by common low-capacity systems which are quite distinct from the high-capacity systems available for neutral amino acids.

Further evidence for different mechanisms in the transport of cysteine and cystine was reported by Segal et al (125): a comparison between incubation experiments on newborn and adult rat kidney slices revealed that the ability of the neonatal cortex slices to take up L-cystine was impaired compared to that of adult slices, at a time when the neonatal slices' ability to accumulate L-cysteine was similar to that of the adult tissue; differences in dependence on oxygen and temperature also pointed to the existence of different transport systems. Aromatic amino acid urinary excretion was analyzed by Lines & Waisman (88) in conscious monkeys made hyperphenylalaninemic and injected with β-2-thienylalanine which competed with both tyrosine and phenylalanine reabsorption, as shown by a significant increase in urinary clearance of these amino acids. Since the urinary output of other amino acids was not consistently affected, this study suggested the presence of a specific mechanism for phenylalanine and tyrosine reabsorption in the monkey kidney. The inhibition of amino acid accumulation by cycloleucine was analyzed in incubated human and rat cortex slices by Holtzapple et al (56). Kinetic experiments demonstrated competitive inhibition of both L-lysine and α-aminoisobutyric acid accumulation by cycloleucine; cycloleucine had similar effects on both the basic and neutral amino acid transport systems.

As far as proline is concerned, at least two transport systems were postulated to exist in kidney cortex in order to account for the observed in vitro accumulation kinetics (53, 99). From competitive inhibition assays, Hillman & Rosenberg (53) deduced that in isolated rabbit kidney tubules a third component of proline transport might exist, characterized by a very low affinity (K_m: 30 mM) and a high capacity. This third system was not found to be shared by either alanine or glycine. It seemed important to recall these results, since the same authors later reported evidence for what they considered specific L-proline binding to a brush border-rich membrane fraction prepared from isolated rabbit renal tubules (54). The fraction was obtained by stirring the tubules in a 5 mM EDTA hypotonic medium, followed by differential centrifugation. Maximum binding of ^{14}C-L-proline to this fraction took place during the first minute of incubation and reached equilibrium within five min; saturation occurred at a medium proline concentration of 75 mM, and the curve suggested an apparent K_m for binding in the range of 30–35 mM. This binding was completely inhibited by PCMB and thermal denaturation. Depletion of Na ions from the incubation medium reduced binding significantly, as did cyanide; DNP and ouabain, on the other hand, had no inhibitory effect. Glycine and L-alanine reduced L-proline binding, whereas L-valine and L-phenylalanine in similar concentrations (50 mM) did not. From these observations, and mainly from the fact that glycine and alanine reduced proline binding as much as they inhibited proline transport in the intact tubules (53), the authors concluded that the binding observed may correspond to a specific interaction of the amino acid with membrane carriers involved in proline transport.

This important conclusion calls for some comment. The kinetics of accumulation in isolated tubules probably measure mainly transport properties of peritubular and not luminal cell membranes; indeed it may well be that the membrane fraction prepared by the authors contained a large proportion of basal membranes as well, so that comparisons remain possible. Apparent K_m values for proline binding to the membrane fraction in the range observed (30–35 mM) are compatible with specific substrate-carrier interaction since a transport system of similar affinity (30 mM) and very high capacity was observed to exist in living tubules; but it is precisely this low-affinity transport system which according to Hillman & Rosenberg (53) is not shared by either glycine or alanine, so that the inhibition of proline binding by these two amino acids is difficult to explain by referring to the in vivo experiments. Although these results look promising, further experiments are necessary before it can be accepted that the binding process observed represents the initial step in the transtubular transport of L-proline as suggested by the authors.

In vivo microperfusion experiments.—Quantitative in vivo microperfusion studies dealing with amino acid transport were published by Silbernagl & Deetjen (129) and Chan & Huang (27). The former authors analyzed glycine reabsorption in rat single proximal tubules microperfused with various ^{3}H or ^{14}C glycine concentrations in the perfused solution. The glycine concentration in the recollected fluid decreased exponentially as a function of the perfused distance. The slope of the line decreased when the glycine concentration in the perfusate or the perfusion rate was increased. From these curves. glycine permeability constants were calculated: the values obtained were independent of the perfusion rate, but varied according to the glycine concentration ($P_{gly} = 22 \times 10^{-5}$ cm/sec from 0.2 to 3mM; $12 - 14 \times 10^{-5}$ cm/sec from 20 to 40 mM). The addition of 5 mM cyanide to the perfusate did not modify the glycine efflux, whereas marked inhibition was noted when cyanide was perfused into peritubular blood capillaries. The proportionality observed between labeled glycine efflux and its concentration in the tubular fluid (in the range of 0.2 to 3mM) strongly suggests either that efflux resulted from simple diffusion out of the lumen or that it was mediated by a low-affinity carrier-mediated system. The fact that fractional reabsorption was markedly reduced when glycine concentration was raised to 20 mM points to the second hypothesis. But simple diffusion may well have contributed to the efflux measured, especially when a large transmural chemical gradient was present. Plasma-to-lumen backflux of radioactivity was noted by Bergeron et al (16, 17) when radioactive L-arginine and L-leucine were microinjected into peritubular capillaries.

Microperfusion studies of tryptophan transport by Chan & Huang (27) led to quantitatively very different results from those obtained by Silbernagl & Deetjen for glycine. When solutions containing either 1 mM labeled D-tryptophan, 5-OH-tryptophan or 5-OH-tryptamin were perfused at a rate of 16 nl/min, the proximal reabsorption rate observed was very low and corresponded to a permeability coefficient for these three tryptophan derivatives ranging from 2 to 3 $\times 10^{-5}$ cm/sec. In contrast, L-tryptophan was found to be rapidly reabsorbed from the perfusate: with a 1 mM tryptophan concentration in the perfused solution, the concentration remaining in the tubular fluid decreased exponentially as a function of the distance perfused; at about 1 mm distance from the perfusion site, about 90% of the perfused amino acid was already reabsorbed. The tubular reabsorption rate of L-tryptophan showed saturation kinetics with a maximum reached at a perfused concentration of 8 mM; the corresponding K_m calculated value was 4 mM, but owing to the quick drop in concentration along the perfused segment, a somewhat higher affinity would probably have been found if the authors had used the mean tubular concentration in place of that in the perfusate in their calculations. Reabsorption was greatly reduced when cold L-phenylalanine (1–10 mM) was added to the perfused solution. Kinetic evidence supports the hypothesis that phenylalanine acted as a competitive inhibitor of tryptophan reabsorption. 1 mM sodium azide as well as 0.1 and even 1 mM DNP in the perfusate only slightly affected L-tryptophan tubular transport. Since it had earlier been observed that DNP completely blocks in vitro tryptophan accumulation in kidney cells (148), Chan & Huang concluded that two different steps are involved and that the transluminal transport mechanism for L-tryptophan does not require energy obtained through oxidative phosphorylation. In addition, this study clearly establishes that L-tryptophan reabsorption by the proximal rat tubule is a T_M-limited process and that phenylalanine and tryptophan share common carrier transport systems.

Freedman & Young (41) reported the results of histidine in vivo microperfusion experiments in the rat, which showed that about 80% of the perfused histidine was reabsorbed by the end of the perfused proximal segment under control conditions. When up to 40 mM cyanide concentration was present in the perfusate, some limited inhibition of histidine reabsorption was noted, but about 70% of the infused load was still reabsorbed by the end of the proximal tubule.

These microperfusion studies raise the important problem of energy coupling mechanisms for amino acid transport at the luminal border of the tubular cells. Since a direct energy supply from oxidative metabolism is perhaps not an absolute prerequisite, alternative mechanisms should be evaluated, such as the Na gradient hypothesis, some other types of coupled transport or countertransport or carrier-mediated facilitated diffusion.

This short analysis of amino acid transport within the kidney has been deliberately limited to some of the contributions to the problem which have appeared since 1969. Readers interested in this question are invited to refer to an excellent critical review recently published by Young & Freedman (152).

Mechanisms of Urine Concentration

It is now generally agreed that the formation of hypertonic urine by the mammalian kidney requires the action of the antidiuretic hormone (ADH) and results from the passive osmotic equilibration of the tubular fluid flowing through the collecting ducts with the surrounding hyperosmotic interstitial fluid of the renal medulla and papilla. The existence of the medullary osmotic pressure gradient is made possible, in the presence of ADH, by two of the structure's main properties, (a) the hairpin shape of the tubular and vascular loops, which function as countercurrent exchangers, and (b) the properties of the tubule cells of the ascending limbs, which have low water permeability and actively reabsorb salt. However, although this general framework is widely accepted, many problems are still unresolved or open to discussion. Among these questions, the following deserve mention: What mechanism is responsible for building up the medullary gradient of osmotic pressure in the presence of ADH? What processes make it possible for tissue osmolarity to increase up to the tip of the papilla? How does the tubular fluid increase in osmotic pressure when flowing along the descending limb of the loop of Henle? What is the exact role of medullary blood flow rate in maintaining or washing out medullary hyperosmolarity? As will appear from this section, none of these problems has been resolved unequivocally during the last two years.

Counter-current flow was also claimed to exist at the surface of the cortex between proximal convolutions and peritubular capillaries. Thus Steinhausen et al (133, 134) systematically analyzed the direction of both fluid and blood flow in a number of convolutions and adjacent capillaries and discovered that opposite flow direction was far more frequent than flow in the same direction. This observation was recently questioned by Solomon (132), and its physiological significance, if any, remains to be established.

Urine osmolarity and the medullary osmotic pressure gradient.—Postnatal development of kidney function was analyzed by Horster et al in the rat (60) and the dog (59, 61). In the dog, GFR increased linearly from 0.13 ml min^{-1} g^{-1} kidney weight 2 days after birth, to 0.91 at 77 days. Urea clearance per unit of renal mass increased with age, whereas the fraction of filtered urea reabsorbed declined during the early part of the postnatal period. This pattern of fractional urea reabsorption may be due mainly to increased medullary recycling of urea and to a rise in reabsorption of water from the medullary collecting ducts. Urine osmolarity was higher than plasma from birth onwards and rose with age. Osmolal equality of collecting-duct fluid and medullary interstitium reflected mature ADH-induced water permeability. The rise observed in urinary concentration was predominantly due to increasing medullary sequestration of urea. Better et al (18) analyzed the maximum urine concentration and dilution capacities in ten uninephrectomized human subjects. The remaining hypertrophic kidney was found to concentrate and dilute urine normally (mean values—1003 and 82 mOsm/kg H_2O).

Apparent discrepancies between anatomical development of the papilla and maximum urinary osmolarity were reported. In the rhesus monkey *Macaca mulatta,* Tisher (137) measured a mean urine osmolality of 1400 mOsm/kg H_2O after one to two days of water deprivation. Morphologically, however, the inner medulla was little developed in the kidney of these animals, representing only 14% of its relative thickness; thus, despite the virtual absence of an inner medulla containing long loops of Henle with ascending thin limbs, this monkey concentrated urine as well as animals with well-developed inner medullary zones. In contrast, a primitive rodent species like the mountain beaver (*Aplodontia rufa*) whose kidney medulla structure roughly resembles that of the rhesus monkey, was found by Schmidt-Nielsen et al (123) to concentrate urine after fluid deprivation up to only 550 mOsm/kg H_2O. It may well be that differences of species in urea handling by the kidney could account for the differences observed in urine maximum osmolarity. Gutman & Beyth (48) noted the opposite discrepancy between concentrating ability and kidney structure in a rodent species, *Chinchilla laniger,* known to tolerate long periods of water deprivation. The bladder urine was collected and analyzed in chinchillas and albino rats submitted to three days of water deprivation. Mean urine osmolality was found significantly higher in the rat (2744 mOsm/kg H_2O) than in the chincilla (2006 mOsm/kg H_2O), although the kidney of this latter species has a voluminous long papilla, protruding into the ureter and similar to that of rodents like the kangaroo rat and the jerboa which have a markedly higher concentrating ability. The relatively low urine osmotic pressure measured by Gutman & Beyth in dehydrated chinchillas might have resulted from inappropriate diet or some other cause, since Weisser et al (146) measured urine osmolalities ranging from 2350 up to 7600 mOsm/liter after water deprivation in the same species (*Chinchilla laniger*). Weisser et al also performed micropuncture experiments at the surface of the cortex in this species, with results roughly similar to those previously obtained in other rodent species; fluid from the distal tubule was persistently hypotonic throughout its entire length (mean *TF/P* Osm = 0.52).

Electrolyte distribution and renal function were analyzed in two hibernating species. Clausen & Storesund (31) compared kidneys removed from active and hibernating hedgehogs. The medullary gradients of both electrolyte (Na and Cl) and urea concentrations were completely abolished during hibernation. In addition, the tissue water content was increased in the papilla and inner medulla, but not in the outer medulla and cortex of the hibernating animals, compared to the active ones. The ground squirrel *Spermophilus columbianus*, on the other hand, was studied by Lesser et al (86) and by Moy (103). Using tissue analysis, Moy did not find urea and Na solute gradients in torpid ground squirrels. In contrast, animals arousing from torpor normally and killed 15 to 40 min after urine began to flow into a catheterized ureter had built up distinct renal urea and Na gradients. It is not really surprising that euthermia and sufficient metabolic rates are prerequisites for the generation of significant medullary gradients of osmotic pressure.

The effect of ADH on the osmotic permeability to water of distal and collecting tubules is well documented, but the possibility that this hormone could directly or indirectly exert additional effects at different sites within the kidney has several times been suggested. The morphology of the rat renal medulla in water diuresis and in vasopressin-induced antidiuresis was examined by Tisher et al (138). All kidneys were preserved in vivo by intraaortic perfusion of hypertonic or hypotonic fixative. Whatever the osmolality of the fixatives used, the following changes were noted two hours after subcutaneous injection of 1 IU vasopressin tannate into diabetes insipidus (*DI*) rats: expansion of the medullary interstitium, widening of the lateral intercellular spaces of medullary collecting ducts, and widening of the basilar and lateral intercellular compartments of the thin descending loops of Henle. The enlargement of collecting-tubule intercellular spaces had already been reported (e.g. 46), and probably indicates that ADH-induced fluid reabsorption occurs at least in part via lateral intercellular channels. Tisher et al noted that in thin descending limbs "the epithelium appeared to be lifted from the basement membranes as a result of expansion of the basal labyrinth and lateral intercellular space. These enlarged spaces were filled with a flocculent material identical in appearance to that of the adjacent, greatly widened interstitium." In addition, it should be stressed that thin segments of the ascending limb failed to exhibit this morphological appearance in ADH treated animals and resembled those of control DI rats. The authors concluded that "because the thin descending limb of the nephron is seemingly already freely permeable to water, there appears to be no reason to postulate a direct action by the hormone at this site."

But types of action other than increasing water permeability remain quite possible in so far as the aspects observed are ADH specific and not indirect effects of artifacts. In a recent electron microscope study of the junctional complexes along the descending thin limb of the loop of Henle, Bulger (23) did not mention any structural modifications similar to those observed by Tisher et al, although she examined kidneys from both hydropenic and water loaded rats, nor did she confirm the earlier report of Darnton (34) indicating that 70 Å (or more) spaces are present within the tight junctions of rabbit descending thin limbs. Dense granules resembling the peroxisomes described in the proximal tubules were also reported to be present in the cells of the loop of Henle and of the distal convoluted tubule; the histoenzymological properties were those expected of peroxysomes and not of lysosomes (28). In addition, Azar et al (9) observed that the solute content (mainly Na) of the renal papilla was correlated to the amount of granules measured in the interstitial cells of the papilla in rats submitted to different versions of prolonged water diuresis.

Changes in the morphology of the vascular bundles in the outer medulla of the rat kidney under conditions of water diuresis and water deprivation, and after administration of ADH, were observed by Creasey & Moffat (33). In addition, experiments using Evans blue as a protein tracer showed that after the dye had been allowed to circulate for 2 min, almost twice as much extravascular dye was found in the medulla of DI rats as in that of ADH treated rats (149). Mucopolysaccharides of the rabbit renal papilla (38) and their turnover as a function of the osmolarity of the incubation medium (39) were studied by Farber et al. Histochemical detection of mucoprotein anionic charges in the renal medulla also revealed reproducible variations in response to ADH administration (100). The physiological importance of all these observations remains difficult to assess at the present time.

A careful systematic analysis of the influence of various doses of lysine-vasopressin (LVP) on the time course of changes in renal tissue and urinary composition in the conscious rat was carried out by Atherton et al (8). LVP 2.5–60 μU/min/100 g body weight was intravenously infused for up to 4½ hr in water-loaded rats. The authors observed that: (a) the dose-dependent changes in medullary composition consisted of graded decreases in water content and graded increases in solute content (mainly Na and urea); (b) the relative contribution of the changes in water, Na, and urea contents varied with time and with dose; Significant increases in papillary urea content occurred for all doses and the magnitude of the changes in urea content were greater than for any other solute; and (c) at low doses (2.5 and 5 μU/min), the changes in urinary flow and osmolality were almost entirely ascribable to a big drop in free-water clearance, with minor changes in medullary composition. At higher doses (15–60 μU/min), the increases in urinary osmolality were accompanied by steep increases in medullary solute concentrations. (*d*) Variable, dose-dependent, transient natriuresis occurred during the phase of increasing medullary Na concentration; the peak natriuresis preceded the times of maximal osmolal and Na concentrations in the papilla and urine. The authors have suggested that several hormone-sensitive sites exist in the kidney, each with its own dose-response and kinetic characteristics. In their experiments, a higher concentration of ADH stimulated the sequestration of Na ions in the tissue of the medulla, in addition to acting on the permeability of the distal tubular segment to water. Many mechanisms could be suggested to account for such an effect of ADH—for instance (*a*) proximal effects resulting in increased Na delivery to the loops; (*b*) vascular effects decreasing blood flow to the medulla; (*c*) increased permeability to solutes of the thin descending limb, favoring the medullary recycling of Na ions; and (*d*) some kind of stimulation of active sodium transport out of the ascending limbs or the medullary collecting ducts. Nevertheless, the distal ADH action cannot be ruled out as being the sole mechanism responsible for the results observed. Some of these mechanisms will be discussed further on.

The fact that neurohypophysial hormones both increase water permeability and stimulate active Na transport in epithelial cells is well established for amphibian skin, bladder, and kidney tubule. This was also recently reported by Ames et al (3) to be the case for the avian kidney. These authors injected small amounts of arginine-vasotocin (*AVT*) into chickens undergoing water diuresis. Less than 30 ng AVT had no significant effect on GFR, but resulted in a tubular antidiuretic effect. Whereas urine osmotic pressure increased up to nearly 300 mOsm/liter, Na and Cl concentrations in the urine, in fact, decreased. At the peak of the effect, Na and Cl excretion per unit GFR fell by approximately 30%, where K and urea excretion were not affected in any regular manner. Thus the renal effects of AVT in the chicken are comparable to those occurring in other nonmammalian tetrapods. No similar effect of ADH on Na tubular reabsorption has been reported in mammals, although vasopressin was observed by Helman et al (51) to cause a transient increase in potential difference without any change in electrical resistance when applied in vitro to perfused rabbit cortical collecting tubules. These authors inferred that ADH could directly increase active ion transport by this segment. As for the loop of Henle, the effects of ADH on distal tubular fluid composition were analyzed by Schnermann et al (124) by using micropuncture techniques on DI rats: they observed no increase in Na reabsorption in response to administration of ADH. However, their results concerned short loops only. In addition, the situation is obscured in the case of the mammalian kidney by the possibility of Na recycling from ascending to descending limbs of the medullary loops. In fact, the overall effect frequently reported in response to ADH administration was a transient increase in urinary Na output. Recently, Humphreys et al (63) reproduced such an effect in hydrated dogs when the endogenous release of

ADH was induced by hemorrhage. Under such conditions, natriuresis could not be ascribed either to extracellular expansion or to enhanced GFR (which in fact was reduced). To explain these findings, the authors suggested that active Na transport out of the ascending limb might have been inhibited as a result of a transient overhydration of the medullary interstitium, due to increased water reabsorption out of the collecting ducts. Martinez-Maldonado et al (97) have suggested, on the contrary, that inhibition of proximal reabsorption could be an explanation for the unilateral natriuretic effect induced by the injection of low doses of vasopressin (20–200 μU) into one renal artery of dogs undergoing hypotonic saline diuresis, since phosphate reabsorption was to some extent simultaneously inhibited and cyclic AMP injections resulted in comparable effects. A series of studies by Atherton et al on the rat (6, 7) clearly showed that the effects of either water loading or ADH administration on both solute excretion into the urine and solute accumulation in the medulla depend largely on the hydration state prevailing at the beginning of the experiment. Similarly, when animals have to be loaded with urea, the results obtained will depend on the amount of water and salt given together with urea (75, 107). On the other hand, rises in renal venous pressure (57) or ureteral pressure (58) were observed to reduce greatly the medullary gradient of osmotic pressure in hydropenic rabbits. Differences in sodium handling in the loop of Henle and the distal tubule among mice of different genetic strains were also recently reported and analyzed by Stewart (135, 136). Sensitivity to vasopressin as well may vary greatly from strain to strain as shown by Kar et al (72) in the rat.

Functioning of the loop of Henle.—As indicated above, the main function of the loop of Henle is to reabsorb salt in excess of water along the ascending limb, and thus (*a*) deliver a large amount of free water to the cortical distal tubule and (*b*) maintain medullary hyperosmolarity. Although this main function of the ascending limb has been established beyond a doubt, important assumptions need to be substantiated in order to evaluate quantitatively the net Na reabsorption along this segment. The use of conditions that produce a maximal diuresis results in maximal reduction of salt and water reabsorption in the distal tubules and collecting ducts, and makes it possible to calculate fractional reabsorption of sodium in the loop of Henle in the following way: It is assumed that urinary fractional Na excretion may be used as an estimation of the rate of Na delivery by the loops to the distal segments and it is assumed that the urinary fractional free water clearance may be used as an estimation of the rate of Na net absorption by the loops. $(C_{H_2O} + C_{Na})/GFR$ is therefore assumed to measure the fractional Na delivery to the loops, and $C_{H_2O}/(C_{H_2O} + C_{Na})$ the fraction of Na entering the loops which is reabsorbed by them. Although a relatively large number of additional studies involving this kind of calculation have recently been published, they will not be analyzed here, since in the reviewer's opinion such an indirect approach does not permit any precise conclusion.

The use of inhibitors to estimate active Na reabsorption by the loops of Henle is also of limited value, since no diuretic in current use has an action restricted to this segment of the nephron. Morgan et al (102) in microperfusion experiments, and Brenner et al (21) and Dirks et al (36) in micropuncture experiments, examined the effects of furosemide. Clearcut proximal effects were noted, in addition to the inhibitory action of the Na transport in the loop of Henle. Ethacrynic acid also reduced proximal Na reabsorption, as shown by Clapp et al (30). On the other hand, Duarte et al (37) observed and analyzed distal effects produced by amiloride and ouabain on Na and K transfers in the rat tubule. Even in the case of more direct experimental approaches such as the micropuncture technique, the rate of Na reabsorption in the medullary segments of the loops cannot be measured directly; thus, the calculation of net transfers along the entire loop from late proximal and early distal micropuncture samples is limited in that (a) only short-looped nephrons are accessible at the surface of the cortex, and (b) net transfers taking place along the *pars recta* of the proximal tubule represent an unknown fraction of the net reabsorption measured. In addition, in order to evaluate the rate of active Na transport by the ascending limb, appropriate measurements at early distal and late proximal levels are not sufficient; estimation of Na delivery to the ascending limb (i.e. at the tip of the loop) is obviously required. Unfortunately, direct measurement is impossible in short loops at present, since the tip of these loops is not accessible to micropuncture. Indirect estimations from late proximal micropuncture data are based on the assumptions that (a) Na and water reabsorption continue in the *pars recta* at the same rate as in the proximal convoluted tubule and (b) no net Na transfer takes place in the thin descending segment. This latter assumption is only reasonable if the thin descending limb is impermeable to Na diffusion, i.e. in so far as the tubular fluid mainly equilibrates its osmotic pressure with that of the hypertonic extratubular fluid by osmotic withdrawal of water, and not by diffusional addition of solutes. The permeability properties of the descending and ascending thin limbs were analyzed by Marsh (95) in micropuncture experiments at the surface of the exposed hamster papilla. Collections were made from two sites of the same single thin limbs. Along the ascending limb, no change in inulin TF/P was noted (over a 1 mm distance), whereas either osmolality or Na and K concentration fell as the tubular fluid flowed from the bend up to the ascending limb. The data confirm the properties expected for this segment. In the descending limb, a net addition of urea to the tubular fluid as it flowed down toward the bend was noted, but the data were inconclusive as far as net movements of Na were concerned. Indeed, the mean change in *TF/P* osmolality between the two puncture sites was very low (10%) in this series of paired collections. In a more direct approach, Kokko (83) carried out in vitro microperfusion experiments of single isolated rabbit thin descending limbs and observed that active Na transport was absent as indicated by the failure to demonstrate either net transport or transmembrane potential difference when perfusing the structure with ultrafiltrate of the same rabbit serum as the bath. The passive permeability coefficient for Na (P_{Na}) was determined from the disappearance rate of ^{22}Na from an isosmolal perfusion solution. P_{Na} was found to be surprisingly low (1.6 × 10^{-5} cm/sec), a figure significantly less than P_{Na} in the proximal convoluted tubule. The reflexion coefficient for NaCl (σ NaCl) was measured by perfusing the tubule with Na-free raffinose solution in a bath of rabbit serum to which sufficient NaCl was added to obtain conditions of zero net fluid movement. The σ NaCl value measured (0.96) is significantly greater than that in the proximal convoluted tubule. The osmotic permeability to water (Lp) was also measured, and the value obtained—about 1.7 × 10^{-4} ml cm^{-2} sec^{-1} atm^{-1}—is much greater than that in the proximal tubule. These observations enabled the author to conclude that low permeability to Na and high permeability to water is consonant with the hypothesis that high interstitial Na concentration in the medulla generates effective osmotic pressure, resulting in the concentration of the fluid as it courses through the descending thin limb, primarily by abstraction of water without significant net entry of NaCl. Permeability to urea was not analyzed in this study nor were the possible effects of adding ADH to the bathing medium tested. The above conclusions are exactly opposed to those previously reported by de Rouffignac et al (115) from *Psammomys papilla* micropuncture experiments and, to a lesser extent, to those reached by Morgan & Berliner (101) in loop microperfusion experiments on excised rat papillae. This point may be important with regard to the way the system functions. If the concentrating mechanism suggested by Kokko, i.e. osmotic equilibration mainly by water subtraction-functions under physiological conditions, one would expect that (*a*) the higher the medullary osmotic pressure, the higher the inulin concentration at the tip of the loops, and (*b*) *TF/P* inulin in early distal fluid would increase as a function of the final osmotic pressure (assuming the ascending limb to be poorly permeable to water osmotic flow). For the reverse hypothesis, i.e. osmotic equilibration mainly by solute addition, *TF/P* inulin ratios, both at the tip of the long loops and the entrance of the distal short loop convolution, should remain constant regardless of tissue and urinary osmotic pressure. Recently published results tend to favor the second hypothesis: thus, Jamison et al (65) punctured descending and ascending limbs near the tip of the exposed papilla of young rats. Although the mean osmolality of the punctured fluid samples was 1.002 Osm, the corresponding *TF/P* inulin value was only 7.01; in addition, no difference in TF/P_{in} was detected between samples punctured in descending, bend, or ascending sites. The data confirmed that single nephron GFR is higher in juxtamedullary than in superficial nephrons. (*TF/P*) Na/inulin was 0.41, indicating that, if no Na net addition occurred in the thin limb, *TF/P* inulin should have been about 2.5 at the end of the *pars recta* of these deep nephrons. In a further loop micropuncture study of young rats, Jamison & Lacy (66) included two control groups of hydropenic rats, which had comparable whole kidney GFR and comparable calculated single nephron GFR for the punctured loops. The main difference observed in the two groups was that the mean osmotic pressure of the fluid collected at the tip of the loops which was 1537 and 1043 mOsm. From inulin and Na measurements, it appears that the rate of tubular flow at the tip of these loops was almost the same in the two groups (15.4 and 17.3% of the filtration rates respectively), whereas the Na delivery rate was definitely greater in the higher osmolality group than in the other (61 and 49% of the filtered load respectively).

Superficial nephron micropuncture and microperfusion experiments led to similar conclusions. Thus, in the long-looped rodent species *Meriones shawii*, Murayama et al (104) perfused nephrons from the last accessible proximal convolution, and recollected the perfusate in the corresponding first distal convolution. No correlation was observed between inulin concentration at the end of the perfused loops and urinary osmotic pressure. More recently Armsen & Reinhardt (4) carried out micropuncture experiments in groups of rats undergoing different degrees of water diuresis, so that urine osmolarity mean values ranged from 233 to 1420 mOsm/liter. No difference in GFR was observed among the groups. TF/P inulin mean value at the end of the proximal was 2.33 in the lower urine osmolarity group and 2.63 in the higher osmolarity group. The corresponding values in early distal samples were 5.5 and 6.1 respectively. Thus, in this study, there was no indication of increased water reabsorption in the descending limb of the loops of Henle as a function of the osmotic pressure in the medulla.

In a previous micropuncture study, Schnermann et al (124) analyzed the effects of ADH on water and salt reabsorption by the superficial loops of DI rats and observed that no effect of ADH on the proximal convoluted tubule could be detected. However, vasopressin increased the delivery of sodium and water to the early distal tubule. Since the Na concentration in the early distal fluid was unchanged by vasopressin but TF/P_{in} decreased, the hormone apparently depressed water reabsorption within the loop but did not change the minimum sodium concentration achieved by reabsorption in the ascending limb. Clearly, enhancement of medullary osmolarity by the hormone did not result in an increase in TF/P_{in} in early distal fluid; in fact, the reverse was observed.

Although indirect, these in vivo observations do not appear to confirm the permeability properties of the thin descending limb as revealed by the direct in vitro measurements carried out by Kokko (83). At this point in the discussion, we would like to suggest a hypothesis which could reconcile many of the above observations. We suggest that, in addition to its main action on the distal tubules and collecting ducts, ADH could increase the permeability of the thin descending limb to solute diffusion (mainly Na and Cl ions and also urea molecules). This hypothesis is compatible with the morphological observations by Tisher et al already discussed (138). As a result of this ADH-induced permeability change, osmotic equilibration along this segment would involve proportionally more net solute addition and less water subtraction than in the DI state, which agrees with the observations of Schnermann et al (124). The resulting recirculation of salt between the ascending and descending limbs of the loops will consequently favor the medullary sequestration of sodium and the building up of the medullary osmotic pressure gradient in the presence of the hormone, as proposed by Atherton et al (8). A relatively constant water flow, combined with increasing solute delivery to the ascending limb as a function of tissue osmotic pressure, will maintain TF/P_{in} relatively constant at the early distal level. Regardless of the osmotic pressure of the urine, the fluid composition will also remain constant, since it is well established that salt reabsorption in the ascending limb is concentration-limited rather than T_M-limited. Depending on the conditions, T_M might be attained in some instances, which would account for the transient natriuretic action of the hormone. But we are fully aware that this proposal needs direct substantiation, for instance, demonstration by in vitro microperfusion experiments that the reflexion coefficient of the thin descending limb drops sharply when ADH is added to the incubation medium.

The permeability of the loop of Henle to urea seems less complex. Recent micropuncture studies in the rat have confirmed earlier observations and produced new data. Armsen et al (5) infused rats with hypertonic urea solutions. Plasma urea concentrations ranged from 5 to 20 mM/liter. GFR was not affected, nor was the fraction of the filtered urea reabsorbed in the proximal tubule (about 54%). Recirculation of urea in the medulla (approximately equal to 50% of the filtered urea) was present at a low urea plasma concentration; when this concentration was raised to 20 mM/liter, the addition of urea to the loop of Henle dropped to approximately zero. Distal urea reabsorption increased more than expected as a function of the plasma concentration. Distal permeability to urea was thus apparently a function of plasma urea concentration.

In a more recent publication, Armsen et al (4) examined urea handling in rats undergoing different degrees of water diuresis and observed that urea medullary recycling vanished at higher urine flow rates (U/P inulin in the range of 15 to 25). In addition, at low U/P inulin values, the late distal urea load in superficial nephrons was found smaller than the excreted fraction in the urine. Thus, under these conditions, the authors admitted that the deep nephrons excreted a higher fraction of their filtered urea compared to superficial nephrons. Joppich et al (67) measured distal permeability to urea in DI rats undergoing different types of diuresis; the value obtained (about 1×10^{-4} mm/sec) was independent of the urea concentration both in the plasma and the distal fluid, thus excluding the suggested possibility that there exists a reabsorption mechanism for urea unrelated to water reabsorption. The permeability to urea of both the proximal tubule and the loop of Henle was estimated by Wilczewski et al (147). The value found was comparable for the two structures (12.5×10^{-4} and 10.4×10^{-4} mm/sec respectively). Urea excretion in response to ADH administration to DI dogs, as reported by Kauker et al (74) showed transient changes which could be related to urea accumulation into or release from a medullary pool. Readers interested in more detailed aspects of urea handling by the kidney should refer to the symposium *Urea and the Kidney* edited by Schmidt-Nielsen and Kerr (122).

Permeability of the collecting tubules.—New information has been obtained from cortical collecting tubules using the in vitro microperfusion technique described by Burg et al (24), and from terminal collecting ducts by micropuncture of the exposed papilla of young rats. Evidence for coupled active transport of both Na (reabsorption) and K (secretion) in rabbit cortical collecting tubules was reported by Grantham et al (45). Earlier observations by Grantham & Burg (44) showed that ADH acts on this segment by increasing both osmotic and diffusional permeability to water, whereas urea permeability was not altered by the hormone. Helman et al (51) recently reported that vasopressin might also stimulate active ion transport in this segment. Aldosterone, on the other hand, has also been claimed to cause a substantial decrease in collecting-duct permeability to Na ions, in tracer efflux experiments reported by Uhlich et al (140). Bowman & Foulkes (20) obtained indirect evidence that ADH might increase the permeability of the collecting ducts to urea by injecting labeled urea during stop-flow experiments in the rabbit. Young DI rats (Brattleboro strain) were used by Jamison et al (64) to measure net movements of water out of the collecting ducts both in the presence and absence of ADH action. The collecting ducts were punctured either at the tip of the exposed papilla or about 1 mm from the tip. As expected, the collecting duct fluid was found to be hypoosmotic to plasma at the papilla tip in the DI control ($TF/P_{Osm} = 0.55$) and hyperosmotic ($TF/P_{Osm} = 2.65$) when vasopressin was infused. Although ADH increased the osmotic permeability of the collecting tubule to water and allowed osmotic equilibrium of the tubular fluid with that of the papillary interstitium, the data showed that the amount of water reabsorbed by the terminal collecting duct was less in antidiuresis (0.58% of the filtered water) than in water diuresis (1.58%). It is difficult to decide whether such a decrease in absolute water reabsorption out of the collecting ducts (as a result of the ADH-mediated increase in cortical free-water reabsorption) is a factor of physiological importance in building up the medullary osmotic pressure gradient, as suggested by several authors in the past. In some instances, when the urine flow rate is very high, osmotic equilibration of the collecting-duct fluid and peritubular medium is no longer reached, even in the presence of ADH, as demonstrated by the experiments of Porush et al (110) in the dog. These authors calculated the papillary tip osmolality from urea, Na, and K tissue measurements in normal dogs and dogs with experimental constriction of the inferior vena cava (caval dogs). Osmotic equilibrium between final urine and papillary tip tissue was noted in the nondiuretic state. When acute sodium diuresis was induced (C_{Na} more than 15 ml/min/ 100 ml GFR), the urine osmolality in the normal dogs was about 100 mOsM lower than that calculated in the papilla. In the caval dogs, the discrepancy was even greater. These observations indicate that, by reducing the transit time in the collecting tubules, high urine flow rates may act as a factor that prevents osmotic equilibrium from being reached. The greater osmotic disequilibrium noted in the caval dogs was not due to a higher urine flow rate, since rates were in fact higher in the normal dogs; it is more likely to have resulted from the delivery to the collecting tubule of a fluid of lower osmotic pressure in the caval than in the control dogs. Indeed, micropuncture experiments by Levy (87) showed that the sodium concentration in distal fluid samples was lower in caval than in normal dogs both under nondiuretic conditions and during volume expansion.

The existence of osmotic disequilibrium between final urine and papillary tip osmolalities was deduced by Rabinowitz from theoretical considerations (111). Thus in dehydrated mammals, the urine may contain more urea and less sodium than does the tissue of the papilla; therefore if the reflexion coefficient of the collecting duct wall is lower for urea molecules than for sodium ions, osmotic equilibrium should no longer be reached. But in that case one would expect higher urine than papillary tip osmolality—i.e. a difference in the opposite direction to that noted by Porush et al (110).

Metabolic and biochemical studies.—Since the osmotic work carried out by the medulla mainly consists of active salt transport out of the ascending limbs of the Henle loop, attempts were made to correlate Na transport to the rate of either total metabolism or more specific enzyme reactions within different areas of the medulla. Martinez-Maldonado et al (96) infused cyanide into the renal artery of dogs undergoing hypertonic mannitol diuresis or water diuresis. Under both conditions, cyanide induced natriuretic responses which were associated with decreased free water clearance, indicating a poisoning effect on Na reabsorption in the cortex and outer medulla. Since these effects were abolished by pretreating the animals with sodium thiosulfate, the authors have suggested that cyanide inhibited Na transport by inhibiting cytochrome oxidase activity: the electron transport system of oxidative metabolism could therefore be of importance in medullary sodium transport. Urbaitis & Kessler (141) analyzed the effects of administering cyanide, DNP, ouabain, and oligomycin to dogs in vivo on the adenine nucleotide content of the renal cortex. Cyanide reduced sodium reabsorption and cortical ATP and ADP content, which is also consistent with in vivo inhibition of oxidative metabolism. Abodeely & Lee (1) measured O_2 consumption and CO_2 production in vitro by slices of rabbit outer medulla in the presence of different substrates and of 0 or 350 mM Na in the incubation medium. In every instance

CO_2 increased about threefold in the presence of Na, suggesting that extracellular Na was of prime importance in determining the rate of outer medullary substrate oxidation, possibly through activation of $(Na + K)$-ATPase. In addition, glucose was shown to be the preferential exogenous fuel for respiration. Using similar techniques, Kannegiesser & Lee (71) analyzed the role of outer medullary metabolism in the concentrating defect of K depletion. Holmes et al (55) showed that the urinary concentrating defect and the exaggerated natriuresis known to occur in hypothyroid rats are associated with a reduced rate of aerobic metabolism in the cortex and of glycolytic metabolism in the inner medulla.

The effects of several diuretics on the metabolism of both the cortex and the outer medulla were recorded in vivo in the dog by Sejersted et al (127) by using an ingenious thermoelectric method. Thermocouples were inserted into the renal cortex and outer medulla of anesthetized dogs and the local metabolic rate was estimated from the initial temperature rise after clamping the renal artery. After several control measurements, ouabain was injected into the renal artery, and cortical and outer medullary metabolic rates fell by averages of 28 and 52% respectively. When ouabain was injected after the intravenous infusion of ethacrynic acid and chlorothiazide (which reduced cortical and outer medullary metabolic rates by 30 and 60% respectively), no further reduction was observed either in Na reabsorption or in the metabolic rate. The authors concluded that ouabain reduced the metabolic rate in vivo mainly by inhibiting active Na transport in the ascending limb of the loops of Henle and in the distal tubules. The same experimental technique was used by Kiil et al (77) to analyze the effects of mannitol and saline infusions on the metabolic rates in vivo. During isotonic or hypertonic saline infusion the metabolic rate increased in the outer medulla and remained constant in the cortex. Mannitol diuresis did not significantly affect the metabolic rates of either the cortex or the medulla; on the other hand, constriction of the renal artery resulted in a decrease in both metabolic rates. These data provide additional direct evidence that variations in active Na transport are closely correlated to variations in the metabolic rate. In addition, Kiil et al's study (77) implies that the net changes in energy utilization coupled to Na transport produced by saline diuresis are greatest in the outer medulla (probably the ascending limb of Henle's loop).

A very large number of publications dealing with kidney $(Na + K)$-ATPase have appeared during the last two years; among these papers, we shall limit our discussion to those directly related to the physiology of Na transport in the renal medulla. Purely biochemical work will not be considered. Improved methods for purification and characterization of $(Na + K)$-ATPase activity from rabbit outer medulla were recently reported by Jørgensen et al (69, 70). Nechay & Nelson (105, 106) analyzed the correlations between active transport of Na in vivo and cortical and medullary $(Na + K)$-ATPase activities in vitro for a variety of animal species and experimental conditions. Ouabain, when infused into the left renal artery of dogs in vivo, inhibited both Na reabsorption and enzyme activity in roughly the same dose range and for similar periods of time. Hendler et al (52), found that the ouabain-inhibited (Na + K)-ATPase activity content is considerably higher in homogenates of the outer medulla than the cortex or papilla. A very careful analysis of the ATPase activity content in different portions of the rat nephron was carried out by Schmidt & Dubach by measuring enzyme activities in single tubule microdissected segments (118, 119). These authors observed that Mg-ATPase activity was of the same order of magnitude in the proximal convoluted tubule, the ascending limb of the loop, and the distal convoluted tubule and it was about twice as great in the glomerulus. On the other hand, (Na + K)-ATPase activity was very low in the glomerulus, intermediate in the proximal tubule, and very high and of comparable magnitude in both the ascending limb of the loop of Henle and the distal convoluted tubule (120). In a recent study, Schmidt & Dubach (121) even separated by microdissection the basal cell border from the apical cell border in isolated proximal tubules; the (Na + K)-ATPase activity per unit dry weight they measured was about 100 times greater in the basal area fragments of the tubules than in the brush border fragments. On the other hand, Mg-ATPase activity was similar in both types of fragments. These studies show that the (Na + K)-ATPase activity is more abundant in those segments of the nephrons which reabsorb sodium against a concentration gradient and, as far as the proximal tubule is concerned, that the ATP-dependent Na transport system is probably almost entirely localized in the basal infolding membrane and absent from the brush border membrane. This latter conclusion was also reached by Kinne et al (78), who used centrifugation on continuous and discontinuous sucrose gradients to separate brush border membrane fractions from basal infolding membrane fractions of rat kidney cortex homogenates.

Since osmotic pressure as well as Na and urea concentrations are normally greater in the kidney medulla than in other tissues, the effects of these parameters on enzyme activity were analyzed by several groups of authors with somewhat conflicting results. When the Na concentration was increased in the incubation medium of microsome fractions of the outer medulla, ouabain-sensitive ATPase activity was found by Cole & Dirks (32) to be little affected in dog preparation within the range of 100 to 300 mM. In guinea-pig preparations, Gutman et al (47) observed significant inhibition when the Na concentration was increased from 100 to 200 mM. The opposite was the case, however, for the rabbit preparations examined by Alexander & Lee (2) who reported a great stimulatory effect when the osmolality of the medium was increased up to 800 mOsm/liter by adding either NaCl, sucrose, or choline chloride. These discrepancies in the data probably resulted from differences in the procedure used for preparing the membrane fractions or from differences in incubation conditions, rather than from differences in animal species. In any case, when compared to (Na + K)-ATPase activities in other tissues, the enzyme activity of the outer medulla of the kidney remained very active in vitro under conditions of high osmolality and high Na concentration roughly similar to those prevailing in vivo.

It is now well established that aldosterone [and even glucocorticoids, as recently shown by Sakai & Murayama (116)] controls active Na reabsorption in the ascending limb of the loops of Henle. However, the molecular mechanisms of the aldosterone action are not yet quite clear. It has not been established whether aldosterone controls the protein synthesis involved (*a*) in the energy supply to active Na transport steps, (*b*) in the carrier-mediated Na entry through the apical border of the epithelial cells, or (*c*) in some other limiting step or steps. Possible correlations between (Na + K)-ATPase activity in the outer medulla and adrenal function therefore aroused great physiological interest and were further investigated. Jorgensen (68) measured Mg and (Na + K)-activated ATPase activities in kidney homogenates and microsomal fractions from uninephrectomized, uninephrectomized-adrenalectomized and sham-operated rats. Whereas adrenalectomy neither impaired compensatory renal growth nor affected Mg-ATPase activity, it significantly reduced the (Na + K)-ATPase content expressed per mg protein or per mg tissue wet weight; thus corticoids apparently control Na transport ATPase activity independently of tissue growth. Schmidt & Dubach (120) analyzed ATPase activities in single isolated proximal and distal rat nephron segments as a function of the time which elapsed after adrenalectomy. Six hours after adrenal enucleation, they noted a 65% reduction of (Na + K)-ATPase activity in the ascending limb of Henle's loop, and an 81% reduction in the distal convoluted portion; at the same time, neither (Na + K) ATPase activity in the proximal tubule, nor Mg-ATPase activities in all the segments analyzed were modified compared to the sham-operated controls. This study shows that distal (Na + K)-ATPase activity rapidly adapts to the modified Na transport in kidney after adrenalectomy. On the basis of kinetic analysis of the enzyme activity in plasma membrane and microsomal fractions prepared from kidneys of adrenalectomized rats with and without steroid hormone substitution, de Santo et al (117) also concluded that the changes observed were due to adaptation to altered renal Na reabsorption, which in turn was regulated by corticosteroids; this adaptation process was observed to vary according to the different subcellular fractions analyzed. The enzyme activity measurements made by Katz & Genant (73), working on kidney extracts from extracellular volume-expanded rats, also suggested that (Na + K)-ATPase activity in the outer medulla may rapidly adapt to changes in the tubular Na load delivered to the ascending limbs. These authors observed that (Na + K)-ATPase specific activity of the outer medulla—but not of the cortex—increased in tissue extracts from the in vivo expanded animals compared to the controls. It seems quite obvious that aldosterone (and other regulatory agents) may indirectly control (Na + K) ATPase activity in vivo, either by changing the concentration of the enzyme substrates or by acting via intermediates which affect the enzyme's K_m and V_{max}. However, it seems more difficult to imagine how such factors could be sufficient to induce changes which persisted when the enzyme activity was measured in isolated membrane fractions using standard constant-medium conditions. Indirect induction of new enzyme synthesis might be an alternative explanation.

LITERATURE CITED

1. Abodeely, D. A., Lee, J. B. 1971. Fuel of respiration of outer renal medulla. *Am. J. Physiol.* 220:1693–1700
2. Alexander, J. C., Lee, J. B. 1970. Effect of osmolality on $Na^+ = K^+ = ATPase$ in outer renal medulla. *Am. J. Physiol.* 219: 1742–45
3. Ames, E., Steven, K., Skadhauge, E. 1971. Effects of arginine vasotocin on renal excretion of Na^+, K^+, Cl^- and urea in the hydrated chicken. *Am. J. Physiol.* 221:1223–28
4. Armsen, T., Reinhardt, H. W. 1971. Transtubular movement of urea at different degrees of water diuresis. *Pfluegers Arch.* 326:270–80
5. Armsen, T., Schad, H., Reinhardt, H. W. 1969. Die Harnstoffkonzentrierung in der Niere. II. Mikropunktions experimente an ratten. *Pfluegers Arch.* 313:222–44
6. Atherton, J. C., Evans, J. A., Green, R., Thomas, S. 1971. Influence of variations in hydration and in solute excretion on the effects of lysine-vasopressin infusion on urinary and renal tissue composition in the conscious rat. *J. Physiol. London* 213:311–28
7. Atherton, J. C., Green, R., Thomas, S. 1970. Effects of 0.9% saline infusion on urinary and renal tissue composition in the hydropaenic, normal and hydrated conscious rat. *J. Physiol. London* 210:45–71
8. Atherton, J. C., Green, R., Thomas, S. 1971. Influence of lysine-vasopressin dosage on the time course of changes in renal tissue and urinary composition in the conscious rat. *J. Physiol. London* 213:291–309

9. Azar, S., Tobian, L., Ishii, M. 1970. Prolonged water diuresis affecting solutes and interstitial cells of renal papilla. *Am. J. Physiol.* 221:75–79
10. Bailey, J. M., Fishman, P. H., Pentchev, P. G. 1970. Studies on muterotases. VI. Enzyme levels and sugar reabsorption in developing rat kidney and intestine. *J. Biol. Chem.* 245:559–63
11. Baines, A. D. 1971. Effect of extracellular fluid volume expansion on maximum glucose reabsorption in Rat and glomerular tubular balance in single rat nephrons. *J. Clin. Invest.* 50: 2414–25
12. Baines, A. D., Morel, F. 1969. Absorption of acidic amino acids from proximal tubule fluid. *4th Int. Congr. Nephrol. (Stockholm)*, Abstr., 293
13. Bank, N., Yarger, W. E., Aynedjian, H. S. 1971. A microperfusion study of sucrose movement across the rat proximal tubule during renal vein constriction. *J. Clin. Invest.* 50:294–302
14. Bergeron, M. 1966. Microinjection tubulaire associée à la radioautographie en microscopie électronique: réabsorption des acides eminés dans le tube contourné proximal du rein. *J. Microsc.* 5:32a.
15. Bergeron, M., Morel, F. 1969. Amino acid transport in renal tubules. *Am. J. Physiol.* 216: 1139–49
16. Bergeron, M., Vadeboncoeur, M. 1971. Microinjections of L-Leucine into tubules and peritubular capillaries of the rat. II. The maleic acid model. *Nephron* 8:367–74
17. Bergeron, M., Vadeboncoeur, M. 1971. Antiluminal transport of L-Arginine and L-leucine

following microinjections in peritubular capillaries of the rat. *Nephron* 8:355–66

18. Better, O. S., Nahir, A. M., Chaimowitz, C., Naveh, Y., Richter-Levin, D. 1971. Urinary concentration, dilution and acid excretion in subjects with a single kidney. *J. Urol.* 105:323–25

19. Bode, F., Baumann, K., Frasch, W., Kinne, R. 1970. Die Bindung von Phlorrhizin an die Bürstensaumfraktion der Rattenniere. *Pfluegers Arch.* 315:53–65

20. Bowman, F. J., Foulkes, E. C. 1970. Antidiuretic hormone and urea permeability of collecting ducts. *Am. J. Physiol.* 218:231–33

21. Brenner, B. M., Keimowitz, R. I., Wright, F. S., Berliner, R. W. 1969. An inhibitory effect of furosemide on sodium reabsorption by the proximal tubule of the rat nephron. *J. Clin. Invest.* 48:290–300

22. Brown, D. M., Michael, A. F. 1971. Effects of Ca^{2+} and Mg^{2+} upon amino acid transport in rat renal cortex slices. *Biochim. Biophys. Acta* 233:215–21

23. Bulger, R. E. 1971. Ultrastructure of the junctional complexes from the descending thin limb of the loop of Henle from rats. *Anat. Rec.* 171:471–76

24. Burg, M., Grantham, J., Abramow, M., Orloff, J. 1966. Preparation and study of fragments of single rabbit nephrons. *Am. J. Physiol.* 210:1293–98

25. Busse, D., Elsas, L. J., Rosenberg, L. E. 1970. D-glucose binding by a brush border fraction from rabbit renal tubules. *J. Clin. Invest.* 49:A15

26. Carneiro, J., Saldanha, R. V. 1969. Incorporation of labeled amino-acids by different segments of the proximal tubules in mice kidneys. *Lab. Invest.* 20:332–37

27. Chan, Y. L., Huang, K. C. 1971. Microperfusion studies on renal tubular transport of tryptophan derivatives in rats. *Am. J. Physiol.* 221:575–79

28. Chang, C. H., Schiller, B., Goldfisher, S. 1971. Small cytoplasmic bodies in the loop of Henle and distal convoluted tubule that resemble peroxisomes. *J. Histochem. Cytochem.* 19:56–62

29. Chinard, F. P., Taylor, R. W., Nolau, F., Enns, T. 1959. Renal handling of glucose in dogs. *Am. J. Physiol.* 196:535–44

30. Clapp, J. R., Nottebohm, G. A., Robinson, R. R. 1971. Proximal site of action of ethacrynic acid: importance of filtration rate. *Am. J. Physiol.* 220:1355–60

31. Clausen, G., Storesund, A. 1971. Electrolyte distribution and renal function in the hibernating hedgehog. *Acta Physiol. Scand.* 83:4–12

32. Cole, C. H., Dirks, J. H. 1971. A comparison of Na^+ activation of ATPase in the red cell, renal cortex and renal medulla. *Can. J. Physiol. Pharmacol.* 49:63–69

32a. Crane, R. K. 1962. Hypothesis for mechanism of intestinal active transport of sugars. *Fed. Proc.* 21:891–95

33. Creasey, M., Moffat, D. B. 1971. The effect of changes in conditions of water balance on the vascular bundles of the rat kidney. *J. Anat.* 109:437–42

34. Darnton, S. J. 1969. A possible correlation between ultrastructure and function in the thin descending and ascending limbs of the loop of Henle of Rabbit kidney. *Z. Zellforsch. Mikrosk. Anat.* 93:516–24

35. Deetjen, P., Boylan, J. W. 1968. Glucose reabsorption in the rat Kidney. Microperfusion studies. *Pfluegers Arch.* 299:18–29

36. Dirks, J. H., Seely, J. F. 1970. Effect of saline infusions and furosemide on the dog distal nephron. *Am. J. Physiol.* 219:114–21

37. Duarte, C. G., Chomety, F., Giebisch, G. 1971. Effect of amiloride, ouabain, and furosemide on distal tubular function in the rat. *Am. J. Physiol.* 221:632–40

38. Farber, S. J., Van Praag, D. 1970. Composition of glycosaminoglycans (mucopolysaccharides)

in rabbit renal papillae. *Biochim. Biophys. Acta* 208:219–26

39. Farber, S. J., Walat, R. J., Benjamin, R., Van Praag, D. 1971. Effect of increased osmolality on glycosaminoglycan metabolism of rabbit renal papilla. *Am. J. Physiol.* 220:880–85

40. Frasch, W., Frohnert, P. P., Bode, F., Baumann, K., Kinne, R. 1970. Competitive inhibition of Phlorizin binding by D-glucose and the influence of sodium: a study on isolated brush border membrane of rat kidney. *Pfluegers Arch.* 320:265–84

41. Freedman, B. S., Young, J. A. 1969. A microperfusion study of L-Histidine transport by the rat nephron. *Aust. J. Exp. Biol. Med. Sci.* 47:10–19

42. Frohnert, P. P., Höhmann, B., Zwiebel, R., Baumann, K. 1970. Free flow micropuncture studies of glucose transport in the rat nephron. *Pfluegers Arch.* 315:66–85

43. Genel, M., Rea, C. F., Segal, S. 1971. Transport interaction of sugars and amino-acids in mammalian kidney. *Biochim. Biophys. Acta* 241:779–88

44. Grantham, J. J., Burg, M. B. 1966. Effect of vasopressin and cyclic AMP on permeability of isolated collecting tubules. *Am. J. Physiol.* 211:255–59

45. Grantham, J. J., Burg, M. B., Orloff, J. 1970. The nature of transtubular Na and K transport in isolated rabbit renal collecting tubules. *J. Clin. Invest.* 49:1815–26

46. Grantham, J. J., Ganote, C. E., Burg, M. B., Orloff, J. 1969. Path of transtubular water flow in isolated renal collecting tubules. *J. Cell. Biol.* 41:562–76

47. Gutman, Y., Katzper-Shamir, Y. 1971. The effect of urea, sodium and calcium on microsomal ATPase activity in different parts of the kidney. *Biochim. Biophys. Acta* 233:133–36

48. Gutman, Y., Beyth, Y. 1970. Discrepancy between concentrating ability and kidney structure. *Life Sci.* 9:37–42

49. Hauser, G. 1969. Myo-Inositol transport in slices of rat kidney cortex. I. Effect of incubation conditions and inhibitors. *Biochim. Biophys. Acta* 173:257–66

50. Hauser, G. 1969. Myo-Inositol transport in slices of rat kidney cortex. II. Effect of ionic composition of the medium. *Biochim. Biophys. Acta.* 173:267–76

51. Helman, S. I., Grantham, J. J., Burg, M. B. 1971. Effect of vasopressin on electrical resistance of renal cortical collecting tubules. *Am. J. Physiol.* 220:1825–32

52. Hendler, E. D., Torreti, J., Epstein, F. H. 1971. The distribution of sodium-potassium-activated adenosine triphosphatase in medulla and cortex of the kidney. *J. Clin. Invest.* 50:1329–37

53. Hillman, R. E., Rosenberg, L. E. 1969. Amino-acid transport by isolated mammalian renal tubules. II. Transport systems for L-Proline. *J. Biol. Chem.* 244:4494–98

54. Hillman, R. E., Rosenberg, L. E. 1970. Amino-acid transport by isolated mammalian renal tubules. III. Binding of L-proline by proximal tubule membranes. *Biochim. Biophys. Acta* 211:318–26

55. Holmes, E. W., Jr., DiScala, V. A. 1971. Oxygen consumption, glycolysis and sodium reabsorption in the hypothyroid rat kidney. *Am. J. Physiol.* 221:839–43

56. Holtzapple, P., Rea, C. F., Genel, M., Segal, S. 1970. Cycloleucine inhibition of amino-acid transport in human and rat kidney cortex. *J. Lab. Clin. Med.* 75:818–25

57. Honda, N., Aizawa, C., Morikawa, A., Yoshitoshi, Y. 1970. Effect of elevated venous pressure on medullary osmolar gradient in rabbit kidney. *Am. J. Physiol.* 218:708–13

58. Honda, N. Aizawa, C., Morikawa, A., Yoshitoshi, Y. 1971. Effect of elevated ureteral pressure on renal medullary osmolar concentration in hydropenic rab-

bits. *Am. J. Physiol.* 221:698–703

59. Horster, M., Kemler, B. J., Valtin, H. 1971. Intracortical distribution of number and volume of glomeruli during postnatal maturation in the dog. *J. Clin. Invest.* 50:796–800

60. Horster, M., Lewy, J. E. 1970. Filtration fraction and extraction of P.A.H. during the neonatal period in the rat. *Am. J. Physiol.* 219:1061–65

61. Horster, M., Valtin H. 1971. Postnatal development of renal function: micropuncture and clearance studies in the dog. *J. Clin. Invest.* 50:779–95

62. Huang, K. C., Woosley, R. L. 1968. Renal tubular secretion of L-glucose. *Am. J. Physiol.* 214:342–47

63. Humphreys, M. H., Friedler, R. M., Earley, L. E. 1970. Natriuresis produced by vasopressin or hemorrhage during water diuresis in the dog. *Am. J. Physiol.* 219:658–65

64. Jamison, R. L., Buerkert, J., Lacy, F. 1971. A micropuncture study of collecting tubule function in rats with hereditary diabetes insipidus. *J. Clin. Invest* 50:2444–52

65. Jamison, R. L. 1970. Micropuncture study of superficial and juxtamedullary nephrons in the rat. *Am. J. Physiol.* 218:46–55

66. Jamison, R. L., Lacy, F. B. 1971. Effect of saline infusion on superficial and juxtamedullary nephrons in the rat. *Am. J. Physiol.* 221:690–697

67. Joppich, R., Deetjen, P. 1971. The relation between the reabsortion of urea and of water in the distal tubule of the rat kidney. *Pfluegers Arch.* 329:172–85.

68. Jørgensen, P. L. 1971. Dissociation between compensatory renal growth and induction of (Na⁺ + K⁺)—ATPase in rat kidney after uninephrectomy. *Experientia* 27:527

69. Jørgensen, P. L.., Skou, J. C. 1971. Purification and characterization of (Na⁺ + K⁺)—ATPase. I. the influence of detergents on the activity of Na⁺ + K⁺) — ATPase in preparations from the outer medulla of rabbit kidney. *Biochim. Biophys. Acta* 233:366–80

70. Jørgensen, P. L., Skou, J. C., Solomonson, L. P. 1971. Purification and characterization of (Na⁺ + K⁺)—ATPase. II. Preparation by zonal centrifugation of highly active (Na⁺ + K⁺)—ATPase from the outer medulla of rabbit kidneys. *Biochim. Biophys. Acta* 233:381–94

71. Kannegiesser, H., Lee, J. B. 1971. Role of outer renal medullary metabolism in the concentrating defect of K depletion. *Am. J. Physiol.* 220:1701–07

72. Kar, K., Sur, R. N., Dhawan, B. N. et al 1970. Sensitivity of male rats of different strains to vasopressin. *Indian J. Exp. Biol.* 8:194–97

73. Katz, A. I., Genant, H. K., 1971. Effect of extracellular volume expansion on renal cortical and medullary Na⁺—K⁺ ATPase. *Pfluegers Arch.* 330:136–48

74. Kauker, M., Hare, R., Hare, K. 1970. The effect of vasopressin on renal transport of urea and water in dogs with experimental diabetes insipidus. *Arch. Int. Pharmacodyn Ther.* 185:174–84

75. Kauker, M. L., Lassiter, W. E., Gottschalk, C. W. 1970. Micropuncture study of effects of urea infusion on tubular reabsorption in the rat. *Am. J. Physiol.* 219:45–50

76. Keyes, J. L., Swanson, R. E. 1971. Dependence of glucose Tm on GFR and tubular volume in the dog kidney. *Am. J. Physiol.* 221:1–7

77. Kiil, F., Johannesen, J., Aukland, K. 1971. Metabolic rate in renal cortex and medulla during mannitol and saline infusion. *Am. J. Physiol.* 220:565–570

78. Kinne, R., Schmitz, J. E., Kinne-Saffran, E. 1971. The localization of the Na⁺—K⁺—ATPase in the cells of rat kidney cortex. A study on isolated plasma membranes. *Pfluegers Arch.* 329:191–206

79. Kleinzeller, A. 1970. The specificity of the active sugar transport

in kidney cortex cells. *Biochim. Biophys. Acta* 211:264–76

80. Kleinzeller, A. 1970. Active sugar transport in renal cortex cell: the electrolyte requirement. *Biochim. Biophys. Acta.* 211:277–92

81. Kleinzeller, A., Ausiello, D. A., Almendares, J. A., Davis, A. H. 1970. The effect of pH on sugar transport and ion distribution in kidney cortex cells. *Biochim. Biophys. Acta* 211:293–307

82. Kleinzeller, A., Kolinska, J., Bines, J. 1967. Transport of monosaccharides in kidney cortex cells. *Biochem. J.* 104:852–60

83. Kokko, J. P. 1970. Sodium chloride and water transport in the descending limb of Henle. *J. Clin. Invest.* 49:1838–46

84. Kolinska, J. 1970. Kinetics of sugar transport in rabbit kidney cortex, in vitro: movement of D-galactose, 2-deoxy-D-galactose and α-methyl-D-glucoside. *Biochim. Biophys. Acta* 219:200–9

85. Kurtzman, N. A., White, M. G., Rogers, P. W., Flynn, J. J., III 1972. Relationship of sodium reabsorption and glomerular filtration rate to renal glucose reabsorption. *J. Clin. Invest.* 51:127–33

86. Lesser, R. W., Moy, R. M., Passmore, J. C., Pfeiffer, E. W. 1970. Renal regulation of urea excretion in arousing and homeothermic ground squirrels (*Citellus columbianus*). *Comp. Biochem. Physiol.* 36:291–96

87. Levy, M. 1970. Proximal and distal tubular function in chronic caval dogs. *Clin. Res.* 18:507–13

88. Lines, D. R., Waisman, H. A. 1970. Renal amino-acid reabsorption in hyperphenylalaninemic monkeys infused with β-2-Thienylalanine. *Proc. Soc. Exp. Biol. Med.* 134:1061–64

89. Loeschke, K., Bauman, K., Renschter, H., Ullrich, K. J. 1969. Differenzierung zwischen aktiver und passiver Komponente des D-Glucosetransports am proximalen Konvolut der Rattenniere. *Pfluegers Arch.* 305:118–38

90. Loeschke, K., Baumann, K. 1969. Kinetische studien der glucose resorption in proximalen Konvolut der Rattenniere. *Pfluegers Arch.* 305:139–54

91. Lowenstein, L. M., Hagopian, L. 1969. Amino acid transport in stored renal medulla. *Transplantation* 8:558–65

92. Lowenstein, L. M., Smith, I., Segal, S. 1968. Amino acid transport in rat renal papilla. *Biochim. Biophys. Acta* 150:73–81

93. Mackenzie, S., Scriver, C. R. 1971. Transport of L-Proline and α-aminoisobutyric acid in the isolated rat kidney glomerulus. *Biochim. Biophys. Acta* 241:725–36

94. Mackenzie, S., Scriver, C. R. 1970. Proline transport into isolated rat glomeruli. *Biochim. Biophys. Acta* 196:110–12

95. Marsh, D. J. 1970. Solute and water flows in thin limbs of Henle's loop in the hamster kidney. *Am. J. Physiol.* 218:824–31

96. Martinez-Maldonado, M., Eknoyan, G., Suki, W. N. 1969. Effects of cyanide on renal concentration and dilution. *Am. J. Physiol.* 217:1363–68

97. Martinez-Maldonado, M., Eknoyan, G. Suki, W. N. 1971. Natriuretic effects of vasopressin and cyclic AMP: possible site of action in the nephron. *Am. J. Physiol.* 220:2013–20

98. McNamara, P., Rea, C. F. Segal S. 1971. Sugar transport: effect of temperature on concentrative uptake of α-methylglucoside by kidney cortex slices. *Science* 172:1033–34

99. Mohyuddin, F., Scriver, C. R. 1970. Amino-acid transport in mammalian kidney: multiple systems for imino acids and glycine in rat kidney. *Am. J. Physiol.* 219:1–8

100. Morard, J. C., Abadie, A. 1968. Fonction des mucopolysaccharides et des mucoïdes acides de la médullaire rénale dans l'élaboration de l'urine: II. Etudes histochimiques au cours de diurèses controlées. *J. Physiol. Paris.* 60:323–56

101. Morgan, T., Berliner, R. W. 1968.

Permeability of the loop of Henle, *vasa recta* and collecting ducts to water, urea and sodium. *Am. J. Physiol.* 215:108–15

102. Morgan, T., Tadokoro, M., Martin, D., Berliner, R. W. 1970. Effect of furosemide on Na^+ and K^+ transport studied by microperfusion of the rat nephron. *Am. J. Physiol.* 218:292–97

103. Moy, R. M. 1971. Renal function in the hibernating ground squirrel *Spermophilus columbianus*. *Am. J. Physiol.* 220:747–53

104. Murayama, Y., de Rouffignac, C., Morel, F. 1971. Etude par microperfusion du fonctionnement de l'anse de Henle chez un rongeur désertique (Meriones Shawii Duvernois). *Actualités Néphrologiques*, ed. Hamburger et al. 91–104. Paris: Flammarion

105. Nechay, B. R., Nelson, J. A. 1970. Renal ouabain-sensitive adenosine triphosphatase activity and Na^+ reabsorption. *J. Pharmocol. Exp. Ther.* 175:717–26

106. Nelson, J. A., Nechay, B. R. 1970. Effects of cardiac glycosides on renal adenosine triphosphatase activity and Na^+ reabsorption in dogs. *J. Pharmacol. Exp. Ther.* 175:727–40

107. Niesel, W., Roeskenbleck, H., Hanke, P., Specht, N., Heuer, L. 1970. Die gegenseitige Beeinflussung von Harnstoff, NaCl, KCl, und Harnfluss bei der Bildung eines maximal konzentrierten Harns. *Pfluegers Arch.* 315:308–20

108. Orloff, J., Burg, M. 1971. Kidney. *Ann. Rev. Physiol.* 33:83–130

109. Pellet, M., Cohen, H., Seigner, C. 1971. L'exrétion rénale de l'acide citrique: régulation de la réabsorption. *J. Physiol. Paris* 63:577–98

110. Porush, J. G. et al 1971. Urinary concentrating operation in caval dogs. *Am. J. Physiol.* 220:1547–52

111. Rabinowitz, L. 1970. Discrepancy between experimental and theoretical urine-to-papilla osmotic gradients. *J. Appl. Physiol.* 29:389–90

112. Rasmussen, S. N. 1970. Renal reabsorption and metabolic conversion of galactose in the cat. *Acta Physiol. Scand.* 80:160–71

113. Robson, A. M., Srivastava, P. L., Bricker, N. S. 1968. The influence of saline loading on renal glucose reabsorption in the rat. *J. Clin. Invest.* 47:329–35

114. Rohde, R., Deetjen, P. 1968. Die Glucoseresorption in der Rattenniere. Mikropunktionsanalysen der tubulären Glucosekonzentration bei freiem Fluss. *Pfluegers Arch.* 302:219–32

115. de Rouffignac, C., Morel, F. 1969. Micropuncture study of water, electrolyte and urea movements along the loops of Henle in Psammomys. *J. Clin. Invest.* 48:474–86

116. Sakai, F., Murayama, Y. 1970. Effects of cortisol on the Henle's loop of adrenalectomized rat's kidney. *Jap. J. Pharmacol.* 20:458–59

117. de Santo, N. G., Ebel, H. Hierholzer, K. 1971. Plasma cell membranes of the rat kidney. II. ATPase activities in adrenalectomized rats with and without steroid hormone substitution. *Pfluegers Arch.* 324:26–42

118. Schmidt, U., Dubach, U. C. 1969. Activity of (Na K)–stimulated adenosine triphosphatase in the rat *Pfluegers Arch.* 306:219–26

119. Schmidt, U., Dubach, U.C. 1969. The behaviour of NaK activated adenosine triphosphatase in various structures of the rat nephron after furosemide application. *Nephron* 7:447–58

120. Schmidt, U., Dubach, U. C. 1971. Sensitivity of NaK adenosine triphosphatase activity in various structures of the rat nephron: studies with adrenalectomy. *Eur. J. Clin. Invest.* 1:307–312

121. Schmidt, U., Dubach, U. C. 1971. NaK stimulated adenosinetriphosphatase: intracellular localisation with the proximal tubule of the rat nephron. *Pfluegers Arch.* 330:265–270

122. Schmidt-Nielsen, B., Kerr, D. N. S., Eds. 1970. *Urea and the Kidney.* Amsterdam: Excerpta Medica Foundation

123. Schmidt-Nielsen, B., Pfeiffer, E. W. 1970. Urea and urinary concentrating ability in the mountain beaver, *Aplodontia Rufa. Am. J. Physiol.* 218: 1370–75

124. Schnermann, J. et al 1969. Micropuncture studies on the influence of antidiuretic hormone on tubular fluid reabsorption in rats with hereditary hypothalamic diabetes insipidus. *Pfluegers Arch.* 306:103–18

125. Segal, S., Smith, I. 1969. Delineation of cystine and cysteine transport systems in rat kidney cortex by developmental patterns. *Proc. Nat. Acad. Sci. USA* 63:926–33

126. Segal, S., Rea, C., Smith, I. 1971. Separate transport systems for sugars and amino acids in developing rat kidney cortex. *Proc. Nat. Acad. Sci. USA* 68: 372–76

127. Sejersted, O. M., Lie, M., Kiil, F. 1971. Effect of ouabain on metabolic rate in renal cortex and medulla. *Am. J. Physiol.* 220: 1488–93

128. Shannon, J. A. 1938. The tubular reabsorption of xylose in the normal dog. *Am. J. Physiol.* 122:775–81

128a. Shannon, J. A., Fischer, S. 1938. The renal tubular reabsorption of glucose in the normal dog. *Am. J. Physiol.* 122:765–74

129. Silbernagl, S., Deetjen, P. 1971. Glycine reabsorption in rat proximal tubules. Microperfusion studies. *Pfluegers Arch.* 323:342–50

130. Silverman, M., Aganon, M. A., Chinard, F. P. 1970. Specificity of monosaccharide transport in dog kidney. *Am. J. Physiol.* 218:743–50

131. Silverman, M., Aganon, M. A., Chinard, F. P. 1970. D-Glucose interactions with renal tubule cell surfaces. *Am. J. Physiol.* 218:735–42

132. Solomon, S. 1971. Is there an effective countercurrent system in the superficial renal cortex? *Proc. Soc. Exp. Biol. Med.* 137: 1019–20

133. Steinhausen, M., Eisenbach, G. M., Galaske, R. 1970. A counter-current system of the surface of the renal cortex of rats. *Pfluegers Arch.* 318:244–58

134. Steinhausen, M., Eisenbach, G. M., Galaske, R. 1970. Counter-current system in the renal cortex in rats. *Science* 167: 1631–33

135. Stewart, J. 1970. Genetic variation in patterns of nephron function during natriuresis in mice. *Am. J. Physiol.* 219:865–71

136. Stewart, J. 1971. Renal concentrating ability in mice: a model for the use of genetic variation in elucidating relationships between structure and function. *Pfluegers. Arch.* 327:1–15

137. Tisher, C. C. 1971. Relationship between renal structure and concentrating ability in the rhesus monkey. *Am. J. Physiol.* 220:1100–6

138. Tisher, C. C., Bulger, R. E., Valtin, H. 1971. Morphology of renal medulla in water diuresis and vasopressin-induced antidiuresis. *Am. J. Physiol.* 220: 87–94

139. Tune, B. M., Burg, M. B. 1971. Glucose transport by proximal renal tubules. *Am. J. Physiol.* 221:580–85

140. Uhlich, E., Halbach, R., Ullrich, K. J. 1970. Einfluss von Aldosteron auf den Ausstrom markierten natriums aus den Sammelrohren der Ratte. *Pfluegers Arch.* 320:261–62

141. Urbaitis, B. K., Kessler, R. H. 1971. Actions of inhibitor compounds on adenine nucleotides of renal cortex and sodium excretion. *Am. J. Physiol.* 220: 1116–23

141a. Vander, A. J. 1967. Control of renin release. *Physiol. Rev.* 47:359–82

142. Van Liew, J. B., Deetjen, P., Boylan, J. W. 1967. Glucose reabsorption in the rat kidney-dependence on glomerular filtration. *Pfluegers Arch.* 295:232–44

143. Walker, A. M., Bott, P. A., Oliver, J., MacDowell, M. C. 1941. The collection and analysis of fluid from single nephrons of the mammalian kidney. *Am. J. Physiol.* 134:580–95

144. Wedeen, R. P. 1969. Autoradiography of freeze dried sections: studies of concentrative transport in the kidney. In *Autoradiography of diffusible substances,* ed. L. J. Roth, W. E. Stumpf, 147. New York: Academic

145. Wedeen, R. P., Thier, S. O. 1971. Intrarenal distribution of nonmetabolized amino acids in vivo. *Am. J. Physiol.* 220:507–12

146. Weisser, F., Lacy, F. B., Weber, H., Jamison, R. L. 1970. Renal function in the chinchilla. *Am. J. Physiol.* 219:1706–13

147. Wilczewski, T. W., Sonnenberg, H., Carrasquer, G. 1970. Permeability of superficial proximal tubules and loops of Henle to urea in rats. *Proc. Soc. Exp. Biol. Med.* 135:609–12

148. Williams, W. K., Huang, K. C. 1970. In vitro and in vivo renal tubular transport of tryptophan derivatives. *Am. J. Physiol.* 219:1468–74

149. Williams, M. M. M., Moffat, D. B., Creasey, M. 1971. The effect of antidiuretic hormone on the permeability of the vessels of the renal medulla of the rat during water diuresis. *Quart. J. Exp. Physiol.* 56:250–56

150. Woosley, R., Huang, K. C. 1967. Renal excretion of some isomeric hexoses in the dog. *Proc. Soc. Exp. Biol. Med.* 124:20–26

151. Woosley, R. L., Kim, Y. S., Huang, K. C. 1970. Renal tubular transport of 2-deoxy-D-glucose in dogs and rats. *J. Pharmacol. Exp. Therap.* 173:13–20

152. Young, J. A., Freedman, B. S. 1971. Renal tubular transport of amino acids. *Clin. Chem.* 17:245–66

Ann. Rev. Physiol. 1973. 35:55–86

HEART: EXCITATION-CONTRACTION COUPLING[1] 1089

G. A. Langer

Departments of Medicine and Physiology, University of California
Center for the Health Sciences, Los Angeles, California

The *Annual Review* chapters devoted to "Heart" in the past two years have concentrated on various topics: Johnson & Lieberman (41) stressed the excitation process and presented a critical review of voltage clamping. Ross & Sobel (92) reviewed biochemical aspects of myocardial cellular function and discussed factors that affect ventricular performance as well as methods used to assess this performance. I will focus my attention upon the excitation-contraction (*EC*) coupling sequence of heart muscle with emphasis upon the location, movement, and control of the cation central to the sequence: Ca^{2+}.

For the sake of perspective, reference will be made to studies that appeared prior to the past two to three years but, pursuant to the policy of the Annual Reviews, emphasis will be placed upon the most recently reported work.

ULTRASTRUCTURAL TECHNIQUES

The fundamental characteristics of myocardial ultrastructure have been elegantly described by Fawcett & McNutt (26). In their discussion they raised a number of points important to the study of myocardial Ca localization and movement.

They drew attention to a structure that, heretofore, has been largely neglected. This structure is the rather homogeneous-appearing layer, approximately 500 Å thick, which coats the sarcolemma. This layer is termed the basement membrane or external lamina and is typical of the surface-coating of cells from many tissues. It is composed of a dense mat of fine filaments and has been studied in myocardial cells from a number of species using histochemical techniques (40). The layer has been found to be rich in carbohydrate with a concentration of acidic residues. This endows it with a high density of negatively charged sites. It is particularly well-stained by lanthanum, a trivalent rare earth cation, and Shea (99) has provided strong evidence that the lanthanum-stainable material is a mucopolysaccharide or mucopolysac-

[1] Supported by Grants HE 11074–05 and HL 11351–06A1 from the USPHS and a Grant from the Bear Foundation.

charide-protein complex. The acid mucopolysaccharides contain a large number of negatively charged sites and are noted for their ability to selectively bind cations (98).

Fawcett & McNutt have reemphasized that the transverse tubular system (*T system*) in heart is about five times the diameter of the system in skeletal muscle. In addition the myocardial T system is lined with a layer of basement membrane material—i.e. as the sarcolemma invaginates to form the T tubule, the basement membrane invaginates with it. This indicates that the T tubules of myocardium are filled with negatively charged mucopolysaccharide. There is, therefore, a very significant amount of negatively charged material coating the sarcolemmal unit membrane of mammalian heart muscle cells. It has been demonstrated (98) that among the physiological cations, the mucopolysaccharide substances have a strong affinity for Ca. I will return to the possible significance of basement membrane structure later, but it is pertinent to keep in mind the first sentence from the recent paper by Whaley et al (112), ". . . there is a growing awareness that many cellular functions are directly influenced or 'controlled' by macromolecules 'outside' the cell, either as components of the plasma membrane, or as cell surface-associated materials, or as components of intercellular matrices."

Fawcett & McNutt have pointed out that the subsarcolemmal cisternae of the sarcotubular system in mammalian heart muscle are "far less capacious and are in apposition to the sarcolemma over a much more limited area than are the terminal cisternae of skeletal muscle." The terminal cisternae of skeletal muscle are considered the major releasing sites for the Ca involved in the coupling process (116). That the capacity of the cisternae and the membrane area apposed to T tubules are much less in cardiac muscle raises the possibility that the source of coupling Ca is different in this tissue. In addition, Fawcett & McNutt noted that skeletal muscle T tubules showed no evidence of mucopolysaccharide material in their lumina.

In addition to the transversely oriented T tubules it has been found that there are longitudinal branches of the system. In the rat heart (29) some of these branches taper to a diameter as small as 350 Å but can still be filled with horseradish peroxidase marker placed in the extracellular space. These finer "longitudinally oriented" T tubules do not seem to contain basement membrane. Large longitudinally oriented T tubules have also been demonstrated in the ventricle of guinea pig (104) and these show abundant basement membrane. These findings indicate that myocardial T tubular volume and basement membrane structure are of considerable magnitude in mammalian ventricle tissue.

Page, McCallister & Power (80a) have made quantitative ultrastructural studies in rat ventricular muscle and compared them with the previous studies by Peachey (81a) in frog sartorius, a fast twitch-type of skeletal muscle. It was found that the fractional volume of the T system of the rat cell was four times that of the skeletal muscle but that the ratio was reversed with respect to total sarcotubular volume, i.e. the skeletal cell had almost four times the fractional volume of the cardiac cell. The difference is even more striking when the rat ventricular cells are compared with guinea pig soleus (21a), a slow twitch muscle. In this case the heart cells have almost ten times the fractional volume of T system and almost an equal amount of total sarcotubular volume. If the fractional volumes of only the lateral cisternal component of the sarcotubules of fast twitch, slow twitch, and ventricular cells are compared then the fractional volume ratio is 18:2.5:1 (21a, 80a, 81a). This suggests that the contribution of internally located lateral cisternal Ca to EC coupling is much greater in skeletal muscle (especially fast twitch) than in mammalian ventricle.

Intracellular localization of calcium in mammalian ventricle was attempted with the use of pyroantimonate as a precipitating agent for Ca (56). Calcium pyroantimonate was concentrated in the lateral cisternae of the sarcoplasmic reticulum and over the sarcomeric I bands. Little precipitate was present over the medial portions of the sarcomere; this is consistent with the radioautographic studies in skeletal muscle (116). Mitochondria did not demonstrate significant amounts of precipitate. It should be noted that localization of precipitate in these studies is as much dependent upon diffusion of pyroantimonate as it is upon local concentration of Ca. The studies are, however, consistent with placement of intracellular storage of Ca within the lateral cisternae of the sarcotubular system in mammalian heart muscle, though as indicated above, the lateral cisternae of heart are of relatively small volume compared to those of skeletal muscle.

Recent ultrastructural work has, then, defined characteristics of mammalian ventricular muscle which might provide important clues to the localization and movement of Ca. Points to be emphasized are: (a) a layer of negatively charged mucopolysaccharide (basement membrane) covering the sarcolemmal unit membrane and filling the T tubules, (b) T tubules of wide diameter (five times the size of skeletal muscle T tubules) with limited area of apposition to the lateral cisternae, and (c) a portion of intracellular Ca storage within the lateral cisternae with little evidence of high concentration in medial components of the sarcotubular system.

In addition to comparison of mammalian ventricular muscle ultrastructure to that of skeletal muscle it is of interest to compare the mammalian ventricle to that of the frog. Staley & Benson (105) emphasized the differences in distribution of cellular membranes in the frog. Cells of small diameter (5 μ), arranged in bundles, are separated by intercellular clefts. The surface of the bundles is lined with basement membrane but this does not extend into the intercellular clefts. Therefore, though the bundle is invested with mucopolysaccharide, the sarcolemmal surface of the cells within the bundle is not. There are no T tubules present and the longitudinal sarcoplasmic reticulum is very sparse. It consists of a few scattered tubules—some subsarcolemmal in location. Staley & Benson emphasized the structural differences among frog ventricle, skeletal muscle, and mammalian ventricle and suggested that there must be significant differences in the manner by which Ca is handled by the different tissues during the course of the EC coupling sequence. Though it is likely that the process of actin-myosin interaction is similar in the three tissues it is quite certain that the quantity, sequence, and control of Ca movements is markedly different. There has been a tendency in the field to generalize and apply experimental results found in one tissue to the definition of the EC coupling sequence in another. It is clear that this cannot be done. Since in many instances the differences between tissues give insight into the complexities of subcellular Ca movement, these differences will be emphasized here.

The study of Niemeyer & Forssmann (77) is an example of the contrast between skeletal and mammalian heart muscle—especially with respect to the T tubular system. In skeletal muscle, treatment with hyperosmolar glycerol and return to normal perfusate disrupts the T system and destroys its continuity with the interstitial space (39). This disruption is coincident with uncoupling of the EC sequence. In addition, there are marked alterations induced in the electrical characteristics of the muscle (22). In mammalian ventricle the T system is not disrupted and no significant electrophysiological changes have been observed (77). Niemeyer & Forssmann suggested that the presence of the basement membrane in the T tubules and their large diameter in heart may account for their resistance to hypertonic shock. They pointed out that little is known about the role of the T system in heart and that the smaller diameter of the heart cell and its prolonged action potential may obviate the need of T tubules for excitation to the depths of the fiber. The paucity of areas of lateral cisternal contact supports this possibility. It is difficult, however, to ascribe a vestigial role to the T system in mammalian heart, especially when its tubules are five times the diameter of those in skeletal muscle and, in addition, are packed with negatively charged basement membrane substance. I will return to the role of the T system later in this chapter.

In summary, a review of recent ultrastructural studies indicates that significant differences are to be expected in the EC coupling sequence in skeletal muscle, frog heart, and mammalian heart. The structural differences are summarized in Table 1.

ELECTROPHYSIOLOGICAL TECHNIQUES

The recent work in this area has made extensive use of voltage clamp techniques. In a recent review, Johnson & Lieberman (41) were critical of the methods used in many studies and the interpretations drawn from them—their criticism was based largely on their contention of spatial inhomogeneity of the clamp in the preparations used. This criticism is, no doubt, valid in certain instances but recent studies indicate that, at least in a qualitative sense, a slow inward current is present and is, in part, attributable to Ca.

Reuter & Beeler (5, 6, 90) described a current which was manifest after the action potential spike. They noted that the magnitude of the current was little affected by removal of Na from the perfusing solution but that it was sensitive to alterations of $[Ca]_o$. The threshold for tension development was

TABLE 1. Structural Comparison

	Mammalian skeletal muscle	Frog ventricle	Mammalian ventricle
Cell diameter (μ)	~100	5	15
Transverse tubules	.04 μ diameter. Located at A-I junctions. No evidence of axial extension	Absent	0.2 μ diameter. Located at Z line. Axial extensions in many species
Sarcoplasmic reticulum	Dense, well-organized. Lateral cisternae of large volume. Extensive apposition to T tubules	Sparse, disorganized. Few subsarcolemmal cisternae	Intermediate, plexiform. Lateral cisternae of small volume. Limited apposition to T tubules
Basement membrane	Present on sarcolemma—Not evident in T tubules	Present on surface of fiber bundles. Absent on cell surface within bundles	Present on sarcolemma and in transverse T tubules
Mitochondria	Relatively sparse	Intermediate in number	Numerous
Glycerol treatment	Disrupts T system (Frog skeletal muscle)	—	No disruption of T system

very near the threshold for the slow inward current—approximately −35 mV. The most plausible explanation for this current is that it is carried, at least in part, by Ca ions. There is evidence in other tissues, however, that all slow inward current is not Ca in origin. In frog atrium (93), sheep ventricle (60), and guinea pig ventricle (78), evidence for a slow Na current was presented. Both of these currents would contribute to the configuration and maintenance of the plateau of the action potential.

If it is accepted that Ca ions contribute to slow inward current, there are some implications which might be drawn from voltage clamp studies about the location and movement of Ca during the EC coupling sequence. Beeler & Reuter (6) noted that, following a quiescent period, the slow inward current attributable to Ca (I_{Ca}) was fully activated with the first depolarization and did not change in magnitude during subsequent depolarizations, despite the fact that contractile force increased steadily (staircase) over 5–8 depolarizations. Though it is necessary that I_{Ca} be demonstrable at mechanical threshold, the magnitude of the force is not proportional to I_{Ca}. Ochi & Trautwein (79) came to the same conclusion—i.e. the tension staircase cannot be directly related to I_{Ca}. On the basis of these studies it is necessary to postulate a store of Ca which increases upon repetitive depolarizations and from which Ca is released, without evidence of current, to the myofilaments.

The relationship of I_{Ca} to contractile force under the conditions of Na-free perfusion is of interest (6). After exposure to Na-free solutions, force development, following a period of quiescence, is maximal with the first depolarization for any particular clamp duration. As is the case with the staircase, there is no discernible increase in slow inward current associated with the increased force. It would seem that Na-free perfusion also augments a store of Ca which is released, without evidence of additional current, to the myofilaments.

Quantitation of Ca influx on the basis of integration of the slow inward current is uncertain since the contribution of simultaneous outward currents and stray inward currents is difficult to evaluate. Beeler & Reuter (6) calculated a net gain in intracellular Ca between 1×10^{-6} and 5×10^{-5} M on the basis of charge transfer during the initial "Ca inward current." This is a 50-fold range and emphasizes the difficulty in quantitation. If the larger value (50 μmoles/Kg) represents the inward movement of Ca with each excitation it is, indeed, nearly enough to saturate the myofilamentous sites (42). If such a large quantity moves across the membrane with each excitation, the "internal store," which may fill over the course of 5–8 beats as the staircase develops (in perfusate which contains Na), is really quite large. It is possible that the same "store" fills upon perfusion with Na-free solution. As noted above, if Ca from this "store" participates in coupling, which seems likely, it is non-electrogenic. It is possible that there are balancing inward anionic or outward cationic movements to explain the absence of demonstrable current.

Mascher (62) also suggested that the augmentation of the contractile response in Na-free solution can be observed in the absence of an increase in the slow component of inward current—i.e. in the absence of any electrogenic Ca influx from the extracellular area. Recent studies (71, 72) by New & Trautwein failed to show any significant change in slow inward current in low Na solution despite marked increase in contractile force. Therefore, as with the staircase phenomenon, there is no evidence of a direct relation between the magnitude of the slow inward current (ascribed to I_{Ca} at least in part) and the tension developed. Again this strongly suggests, in mammalian heart, the existence of a pool of Ca, not extracellular in location, which supplies the Ca released to the myofilaments. Influx of Ca from this pool is not electrogenic and therefore its movement is not discernible with voltage clamp techniques.

In frog ventricle (67) inward Ca flux seems to be directly controlled by the membrane potential. When the ventricle is clamped to the level of the plateau of the action potential for less than 80–100 msec no tension is developed. In addition, the level of holding potential (-60 to -110 mV) has no effect on the tension developed with subsequent depolarization. The tension developed depends solely on the absolute magnitude of the potential and rises almost linearly between -50 mV and $+80$ mV. There is no evidence of a triggered release of a "separate store" of Ca not under direct control of the membrane. If the frog action potential is suddenly terminated by "clamping down" to the resting potential contraction is abruptly terminated. All of this indicates a meager "internal" store of Ca in the frog ventricle and that the coupling Ca is at a site or sites which are under direct control of the potential across the sarcolemma. In the frog the voltage clamp studies imply that the Ca which is released to the myofilaments is in very close association with the sarcolemma and, relative to mammalian ventricle, of small quantity. Prolonged depolarizations produce sustained tension responses indicating continuous and maintained influx of Ca from the extracellular space across the sarcolemma to the myofilaments.

It is also appropriate to review the effects of other cations on the slow inward current and contractile response. This information will be correlated with effects upon Ca flux in a later section. Mascher (61), and Vitek & Trautwein (108) found that manganese (Mn^{2+}) ions caused a shortening of the action potential and blocked the slow inward current. It also eliminated force development (61). The rare earth element lanthanum (La^{3+}) is also a very potent inhibitor of slow inward current (91) and eliminates contractile force at low concentrations. La has proven to be a very valuable tool in the definition of the locus of Ca. Mn, under certain conditions, is capable of contributing a small, slow inward current (78) and therefore enters the cell. La, on the other hand, seems to be limited to the "exterior" of the cell, i.e. it does not penetrate beyond the sarcolemma. These properties have made La useful in the correlations among ultrastructural, electrophysiological and flux characteristics in heart muscle (see following section).

The electrophysiological studies of mammalian and frog ventricle both indicate that attainment of mechanical threshold depends upon the activation of a current which is, at least in part, attributable to inward movement of Ca. In the situation of a normal twitch with an action potential of normal duration the Ca is directed to the myofilaments largely from sites on or within the sarcolemma or in close juxtaposition to the sarcolemma. The total capacity of these "superficial sites" is much less in frog ventricle than in mammalian ventricle. This may be related to structural differences summarized in Table 1 —i.e. absence of T tubules and the paucity of basement membrane in the frog. In mammalian ventricular and Purkinje fibers a release of Ca can be achieved by brief (5–10 msec) depolarizations (31, 65). This may be a manifestation of increased quantity of Ca in the membrane pool or compartment. The quantity of Ca in this compartment can be augmented during the staircase and by low Na perfusion. This compartment is present in the frog but is of much less capacity. An 80–100 msec depolarization is not sufficient to release enough Ca to achieve mechanical threshold and more prolonged excitation is required. Referring to Table 1 again, it might be expected that skeletal muscle activation would be less dependent on superficial stores of Ca. The well-developed, capacious intracellular sarcotubular system serves as the source of coupling Ca in this tissue.

On the basis of measurements of the reversal potential (that potential at which an ion moves neither inward nor outward across the cell membrane) for the slow inward current it seems very likely that inflowing Ca is not distributed directly to a homogeneous pool about the myofilaments. The problem is comparing experimentally measured values of reversal potential with a derived Nernst equilibrium potential is that $[Ca]_i$ changes significantly with depolarization. The $[Ca]_i$ during diastole is 10^{-7} M or less and in the range of 10^{-5} M with the heart in full contracture. Thus with $[Ca]_o$ of 1.8×10^{-3} M the equilibrium potential for Ca, E_{Ca} is about $+130$ mV during diastole and about $+70$ mV at full stimulation of the contractile apparatus. Thus one would expect a marked variation in driving force for Ca entry as the cell depolarizes and contraction develops. Morad & Orkand (67) found that the voltage-tension curve rises almost linearly from $+5$ to $+80$ mV in frog heart and this is not consistent with E_{Ca} acting as the sole determinant of Ca entry. If it were, the Δ tension would progressively decrease as voltage approached E_{Ca}.

The studies of New & Trautwein (71, 72) also indicated that the slow inward current system does not conform to a simple Nernstian system. They found that a fourfold reduction in $[Ca]_o$ (from 3.6 to 0.9 mM) produced a decline in reversal potential from $+80$ mV to about $+40$ mV. If $[Ca]_i$ remained unchanged a decline of only 18 mV would be expected. Since tension decreased to less than 30% as $[Ca]_o$ was reduced from 3.6 to 0.9 mM, $[Ca]_i$ at the myofilaments was certainly reduced. This would result in a decline of E_{Ca} less than 18 mV, not 40 mV as measured. These results suggest that the value of E_{Ca} derives from Ca distributed within a restricted area of the cell and does not give a measure of the free Ca concentration distributed about the myofilaments or of Ca distributed homogeneously in cell water.

Reuter (91) also reported on studies of reversal potential for slow inward current. These indicated that there has to be a small distribution space for Ca in juxtaposition to the membrane to account for the large changes in reversal potential which occur with variation in the duration of clamp steps (a means of altering total Ca current). Reuter estimated that the distribution volume is of the order of only 1% of the total cell volume and that the Ca concentration in this restricted region would have to be two orders of magnitude greater than the free concentration around the myofilaments in the relaxed state. This would indicate a remarkable compartmentalization.

Therefore the tension-voltage studies lend support to the idea that slow inward current in heart muscle does not represent Ca which simply flows from the extracellular space across the sarcolemma to distribute itself homogeneously in tissue water about the myofilaments. There is evidence for an intermediate juxtasarcolemmal site of storage or binding which is in rapid equilibrium with Ca in the interstitial space. It is this Ca which may be involved directly in the coupling process.

FLUX AND PERFUSION STUDIES

Studies in frog heart ventricle (13, 14) have been interpreted to indicate that two "Ca compounds" are involved in the final determination of contractile force. Upon a reduction in $[Ca]_o$ it was found that the decline of force could be described in two phases: a rapid phase (t ½ of 3–10 sec) and a slow phase (t ½ of 80–180 sec). It was proposed that Ca from the extracellular space associates to form a compound which initiates the twitch. This compound was designated Ca_1. Relaxation is assumed to occur when Ca_1 dissociates. Ca is assumed to reach Ca_1 in combination with a carrier R. An unknown substance I is proposed to control the rate by which CaR contributes to the formation of Ca_1. Ca dissociating from Ca_1 is visualized either to return to the extracellular space or to combine with "other cellular sites" designated as Ca_2. The rate of turnover of Ca_2 is much less rapid than that of Ca_1 and contributes to a fraction of force developed. Chapman & Niedergerke (13, 14) have added to their basic model a number of modifications which have increased its complexity. It is difficult to relate these functional studies and their interpretation to other ultrastructural, electrophysiological, and flux data. Chapman & Niedergerke have raised a number of possibilities, none of which are completely satisfactory. It is, however, interesting that they find it necessary to propose two components of Ca (Ca_1, Ca_2) which contribute to tension, a transmembrane carrier (R) and an intermediate controller (I) for the rate of formation of the rapidly exchanging Ca component (Ca_1). The voltage clamp studies on frog ventricle (67) indicate that the major source of coupling Ca would enter as CaR in Niedergerke's scheme and form Ca_1. It would seem that a depolarization of at least 80–100 msec is required to activate the controller (I) so that mechanical threshold is reached. The contribution of Ca_2 would be predicted to be nil since "clamping down" the transmembrane potential to resting level abruptly terminates the contraction—indicating little contribution from the intracellularly placed Ca_2. The possibility remains that Ca_1 acts as a "primer" to promote Ca release to the myofilament from Ca_2, and thus termination of Ca flow through Ca_1 would terminate release from Ca_2. The foregoing discussion indicates the difficulty in correlating the functionally derived Niedergerke model with the data from voltage clamp studies.

Difficulties in correlation are further emphasized by examination of another proposal by Chapman & Niedergerke (13). It is proposed, as indicated above, that "some part of the calcium which combines with contractile protein enters the cell during the action potential from the outside medium." This, it is stated, is consistent with the fact that extra Ca influx is associated with each action potential and dependent on external Ca and Na concentrations. Thus low Na perfusion is associated with an increased Ca influx. It was pointed out earlier in this review that in all the voltage clamp studies no increase in slow (Ca) inward current is discernible in low Na media. It is true that these studies used mammalian tissue but they do not support the contention (13) that, with low $[Na]_o$, "additional Ca enters the cell during the action potential from the *outside medium*."

Although there remain, at present, a large number of discrepancies between functional and electrophysiological studies, some agreement exists on certain aspects of the model for Ca movements as derived from electrophysiological and functional studies in the frog heart:

1. The major source of contractile-dependent Ca is derived from the extracellular space or from sites in rapid equilibrium with it. This Ca does not simply flow directly from extracellular space to the myofilaments but is bound, at least transiently, to a carrier or some juxtasarcolemmal site.

2. There is a second pool of cellular Ca which contributes very much less to force development. This is not in rapid equilibrium with the extracellular

space and seems to be the region of Ca sequestration upon which relaxation is dependent.

3. There are, then, three Ca components to be considered: (a) Ca in the extracellular space, (b) an intermediate carrier or juxtamembrane bound form, and (c) a deeper cellular bound or stored form. A similar three component system has been proposed by Chapman & Tunstall (15) from results obtained in perfused frog ventricular trabeculae. Chapman (16) proposed a morphological localization for the three components. He suggested a sequential release of activating Ca from b and c (Ca$_{II}$ and Ca$_2$ respectively in his terminology). This release is "triggered" by Ca entering from a (Ca$_I$) during depolarization of the sarcolemma. He placed the three components in series and suggested that a is located on the outer surface of the membrane (essentially extracellular), b on the inner surface of the sarcolemma, and c on sites in the sarcoplasm—possibly sarcoplasmic reticulum or mitochondria.

Recent studies of Ca flux in the frog heart are in general agreement: Direct measurements of ^{45}Ca uptake in the perfused papillary muscle of mammalian (dog) heart done by Langer & Brady (43) demonstrated that increased frequency of contraction was associated with a net uptake of Ca. Similar findings have been found in frog heart (75, 76, 96) and the extra influx per beat calculated to be 1 μmole Ca/kg or less wet tissue. This amount is about 2% of that needed to saturate the troponin sites in the frog. It requires a number of beats following a sudden increase in frequency of stimulation to "ascend the staircase" and reach steady-state contractile force. This is consistent with the proposal that an intermediary Ca pool (Site b above), from which Ca is released to the troponin, is progressively augmented from the extracellular space at a rate of about 1 μmole Ca/kg/beat until steady-state is reached. This quantity of Ca is small but should be recognizable as an augmentation of slow inward current, I$_{Ca}$, by voltage clamp technique. As previously indicated, no change in slow inward current, at least in mammalian tissue, can be found in association with the positive staircase phenomenon—i.e. the magnitude of force is not proportional to I$_{Ca}$. This fact makes it difficult to reconcile voltage clamp, functional, and flux data, and will be discussed further in a later section.

A comparison of Ca kinetics in frog and dog heart was undertaken by Sopis & Langer (103). The general kinetic pattern was found to be similar, but interesting quantitative differences were found—especially in the component that exchanges next most rapidly after the extracellular space and has been termed phase 2. The Ca content of this component is specifically increased in both dog (44) and frog ventricle when these tissues are perfused with solution low in [Na]$_o$. At the point where each tissue first showed evidence of contracture (inability to relax completely after contraction) with low [Na]$_o$, the phase 2 component of the dog contained seven times more Ca. It has been suggested that phase 2 represents Ca localized, at least in part, to the sarcoplasmic reticulum (47). This is consistent with the ultrastructural studies (105) demonstrating sparseness of SR in frog ventricle and, hence, a diminished ability to sequester and store large amounts of Ca. Upon return to normal $[Na]_o$ perfusion, some 15–20 min are required to eliminate the accumulated Ca in phase 2 from the muscle in both the dog and frog ventricle, despite the fact that contractile force declines to control values much more rapidly. This again emphasizes the fact that the site or sites of "internal" Ca storage in both tissues probably play little role in the release of activator Ca to the myofilaments.

A number of studies in mammalian heart emphasize the fact that coupling Ca is derived from a superficial site. The studies of Bailey & Dresel (2) using isolated, gas-perfused (water-saturated mixture of 95% O_2 and 5% CO_2) cat hearts found that force declined at the same rate as Ca was cleared from a kinetically defined component, Ca_{II} in their terminology. Ca_{II} exchanged with a half-time of 43 sec and would seem to represent, at least in part, Ca in the interstitial space. Shine, Serena & Langer (100) reached the same conclusion using the arterially perfused isolated rabbit interventricular septum. It was shown that the Ca content of their kinetically defined phase 1 component was linearly proportional to the $[Ca]_o$ in the perfusion medium over the range of 0.5 to 12.0 mM $[Ca]_o$. In addition the Ca content of phase 1 was consistent with the amount expected to be distributed within the interstitium and its exchange was perfusion limited even at perfusion rates 2–3 times physiological (up to 3.2 ml g^{-1} mm^{-1}). These characteristics indicated that their phase 1 Ca was located within the interstitial space and/or at sites in rapid equilibrium with this space. The half-time for exchange of phase 1 was 83 sec. When the septum was perfused with solution of 0 $[Ca]_o$ contractile force fell with a half-time of 72 sec. The values are not very different from those found by Bailey & Dresel in the gas-perfused cat heart when differences in perfusion rate and technique are considered—i.e. Ca_{II} and phase 1 are probably one and the same. This indicates that Ca in the interstitial space, or at sites in such rapid equilibrium with this space that it cannot be separated kinetically, is crucial to the EC coupling process in mammalian heart. The study of Saari & Johnson (94) in the Langendorff perfused rabbit heart came to the same conclusion. An earlier study by Langer (45) in the arterially perfused dog papillary muscle indicated that force declined proportionally to the decline in Ca content of a kinetically-defined component (phase 2) with a half-time of 6 min. The conditions of perfusion of this preparation made it more likely that it was more heavily loaded with Ca. It has been shown that myocardium in which intracellular Ca levels are considerably above those in the physiological range (with some element of contracture present) are less dependent on extracellular Ca for their force development (48) and demonstrate a less rapid decline in force upon perfusion with Ca-free solutions. The later studies (100) are certainly more physiological.

Little & Sleator (57) indicated that the major portion of activating Ca does not come directly from the extracellular space in guinea pig atrium. At close to maximal tension (120 beats/min, 2.5 mM $[Ca]_o$) they estimated that Ca entry was 15 μmoles/kg cells/beat. Although they assumed that heart and skeletal muscle require essentially equal quantities of Ca to saturate the contractile system [heart requires approximately ⅓ as much Ca per mass total tissue as that required by skeletal muscle (42)], 15 μmoles represents only about 25% the amount of Ca needed. In addition they found that the Ca entry per beat was not significantly different at heart rates of 60 and 120—although peak tension was 65% greater at 120/min. The conclusion is, therefore, that direct entry of extracellular Ca to the myofilaments with each beat does not occur. They noted, however, that average Ca influx and efflux values are about twofold greater when contractile frequency is doubled—indicating an increase in mean Ca content somewhere in the tissue. It is likely that a portion of this increment is involved in the coupling process and, though not extracellular, is bound at sites in rapid equilibrium with the extracellular space.

The dependence of force development upon Ca which is in rapid equilibrium with extracellular Ca in myocardium is in sharp contrast to the situation in skeletal muscle. Early studies (21) in which tension responses were recorded from single skeletal muscle fibers in Ca free solutions indicated that force declined with a half-time of two hours or more. These studies were done at low temperature (0.5–2.0°C) and it might be said that this contributed to the slowness of the decline. This is not, however, a satisfactory explanation since, in our laboratory, arterial perfusion of guinea-pig semimembranosus muscle with Ca-free solutions at 24°C produced a decline in a significant component of total force with a half-time of 40–60 minutes (Dr. Terrell Rich, unpublished observation). This is many times slower than in myocardium and again emphasizes the marked differences in the EC coupling sequence of the two tissues.

Further information on the locus of the coupling Ca has been provided through the use of the trivalent rare earth cation, La. This element has an atomic weight of 139 and a hydrated radius of 3.1 Å—close to that of hydrated Ca at 2.8 Å. It is electron-dense and therefore can be localized ultrastructurally. Sanborn & Langer (95) described the effect of adding La to the solution perfusing rabbit ventricular muscle. The addition of as little as 40 μM [La]$_o$ essentially abolished force development at a time when only minimal alterations were induced in the configuration of the action potential. Coincident with its uncoupling action La produced a displacement of Ca from the tissue. On the basis of these findings it was proposed that contractile dependent Ca was derived from "superficially" located sites on the myocardial cell. As reviewed previously, La does not penetrate intracellularly, has great affinity for mucopolysaccharide material at the cell surface (99), and eliminates the slow inward current in heart muscle (91).

The application of La to skeletal muscle preparations once again emphasizes the differences in the EC coupling sequence in the two tissues. As indicated, addition of La to the arterially perfused skeletal muscle has very much less effect upon twitch tension than it does in myocardium. Weiss (111) noted in frog sartorius, however, that La inhibited tension responses to hyperkalemic perfusion and concluded that La acts at superficial sites to displace Ca and prevent the hyperkalemic contracture. This indicates that an extracellular flux of Ca is required to support K contracture but that a significant component of the twitch response can be supported by an intracellular cycling of the ion. Such is clearly not the case for the myocardium.

There are a few skeletal muscles which are different in their response when compared to the majority of skeletal muscle. These differences are instructive: One such muscle is the myotome of amphioxus studied by Hagiwara, Henkart & Kidokoro (36). Their results show that there are two sources of Ca in amphioxus muscle cells. One component is directly related to the initiation of the twitch and this Ca is replaced by La. La was found only at the surface of the cells and, as in myocardium, eliminated twitch tension. These muscles contain a sparse SR and they concluded that this is the locus of the second Ca component which contributed practically not at all to the twitch tension. The striated muscle of amphioxus is, then, similar to myocardium in its EC coupling response—i.e. dependent upon a superficial store of Ca for its twitch response. It is much like heart ultrastructurally with a much less capacious SR storage and release system.

These studies strongly suggest that La acts as it binds to a cellular surface component as has been directly demonstrated in myocardial tissue culture (53). In this preparation La also specifically uncoupled excitation from contraction. This action was associated with displacement of a component of rapidly exchangeable Ca and, in addition, with marked inhibition of Ca influx and efflux—i.e. Ca exchange virtually ceased. While this occurred La bound exclusively to the superficial surface of the cells. La heavily saturated the basement membrane and was not found internal to the sarcolemma.

The results derived from the La experiments suggest that the presence of fixed negatively charged sites located in the mucopolysaccharide substance on the sarcolemma and within the T tubules may play an important role in the control of Ca movements in the myocardium. If so, it would be expected that this region would function, in many respects, as a cation exchanger. Evidence for such a process comes from Busselen (11). He experimented with K-induced contractures in the presence of strontium (Sr^{2+}) and Ca in rabbit atria. He found that the relation of contracture tension to external Sr concentration (1 to 10 mM) was hyperbolic and yielded a straight line on a Lineweaver-Burk plot. When 0.5 mM Ca was added to the Sr solutions, contractures were markedly reduced and the plot indicated a system in which the affinity was 50–100 times larger for Ca than for Sr. It is possible that the cation affinity sequence is based upon the negatively charged surface material.

Another method of uncoupling excitation from contraction also indicates the presence of an intermediate binding site from which Ca is released. The refractory period of rat heart is extremely short so that a second, essentially normal action potential can be generated as little as 50–80 msec after a primary excitation. Mainwood & Lee (59) found that as the interval between action potentials was progressively decreased the mechanical response became smaller until at pulse intervals of 80 to 100 msec contractile force was virtually undetectable. This indicated to them that a finite period of time is required for Ca to be replenished at the sites from which it is released to the contractile elements. The amount of Ca at the sites was dependent upon the external Ca concentration—indicating that they are in rapid equilibrium with the interstitial space.

Other sites have been suggested as being important in Ca release and sequestration in the myocardium. Patriarca & Carafoli (81) indicated that a large fraction of cellular Ca is located within the mitochondria and considered the possibility that cyclic release to the myofilaments might occur from mitochrondia and play a role in the coupling process. In addition, it was proposed that they also function in the sequestration of Ca. Williamson (114), on the other hand, doubted that the mitochondria play a significant role in the EC coupling process. He cited the study of Legato & Langer (56) indicating that in the intact cell the larger concentrations of Ca are extramitochondrial and only under conditions of very high Ca-loading are calcium deposits found in the mitochondria. Williamson suggested that upon disruption of tissue preliminary to localizing Ca in mitochondria, the Ca is released from its binding sites on the myofibrils and SR and is rapidly taken up by the mitochondria. The Ca found to be associated with the mitochondria would then be largely a result of shifts that occurred during their preparation.

There is little doubt that under appropriate circumstances mitochondria can bind and accumulate large amounts of Ca (19, 64) and the abundance of mitochondria in mammalian myocardium as well known (26). It is possible that the mitochondria function as additional storage depots in heart muscle—especially under conditions of high Ca-loading (56) or under circumstances in which the uptake of the SR is inhibited, as with caffeine (9, 101). Whether the mitochondria function in the cyclic release of Ca attendant upon membrane depolarization is questionable. The close association of the mitochondria with T system and SR membrane has been pointed out (19) but no firm evidence has been presented to support the idea of electrical coupling of mitochondrial membrane, either directly or indirectly, with sarcolemmal depolarization.

The foregoing discussion summarized the data leading to the conclusion that a rapidly exchangeable, superficial store of Ca is important in the EC coupling sequence in amphibian and mammalian heart muscle. It is now appropriate to consider present theories as to how this Ca functions in the process of initation and maintenance of contractile force. The question is: Does this Ca move directly to troponin sites or does it serve only as a "primer" for regenerative release of Ca from deeper stores, e.g. the SR, which then moves to the troponin?

Information gained from skinned skeletal muscle fibers (fibers from which the sarcolemma has been stripped) has indicated that Ca induces release of

Ca from the SR (23, 28). The skinned fibers were allowed to accumulate Ca for a short period or were exposed to caffeine. Upon application of subthreshold concentrations of Ca a contraction was elicited—clearly indicating a release of additional Ca from internal stores—presumably the SR. It was implied that this regenerative Ca release was a physiological mechanism and occurred upon excitation with membrane intact. There is some difficulty, however, in reconciling this idea with the lack of rapid effect of La or perfusion with Ca-free solutions on a significant fraction of skeletal muscle twitch tension. If the "priming" Ca is derived from external superficial stores, why is La or zero $[Ca]_o$ perfusion incapable of rapidly uncoupling the EC sequence in skeletal muscle? It might be proposed that the source of the primer is intracellular but then one has to propose a mechanism which includes a means of release for the primer or "a primer for the primer."

Various "skinned" heart cell preparations have been reported recently. Membrane permeability to Ca was increased by 15 min exposure to EDTA (117), or segments of the membrane were removed by mechanical mincing or homogenization (10, 25). Subsequent to EDTA treatment graded contractures could be achieved by application of solutions containing Ca at concentrations between 10^{-6} and $10^{-5}M$. The relation of maximum tension to pCa (negative logarithm of Ca concentration) is very similar to the relation of myofibrillar ATPase to pCa recorded for heart muscle (42). The EDTA "partially skinned" preparation was not used to examine the possibility of regenerative release in heart muscle. Homogenized skinned preparations were, however, employed to study this possibility (25). Skeletal muscle produced contractions only after pretreatment with caffeine. Rat ventricular muscle, however, developed oscillatory contractions upon addition of Ca. Skinned frog ventricular muscle failed to respond with an oscillating contraction response upon exposure to Ca. These variations in response were attributed to the differences in SR content of the various tissues. It was proposed that the applied Ca produced a cyclic release of Ca from the SR in rat ventricle but not in frog ventricle because of the sparse SR in the latter. It was thought that caffeine was required in skeletal muscle to partially inhibit sequestration or promote release of Ca in the capacious SR and thus prevent all of the administered Ca from simply being stored. The proposal seems logical enough but again the question arises as to whether the results can be extended to the myocardium with an intact sarcolemma. Electron microscopic examination of the sarcotubular system in both the EDTA-treated and mechanically skinned mammalian ventricular fibers has demonstrated a hugely dilated SR. The reason for the dilation is not clear but raises the possibility that regenerative Ca release and the production of oscillatory force development is a property of a dilated sarcotubular system. The oscillatory tension response brings to mind the oscillatory after-contractions which occur in heart muscle (with intact sarcolemma) in a highly Ca-loaded state. A possible basis for these oscillations was presented by Posner & Berman (83). In their model it was proposed that under normal circumstances relaxation to rest tension occurs smoothly, with the process heavily damped. In the presence of high Ca however, oscillations (after-contractions), should appear. Ultrastructural examination of highly Ca-loaded ventricular myocardium discloses a dilated sarcotubular system (55) similar to that found in the skinned preparations. It remains to be proven that regenerative Ca release in heart muscle is not a property of SR in either an overloaded state or a condition in which normal uptake is otherwise inhibited. The foregoing examination of the proposal for regenerative Ca release again illustrates the difficulty in the attempt to consider skeletal and cardiac muscle function in essentially the same manner with respect to Ca movements.

In summary, the majority of flux and perfusion studies have indicated a superficial, rapidly exchangeable Ca store which is critical in the maintenance of EC coupling in heart tissue. This store does not seem to be simply the free Ca in the interstitial space nor the bulk of Ca stored in the sarcotubules or mitochondria. Voltage clamp studies also support the existence of this Ca component. Its locus on or within the cell has not been defined but the possibility that the basement membrane with its negatively charged sites may, in some way, be linked to the component is under consideration. This sequence is similar to that defined in a previous review (47) as an "Alternative Hypothesis" and has recently been discussed further (49, 50).

PHARMACOLOGICAL TECHNIQUES

This section is not intended to be a comprehensive review of the effects of pharmacological agents on Ca movements and the EC coupling sequence. Recent studies employing drugs have, however, given some additional insight or emphasized different theories with respect to Ca movement. A brief discussion of some of these is pertinent here.

Catecholamine.—Previous studies in auricular tissue (35, 88) indicated that catecholamines produced an increment in Ca influx. This is supported by the effect of epinephrine on the action potential recorded from Purkinje fibers (12, 89). The plateau of the action potential was shifted to more positive potential values by epinephrine in a manner very similar to the change induced by elevation of $[Ca]_o$. This change is consistent with an augmentation of slow inward current, presumably carried by Ca; such augmentation was demonstrated in voltage clamp experiments (71, 89). These findings implicate an effect of the catecholamines on Ca movements as important in their production of increased contractile force.

Williamson (114) reviewed evidence that the catecholamines influence Ca movements through a primary effect of cyclic AMP. He noted: (*a*) that cyclic AMP levels increase prior to or with increased contractile force after epinephrine, (*b*) that the ability of the catecholamines to stimulate cyclic AMP production matches the potency of their inotropic effects (isoproterenol > epinephrine > norepinephrine), (*c*) that agents which enhance or inhibit the degradation of cyclic AMP (by their effect on phosphodiesterase) decrease or increase, respectively, the inotropism of the catecholamines, and (*d*) that β receptor blockade blocks both inotropism and increments in cyclic AMP by the catecholamines. Though the mobilization of both Ca and cyclic AMP are concurrent effects of the catecholamines and seem to coordinate in some way to produce a positive inotropic result, the link between cyclic AMP and Ca movements remains to be defined.

An indication that catecholamines may act, at least in part, by mobilizing internal stores has been presented by Schaffer & Williamson (97). In rat ventricle in which the EC coupling sequence was interrupted by perfusion with ruthenium red (a cationic dye which is lanthanum-like in action) or EGTA (chelation of extracellular Ca) norepinephrine addition increased force development. This response indicates that norepinephrine is capable of inducing a release of intracellular Ca not normally available or of increasing the sensitivity of Ca receptor sites at the contractile protein level. It would be interesting to determine if norepinephrine is capable of restoring any fraction of the slow inward current which is eliminated by agents such as La.

The catecholamines, in addition to their effect upon force development, also produce an earlier and more rapid relaxation. The role of the catechols in the relaxation process was emphasized by Morad (66). He first described the different sensitivity of mammalian and frog ventricle to the application of high $[K]_o$. Contracture is readily produced in the frog whereas mammalian ventricles respond not at all or with a minor contracture transient. If, however, the mammals are pretreated with reserpine (depleting endogenous catechols) or the ventricular muscle is incubated in the presence of propranolol (blocking the beta receptors), marked and sustained contractures are produced upon application of solutions high in $[K]_o$. If epinephrine is added at the peak of the contracture, partial relaxation immediately occurs. The presence of epinephrine in the perfusate prevents K-induced contracture. Morad & Rolett (68) have suggested that the catecholamines increase the Ca sequestration rate of the sarcolemma and/or sarcotubules. Support for this suggestion has come from Entman, Levey & Epstein (24). They demonstrated that, in isolated cardiac sarcoplasmic reticulum, Ca uptake was stimulated by epinephrine, glucagon, and cyclic AMP. This fits the hypothesis, but other studies (17, 20) have failed to find an effect of the catechols on Ca uptake by isolated SR. As with the effect of catecholamines on force development, the mechanism of action of catecholamines on relaxation remains to be more completely defined. These agents almost certainly operate via their effects upon Ca movements, but the sequence of action and the intermediates involved continue to be appropriate subjects for future investigation.

Caffeine.—Caffeine produces striking effects upon myocardial force development. Two studies on mammalian heart reported the effects of caffeine on rabbit ventricle (101) and on kitten atria and ventricle (9). In both studies an initial and rapid increase in tension and its first derivative, d*P*/d*t* occurred followed by a short period of decline and then a gradual secondary increase in both parameters. In the kitten, diastolic tension did not increase over a large range of caffeine concentration. In the rabbit, even the smallest dose of caffeine (1 mM) induced a small but significant elevation of diastolic tension. The other major difference in the two studies is that caffeine always increased the time to peak tension in kitten heart, but in 8 of 10 rabbit preparations time to peak tension decreased. The effect of caffeine upon action potential duration was examined in the rabbit heart and the duration was found to decrease by 27% as time to peak tension decreased by the same amount. By contrast a previous study on papillary muscles from kittens (18) disclosed that caffeine increased action potential duration by 10–20% at a heart rate of 20/min. The difference in duration of active state might, then, be attributed to dissimilar electrical effects in different species of different age.

The effects of caffeine on force development in myocardium are consistent with the effects of the drug upon isolated sarcoplasmic reticulum with respect to Ca movement. Weber & Herz (109) noted that caffeine produced a release and inhibited the uptake of Ca in frog and rabbit skeletal muscle reticulum. The releasing action is consistent with the production of the initial transient increase in force; such a releasing action is supported by the study of Blinks et al (9) in which procaine was used in association with caffeine. Procaine antagonized the caffeine-induced prolongation of tension development but did not affect the initial rapid increase in dP/dt and peak tension. Thus caffeine is capable of inducing a Ca release (procaine insensitive) as well as inhibiting its sequestration (procaine sensitive). The subsequent more prolonged increase in force would be associated with the inhibition of uptake by caffeine in that Ca binding to the myofilaments would be augmented in the presence of inhibited SR sequestration—i.e. less active uptake by SR would result in a greater proportion of the Ca released upon excitation to be bound to the competing group of sites, troponin. The differences in response (TPT and diatolic tension) among species may reflect differences in the relative sensitivities to caffeine of the membrane system involved. It should be noted that Weber (110) found that caffeine had no effect on the Ca uptake system of mitochondria. Nayler (69) had previously shown an inhibitory effect on Ca flux of mitochondria. ^{45}Ca flux studies and electronmicroscopy (101) suggest, however, that if a mitochondrial effect is present, it is considerably less than the SR effect.

The ^{45}Ca flux studies of Shine & Langer (101) support these concepts concerning the movements of Ca and the effects caffeine has upon these movements. Caffeine consistently produced a net uptake of ^{45}Ca in the perfused rabbit interventricular septum. This net uptake was associated with a striking decrease in ^{45}Ca efflux rate, which rapidly returned to control when caffeine was removed from the perfusing solution. Of particular interest was the demonstration that caffeine seemed to induce a specific block to Ca efflux in whole tissue. Though the muscle was accumulating Ca, this Ca could not be eliminated as long as caffeine was present in the perfusate. There does not seem to be an alternative pathway by which the caffeine-induced block to efflux can be bypassed. Electronmicroscopy of the Ca-loaded tissue disclosed that the mitochondria seemed to be increased in volume but that the sarcotubules were not dilated as they appear in other Ca-loaded states (55). These results support the proposal that caffeine inhibits uptake of Ca by the SR with little effect upon mitochondria. This inhibition will lead, initially, to increased force development and slowed relaxation. As Ca continues to accumulate diastolic tension increases and contracture develops. It would seem that the mitochondria may serve to store a portion of the Ca which does not enter the inhibited SR, but that in order for Ca to be eventually eliminated from the cell it has to pass through the SR system.

In addition to its effects upon Ca movement, caffeine belongs to a group of drugs which inhibit phosphodiesterase, the enzyme responsible for the degradation of cyclic AMP. It is possible that a component of its inotropic effect is related to elevation of cyclic AMP levels in the myocardium (114).

Digitalis.—The literature on the effects of the digitalis glycosides is voluminous and contradictory. This has been recently reviewed by Lee & Klaus (54) in a very comprehensive manner. Their conclusions concerning the basis for digitalis-induced inotropism differ from those of the author (52), but all agree that Ca movements are affected by the glycosides and play a crucial role in their mode of action. It is generally agreed that doses of glycoside in the toxic range (leading to contracture) are associated with a net uptake of Ca by the myocardium (38). It has also been demonstrated that nontoxic doses increase the exchangeability or "turnover" of Ca, but it is more difficult to validate a net gain of Ca by the cell (35, 58). A recent study from the author's laboratory (48) indicated that a net gain in tissue Ca is associated with pretoxic glycoside-induced inotropism. The net uptake was small— amounting to 100–150 μmoles/kg wet weight or 3% of the total myocardial Ca.

Bailey & Sures (3), using the gas-perfused cat heart, demonstrated both an increased rate of Ca uptake and an increased total Ca at a time when contractile force had been increased by greater than 20% with no evidence of toxicity. Though uptake and total Ca were increased, the content of the rapidly exchangeable (Ca_{II} fraction [which had been related directly to support of contractile force (2)] was not increased by ouabain. Therefore it was proposed that bulk influx of Ca was increased with each excitation, without augmenting the content of the superficial Ca storage site. They suggested that glycoside may have "activated a hitherto inactive Ca carrier for the movement of extracellular Ca into the cell with each depolarization." The net uptake found by Bailey & Sures (3) following ouabain was over 900 μmoles/kg wet weight or many times that found by Langer & Serena (48).

A recent study by Nayler (70) differs from that of Bailey & Sures in that she found that inotropic (no contracture induced) doses of ouabain significantly increased the amount of ^{45}Ca which could be displaced by La. As noted previously, the action of La is limited to surface sites (53). The increment in La-displaceable Ca was not quantitated by Nayler, but the study indicated that a component of surface-bound Ca is increased by glycoside coincident with the positive, nontoxic inotropic effect. It is probable that some of this Ca is rapidly exchangeable, and one might have expected it would have been demonstrable in the Bailey & Sures study.

The studies support the contention that by some mechanism, as yet undefined, the glycosides augment Ca influx through the sarcolemmal membrane. There is little evidence in any of these studies that efflux is greatly affected. This implies that the glycosides have no or very minor effects on the SR system. This implication is supported by studies indicating that Ca movements on and through isolated SR membranes are not affected by glycoside (7, 17, 82). The mitochondrial transport of Ca seems also not to be affected (7). These studies clearly show that the glycosides affect Ca movements through a completely different mechanism than was defined for the methylxanthines as typified by caffeine.

The action of glycosides at the cell surface is supported by recent studies using albumin-bound glycoside (1) or glycoside-specific antibodies (102). Digitoxin covalently bound to human serum albumin produced an inotropic response of guinea pig myocardium as large as that produced by free digitoxin (1). No evidence was found for unbinding of the digitoxin-albumin complex upon exposure to the heart muscle. Since the complex was deemed incapable of gaining access to intracellular sites, it was concluded that the glycoside acts at the cell membrane. Similar conclusions were reached with the use of digoxin antisera (102). It was found that the antisera prevented or reversed the inotropism induced by digoxin in cat papillary muscles. Since it is assumed that the size of the antibody precludes its entry into the cell, these results strongly suggest that the inotropic actions of the glycoside are mediated at a receptor site located on the surface of the cell.

Since the glycosides augment Ca influx and seem to be operative at the cell surface, it would be of interest to know what effect, if any, they have on the slow inward currents as measured by voltage clamping techniques. To the author's knowledge, nothing has yet been reported on this subject.

In summary, recent data on the effects produced by three groups of drugs —catecholamines, methylxanthines, and glycosides—has provided further insight into the movements of Ca in the myocardium. The catechols may act at both cell surface and SR, caffeine predominatly at the SR, and the glycosides at the sarcolemmal surface. The varying effect of these agents on Ca flux and contractile function aid in the definition of the EC sequence and will be referred to in the last section of this review.

THE CONTROL OF THE QUANTITY OF CA MOVEMENT

Under the condition of unchanged resting (diastolic) length there are two basic mechanisms by which contractile force is modified in heart muscle. These are best expressed in terms of the two characteristics of active state— its intensity and its duration. The intensity refers to the instantaneous rate of its development. Changes in this parameter affect the magnitude of the force and the rate at which it is developed. The duration refers to the period of time during which the processes which lead to active force development are, so to speak, "turned on." Changes in duration also affect the magnitude of force but through processes which alter the total period during which acto-myosin bridges are formed.

Duration of active state is determined by the balance between the time course of Ca influx and the activity of the Ca sequestration system. Prolongation of the former with no change in the latter will prolong the active state and lengthen the period of force development. A simple prolongation of the action potential will accomplish this. On the other hand, if the process of sequestration is augmented in terms of the quantity of Ca sequestered per unit time and duration of influx remains unchanged, then active state will be shortened, relaxation will occur sooner, and the period of force development will be shortened. Changes in temperature greatly modify the duration of active state. Cooling prolongs influx and decreases sequestration activity, prolongs active state, and usually increases peak force. However, significant changes in temperature usually do not occur in mammalian species unless imposed in an experimental situation. Aside from temperature alteration there are few interventions which result in increased force that are based upon prolongation of the active state. Most physiological and pharmacological interventions alter contractile force by altering the intensity of the active state. In fact they induce positive inotropy in the face of a decrease in active state duration. This means that the positive effect upon intensity outweighs the negative effect upon duration. Increased frequency of stimulation, increased $[Ca]_o$, decreased $[Na]_o$, digitalis glycoside, and the catecholamines are all examples of positive inotropic interventions in which increased intensity more than compensates for a decreased duration. (As discussed, caffeine is, in some instances, an agent which induces increased force through prolongation of active state).

The intensity of the active state is determined by the quantity and rate of arrival of Ca at the troponin sites. The more Ca which binds per unit time, the more force-generating bridges are formed per unit time, and the more rapidly force is developed. If duration is not drastically shortened, increased peak force results.

It is probable that the movement of Ca from releasing sites to troponin occurs by diffusion down its steep concentration gradient. The rate of this movement is extremely rapid and likely not greatly altered over a wide range of conditions. This means that the major determinant of active state intensity is the absolute quantity of Ca which moves following excitation. This quantity is, in turn, determined by the amount located at the releasing sites immediately prior to excitation. Therefore a consideration of Ca-mediated inotropisms focuses upon the mechanisms by which the quantity of Ca at the releasing sites is controlled. It appears that there are a number of factors which might affect this quantity.

$[Ca]_o$.—The early study of Winegrad & Shanes (115) showed that as $[Ca]_o$ was increased, Ca influx was augmented. The voltage clamp studies reviewed earlier (5, 6, 60, 71, 72, 78, 79, 90, 93) indicated that slow inward current increased as $[Ca]_o$ increased and correlated with augmented force development. It was demonstrated, however, that Ca influx did not increase linearly with $[Ca]_o$ in mammalian myocardium (100). Though interstitial Ca was linearly related to $[Ca]_o$ over the 0.5 to 12 mM range, cellular Ca increased by a relatively small amount as $[Ca]_o$ was increased above 4–5 mM. The study indicated that this was due to a progressive limitation of influx at the higher $[Ca]_o$ values. This could not be due to an accumulation of free Ca in the cell, which would diminish the concentration gradient outside to inside, since diastolic tension did not increase even at 12 mM $[Ca]_o$. This indicates that no accumulation of Ca about the myofilaments had taken place. The study indicated that the membrane sites from which Ca is released to enter the cell approach saturation as $[Ca]_o$ rises, and limit further influx. Such saturation would be a property of negatively charged sites on or within the cell membrane. The layer of negatively charged mucopolysaccharide discussed previously could function in this manner.

$[K]_o$.—It has been known for some time that a decrease in $[K]_o$ is positively inotropic. This inotropism is associated with an increase in Ca uptake (106). Fleckenstein & Kaufmann (27) have proposed that the increase in $[K]_i/[K]_o$ gradient enhances K efflux and that inward movement of Ca is coupled to the outward movement of K. This is an attractive hypothesis since the inotropisms following increased frequency of contraction and glycoside administration are associated with a net K loss from the myocardium (47). The study of Reiter, Seibel & Stickel (86) indicates, however, that the mechanism may not be primarily dependent upon the enhanced K efflux. They first ruled out the possibility that membrane hyperpolarization could account for the inotropic effect of reduced $[K]_o$. They found that the inotropic effect depended on the extracellular Na concentration, $[Na]_o$. Decrease in $[Na]_o$ (with maintenance of $[Ca]_o/[Na]_o^2$ ratio constant so as to obviate consideration of the external Na-Ca competitive effect) greatly reduced or prevented the inotropic effect of decreased $[K]_o$. Reiter et al have proposed that reduced $[K]_o$ inhibits active Na transport. The effect of $[K]_o$ on Na-pumping systems, including heart muscle, is well known (34, 80, 113). If $[Na]_o$ is high, this inhibition would lead to an accumulation of Na intracellularly. This intracellular accumulation would be much less in the presence of low $[Na]_o$ since Na influx is reduced as $[Na]_o$ is reduced. Reiter, et al have suggested that the increase in $[Na]_i$ stimulates Ca influx and thereby is primarily responsible for the inotropism. Evidence is rapidly accumulating for a significant role of $[Na]_i$ in the regulation of Ca flux and contractile tension. This will be reviewed in a later section.

A primary effect on contractile force of K, through a K-Ca exchange system, in mammalian heart is brought further into question by the study of Reiter & Stickel (85). Increase in $[K]_o$ from 4.8 to 9.6 mM (guinea pig papillary muscle) produced no effect on force development. Morad (personal communication) has observed augmentation of contractile force upon elevation of $[K]_o$ in frog ventricle and is presently proposing a K-Ca exchange system as operative in the frog. Such an inotropic effect cannot be found in rabbit ventricle, nor is there any discernible effect on ^{45}Ca efflux upon elevation of $[K]_o$ from 4 to 10 mM (unpublished observation).

The weight of evidence, at present, indicates that the effects of $[K]_o$ on Ca flux and force in mammalian heart may not be direct but operative through Na.

$[Na]_o$.—It is generally accepted that alterations in $[Na]_o$ affect force development by affecting Ca movements (44, 73, 74). It is believed that Na and Ca compete for superficial sites which bind $2Na^+$ for $1Ca^{2+}$. Applying the law of mass action to the Na-Ca relationship, force is found to be proportional to $[Ca]_o/[Na]_o^2$ over a large range of concentrations. The competition for binding sites could well be on the basis of ionic charge. As suggested previously, a layer of negatively charged mucopolysaccharide near the cell surface might represent the region of Na-Ca competition. A reduction of $[Na]_o$ at this area would permit additional Ca to bind and lead to augmentation of Ca released to the myofilaments upon excitation.

$[Na]_i$.—The possibility that intracellular Na content or concentration might play a significant role in the control of Ca movement in heart muscle has been the subject of increasing investigation since it was suggested less than ten years ago (45, 87). Evidence for such a role in any biological system was indirect until the very significant study on the perfused squid axon (4). This preparation consists of an axon from which the axoplasm has been removed, leaving a tube of membrane which can then be perfused both externally and internally. Decrease in $[Na]_o$ increased Ca influx across the membrane—a response similar to that defined in heart muscle. Of particular interest, however, was the demonstration that an increase of $[Na]_i$ also produced a striking increase in Ca influx. It seems quite possible that this represents a general property of excitable membranes. Baker et al have proposed a carrier system based upon Na-Ca coupling. I have incorporated such a system in a recently proposed myocardial membrane model (50) (see later discussion).

Evidence for a role of $[Na]_i$ in Ca movement is increasing. Glitsch, Reuter & Scholz (33) found that ^{45}Ca influx increased in guinea-pig auricles when $[Na]_i$ was increased either by cooling or by very rapid stimulation (300/min) of the preparation. They found that contractile force was increased when $[Na]_i$ was high. It was suggested that the Na-Ca carrier system was far from saturation at normal inside ionic concentrations, and increased $[Na]_i$ was capable of stimulating a significant Ca inward movement. It is to be noted, however, that the methods used to induce elevation of $[Na]_i$

(cooling and high rate of stimulation) cause a decrease in $[K]_i$. It is possible, though more difficult, to ascribe the Ca movement in terms of a K-Ca coupling. To resolve this problem, it would be desirable to induce a gain in $[Na]_i$ without inducing a reduction in $[K]_i$.

Hercus, McDowall & Mendel (37) noted over 15 years ago that upon exposure of rat ventricle to high $[Na]_o$ (177 mM) cellular Na uptake was increased but there was "unexpectedly no increased loss of potassium." The functional response induced by high $[Na]_o$ was complex (63). These findings seemed of particular interest from the point of view of further definition of the role of $[Na]_i$, and we have just completed a study of the functional and ionic flux effects of increasing $[Na]_o$ to 200 mM (107).

The initial response upon perfusion with 200 mM hyperosmolar $[Na]_o$ is a 20% depression in force. This would be expected on the basis of the "superficial" Na vs Ca competition discussed previously. This depression is complete within 2 min of the onset of 200 mM $[Na]_o$ perfusion. Over the next 7 min, despite maintenance of 200 mM $[Na]_o$, force returns to control level and remains at this level until 142 mM $[Na]_o$ is reinstituted. Upon reinstitution of 142 mM $[Na]_o$, force "overshoots" by 20% above control within 2 min and then returns over the next 8–10 min. The time course of tissue dehydration following 200 mM $[Na]_o$ has been defined and cannot be implicated as the basis for return to control tension or for the "overshoot" upon return to 142 mM $[Na]_o$. In addition we have confirmed that there is no K loss. The course of events correlates most closely with changes in $[Na]_i$ and indicates that increased $[Na]_i$ can compensate for the effects of increased $[Na]_o$ on Ca influx—i.e. as $[Na]_i$ increases, Na-outward/Ca-inward coupled flux is augmented.

Studies in diverse tissues using diverse techniques support the existence of a Na-Ca coupled flux system. Whether or not this plays a physiological role in Ca-mediated control of contractile force in myocardium remains controversial at this time. At least two recent studies tend to discount the importance of $[Na]_i$ in the control of contractile force in the heart.

Gilmore, Nizolek & Jacob (32) examined net K movements associated with alterations in contraction frequency in the Langendorff perfused dog heart preparation. They found that the total net K loss associated with a standard increment in frequency was the same whether this increment was abruptly induced (within less than a second) or slowly induced (over a two minute period). They interpreted these results to reject as untenable the hypothesis (46, 47) which proposes that the Bowditch staircase response is dependent upon a gain in $[Na]_i$ secondary to a lag in Na transport. Their logic was based on the premise that an increment in frequency induced rapidly should produce a greater total net K loss (at final steady-state) than the same increment induced slowly, if the proposed (46, 47) lag in response of the Na pump occurred. Langer (51) examined this premise in light of the currently accepted model for the feedback control of active Na transport and concluded that no difference in total net K loss was to be expected in the Gilmore et al study. Moreover, the change in force (at steady-state) induced by rapid and slow alterations in frequency was not significantly different. Since the net loss of K was also essentially the same, this indicated that equivalent net gains in $[Na]_i$ (equal to net losses of K) were associated with equivalent steady-state contractile forces—i.e. which would be expected in a system in which $[Na]_i$ was an important control factor.

Gadsby, Niedergerke & Page (30) also examined K movements in frog ventricles associated with alterations in contractile frequency, $[K]_o$, and acetylstrophanthidin administration. They found that the inotropic responses were not proportional to net K changes nor was the time course of net K movement and inotropic events comparable. For example, they found that perfusion with acetylstrophanthidin ($4 \times 10^{-7}M$) produced a net K loss continuing over 40 min whereas peak tension rose to stable levels within 20 min. They reported that this was a submaximal dose of strophanthidin, and higher peak tensions could be obtained with higher doses. The loss of K induced by the "submaximal" dose reduced the concentration of K in the cell water by some 15 mM. This means that there was a loss of at least 7–8 mmoles K/kg tissue at a time when full inotropism was not yet achieved. Comparable losses were reported with changes in $[K]_o$ and frequency. These are extraordinarily large net losses. Most studies (47, 52, 84) have indicated full inotropic effects associated with losses in the range of 1–3 mmoles/kg tissue. Mammalian ventricles demonstrate clear evidence of glycoside toxicity when net K loss exceeds 3–4 mmoles/kg tissue (48).

On the basis of their study Gadsby et al (30) concluded that cellular K for Na exchanges could not make substantial contributions to the regulation of contractile force. It would seem, however, that their experimental preparation was quite unique in a number of respects. Comparable K loss in other preparations is clearly far outside the physiological range and it is difficult to draw general conclusions about Na, K effects on force development from the Gadsby study. Evidence in support of the importance of the Na-Ca coupled system in the inotropic action of the cardiac glycosides has recently been reviewed (52).

In a qualitative sense it seems to be true that the hearts from most species which demonstrate a positive staircase also demonstrate a net K loss (and net Na gain). Whether or not there is a cause and effect relationship through an enhanced Na-Ca transport system has been reviewed above. The rat heart, however, ordinarily does not demonstrate a positive tension response upon an abrupt increase in stimulation frequency in the range between 15 and 150/min. It is pertinent to note that under conditions in which frequency is increased with little or no positive tension staircase, no net K loss was found (8). This indicates no net Na gain and, presumably, no stimulation of Na-Ca coupled flux which could explain the absence of the tension staircase phenomenon.

At the present time I believe the weight of evidence favors a significant role for Na in the physiological and pharmacological regulation of Ca movement in myocardium.

CONCLUSION

The theme of this review has been an evaluation of the EC coupling sequence in heart muscle through analysis of the movements of Ca. I elected to divide the presentation on the basis of the diverse techniques used. In many cases the results derived from the use of one technique or approach are reconcilable with those derived from another; in other cases this is not so. It is clear that before the EC sequence is completely understood, structural, electrophysiological, flux, and pharmacological results must be compatible. In conclusion I would like to reemphasize areas which I believe to be of particular interest for the future:

1. Further consideration of the surface structure of myocardial cells with particular attention to the role played by negatively charged mucopolysaccharide material.

2. Further correlation of voltage clamp results with flux and structural data. Most important is the definition of the juxtamembrane locus of the "superficial Ca compartment" involved in the EC coupling sequence. It is obvious that more knowledge about subcellular compartmentalization of ions will provide a great deal of insight into control of Ca movements.

3. Further direct comparative studies of cardiac and skeletal muscle EC coupling. It is clear that untested extrapolations from the one tissue to the other can be very misleading.

4. Further definition of the relationship between Na-K coupled flux and Na-Ca coupled flux. It is clear that cationic movements are closely interrelated both in the determination of electrophysiological and mechanical characteristics. Again correlation of voltage clamp and flux studies is required to synthesize a more complete picture. Myocardial tissue culture techniques should prove to be very useful in this area.

5. Further use of "unphysiological" ions and pharmacological agents which have specific functional effects in association with voltage clamping and flux studies. This will permit correlation among mechanical, electrical, and biochemical events.

ACKNOWLEDGMENTS

The author expresses his appreciation to Drs. A. J. Brady, K. I. Shine, and J. H. Tillisch for their many helpful comments and suggestions.

LITERATURE CITED

1. Bahl, O., Oliver, C. 1971. Extracellular myocardial action of digitalis. Abstr. *Circulation* 44:II–117
2. Bailey, L. E., Dresel, P. E. 1968. Correlation of contractile force with a calcium pool in the isolated cat heart. *J. Gen. Physiol.* 52:969–982
3. Bailey, L. E., Sures, H. A. 1971. The effect of ouabain on the washout and uptake of calcium in the isolated cat heart. *J. Pharmacol. Exp. Ther.* 178: 259–70
4. Baker, P. F., Blaustein, M. P., Hodgkin, A. L., Steinhardt, R. A. 1969. The influence of calcium on sodium efflux in squid axons. *J. Physiol. London* 200: 431–58
5. Beeler, G. W., Jr., Reuter, H. 1970a. Membrane calcium current in ventricular myocardial fibers. *J. Physiol. London* 207: 191–209
6. Beeler, G. W., Jr., Reuter, H. 1970b. The relation between membrane potential, membrane currents and activation of contraction in ventricular myocardial fibers. *J. Physiol. London* 207:211–29
7. Besch, H. R., Allen, J. C., Glick, G., Schwartz, A. 1970. Correlation between the inotropic action of ouabain and its effects on subcellular enzyme systems from canine myocardium. *J. Pharmacol. Exp. Ther.* 171:1–12
8. Blesa, E. S., Langer, G. A., Brady, A. J., Serena, S. D. 1970. Potassium exchange in rat ventricular myocardium: its relation to rate of stimulation. *Am. J. Physiol.* 219:747–54
9. Blinks, J. R., Olson, C. B., Jewell, B. R., Braveny, P. 1972. Influence of caffeine and other methylxanthines on mechanical properties of isolated mammalian heart muscle. *Circ. Res.* 30:367–92
10. Bloom, S. 1971. Requirements for spontaneous contractility in isolated adult mammalian heart muscle cells. *Exp. Cell Res.* 69: 17–24
11. Busselen, P. 1971. Potassium chloride contractures in rabbit auricles: Interaction of Sr^{++} and Ca^{++}. *Arch. Int. Physiol. Biochim.* 79:809
12. Carmeliet, E., Vereecke, J. 1969. Adrenaline and the plateau phase of the cardiac action potential. Importance of Ca, Na and K conductance. *Pfluegers Arch.* 313:300–15
13. Chapman, R. A., Niedergerke, R. 1970a. Effects of calcium on the contraction of the hypodynamic frog heart. *J. Physiol. London* 211:389–421
14. Chapman, R. A., Niedergerke, R. 1970b. Interaction between heart rate and calcium concentration in the control of contractile strength of the frog heart. *J. Physiol. London* 211: 423–43
15. Chapman, R. A., Tunstall, J. 1971. The dependence of the contractile force generated by frog auricular trabeculae upon the external calcium concentration. *J. Physiol. London* 215: 139–62
16. Chapman, R. A. 1971. Experimental alteration of the relationship between the external calcium concentration and the contractile force generated by auricular trabeculae isolated from the heart of the frog, Rana pipiens. *J. Physiol. London* 218:147–61
17. Chimosky, J. E. Gergely, J. 1968. Effect of norepinephrine, ouabain, and pH on cardiac sarcoplasmic reticulum. *Arch. Int. Pharmacodyn. Ther.* 176:289–97
18. Clark, A., Olson, C. B. 1968. Effects of caffeine on action potentials of mammalian ventricular cells. (Abstract) *Fed. Proc.* 27:304
19. Dhalla, N. S., McNamara, D. B., Sulakhe, P. V. 1970. Excitation-contraction coupling in heart. V. Contribution of mitochondria and sarcoplasmic reticulum in the regulation of calcium concentration in the heart. *Cardiology* 55:178–91
20. Dhalla, N. S., Sulakhe, P. V., Khandelwal, R. L., Hamilton,

I. R. 1970. Excitation-contraction coupling in heart. II. Studies on the role of adenyl cyclase in the calcium transport by dog heart sarcoplasmic reticulum. *Life Sci.* 9:625–32

21. Edman, K. A. P., Grieve, D. W. 1964. On the role of calcium in the excitation-contraction process of frog sartorius muscle. *J. Physiol. London* 170:138–52

21a. Eisenberg, B., Kuda, A., Peter, J. B. 1972. Morphometric analysis of the slow-twitch fibers of the guinea pig. *Proc. Elec. Microsc. Soc. Am.* 30:36

22. Eisenberg, R. S., Gage, P. W. 1967. Frog skeletal muscle fibers: Changes in electrical properties after disruption of transverse tubular system. *Science* 158:1700–01

23. Endo, M., Tanaka, M. Ogawa, Y. 1970. Calcium induced release of calcium from the sarcoplasmic reticulum of skinned skeletal muscle fibers. *Nature* 228:34–36

24. Entman, M. L., Levey, G. S., Epstein, S. E. 1969. Mechanism of action of epinephrine and glucagon on the canine heart. Evidence for increase in sarcotubular calcium stores medicated by 3′,5′-AMP. *Circ. Res.* 25:429–38

25. Fabiato, A., Fabiato, S., Sonnenblick, E. H. 1972. Calcium dependent cyclic contractions of cardiac and skeletal muscle cells with disrupted sarcolemmae. *Abstr. Fed. Proc.* 31:373

26. Fawcett, D. W., McNutt, N. S. 1969. The ultrastructure of the cat myocardium. I. Venticular papillary muscle. *J. Cell Biol.* 42:1–45

27. Fleckenstein, A., Kaufmann, R. 1966. Über den Einfluss der extracellulären K⁺-Konzentration auf das mechanische Verhalten des isolierten Warmblüter-Myokards (Papillarmuskeln von Rhesus-Ayen). *Pfluegers Arch.* 298:R17–R18

28. Ford, L. E., Podolsky, R. J. 1970. Regenerative calcium release within muscle cells. *Science* 67:58–59

29. Forssmann, W. G., Girardier, L. 1970. A study of the T-system in rat heart. *J. Cell. Biol.* 44:1–19

30. Gadsby, D. C., Niedergerke, R., Page, S. 1971. Do intracellular concentrations of potassium or sodium regulate the strength of the heart beat? *Nature* 232:651–53

31. Gibbons, W. R., Fozzard, H. A. 1971. Voltage dependence and time dependence of contraction in sheep cardiac Purkinje fibers. *Circ. Res.* 28:446–60

32. Gilmore, J. P., Nizolek, J. A., Jr., Jacob, R. J. 1971. Further characterization of myocardial K⁺ loss induced by changing contraction frequency. *Am. J. Physiol.* 221:465–69

33. Glitsch, H. G., Reuter, H., Scholz, H. 1970. The effect of the internal sodium concentration on calcium fluxes in isolated guinea-pig auricules. *J. Physiol. London* 209:25–43

34. Glynn, I. M. 1962. Activation of adenosinetriphosphatase in a cell membrane by external potassium and internal sodium. *J. Physiol. London* 160:18–19P

35. Grossman, A., Furchgott, R. F. 1964. The effects of various drugs on calcium exchange in the isolated guinea-pig left auricle. *J. Pharmacol. Exp. Ther.* 145:162–72

36. Hagiwara, S., Henkart, M. P., Kidokoro, Y. 1971. Excitation-contraction coupling in amphioxus muscle cells. *J. Physiol. London* 219:233–51

37. Hercus, V. M., McDowall, R. J. S., Mendel, D. 1955. Sodium exchanges in cardiac muscle. *J. Physiol. London* 129:177–83

38. Holland, W. C., Sekul, A. A. 1959. Effect of ouabain on Ca⁴⁵ and Cl³⁶ exchange in isolated rabbit atria. *Am. J. Physiol.* 197:757–60

39. Howell, J. N., Jenden, P. J. 1967. T tubules of skeletal muscle: morphological alterations which interrupt excitation-contraction coupling. *Fed. Proc.* 26:553

40. Howse, H. D., Ferrans, V. J., Hibbs, R. G. 1970. A comparative histochemical and electronmicroscopic study of the surface coatings of cardiac muscle cells. *J. Mol. Cell. Cardiol.* 1:157–68

41. Johnson, E. A., Lieberman, M.

1971. Heart: excitation and contraction. *Ann. Rev. Physiol.* 33:479–532

42. Katz, A. M. 1970. Contractile proteins of the heart. *Physiol. Rev.* 50:63–158

43. Langer, G. A., Brady, A. J. 1963. Calcium flux in the mammalian ventricular myocardium. *J. Gen. Physiol.* 46:703–20

44. Langer, G. A. 1964. Kinetic studies of calcium distribution in ventricular muscle of the dog. *Circ. Res.* 15:393–405

45. Langer, G. A. 1965. Calcium exchange in dog ventricular muscle: Relation to frequency of contraction and maintenance of contractility. *Circ. Res.* 17:78–90

46. Langer, G. A. 1967. Sodium exchange in dog ventricular muscle: Relation to frequency of contraction and its possible role in the control of myocardial contractility. *J. Gen. Physiol.* 50:1221–39

47. Langer, G. A. 1968. Ion fluxes in cardiac excitation and contraction and their relation to myocardial contractility. *Physiol. Rev.* 48:708–57

48. Langer, G. A., Serena, S. D. 1970. Effects of strophanthidin upon contraction and ionic exchange in rabbit ventricular myocardium: relation to control of active state. *J. Mol. Cell. Cardiol.* 1:65–90

49. Langer, G. A. 1971a. Coupling calcium in mammalian ventricle: its source and factors regulating its quantity. *Cardiovasc. Res. Suppl.* 1:71–75

50. Langer, G. A. 1971b. Physiology in medicine: The intrinsic control of myocardial contraction —ionic factors. *N. Eng. J. Med.* 285:1065–71

51. Langer, G. A. 1972a. Myocardial K⁺ loss and contraction frequency. *J. Mol. Cell. Cardiol.* 4:85–86

52. Langer, G. A. 1972b. The effects of digitalis on myocardial ionic exchange. *Circulation* 45:180–87

53. Langer, G. A., Frank, J. S. 1972. Lanthanum in heart cell culture: Effect on calcium exchange correlated with its local-ization. *J. Cell Biol.* 54:441–55

54. Lee, K. S., Klaus, W. 1971. The subcellular basis for the mechanism of inotropic action of cardiac glycosides. *Pharm. Rev.* 23:193–261

55. Legato, M. J., Spiro, D., Langer, G. A. 1968. Ultrastructural alterations produced in mammalian myocardium by variation in perfusate ionic composition. *J. Cell. Biol.* 37:1–12

56. Legato, M. J., Langer, G. A. 1969. The subcellular localization of calcium ion in mammalian myocardium. *J. Cell Biol.* 41:401–23

57. Little, G. R., Sleator, W. W. 1969. Calcium exchange and contraction strength of guinea pig atrium in normal and hypertonic media. *J. Gen. Physiol.* 54:494–511

58. Lullman, H., Holland, W. C. 1962. Influence of ouabain on an exchangeable calcium fraction, contractile force and resting tension of guinea pig atrium. *J. Pharmacol. Exp. Ther.* 137:186–92

59. Mainwood, G. W., Lee, S. L. 1969. Rat heart papillary muscles: Action potentials and mechanical response to paired stimuli. *Science* 166:396–97

60. Mascher, D., Peper, K. 1969. Two components of inward current in myocardial muscle fibers. *Pfluegers Arch.* 307:190–203

61. Mascher, D. 1970. Electrical and mechanical responses from ventricular muscle fibers after inactivation of sodium carrying system. *Pfluegers Arch.* 317:359–72

62. Mascher, D. 1971. Electrical and mechanical events in depolarized cardiac muscle fibers during low sodium perfusion. *Pfluegers Arch.* 323:284–96

63. McDowall, R. J. S., Munro, A. F. Zayat, A. F. 1955. Sodium and cardiac muscle. *J. Physiol. London* 130:615–24

64. Mela, L. 1969. Inhibition and activation of calcium transport in mitochondria. Effect of lanthanides and local anesthestic drugs. *Biochemistry.* 8:2481–86

65. Morad, M., Trautwein, W. 1968. The effect of the duration of the

action potential on contraction in the mammalian heart muscle. *Pfluegers Arch.* 299:66–82

66. Morad, M. 1969. Contracture and catecholamines in mammalian myocardium. *Science* 166:505–6
67. Morad, M., Orkand, R. K. 1971. Excitation-contraction coupling in frog ventricle: evidence from voltage clamp studies. *J. Physiol. London* 219:167–89
68. Morad, M., Rolett, E. 1972. Relaxing effects of catecholamines on mammalian heart. *J. Physiol. London.* 224:537–58
69. Nayler, W. G., Hasker, J. R. 1966. Effect of caffeine on calcium in subcellular fractions of cardiac muscle. *Am. J. Physiol.* 211:950–54
70. Nayler, W. G. 1972. An effect of ouabain on superficially-located stores of calcium in cardiac muscle cells. Unpublished
71. New, W., Trautwein, W. 1972a. Inward membrane currents in mammalian myocardium. *Pfluegers Arch.* 334:1–23
72. New, W., Trautwein, W. 1972b. Ionic nature of slow inward current and its relation to contraction. *Pfluegers Arch.* 334:24–38
73. Niedergerke, R. 1957. The rate of action of calcium ions on the contraction of the heart. *J. Physiol. London* 138:506–15
74. Niedergerke, R. 1959. Calcium and activation of contraction. *Experientia* 15:128–30
75. Niedergerke, R. 1963. Movements of calcium in beating ventricles of the frog heart. *J. Physiol. London* 167:551–80
76. Niedergerke, R., Page, S., Talbot, M. S. 1969. Determination of calcium movements in heart ventricles of the frog. *J. Physiol. London* 202:58–60P
77. Niemeyer, G., Forssmann, W. G. 1971. Comparison of glycerol treatment in frog skeletal muscle and mammalian heart. *J. Cell. Biol.* 50:288–99
78. Ochi, R. 1970. The slow inward current and the action of manganese ions in guinea-pig's myocardium. *Pfluegers Arch.* 316:81–94
79. Ochi, R., Trautwein, W. 1971. The dependence of cardiac contraction on depolarization and slow inward current. *Pfluegers Arch.* 323:187–203

80. Page, E., Goerke, R. J., Storm, S. R. 1964. Cat heart muscle in vitro. IV. Inhibition of transport in quiescent muscles. *J. Gen. Physiol.* 47:531–43
80a. Page, E., McCallister, L. P., Power, B. 1971. Stereological measurements of cardiac ultra-structures implicated in excitation-contraction coupling. *Proc. Nat. Acad. Sci.* 68:1465–66
81. Patriarca, P., Carafoli, E. 1968. A study of the intracellular transport of calcium in rat heart. *J. Cell. Physiol.* 72:29–37
81a. Peachey, L. D. 1965. The sarcoplasmic reticulum and transverse tubules of the frog's sartorius. *J. Cell. Biol.* 25:209–31
82. Pretorius, P. J., Pohl, W. G., Smithen, C. S., Inesi, G. 1969. Structural and functional characteristics of dog heart microsomes. *Circ. Res.* 25:487–99
83. Posner, C. J., Berman, D. A. 1969. Mathematical analysis of oscillatory and non-oscillatory recovery of contractility after a rested-state contraction and its modification by calcium. *Circ. Res.* 25:725–33
84. Regan, T. J., Markov, A., Oldewurtel, H. A., Harman, M. A. 1969. Myocardial K+ loss after countershock and the relation to ventricular arrhythmias after non-toxic doses of acetylstrophanthidin. *Am. Heart J.* 77:367–71
85. Reiter, M., Stickel, F. J. 1968. Der Einfluss der Kontraktionsfrequenz auf das Aktions potential des Meerschweinchen-Papillarmuskels. *Naunyn-Schmiedebergs Arch. Pharmakol. Exp. Pathol.* 260:342–65
86. Reiter, M., Seibel, K., Stickel, F. J. 1971. Sodium dependence of the inotropic effect of a reduction in extracellular potassium concentrations. *Naunyn-Schmiedebergs Arch. Pharmakol. Exp. Pathol.* 268:361–78
87. Repke, K. 1964. Über den biochemischen Wirkingsmodus von Digitalis. *Klin. Wochenschr.* 41:157–65
88. Reuter, H. 1965. Über die Wirkung

von Adrenalin auf den cellulären Ca-Umsatz des Meerschweinchenvorhofs. *Neunyn-Schmiedebergs Arch. Exp. Pathol. Pharmakol.* 251:401–12

89. Reuter, H. 1967. The dependence of slow inward current in Purkinje fibers on the extracellular calcium concentration. *J. Physiol. London* 192:479–92

90. Reuter, H., Beeler, G. W., Jr. 1969. Calcium current and activation of contraction in ventricular myocardial fibers. *Science* 162:399–401

91. Reuter, H. 1972. Divalent cations as charge carriers in excitable membranes. *Progr. Biophys. Mol. Biol.* In press

92. Ross, J., Jr., Sobel, B. E. 1972. Regulation of cardiac contraction. *Ann. Rev. Physiol.* 34:47–90

93. Rougier, O., Vassort, G., Garnier, D., Gargouil, Y. M., Coraboeuf, E. 1969. Existence and role of a slow inward current during the frog atrial action potential. *Pfluegers Arch.* 308:91–110

94. Saari, J. T., Johnson, J. A. 1971. Decay of calcium content and contractile force in the rabbit heart. *Am. J. Physiol.* 221:1572–75

95. Sanborn, W. G., Langer, G. A. 1970. Specific uncoupling of excitation and contraction in mammalian cardiac tissue by lanthanum. *J. Gen. Physiol.* 56:191–217

96. Sands, S. D., Winegrad, S. 1970. Treppe and total calcium content of the frog ventricle. *Am. J. Physiol.* 218:908–10

97. Schaffer, S. W., Williamson, J. R. 1972. The calcium cycle and myocardial contractility. Abstr. *Fed. Proc.* 31:373

98. Scott, J. E. 1968. Ion binding in solutions containing acid mucopolysaccharides. *Chemistry. and Physiology of Mucopolysaccharides,* ed. G. Quintarelli, 171–87. Boston: Little-Brown

99. Shea, S. M. 1971. Lanthanum staining of the surface coat of cells. Its enhancement by the use of fixatives containing Alcian Blue or Cetylpyridinium Chloride. *J. Cell Biol.* 51:611–20

100. Shine, K. I., Serena, S. D., Langer, G. A. 1971. Kinetic localization of contractile calcium in rabbit myocardium. *Am. J. Physiol.* 221:1408–17

101. Shine, K. I., Langer, G. A. 1971. Caffeine effects upon contraction and calcium exchange in rabbit myocardium. *J. Mol. Cell. Cardiol.* 3:255–70

102. Skelton, C. L., Butler, V. P., Schmidt, D. H., Sonnenblick, E. H. 1971. Immunological studies on the cellular site of action of digitalis. Abstr. *Circulation* 44:II—117

103. Sopis, J. A., Langer, G. A. 1970. Calcium kinetics in frog heart. *J. Mol. Cell. Cardiol.* 1:291–305

104. Sperelakis, N., Rubio, R. 1971. An orderly lattice of axial tubules which interconnect adjacent transverse tubules in guinea-pig ventricular myocardium. *J. Mol. Cell. Cardiol.* 2:212–20

105. Staley, N. A., Benson, E. S. 1968. The ultrastructure of frog ventricular cardiac muscle and its relationship to mechanisms of excitation-contraction coupling. *J. Cell. Biol.* 38:99–114

106. Thomas, L. J., Jr. 1960. Increase of labelled calcium uptake in heart muscle during potassium lack contracture. *J. Gen. Physiol.* 43:1193–1206

107. Tillisch, J. H., Langer, G. A. 1972. Myocardial electromechanical responses and ionic exchange in elevated sodium perfusate. Unpublished

108. Vitek, M., Trautwein, W. 1971. Slow inward current and action potential in cardiac Purkinje fibers. The effect of Mn^{++} ions. *Pfluegers Arch.* 323:204–18

109. Weber, A., Herz, R. 1968. The relationship between caffeine contracture of intact muscle and the effect of caffeine on reticulum. *J. Gen. Physiol.* 52:750–59

110. Weber, A. 1968. The mechanism of action of caffeine on sarcoplasmic reticulum. *J. Gen. Physiol.* 52:760–72

111. Weiss, G. B. 1970. On the site of action of lanthanum in frog sartorius muscle. *J. Pharmacol. Exp. Ther.* 174:517–26

112. Whaley, W. G., Dauwalder, M., Kephart, J. E. 1972. Golgi apparatus: influence on cell surfaces. *Science* 175:596–99

113. Whittam, R. 1962. The asymmetrical stimulation of a membrane adenosine triphosphatase in relation to active cation transport. *Biochem. J.* 84:110–18

114. Williamson, J. R. 1972. Effects of epinephrine on glycogenlysis and myocardial contractility. *Handbook of Physiology:* *Adrenal.* Washington, DC: Am. Physiol. Soc.

115. Winegrad, S., Shanes, A. M. 1962. Calcium flux and contractility in guinea pig atria. *J. Gen. Physiol.* 45:317–94

116. Winegrad, S. 1968. Intracellular calcium movements of frog skeletal muscle during recovery from tetanus. *J. Gen. Physiol.* 51:65–83

117. Winegrad, S. 1971. Studies of cardiac muscle with a high permeability to calcium produced by treatment with ethylenediaminetetraacetic acid. *J. Gen. Physiol.* 58:71–93

Ann. Rev. Physiol. 1973. 35:87–116

HEMODYNAMICS 1090

M. G. TAYLOR

Department of Physiology, University of Sydney, Australia

Since the previous review in this series (99) two very useful surveys have appeared: an extensive text on arterial dynamics by Wetterer & Kenner (216), and a briefer but more recent review by Bergel & Schultz (29). We await with great interest the new edition of McDonald's influential *Blood Flow in Arteries* (133) which is in preparation, and the *Handbook of Cardiovascular Fluid Dynamics* which is soon to be published (28).

It is not easy to fulfil the Editor's invitation to provide a statesman-like survey of the whole field, and doubtless quite a lot of material will unfortunately remain "unobserved publications." But bearing in mind the availability of the detailed and authoritative texts cited above, I have felt free to devote some attention to a few topics which are not always included in discussion of hemodynamics—for example, the elastic properties of the ventricle and the indicator-dilution method of measuring blood flow. For reasons of space, and with regret, I have not discussed the very interesting developments in blood rheology and the microcirculation; these are, however, dealt with by Schmid-Schönbein & Wells (185), and in the chapter by Zweifach in this volume. As a matter of policy I have not included any material which has appeared only in abstract, as this is seldom detailed enough for critical appraisal. Likewise, I have only rarely made use of material from specialized symposia unless full published texts were readily available. The sources of the review are therefore almost entirely confined to major international journals published during the years 1968 through 1971.

THE HEART

Methods.—The preferred technique for recording the motions of the heart seems to be cineangiography in either one or two planes, but some other methods have also been used. The radiographic technique applied to man normally uses radio-opaque dye injection to fill the ventricle with contrast medium and thus outline its shape, but this may be avoided in the chronic animal preparation by attaching metal markers at different points on the ventricular wall (38, 148, 217). Ultrasonic techniques have also been used to measure either the minor axis of the heart (159) or the motion of the posterior left ventricular wall (120), where it was concluded that the method

87

warranted continued exploration. A rather special use of ultrasound is in measuring the distance between two transducers spaced along a catheter which, forming an arc inside the ventricle, is springy enough to press against the wall and thus follow its motion; the transducers are spaced so that they lie on approximately the minor diameter of the ventricle (106).

Most angiographic studies have used biplane X rays. With suitable correction and planimetry of the areas of these images, and assuming an ellipsoidal form for the ventricle, quite reasonable correlation (R = 0.8) was found between stroke volumes so determined and those determined by use of the Fick method (163). On the other hand, single-plane angiography would be preferable as a matter of convenience, and the dimensions of the heart can apparently be fairly well characterized by a single measurement. For instance, a single silastic gauge sewn to the left ventricle of the dog gave a reasonably linear correlation with ventricular volume over the range 10–50 ml (86). A comparison of ventricular dimensions as estimated by biplane angiocardiogram and by single plane antero-posterior X ray showed that the volume calculated from the antero-posterior data exceeded the "true" volume by only a few percent (181). Comparison between the ventricular volumes estimated from single plane cineangiography and by indicator dilution techniques (58) have shown a very good correlation (R = 0.98) between angiogram volume (right anterior oblique) and indicator dilution volume. The theory of indicator mixing in the ventricle has also been carefully studied (89). The availability of high-speed filming (270 to 540 frames/sec) (131) makes possible quite detailed analyses of ventricular movement and dimensions. There is a fair amount of "noise" on such records but suitable digital filtering (34) can overcome this.

Elastic behavior of the ventricular wall.—There has been considerable interest in the detailed analysis of the dimensional changes in the left ventricle caused by changes in intraventricular pressure. First, the distribution of stresses within the thickness of the ventricular wall has important effects on myocardial perfusion, particularly in the left ventricle. Next, there is the relationship between the lengths of individual muscular elements and the tensions which they may sustain or develop at various points in the myocardium. Finally, there is the problem of the orientation and arrangement of fibers in the ventricular wall, since it is not a homogenous isotropic elastic body.

The interpretation of pressures within the thickness of the myocardium must be made cautiously, because of the unavoidable objection that the insertion of the measuring device may have distorted the normal situation. Using a catheter with a continuous slow infusion so that a small "fluid pocket" was created, it was found that during systole the pressure in the wall of the left ventricle of the dog increased linearly with depth, being zero at the epicardial surface and equal to intraventricular pressure at the endocardial surface (32). Somewhat similar results were observed (12) when a small flat pressure-sensitive probe, inserted into the wall of the left ventricle, was used. The pressures found in the outer layers were less than those in deeper layers; both norepinephrine and stellate ganglion stimulation caused increases in intramural pressures, but the effects were not identical. By considering the ventricular wall to be composed of layers of muscle each developing hoop tension, systolic tension in the outer and inner regions was estimated to be 3.3×10^5 dynes/cm^2 and 2.2×10^5 dynes/cm^2.

Studies of the elastic behavior of thick shells, as models of the left ventricle, can be divided into those which assume that the wall is composed of isotropic and homogenous material, and those which make allowance in various ways for the special characteristics and orientation of myocardial fibers. It does not seem to matter greatly what geometrical form is assumed for the ventricle. Attention has, however, been directed to the influence of changing wall thickness during ventricular contraction (47, 51). This is particularly important in those instances where mean wall stress is being determined (91, 92). The effect of changes in wall thickness as a result of hypertrophy is of course also important and, as has been pointed out (224), quite a small increase in thickness as a "compensation" for the load in hypertension will keep the maximum wall stress at a normal level. It is perhaps a little surprising that the mean equatorial stress in the left ventricle (92) was overestimated only by approximately 10% when the thin wall model was used instead of the thick walled ellipsoid. In this same study, normal and abnormal states were compared and the peak systolic average stress seemed to be remarkably similar in normal hearts and those having developed a thick wall in compensation for a pressure overload.

In studies of the stresses in particular regions of the ventricular wall, calculations based on the isotropic elastic properties of a variety of geometrical forms have shown that stresses in the ventricular will be maximal at the inner layers, and decrease towards the outer surface (146). Further, because of the varying radius of curvature and the varying thickness of the wall, the stresses will be greatest at the equator of an ellipsoid model of the ventricle, and least at the pole or apex. The changing wall thickness may in fact compensate for effects of change in radius of curvature from base to apex of the heart, and so keep wall stress approximately constant throughout (31). In a very interesting study (35), comparisons were made between measured stresses in various parts of the left ventricular wall of the dog and stresses computed on the basis of either a thick walled spherical model or a thick walled ellipsoidal model; the wall material was assumed to be isotropic. It was found necessary to take account of the changing wall thicknesses during the cardiac cycle, but even so the calculated peak stresses were greater than those measured. The ellipsoidal model was shown to be preferable to the spherical one.

A more accurate representation of the physical structure of the left ventricle requires that the orientation of the fibers in various parts of the wall be taken into account. Once the system is thus made anisotropic (147), it no longer automatically follows that the stresses will have a maximum at the inner wall and decrease to a minimum at the outer surface of the ventricle.

The maximum may occur at some point within the thickness of the wall, and indeed, it may be possible to get compressive forces near the inner wall, causing folding. The orientation of fibers in the myocardium may be expressed as a parabolic variation in circumferential elastic modulus across the thickness of the wall (147), as a variation in orientation of helical fibers with respect to the long axis of the heart (211–213), as nested shells with random attachments (202), or as helical fibers arranged over an infinitely thin shell (180). These models rest principally on earlier work (76, 200) in which the myocardial wall was described as a continuum of muscle fibers which show a progressive variation in their orientation, from endocardium to epicardium, with the middle layers running more or less circumferentially.

In fact, from endocardium to epicardium there was observed (201) an S-shaped distribution of the angles made by the direction of the fibers in relation to the long axis of the heart; this distribution varied relatively little between systole and diastole. Even this model may represent an oversimplification, since it has further been shown (11) that the interdigitating fibers of ventricular muscle form a continuum which is not sharply delineated into separate muscle bands; moreover, although orientation of fibers varies from one region to another, there is a "principle fiber direction," shown by the bulk of ventricular fibers, which is generally oblique to a vertical axis from base to apex of the heart. The concept of the spiral fibers originating in the fibrous skeleton at the base of the heart, passing spirally down the epicardium through the apex, and finally reentering the fibrous skeleton via the papillary muscles and the cordae is itself an oversimplification, since a significant portion of the muscle strands do not pass from base to apex but swing deeply from the epicardium to the endocardium at all vertical levels.

Models which are still closer to the actual situation involve the consideration of variations in sarcomere length in the muscle. For example, while ejection fractions in excess of 50% are common for the left ventricle, even a 20% shortening of circularly oriented "constrictor" fibers would eject only 49% from a spherical model of the ventricle or 36% from a cylindrical or ellipsoidal model (180). Helical orientation of the fibers around an ellipsoid, with realistic pitch angles, can give 60% ejection for only 20% shortening. Taking the active tension developed as a function of sarcomere length, the total behavior of the ventricle depends to a considerable extent upon which model is employed. If the wall is considered isotropic and homogenous (225), then hypertrophy of the ventricle will be predicted to lead to the development of maximum active tension at higher filling pressures. On the other hand, structural changes which may accompany long standing myocardial conditions cannot be ignored. In a very important paper (177) it was shown, in chronic dilatation of the left ventricle of the dog, that not only does the geometrical form of the ventricle have almost a normal configuration, differing from that found with acute dilatation, but also that in chronically dilated hearts the z lines of the muscle cells are out of register, although the individual sarcomeres are not overstretched. This observation thus makes questionable the involvement of the so-called "descending limb of the Starling curve" in the impaired contractility of the dilated ventricle.

Although most attention has been devoted to behavior of the left ventricle, it has also been demonstrated (126) that cylindrical and spherical models are equally good in relating right ventricular volume to a characteristic fiber length. Further, while in the left ventricle maximum active tension would be attained at the sarcomere length of 2.24 μ produced by a left ventricular filling pressure of 12 mm Hg, the maximum would be developed for the right ventricle at the lower filling pressure of 7 mm Hg. In another study (13), where strain gauges were placed on various parts of the surface of the right ventricle, the regional intraventricular pressures developed were shown to be highly dependent on anatomical structure and, since they appeared to differ in response to inotropic influences, on the autonomic innervation also.

The dynamic properties of the myocardium.—Many of the measurements made of ventricular pressure-volume relations and of the time course of ventricular pressure and diameter changes have been aimed at evaluating the contractile properties of the myocardium and, in particular, at assessing its function in the presence of disease. It would, however, be inappropriate in this review to pursue in detail such aspects of myocardial physiology. Some observations, however, have been reported which refer to variations in the physical properties of the heart at various phases of the cardiac cycle. For instance, by imposing isovolumic left ventricular oscillations at frequencies up to 30 Hz on top of normal contractions (205), it was found that both the volume stiffness and the effective viscosity of the ventricle increased during systole; left ventricular diastolic distensibility was uninfluenced by either vagal stimulation, norepinephrine, or beta-blockade (218, 219). Further, an attempt has been made (67, 68) to study the time-varying elastic properties of the myocardium by assuming that the frequency-components of the first and third heart sounds arise from the various modes of oscillation of a fluid-filled spherical elastic shell. While in theory this proposal may have some validity (132), any parameters obtained in practice would be exceedingly difficult to interpret.

Finally, since the heart is coupled to the vascular system, it is important to be aware of their interaction. Ventricular pressure during systole will vary depending on the frequency characteristics of the vascular system (49, 121, 158). By measuring ventricular pressure and aortic flow, it is possible to compute the ventricular forcing impedance (5) which is said to have the same frequency characteristics as that of the aortic impedance. Unfortunately, in this study the model from which the ventricular impedance was calculated included a lumped element for the systemic impedance which does not have the phase characteristics of the aortic impedance over the range of frequencies employed.

Another aspect of the heart's relationship to the vascular system is the work expended by the left ventricle in producing the cardiac output. As far as the myocardium is concerned, energy is expended not only in moving the blood against the peripheral resistance and imparting kinetic energy to it, but also in developing and maintaining tension during the isovolumetric phases. Even assuming the considerably simplified model of the left ventricle as a spherical shell with an isotropic, homogenous wall of uniform thickness, it has been possible to obtain reasonable agreement with data on the energy expended in the contracting left ventricle (223).

PRESSURE AND FLOW IN THE ARTERIAL SYSTEM

The measurement of pressure.—Intravascular pressure is usually measured either by means of a fluid filled catheter, or directly by a catheter-tip transducer. The presence of the catheter may itself influence the pulsatile events in the artery, (103) but usually the errors so produced are small. In any case, the frequency characteristics of the whole pressure measuring system must be considered; fluid filled catheter systems are particularly liable to error since the smallest air bubble will severely degrade the fidelity of the recording (191). For accurate work one must obtain the frequency response of the entire system by subjecting it either to a sudden step in pressure (the so-called "pop" technique) or to sinusoidal pressure variations generated by some mechanical or electromechanical device (54, 122, 192). Once the frequency characteristics of the system have been thus determined, all subsequent recordings may be corrected either by the application of suitable modulus and phase corrections to frequency components obtained by Fourier analysis, or by the use of a special purpose analog computer (142). In sampled data systems, where subsequent analysis is to be carried out by digital computer, it is important to choose a sampling rate which is appropriate to the frequency components of the signal; 100 samples per second is adequate for most purposes (135).

An interesting recent development has been the use of fiber optics to measure the deflection of a flexible membrane at the end of a catheter and thereby to determine the intravascular pressure. Two examples have been reported; in one, the membrane was a polyester and the frequency response good up to 1600 Hz (169); in the other, the membrane was of glass and gave the instrument a higher frequency response up to 15 kHz (128). Such instruments will be useful for the simultaneous registration of intravascular pressure and sound.

Most measurements of blood pressure in man are still made by the auscultatory method, using the Korotkoff sounds as indicators of systolic and diastolic levels. A slight modification has recently been reported (108): a Doppler ultrasonic flowmeter was placed over the radial artery and, as the cuff-pressure was lowered, the first appearance of pulsatile flow was taken to indicate systolic pressure, while the diastolic pressure was that at which arterial flow remained above zero for the whole cycle. The values obtained for systolic and diastolic pressure by this method correlated very highly with those obtained by direct arterial puncture. The method reportedly worked better than the auscultatory method in shocked patients with very low systolic blood pressures.

The measurement of arterial blood flow.—While the electromagnetic flowmeter retains its deserved popularity, there has been considerable development of intravascular flow probes. Because the extravascular flow probe requires the surgical exposure of the artery for its application, it is of limited use in human medicine—hence the further development of intravascular flow probes for the continuous monitoring of circulatory state. These probes may be electromagnetic or ultrasonic, or may employ hot film techniques.

Electromagnetic flowmeters: A comprehensive review of the use of electromagnetic flowmeters was provided by the proceedings of a 1968 symposium (37). Since then, a very promising development in standard extravascular flow probes has been the use of silicone rubber in their construction (53). This more compliant material is reported to reduce greatly the risk of erosion of the vessel and thus to ensure much longer survival of chronically implanted probes. While the electromagnetic flowmeter normally sets up a magnetic field across a vessel by means of an extravascularly applied magnet or coil, it is also possible to apply an extracorporeal magnetic field by means of a large coil or permanent magnet, and to detect, by intravascular electrodes, the potentials due to the motion of the blood (116–118, 154).

It is well recognized that the frequency characteristics of pressure recording systems must be determined and allowed for; but until relatively recently, little attention was paid to those of the electromagnetic flowmeter. These frequency characteristics are very largely governed by the output filters used to smooth the signal and remove the carrier frequency (72); it is certainly important that they be determined, either by subjecting the transducer to known oscillatory flow or by applying suitably modulated signals directly to the electrodes (80). The electromagnetic flowmeter gives a signal which is proportional to the average velocity of the stream, and does not depend on the form of the velocity profile, provided that it is axisymmetric. However, the influence of the surrounding medium (226) and the degree of uniformity of the magnetic field itself (102) cannot be ignored. For the most accurate work, account must also be taken of the small changes in sensitivity which accompany changes in hematocrit (45).

As mentioned above, one modificaiton of the electromagnetic flowmeter technique which has recently become popular has been the development of miniature intravascular flow probes. The weak magnetic fields set up by such flow probes enable them to sense flow velocity over only a relatively small annulus of fluid surrounding the catheter, and therefore, to determine volume flow through the vessel, one needs to know not only its diameter but also the form of the velocity profile. Fortunately, in a vessel of major interest, namely the aorta, the velocity profile is almost flat, and, provided the flow probe is located somewhere near the axis, very respectable estimates of flow may be obtained (62, 115, 137, 214).

Ultrasonic flowmeters: A previous method of finding blood flow velocity was to measure the difference between the transit times of an ultrasonic pulse with and against the stream, but most instruments today use instead an application of the Doppler effect: when a beam of ultrasound is directed into a stream of blood the echoes returning from the particles in the stream are shifted in frequency in proportion to the velocity. Despite this instrument's attractive simplicity both in construction and in application, the interpretation of its output does not rest on as clear a theoretical foundation as does that of the electromagnetic flowmeter. Provided the magnetic field is uniform and the flow velocities are axisymmetric, the electromagnetic flowmeter will give a signal proportional to the true average velocity of flow in the vessel, but this is not the case for the ultrasonic flowmeter. The signal which it gives is not independent of the velocity profile, and it is by no means simple to determine the exact relation between the details of the flow and of the output signal (50, 66). The manner in which the flow velocities will be weighted in determining the output of the Doppler system depends on the nature of the ultrasound field which is generated in the stream, and this in turn depends on the relationship between the size of the ultrasonic transducer and the dimensions of the vessel (52). On theoretical grounds a suitable means of deriving flow velocity from the Doppler flowmeter signal would be to use the zero-crossing frequency, but only if the time constant of the smoothing system is long enough to obtain information on the averaged flow. The suggestion has been made that it would be advantageous to design the ultrasonic beam so as to give greatest energy in the center of the stream.

Despite these fundamental uncertainties, the ultrasonic flow probe is undoubtedly an extremely useful device, both when directly applied to the vessel and when inserted in the stream on the end of the catheter. Normally, the ultrasonic flowmeter does not distinguish forward from reverse flow (26, 27, 143, 207). However, when suitable circuitry is employed, those frequency components which indicate forward and reverse velocities can be separately identified. Signals can thus be obtained which may indicate that forward and reverse flow is occurring simultaneously in the same blood vessel (175, 199). This, however, should occasion no surprise since such inflections in the velocity profile are characteristic of oscillatory flow.

Heated film velocity probes: The principle of hot film anemometry has been applied to the measurement of blood flow in arteries. The heated films may be either on the end of an intra-arterial catheter or on a hypodermic needle; by means of the latter, velocity distributions have been mapped across the lumen (25, 129, 187–189). Since one is dealing with the thermal properties of a thin boundary layer of fluid in the neighborhood of the needle or probe, details of streaming in the region of the probe are important (44). The responses of these instruments are very similar in blood and water (188, 189) but the "over temperature," on which the sensitivity of the instrument depends, must be very low in order to avoid damage to the blood. These instruments may be made direction-sensitive by using more than one film, but attention must be given to the linearity and the time constants of the amplifiers involved. The instruments to which reference is made here seem to have quite adequate frequency responses (up to 8 Hz) and to be small and sensitive enough to allow the recording of details of oscillatory blood flow (78, 173).

Oscillatory pressure-flow relations.—In a recent extensive review (17), particular attention was devoted to comparing the linear methods using Fourier analysis of pressure and flow with the method of characteristics which enables nonlinear relationships to be included in the equation. Theoretical predictions of velocity profiles for laminar oscillating flow in tubes (82, 83) have been given further experimental confirmation, if that is needed. An interesting study of the entry flow of blood into a tube shows that, for Reynolds numbers less than 100 (124), it is possible to predict the subsequent behavior of the flow, once arbitrary radial and axial velocities have been prescribed at the origin. An ingenious method of approximation was employed, and the results were also applicable to the motion of the column of plasma in front of moving red cells in a capillary. More general studies of the blood flow through the circulatory system have also been made. These range from a treatment so general (94) that the authors themselves stated that the computations would be too elaborate and expensive to be carried out, to more realistic studies of flow through branching sets of tubes. One (119) employed an arbitrary relationship between the length and diameter of segments of a branching system, while another (96) used data derived from measurements made on animal specimens.

If the pressure gradient acting over a short segment of an unbranched blood vessel is known, the pulsatile flow through that segment can, in principle, be calculated. In practice it is probably impossible to determine accurately the mean pressure difference over a very short segment, but when the vessel concerned is the root of the aorta, "zero flow" can be determined in diastole, thus obviating the need to determine the steady pressure gradient. The recording of the pulsatile pressure gradient acting over a short segment in the arch of the aorta is not without technical difficulty, and the alternative use of the time derivative of the pressure at a single point has occasionally been proposed (77). But this method does not work in the presence of reflected pressure waves, and the use of a simple analog device for computing flow under these conditions is not straightforward.

Studies of nonlaminar flow have included both theoretical and practical (56, 57) examination of the flow of liquids in a converging-diverging tube. Theoretical and experimental studies were made of the stresses which might be induced on the walls of blood vessels in the presence of occlusive vascular disease and of the conditions under which flow separation would occur. A somewhat similar study (79) used X rays and a radio-opaque contrast medium to show the separation of flow at the inner border of a sudden angle in a tube. Oscillatory flow in such a region produced very disturbed patterns in the boundary layer. As yet another example of abnormal flow in the arteries, it was found that where a jet issues from a stenosed aortic valve, it is directed into the innominate artery and thus generates an excess pressure there (71). This was confirmed in model experiments when the jet was made visible by a dye stream. Experiments to determine the criteria for the onset of vasular murmurs have shown good agreement between the duration of the murmur and the duration of the "super-critical" flow through a variable stenosis (179). The critical Reynolds number in this situation was best given as $2384 (d/D)^2$ where d and D are the diameters of the orifice and the vessel respectively. In experiments of a more general kind (85) the critical Reynolds number increased with decreasing bore of the tube, which suggested that a relatively larger laminar sublayer had a more stabilizing effect in the smaller tubes. While usually the turbulence and its associated sounds are undesirable, detection of audio signals from chronically installed arteriovenous shunts has been suggested as a useful way of monitoring their patency (73). Finally, as an example of possible benefits of the vortex generations in arteries, the presence of the sinuses of Valsalva, with their trapped vortices during forward blood flow, was found to aid in the closure of the aortic valve (24). In a model with sinuses present, the valves closed with a reverse flow of 4% forward flow; without sinuses, the reverse flow amounted to 35% of the forward flow.

The special problems of flow in veins and other collapsible vessels have not received a great deal of attention although there is an excellent series of papers from a symposium on the subject (152). An interesting series of model experiments and associated theoretical studies carried out on a hybrid computer has dealt with flow through a collapsible tube under variations of transmural pressure (107). A particularly interesting feature found in the experiment and reproduced by the theoretical model was the oscillation of pressure during the phase of decreasing resistance, that is, as the transmural pressure increased. It should be noted, however, that the ends of the vessel in these experiments were held open by the rigid mounting; due caution would have to be observed before drawing immediate anatomical parallels.

Arterial Elasticity

Comprehensive reviews of arterial elasticity have recently appeared (29, 61). The pulsatile events of the cardiovascular system, including the heart, are largely determined by the elastic properties of the arterial walls because of the effect of these properties on impedance and on wave propagation. It is probably not going too far to claim that we can understand most of the pulsatile phenomena in the arterial system on the basis of current knowledge of the elastic properties of arteries. There is, however, the inverse problem—to find ways of evaluating pulsatile or oscillatory events within the cardiovascular system, either naturally occurring or artificially imposed, so as to derive diagnostic information about the elastic properties of the vessels. In view of the pathological changes which arteries may undergo, these attempts are very understandable, but the problem cannot yet by any means be regarded as solved.

Large deformations.—Because of the large variations in operating pressure which may occur in the arteries, it is desirable to have some way of following their elastic behavior over the full range of their diameters. The classically defined Young's modulus of the arterial wall is well known to increase with increasing diameter; measuring it and defining it in the usual way, for small increments in the pressure and diameter, requires that the changes in elastic modulus with larger changes in diameter be expressed by some empirically determined function. The theory of large deformations of elastic bodies, which employs the so-called strain-energy function, permits material such as arterial wall to be characterized over its whole working range (93). Experimental studies of biaxial deformation of various sheets of tissue such as mesentery, pleura, pericardium, etc. (87, 88), have been found to apply also to the analysis of arterial elasticity (194), where in states of biaxial stress, a significant tangential stress gradient may be present in the walls of arteries, and may be a significant force acting on the vasa vasorum. Experiments on the elastic symmetry of arterial segments (160) have shown, however, that in the normally extended state of arteries in vivo, the torsion generated in the wall by changing intravascular pressure is very small and would have little influence on intramural blood vessels or the orifices of vasa vasorum.

Viscoelastic properties of arteries.—The measurement of viscoelastic properties of the arteries is usually made by finding the modulus and phase relations between sinusoidal variations in pressure and diameter, or in force and length, of isolated specimens. Determination of the dynamic elastic modulus in vivo requires very careful attention to the calibration of the manometer, and the application of sensitive but nonloading procedures for the recording of diameter. (The dynamic elastic modulus is frequently written in complex form as $E_{dyn} = E^1 + i\eta\omega$, where E^1 is the real part, η is a viscosity term, and $\omega = 2\pi f$ where f is the frequency.) When the pressure-diameter relations were subsequently resolved into Fourier series for the determination of elastic moduli, frequency by frequency, it was shown (75) that the nonlinear elastic properties of the artery may introduce small but troublesome harmonic distortions and, by leading to errors in phase angle determination, severely distort the measurement of the viscous term in the dynamic elastic constant. There appears now to be general agreement that the phase angle of the complex elastic modulus, except over very low frequency ranges, is almost constant (of the order of 0.1 radians) so that the viscous parameter η decreases with increasing frequency. Measurement of the dynamic elastic properties of the aorta in the radial direction (162) showed, on the other hand, an apparently constant value for η. In one study of the elastic properties of rings of tissue from the aorta, "resonance" at about 10 Hz was reported (10), but this had not been seen in animal experiments (19, 75) or in other experiments (81) on isolated rings of arterial wall, so the original suggestion that this may have been due to an artifact is therefore probably correct.

In a subsequent section the influence of vascular smooth muscle on the static elastic modulus will be discussed. With regard to the internal viscosity of arterial wall, it has been found (81) that the elastic modulus of the carotid and mesenteric arteries of the cow is proportional to the tension regardless of whether this results from stretching the vessel or from inducing a tonic contraction of the muscle within it. The viscosity term was almost constant in the range of Young's modulus 1–2.5 × 10^6 dynes/cm^2 but decreased below this range. Studies of the dynamic behavior of elastomers (139) have shown that at a given frequency the viscous term η was constant up to elongations of about 1.7, after which it slightly decreased, while the dynamic modulus itself rapidly increased at the greater elongations.

Measurements have been made of the elastic properties of peripheral arteries, in particular the common carotid and coronary arteries. Observations with an ultrasonic device in conscious subjects (14) indicated the elastic modulus of the common carotid artery to be only about one tenth that found in excised specimens and the pulse wave velocity to be quite low (4.6 m/sec). A somewhat similar difference between the elastic properties in exposed and unexposed vessels was found for the pressure-diameter relations of the cat's aorta, determined radiographically (15). Again, no clear reason could be found for the difference between properties of the exposed and unexposed vessels. Such discrepancies were not always observed; results obtained by means of an intravascular diameter-measuring device (19) agreed quite well with those obtained by an extravascular caliper. Surgical exposure of an artery may lead to departures from its physiological state, but excision of the specimen (123) does not in itself seem to change the elastic properties; in many instances the pulse wave velocities determined from arterial pressure records agreed well with elastic constants determined subsequently on excised specimens. A similar difference between elastic properties of exposed and unexposed arteries may underly the results reported for volume-elasticity of the coronary arteries; these were 1.2 × 10^6 dynes/cm^5 for the unexposed artery (125) and 3.4 × 10^6 dynes/cm^5 for the exposed artery (161).

The role of vascular smooth muscle.—The general physiology of vascular smooth muscle has been well reviewed (195), and although it has been suggested that smooth muscle cells may have several other functions in the arterial wall (220), there is no doubt that their activity may change the elastic properties of blood vessels (81). The effect of the muscle upon the Young's modulus of the vessel wall depends upon the orientation of the fibers with respect to the direction in which the modulus is being determined (18, 209, 210): strips cut at various angles to the transverse axis of the vena cava were influenced to a greater or lesser extent by norepinephrine depending on whether the muscle fibers were orientated along or across the strip. In general, it appears that for vessels in situ their longitudinal tension is borne by elastic rather than by muscular tissue; this applies as much to a relatively "untethered" artery such as the carotid artery (48) as it does to "tethered" vessels such as the vena cava and the aorta of the rabbit (168). Even the larger peripheral arteries are capable of quite substantial changes in diameter and in elastic properties, as a consequence of reflex or local influences, and show increased Young's modulus at larger diameters (65, 74, 97, 127). These variations in diameter are insignificant in the regulation of flow, since the resistance of these vessels is relatively small. Observations of the aortic pressure-diameter relations in intact dogs have revealed that even here the elastic properties may be varied, presumably by reflex mechanisms (150, 165). These changes may be significant in relation to the impedance matching in the arterial system (165).

Pathological changes in the arterial wall.—The very interesting question of poststenotic dilatation of arteries has been further investigated. The application of random vibrations to isolated segments of arteries (55) sometimes showed resonance at frequencies around 115 and 300 Hz; these same frequencies were prominent when flow was induced through a stenosis in that artery. On the other hand (30), although the application of frequencies between 30 and 400 Hz to isolated perfused human iliac arteries caused dilatation, the critical frequencies for this appeared to vary from artery to artery, and there was no evidence of "resonance." The dilatation was presumed to be due to damage to the elastic network, but no histological change could be demonstrated. Whatever this damage may be, it is apparently reversible (176), since in experiments in dogs where the artery could be visualized by X ray, it returned to normal diameter in 6–8 hours after removal of the stenosis and disappearance of the murmur. It was suggested that this must be due to some change in elastin associated with fatigue under vibration, since the time was too short for any new elastin to have formed.

The important question of the relation between intravascular pressures and flows and the development of atherosclerosis still yields some difference of opinion. On the one hand, experiments (59, 60) have shown that if the wall stress in an artery is sufficiently great (about 400 dynes/cm²) the endothelial cells may yield, and that with increasing wall stress there are progressive changes in permeability of the intima. These changes manifest themselves first as an increased permeability to Evans Blue dye and the appearance of abnormal endothelial cells; next as the loss of normal cells and a somewhat higher ingress of dye; and finally as the loss of endothelial tissue altogether, the deposition of fibrin and fat, and a still greater permeability to Evans Blue. The critical yield stress for endothelium was independent of the duration of its application; for erosion to occur, higher values of stress were required (500–1500 dynes/cm²) but the effects varied with its duration. In these areas in the vascular system where high wall stresses are generated, one may thus expect endothelial damage and consequently an increased risk of atherosclerotic disease.

In a theoretical study of the flow associated with a plaque projecting into the stream in an artery, it was calculated that maximum stress would occur at the upstream end of the plaque (170). On the other hand, vibratory stresses associated with a turbulent flow downstream of an artificial stenosis did not influence the extent or the intensity of atheroma in cholesterol-fed rabbits (4). In these experiments the poststenotic dilatation was not influenced by cholesterol feeding.

A rather different view of this problem was taken in a theoretical study of the effect of arterial wall shear on the transfer of materials such as cholesterol (39). The cholesterol which is synthesized in the arterial wall may accumulate in regions of low mean shear because it cannot diffuse as readily into the blood as it can from regions of higher shear.

The resolution of this conflict must await further experimental work. However, one may observe that the applicability of the shear-dependent mass-transfer model is contingent on first, mass-transfer dependence upon the mean rate of shear, and second, the assumption that permeability of the vascular wall is constant in all situations. As previous work (59, 60) has shown, the endothelium is sensitive to the maximum wall stress, and therefore one might expect its permeability to be affected in regions where peak wall stress was high, even though, in the same regions, the average wall stress was low—namely in the aorta. Since maximum wall stress depends on the pulsatile flow patterns, the relationship between amplitude of flow oscillation and peak wall stress will depend upon the velocity profile and hence on Womersley's parameter α. [α equals $R (2 \pi f/v)^{\frac{1}{2}}$, where R is the vessel radius, f is the frequency of oscillation, and v is the kinematic viscosity of fluid.] For any given amplitude of flow, the wall stress becomes less as α decreases; this occurs with progressive divisions of the arterial system.

Elastic properties of pulmonary artery.—In the general treatment of the elastic deformation of orthotropic vessels (140, 141) and in particular that of the pulmonary artery, the changes in cross section and perimeter of noncircular vessels under increasing distension have been studied both theoretically and in latex models. A quite satisfactory agreement was observed between theory and experiment. It was also found that the elastic behavior of the pulmonary artery, which is noncircular in its unstressed state, is profoundly influenced by its attachments and tethering; in particular, removal of the pericardium seems to free the artery from its constraints.

Measurements in the pulmonary artery in dogs and in humans have shown that its distensibility decreases with increasing distending pressure (98, 172, 174). Also, with increasing age the distensibility of the human pulmonary artery decreases, although its initial volume, at a low distending pressure of 2 mm Hg, increases (114). In these characteristics, the pulmonary artery thus appears to be quite similar to the aorta.

Elastic properties of baroreceptor regions.—The volume distensibility of the carotid sinus region when fixed in situ in dogs, cats, and rabbits (206) was found to be about the same as that of the aorta at low distending pressures, but was greater at higher pressures than that of other arteries of elastic type. Electronmicroscopic studies of the carotid sinus region (171) showed rather sparse collagen in its wall, but chemical analysis (21) has shown that the collagen-elastin ratio was not substantially different from that found in the common or internal carotid artery. It was concluded from these studies that "the dilatation of the internal carotid artery in the development of carotid sinus is more important than the modification of the tunica media." Studies of the elastic properties of aortic strips from hypertensive rabbits suggest that the "resetting" of the aortic baroreceptor system may be due to the increased stiffness of the aortic wall which can be demonstrated 3 to 15 days after onset of hypertension (1–3).

Wave Velocity and Arterial Impedance

The problem of wave transmission in an elastic system such as that of the arteries continues to attract attention, and a number of studies have been made. My own view is that these analyses of wave motion have now been carried to a point where it seems unlikely that further refinement will provide added physiological insight. But this is not to diminish the importance of the inverse problem, alluded to earlier, of obtaining, by measurements of transmission or other characteristics of arterial wave motion, information concerning the state of the arterial wall, particularly in disease.

The wave equation.—Womersley's treatment of the propagation of pressure disturbances in the elastic tube, though not the first, has been the starting point for much recent work (221). His basic model was of the propagation of oscillations in a thin walled, perfectly elastic circular tube filled with a viscous fluid. As a model of the situation in arteries, this has some obvious limitations. First, the arteries are generally not free to move very much longitudinally; second, their elastic properties may not be isotropic; third, the wall is viscoelastic; and finally, there may be special effects due to non-Newtonian behavior of the blood. Although Womersley carried out some analysis of the influence of a viscoelastic wall on wave propagation, his more important result was the remarkable simplification made by taking into account the constraints on longitudinal motion—the so-called "tethered-tube" model (222).

Womersley did not pursue the behavior of modes of vibration other than the radial mode. Recent work has extended the study of propagated disturbances to include the effects of finite wall thickness, viscoelastic wall material, various forms of tethering or loading by peripheral attachment to surrounding tissues, and modes of oscillations other than radial. The radial mode of oscillation which Womersley investigated has a lower wave velocity than the axial mode, and indeed the axial and circumferential modes may exhibit cutoff frequencies below which they are not transmitted (138). The influence of viscoelasticity in the wall, upon both radial and axial modes of oscillation, has also been studied (41, 100, 101), and, while at the frequencies employed in these experiments (40–130 Hz) the presence of viscoelasticity in the wall has little effect on the wave velocity of either, both were substantially attenuated by it, and their transmission per wavelength decreased. It is certainly the case that the attenuation of oscillations travelling in arteries cannot be ascribed solely to the effects of the viscosity of the blood; in fact, the viscous losses in the wall are more significant. However, it has been found both theoretically and experimentally (16, 100, 101) that distributed external constraint of an elastic vessel greatly increases the influence of fluid viscosity on the attenuation of axial waves. The suggestion has been made that this may be why such waves are not detected in arteries under natural conditions.

When it is desired to take into account the nonlinear characteristics of fluid motion in elastic tubes, resulting from either large excursions or variations of properties from point to point, the method of characteristics has proved most convenient. It has been used to compute pulsatile wave propagation in branching tubes (36) and to analyze pressure and flow pulses in the aorta (7, 8). In these latter studies, the elastic and diameter variations of the aorta along its course were prescribed, and allowances made for the variable amount of outflow from the aorta at each point along it. The realism of this latter feature is questionable, since the aorta is not just a tube of variable porosity but possesses branches from which reflections return to influence the course of intra-aortic pressure. While it is true that the wave velocities and dimensions of the arterial system are such that for travelling oscillations its nonuniform elastic properties do result in a substantial uncoupling of the peripheral resistance from the input, it is very unsafe to neglect (186) reflections which arise from its terminations.

The objection is sometimes raised that the inherently nonlinear nature of the equations governing pressure and flow in the arterial system makes linear methods such as Fourier analysis inapplicable. There are indeed situations where nonlinear effects disturb linear methods of analysis (75), but it seems that for most purposes a linear model works very well. When the arterial system of a dog was perfused by two pumps operating at different frequencies (46), spectral analysis of the arterial wave form showed that less than 2% of the total oscillatory pressure energy appeared at intermodulation frequencies. Encouraging agreement between experimental results and calculations based on linear models has also been obtained (42): flow computed on the basis of differential pressure measurements in the femoral artery of the dog agreed well with that recorded by the electromagnetic flowmeter.

Wave velocity in the arterial system may be measured either by timing the passage of an identifiable signal over a known distance (6) or by determining the phase shift of a propagated oscillation. By applying the first method, pulse wave velocities were obtained in the various parts of the arterial tree of the dog (134) and confirmed the general increase from low values (4.1–4.7 m/sec) in the thoracic aorta to high values (8.3–10.3 m/sec) in the femoral artery. When phase differences are used, however, the matter is complicated by reflected components; the value obtained will then not be the true phase velocity, but the so-called "apparent phase velocity." This varies in a complex way, depending on the phase relations between the incident and reflected components at the site of measurement. By use of additional measurements (flow and diameter), the effect of reflections can be eliminated and "true" phase velocities estimated; values found by this means (43) for phase velocities in the femoral artery of the dog agreed well, at comparable blood pressures, with those quoted above. An attractive three-dimensional display of pressure vs time vs distance along the aorta has also been published (155). While the measurement of arterial pulse wave velocity is relatively commonplace, it is interesting to note that pulse wave velocity in veins has also been recorded. In the inferior vena cava and arm veins of man (151) the velocities were 1.15 and 2.05 m/sec, while for high frequency oscillations in the inferior vena cava of the dog (9) the velocity was between 1 and 3.5 m/sec. The damping in this instance was considered to be due almost entirely to the viscoelastic properties of the wall of the vena cava.

Arterial impedance.—Earlier work has been summarized by Bergel & Schultz (29); there appears to be very satisfactory agreement among the impedance patterns reported by numerous workers for different vascular beds. The characteristic feature of arterial impedance patterns as a function of increasing frequency is the very marked fall of the modulus from the steady-flow or "DC" resistance value to a minimum, after which it may rise again and show small oscillations but never regains its DC value. The phase angle of arterial impedance is initially negative at low frequencies, passes through zero at the minimum value of the modulus, and then usually remains positive or oscillates around zero. The explanation of this form rests on the combined effect of the elastic nonuniformity in the system and the interference and cancellation of reflected waves from scattered terminations, when the distances involved become appreciable fractions of a wavelength. It has been shown that in some senses such a system can provide an optimum solution to the problem of minimizing the pulsatile cardiac work while at the same time minimizing the overall distensibility of the arterial system (204).

The transformations of pressure and flow pulses which are associated with the impedance patterns of the vascular system have been extensively studied in man (144). This has been done with particular reference to the changes associated with cardiovascular abnormalities (156, 157) such as coarctation of the aorta, in which the altered reflection conditions lead not only to marked changes in the aortic pressures and flow patterns, but also to changes in aortic input impedance with associated increases in the ratio of pulsatile to total external cardiac work.

Among the special features of the pulmonary circulation is the fact that capillary flow is pulsatile (104, 105), and it is interesting that even though the pulmonary vascular bed is much shorter than the corresponding systemic one, the lower wave velocity in the pulmonary arteries (1.7 m/sec in normal man) (145) so scales the impedance pattern that once again the right ventricle is presented with optimum relations. The influence of the many scattered terminations of the pulmonary arterial tree may be of particular significance in this organ (166).

Input impedance of particular vascular beds.—If the properties of a vascular bed can be characterized in terms of a model composed of capacitors and resistors, the input-output relations studied as a function of frequency can be used to evaluate the constants of the model (183), or an adaptive analog system can be used to vary the constants of the model until its behavior matches that of an animal experiment (178).

The impedance presented by the coronary artery (109, 110) is complicated by the periodic systolic obstruction of the outflow. This makes the impedance negative at some frequencies so that the vascular bed behaves as though it contains an amplifier. Some anomalies have also been reported in the low frequency behavior of the input impedance of the kidney (23, 111). Pressure was found to lead flow at very low frequencies (0.001 Hz) but to be in phase again at 0.01 Hz; at 0.02 Hz, pressure once more led flow, and after this the phase angle decreased with further increase in frequency. Such changes in phase angle were not seen in the impedances of the mesenteric bed or of the dog's forelimb. These anomalies appear to be due to autoregulatory responses of vascular smooth muscle (22) which are abolished by papaverine.

THE USE OF INDICATOR DILUTION METHODS

The indicator dilution technique is extensively used in the measurement of both regional and total systemic blood flow. In a system in which there is no recirculation and no loss or generation of indicator in passage through it, integration of the washout concentration curve, no matter what its form, will give a measure of the flow through the system. In the actual situation, however, recirculation of dye or indicator almost always occurs before the washout concentration has reached negligible values. Many attempts have therefore been made to devise procedures which will characterize the initial undisturbed portions of the washout curve, so that its extrapolation may be accurately made, even though in its later extent recirculation distorts it. A very comprehensive survey has been given of 25 simplified or automated methods currently employed (196). These depend in various ways on the assumptions about the nature of the underlying process, and their success or failure depends on the degree to which the model in fact matches the important features of the real situation (84). In view of the complexity of a vascular bed, it is surprising and gratifying that the assumption of exponential washout appears so satisfactory and permits the relatively simple extrapolation of the indicator dilution curve.

One apparently successful method which correlates well with the ordinary method assumes a gamma distribution function for the primary washout curve, evaluates the three constants of the distribution function from the early part of the washout curve, and thus enables the immediate calculation of its integral either from tables (198) or by computer (197, 227). One model of the process supposes successive mixing chambers (190); another assumes that the flow within and through the vascular bed resembles a random walk diffusion process (153). In one model of blood flow through the kidney, the distribution was taken to have one fast and one slow component, both being log-normal. The constants in this expression required an iterative computer program for their evaluation (203). A convection-diffusion model (164) has also been found appropriate for describing the transport of a diffusible material through the kidney, where there may be effectively an extravascular bypass.

In addition to their use in the measurement of flow, indicator dilution techniques may also provide information on the circulatory processes in the region through which flow is occurring. If the time course of dye concentration in blood entering and leaving an organ is recorded, then by taking Fourier or Laplace transforms of input and output dye curves, one may obtain a transfer function (40) or a frequency function of transit times such as has been found for the pulmonary circulation (113, 136). These latter investigations led to the hypothesis that the lung behaves as a parallel pathway system which becomes relatively more uniform and less dispersive as the rate of flow increases. Because it appears that the frequency function for distribution times through the pulmonary circulation is skewed, calculations based on extrapolation of a monoexponential function can be misleading, particularly if the recirculation of indicator appears at concentrations of 20% of the peak or greater. Where recirculation occurs, the primary dilution curve must be regarded as truncated, and thus only a part of it is available for the evaluation of parameters of models. It has been suggested that the Z transform (149) is more satisfactory than the Laplace or Fourier transforms; however, if parameters are to be fitted by least squares, some results (112) suggest that this is best done in the frequency domain rather than in the time domain since the transforms are often simpler functions with which to deal.

Technical problems with the indicator dilution method.—The use of indicator-dilution techniques to measure ventricular volume requires a high response speed in the sampling system. An analog system has been described (70) which compensates for the distortion in the recording introduced by the sampling catheter. Despite its use over many years, questions have recently arisen about the stability of indocyanine green solutions. It has been found, for instance, that the dye method consistently overestimated flow when compared with the electromagnetic flowmeter (90, 184); this was ascribed to a difference in the absorption spectrum at different concentrations. Also a slow change on dilution was found, and it was recommended that to avoid these difficulties the appearance time of the dye should not be less than 6 sec. Under some conditions the dye appeared to undergo metachromasia (193); initially the solution appeared less dense at high concentrations, but the opacity then increased gradually over approximately 5 hr. The departure from Beer's law was greater with plasma, but the variation with time was less. Indocyanine green in triple distilled water was stable in darkness but not in direct light (64). It was, however, very stable in 2–4% protein solution. For accurate work, therefore, considerable care must be exercised in the handling of solutions and samples containing this indicator. A method which avoids drawing samples through an external densitometer employs fiberoptics and makes the measurement intravascularly (95).

Thermal dilution.—The thermal dilution technique by which a small volume of fluid, either iced or at room temperature, is injected, usually into the right atrium, remains popular. The temperature of the injectate is measured by a thermistor as it leaves the catheter, and the blood temperature downstream, usually in the pulmonary artery or in the aorta, is measured subsequently. The flow, computed then by any of the standard techniques, has been found to compare favorably both with the indocyanine green dilution technique (63, 215) and with the electromagnetic flowmeter (182). Errors may be introduced, however, by changes in blood temperature due to changes in respiratory activity, or by placing the probe too close to the arterial wall. The recommended method (215) is to inject into the right atrium and sample in the pulmonary artery. It was shown that sufficient mixing of the indicator occurs over this pathway (208); thermal dilution curves in right and left pulmonary arteries were identical. The oscillatory nature of the flow does not appear to invalidate the use of this method (130), provided that the time constant of the temperature recording system is fast compared with the apparent time constant of mixing, i.e., the volume divided by the flow rate through the region. The presence of oscillatory flow causes variations in the apparent volume of the mixing chamber, but flow through it can be measured accurately.

Other methods of determining cardiac output.—Diethyl and dimethyl ether dissolved in saline have recently been used for the determination of cardiac output. The ether is infused at a constant rate and the alveolar tension estimated by a rebreathing method (20). Values obtained were within 6% of those obtained by the direct Fick method using oxygen. The advantage of the method is that since there is a continuous infusion of the indicator, the cardiac output can be determined continuously and directly from the downstream concentration. The starting up of the process can be accelerated by augmenting the continuous injection with an initial bolus of indicator (33).

A method which employs rapid gas analysis (N_2 and CO_2) of a single slow exhaled breath (69) was found to correlate well with values obtained by the indicator dilution technique. This method has the advantage of quick measurement, but the subsequent calculations are complex and require a computer. The use of ultrasound to measure variations in the diameter of the ventricular cavity gave estimates of cardiac output which correlated well with values obtained by the indicator dilution technique (167). The method was employed in a group of patients with myocardial infarction, but in about a third of them the ultrasonic echograms were not satisfactory.

LITERATURE CITED

1. Aars, H. 1968. Static load-length characteristics of aortic strips from hypertensive rabbits. *Acta Physiol. Scand.* 73:101–10
2. Aars, H. 1969. Relationship between blood pressure and diameter of ascending aorta in normal and hypertensive rabbits. *Acta Physiol. Scand.* 75:397–405
3. Aars, H. 1969. Relationship between aortic diameter and aortic baroreceptor activity in normal and hypertensive rabbits. *Acta Physiol. Scand.* 75:406–14
4. Aars, H., Solberg, L. A. 1971. Effect of turbulence on the development of aortic atherosclerosis. *Atherosclerosis* 13:283–87
5. Abel, F. L. 1971. Fourier analysis of left ventricular performance. Evaluation of impedance matching. *Circ. Res.* 28:119–35
6. Anliker, M., Histand, M. B. 1968. Dispersion and attenuation of small artificial pressure waves in the canine aorta. *Circ. Res.* 23:539–51
7. Anliker, M., Rockwell, R. L., Ogden, E. 1971. Nonlinear analysis of flow pulses and shock waves in arteries. Part I: derivation and properties of mathematical model. *Z. angew. Math. Phys.* 22:217–46
8. Anliker, M., Rockwell, R. L., Ogden, E. 1971. Nonlinear analysis of flow pulses and shock waves in arteries. Part II: parametric study related to clinical problems. *Z. angew. Math. Phys.* 22:563–81
9. Anliker, M., Yates, W. G., Ogden, E. 1971. Transmission of small pressure waves in the canine vena cava. *Am. J. Physiol.* 221:644–51
10. Apter, J. T., Marquez, E. 1968. of sinusoidal forcings at low and at resonant frequencies. Correlation of visco-elastic properties of large arteries with microscopic structure. V. Effects *Cir. Res.* 22:393–404
11. Armour, J. A., Randall, W. C. 1970. Structural basis for cardiac function. *Am. J. Physiol.* 218:1517–23
12. Armour, J. A., Randall, W. C. 1971. Canine left ventricular intramyocardial pressures. *Am. J. Physiol.* 220:1833–39.
13. Armour, J. A., Pace, J. B., Randall, W. C. 1970. Interrelationship of architecture and function of the right ventircle. *Am. J. Physiol.* 218:174–79
14. Arndt, J. O., Klauske, J., Mersch, F. 1968. The diameter of the intact carotid artery in man and its change with pulse pressure. *Pfluegers Arch.* 301:230–40
15. Arndt, J. O., Stegall, H. F., Wicke, H. J. 1971. Mechanics of the aorta in vivo. A radiographic approach. *Circ. Res.* 28:693–704
16. Atabek, H. B. 1968. Wave propagation through a viscous fluid contained in a tethered, initially stressed, orthotropic elastic tube. *Biophys. J.* 8:626–49
17. Attinger, E. O. 1968. Analysis of pulsatile blood flow. *Advances in Biomedical Engineering and Medical Physics*, ed. S. N. Levine, 1–59. New York: Interscience
18. Attinger, F. M. L. 1968. Two-dimensional in-vitro studies of femoral arterial walls of the dog. *Circ. Res.* 22:829–40
19. Baan, J., Iwazumi, T., Szidon, J. P., Noordergraaf, A. 1971. Intravascular area transducer

measuring dynamic local distensibility of the aorta. *J. Appl. Physiol.* 31:499–503

20. Bachofen, H., Bloom, D. A., Farhi, L. E. 1971. Determination of cardiac output by ether dilution. *J. Appl. Physiol.* 30:131–35

21. Bagshaw, R. J., Fischer, G. M. 1971. Morphology of the carotid sinus in the dog. *J. Appl. Physiol.* 31:198–202

22. Basar, E., Weiss, C. 1968. Analyse des Frequenzganges druckinduzierter Änderungen des Strömungswiderstandes isolierter Rattennieren. *Pfluegers Arch.* 304:121–35

23. Basar, E., Ruedas, G., Schwarzkopf, H. J., Weiss, C. 1968. Untersuchungen des zeitlichen Verhaltens druckabhängiger Änderungen des Strömungswiderstandes im Coronargefässsystem des Rattenherzen. *Pfluegers Arch.* 304:189–202

24. Bellhouse, B. J., Bellhouse, F. H. 1968. Mechanism of closure of the aortic valve. *Nature* 217:86–87

25. Bellhouse, B. J., Bellhouse, F. H., Gunning, A. J. 1969. A straight needle-probe for the measurement of blood velocity. *J. Sci. Instrum. (Ser. 2)* 2:936–38

26. Benchimol, A., Stegall, H. F., Gartlan, J. L. 1971. New method to measure phasic coronary blood velocity in man. *Am. Heart J.* 81:93–101

27. Benchimol, A., Stegall, H. F., Maroko, P. R., Gartlan, J. L., Brener, L. 1969. Aortic flow velocity in man during cardiac arrhythmias measured with the Doppler catheter-flowmeter system. *Am. Heart J.* 78:649–59

28. Bergel, D. H., Ed. 1973. *Handbook of Cardiovascular Fluid Dynamics.* London: Academic. In press

29. Bergel, D. H., Schultz, D. L. 1971. Arterial elasticity and fluid dynamics. *Progr. Biophys. Mol. Biol.* 22:3–36

30. Boughner, D. R., Roach, M. R. 1971. Effect of low frequency vibration on the arterial wall. *Circ. Res.* 29:136–44

31. Bove, A. A., Lynch, P. R. 1970. Measurement of canine left ventricular performance by cineradiography of the heart. *J. Appl. Physiol.* 29:877–83

32. Brandi, G., McGregor, M. 1969. Intramural pressure in the left ventricle of the dog. *Cardiovasc. Res.* 3:472–75

33. Brody, A. W., Connolly, T. C., Lyons, K. P., McGill, J. J., Johnson, J. R. 1971. Bolus-augmented continuous injection of indicators for cardiac output. *J. Appl. Physiol.* 31:117–24

34. Brooks, R. C., VandeLinde, V. D., Hammermeister, K. E., Warbasse, J. R. 1971. Digital filtering of left ventricular heart volume and calculation of aortic valve blood flow. *Comput. Biomed. Res.* 4:340–54

35. Burns, J. W., Covell, J. W., Moyers, R., Ross, J., Jr. 1971. Comparison of directly measured left ventricular wall stress and stress calculated from geometric reference figures. *Circ. Res.* 28:611–21

36. Campbell, J. L., Yang, T. 1969. Pulsatile flow behavior in elastic systems containing wave-reflection sites. *J. Basic Eng.* 91:95–102

37. Cappelen, C., Ed. 1968. *New Findings in Blood Flowmetry.* Oslo: Oslo Univ. Press

38. Carlsson, E. 1969. Experimental studies of ventricular mechanics in dogs using the tantalum-labeled heart. *Fed. Proc.* 28:1324–29

39. Caro, C. G., Fitz-Gerald, J. M., Schroter, R. C. 1971. Atheroma and arterial wall shear. Observation, correlation and proposal of a shear dependent mass transfer mechanism for atherogenesis. *Proc. Roy. Soc. London B.* 177:109–59

40. Coulam, C. M., Warner, H. R., Marshall, H. W., Bassingthwaite, J. B. 1967. A steady-state transfer function analysis of portions of the circulatory system using indicator dilution techniques. *Comput. Biomed. Res.* 1:124–38

41. Cox, R. H. 1968. Wave propagation through a Newtonian fluid contained within a thick-walled, viscoelastic tube. *Biophys. J.* 8:691–709

42. Cox, R. H. 1970. Blood flow and pressure propagation in the ca-

nine femoral artery. *J. Biomech.*
3:131–49

43. Cox, R. H. 1971. Determination of the true phase velocity of arterial pressure waves in vivo. *Circ. Res.* 29:407–18

44. Crowe, W. J., Krovetz, L. J. 1970. Analysis of three dimensional flow birefringence models, with a note on the effects of catheters and needles on vessel flow. *IEEE Trans. Bio-Med. Eng.* 17: 199–206

45. Dennis, J., Wyatt, D. G. 1969. Effect of haematocrit value upon electromagnetic flowmeter sensitivity. *Circ. Res.* 24:875–86

46. Dick, D. E., Kendrick, J. E., Matson, G. L., Rideout, V. C. 1968. Measurement of nonlinearity in the arterial system of the dog by a new method. *Circ. Res.* 22:101–11

47. Dieudonné, J.-M., 1969. The left ventricle as confocal prolate spheroids. *Bull. Math. Biophys.* 31:433–39

48. Dobrin, P. B., Doyle, J. M. 1970. Vascular smooth muscle and the anisotropy of dog carotid artery. *Circ. Res.* 27:105–19

49. Eckermann, P., Millahn, H. P., Bartsch, H.-J. 1969. Modelluntersuchungen über die Bedeuting der Abstimmung zwischen Herzfrequenz und Frequenz der arteriellen Grundschwingung. *Z. Kreislaufforsch.* 58:845–52

50. Fahrbach, K. 1969. Ein Beitrag zur Blutgeschwindigkeitsmessung unter Anwendung des Dopplereffektes. *Elektromedizin* 14:233–46

51. Falsetti, H. L., Mates, R. E., Grant, C., Greene, D. G., Bunnell, I. L. 1970. Left ventricular wall stress calculated from one-plane cineangiography. *Circ. Res.* 26:71–83

52. Flax, S. W., Webster, J. G., Updike, S. J. 1970. Statistical evaluation of the Doppler ultrasonic blood flowmeter. *Biomed. Sci. Instrum.* 7:201–22

53. Folts, J. D., Rowe, G. G. 1971. A nonerosive electromagnetic flowmeter probe for chronic aortic implantation. *J. Appl. Physiol.* 31:782–84

54. Foreman, J. E. K., Hutchison, K. J. 1970. Generation of sinusoidal fluid pressures of relatively high frequency. *J. Appl. Physiol.* 29:511–16

55. Foreman, J. E. K., Hutchison, K. J. 1970. Arterial wall vibration distal to stenoses in isolated arteries of dog and man. *Circ. Res.* 26:583–90

56. Forrester, J. H., Young, D. F. 1970. Flow through a converging-diverging tube and its implications in occlusive vascular disease. I. Theoretical development. *J. Biomech.* 3:297–305

57. Forrester, J. H., Young, D. F. 1970. Flow through a converging-diverging tube and its implications in occlusive vascular disease. II. Theoretical and experimental results and their implications. *J. Biomech.* 3:307–16

58. Frank, M. J., Cundey, P. E., Crews, T. L., Lewis, W. J. 1971. Comparison of left ventricular volumes by single-plane cineangiography and by indicator dilution. *J. Lab. Clin. Med.* 77:580–93

59. Fry, D. L. 1968. Acute vascular endothelial changes associated with increased blood velocity gradients. *Circ. Res.* 22:165–97

60. Fry, D. L. 1969. Certain histological and chemical responses of the vascular interface to acutely induced mechanical stress in the aorta of the dog. *Circ. Res.* 24: 93–108

61. Fung, Y. C. 1968. Biomechanics. *Appl. Mech. Rev.* 21:1–20

62. Gabe, I. T. et al 1969. Measurement of instantaneous blood flow velocity and pressure in conscious man with a catheter-tip velocity probe. *Circulation* 40:603–14

63. Ganz, W., Donoso, R., Marcus, H. S., Forrester, J. S., Swan, H. J. C. 1971. A new technique for measurement of cardiac output by thermodilution in man. *Am. J. Cardiol.* 27:392–96

64. Gathje, J., Steuer, R. R., Nicholes, K. R. K. 1970. Stability studies on indocyanine green dye. *J. Appl. Physiol.* 29:181–85

65. Gerová, M., Gero, J. 1967. Changes in size of a conduit vessel during baroreceptor stimulation. *Physiol. Bohemoslov.* 16: 297–304

66. Gessner, U. 1968. The performance of the ultrasonic flowmeter in complex velocity profiles. *IEEE Trans. Bio-Med. Eng.* 16: 139–42

67. Ghista, D. N., Vayo, H. W. 1969. The time varying elastic properties of the left ventricular muscle. *Bull. Math. Biophys.* 31: 75–92

68. Ghista, D. N., Advani, S. H., Gaonkar, G. H., Balachandran, K., Brady, A. J. 1971. Analysis and physiological monitoring of the human left ventricle. *J. Basic Eng.* 93: 147–61

69. Gilbert, R., Auchincloss, J. H., Jr. 1970. Comparison of single-breath and indicator-dilution measurement of cardiac output. *J. Appl. Physiol.* 29: 119–22

70. Glassman, E., Blesser, W., Mitzner, W. 1969. Correction of distortion in dye dilution curves due to sampling systems. *Cardiovasc. Res.* 3: 92–99

71. Goldstein, R. E., Epstein, S. E. 1970. Mechanism of elevated innominate artery pressures in supravalvular aortic stenosis. *Circulation* 42: 23–29

72. Goodman, A. H. 1968. Low-pass filters for electromagnetic flowmeters. *Med. Biol. Eng.* 6: 477–86

73. Gosling, R. G., King, D. H. 1969. Audio signals in arteriovenous shunts: use in flow monitoring and possible relevance to clotting. *J. Appl. Physiol.* 27: 106–11

74. Gow, B. S. 1970. Viscoelastic properties of conduit arteries. *Circ. Res.* 26: Suppl. II, 113–22

75. Gow, B. S., Taylor, M. G. 1968. Measurement of viscoelastic properties of arteries in the living dog. *Circ. Res.* 23: 111–22

76. Grant, R. P. 1965. Notes on the muscular architecture of the left ventricle. *Circulation* 32: 301–8

77. Greenfield, J. C., Starmer, C. F., Walston, A. 1971. Measurement of aortic blood flow in man by the computed pressure derivative method. *J. Appl. Physiol.* 31: 792–95

78. Gutstein, W. H., Farrell, G. A., Schneck, D. J. 1970. In vivo demonstration of junctional blood flow disturbance by hot wire anemometry. *Atherosclerosis* 11: 485–96

79. Gutstein, W. H., Schneck, D. J., Marks, J. O. 1968. In vitro studies of local blood flow disturbance in a region of separation. *Atherosclerosis* 8: 381–88

80. Hainsworth, R., Ledsome, J. R., Snow, H. M. 1968. Dynamic testing of electromagnetic flowmeters by mechanical and electronic methods. *J. Appl. Physiol.* 25: 469–72

81. Hardung, V. 1970. Dynamische Elastizität und innere Reibung muskulärer Blutgefässe bei verschiedener durch Dehnung und tonische Kontraktion hervorgerufener Wandspannung. *Arch. Kreislaufforsch.* 61: 83–100

82. Harris, J., Maheshwari, R. 1971. The measurement of amplitude and phase in oscillatory flow in a tube. *J. Sci. Instrum.* (*Ser. 2*) 4: 973–76

83. Harris, J., Peev, G., Wilkinson, W. L. 1969. Velocity profiles in laminar oscillatory flow in tubes. *J. Sci. Instrum.* 2: 913–16

84. Harris, T. R., Newman, E. V. 1970. An analysis of mathematical models of circulatory indicator-dilution curves. *J. Appl. Physiol.* 28: 840–50

85. Hershey, D., Gupta, B. P. 1968. The effect of tube diameter on the laminar regime transition for a non-newtonian suspension (blood). *Biorheology* 5: 313–21

86. Hewitt, R. L., Meistrell, M. L., Drapanas, T. 1971. Continuous determination of left ventricular volume by measurement of a single external dimension. *J. Appl. Physiol.* 30: 569–74

87. Hildebrandt, J., Fukaya, H., Martin, C. J. 1969. Simple uniaxial and uniform biaxial deformation of nearly isotropic incompressible tissues. *Biophys. J.* 9: 781–91

88. Hildebrandt, J., Fukaya, H., Martin, C. J. 1969. Stress-strain relations of tissue sheets undergoing uniform two-dimensional stretch. *J. Appl. Physiol.* 27: 758–62

89. Homer, L. D., Krayenbuehl, H. P. 1967. A mathematical model for the estimation of heart volumes from indicator dilution curves. *Circ. Res.* 20: 299–305

90. Homer, L. D., Moss, G. S., Herman, C. M. 1969. Errors in measurement of cardiac output with dye-dilution curves in shock. *J. Appl. Physiol.* 27: 101–03

91. Hood, W. P., Rackley, C. E., Rolett, E. L. 1968. Wall stress in the normal and hypertrophied human left ventricle. *Am. J. Cardiol.* 22:550–58

92. Hood, W. P., Thomson, W. J., Rackley, C. E., Rolett, E. L. 1969. Comparison of calculations of left ventricular wall stress in man from thin-walled and thick-walled ellipsoidal models. *Circ. Res.* 24:575–82

93. Hoppmann, W. H., Wan, L. 1970. Large deformations of elastic tubes. *J. Biomech.* 3:593–600

94. Huckaba, C. E., Hahn, A. W. 1968. A generalised approach to the modeling of arterial blood flow. *Bull. Math. Biophys.* 30: 645–62

95. Hugenholz, P. G., Wagner, H. R., Gamble, W. J., Polanyi, M. L. 1969. Direct read-out of cardiac output by means of the fiberoptic indicator dilution method. *Am. Heart J.* 77:178–86

96. Iberall, A. S. 1967. Anatomy and steady flow characteristics of the arterial system with an introduction to its pulsatile characteristics. *Math. Biosci.* 1: 375–95

97. Ingebrigtsen, R., Leraand, S. 1970. Dilatation of a medium-sized artery immediately after local changes of blood pressure and flow as measured by ultrasonic technique. *Acta Physiol. Scand.* 79:552–58

98. Jarmakani, J. M. M., Graham, T. P., Benson, D. W., Canent, R. V., Greenfield, J. C. 1971. In vivo pressure-radius relationships of the pulmonary artery in children with congenital heart disease. *Circulation* 43:585–92

99. Johnson, P. C. 1969. Hemodynamics. *Ann. Rev. Physiol.* 31:331–52

100. Jones, E., Anliker, M., Chang, I.-D. 1971. Effects of viscosity and constraints on the dispersion and dissipation of waves in large blood vessels. I. Theoretical analysis. *Biophys. J.* 11: 1085–1120

101. Jones, E., Anliker, M., Chang, I.-D. 1971. Effects of viscosity and constraints on the dispersion and dissipation of waves in large blood vessels. II. Comparison of analysis with experiments. *Biophys. J.* 11:1121–34

102. Kanai, H. 1969. The effects upon electromagnetic flowmeter-sensitivity of non-uniform fields and velocity profiles. *Med. Biol. Eng.* 7:661–76

103. Kanai, H., Iizuka, M., Sakamoto, K. 1970. One of the problems in the measurement of blood pressure by catheter insertion: Wave reflection at the tip of the catheter. *Med. Biol. Eng.* 8: 483–96

104. Karatzas, N. B., Phil, D., Lee, G. de J. 1969. Propagation of blood flow pulse in the normal human pulmonary arterial system. *Circ. Res.* 25:11–21

105. Karatzas, N. B., Noble, M. I., Saunders, K. B., McIlroy, M. B. 1970. Transmission of the blood flow pulse through the pulmonary arterial tree of the dog. *Circ. Res.* 27:1–9

106. Kardon, M. B., O'Rourke, R. A., Bishop, V. S. 1971. Measurement of left ventricular internal diameter by catheterisation. *J. Appl. Physiol.* 31:613–15

107. Katz, A. I., Chen, Y., Moreno, A. H. 1969. Flow through a collapsible tube. *Biophys. J.* 9: 1261–79

108. Kazamias, T. M., Gander, M. P., Franklin, D. L., Ross, J. 1971. Blood pressure measurement with Doppler ultrasonic flowmeter. *J. Appl. Physiol.* 30:585–88

109. Kenner, T. 1969. Der Eingangswiderstand der Koronararterien. *Arch. Kreislaufforsch.* 60: 215–20

110. Kenner, T. 1969. The dynamics of pulsatile flow in the coronary arteries. *Pfluegers Arch.* 310: 22–34

111. Kenner, T., Ono, K. 1971. The low frequency input impedance of the renal artery. *Pfluegers Arch.* 324:155–64

112. Kim, B. M., Harris, T. R. 1970. The identification of transport parameters from truncated physiological tracer curves. *Bull. Math. Biophys.* 32:355–75

113. Knopp, T. J., Bassingthwaite, J. B. 1969. Effect of flow on transpulmonary circulatory transport functions. *J. Appl. Physiol.* 27: 36–43

114. Kolb, P., Hägele, U. 1968. Die Volumen-Druck-Beziehung des extrapulmonalen Abschnittes der menschlichen Lungenschlagader und ihre Zuordnung zu Lebensalter, Körperlänge und Herzgewicht. *Z. Kreislaufforsch.* 57: 641–47

115. Kolin, A. 1968. A radial field electromagnetic intravascular flow sensor. *IEEE Trans. Bio-Med. Eng.* 16:220–21

116. Kolin, A. 1970. A new approach to electromagnetic blood flow determination by means of a catheter in an external magnetic field. *Proc. Nat. Acad. Sci. USA* 65:521–27

117. Kolin, A., Grollman, J. H., Steckel, R. J., Snow, H. D. 1970. Determination of arterial blood flow by percutaneously introduced flow sensors in an external magnetic field. I. The method. *Proc. Nat. Acad. Sci. USA* 67:1769–74

118. Kolin, A., Grollman, J. H., Steckel, R. J., Snow, H. D. 1971. Determination of arterial blood flow by percutaneously introduced flow sensors in an external magnetic field. II. Implementation of the method in vivo. *Proc. Nat. Acad. Sci. USA* 68:29–33

119. Kraemer, K. 1967. Der Druckabfall in einem laminar durchströmten regelmässig verzweigten Rohrleitungssystem mit Anwendung auf den Blutkreislauf des Menschen. *Arch. Kreislaufforsch.* 52:79–85

120. Kraunz, R. F., Ryan, T. J. 1971. Ultrasound measurements of ventricular wall motion following administration of vasoactive drugs. *Am. J. Cardiol.* 27:464–73

121. Kühn, P., Brachfeld, N. 1969. Zur Beeinflussung der Ventrikelmechanik durch den arteriellen Windkessel. *Z. Kreislaufforsch.* 58:233–43

122. Latimer, K. E., Latimer, R. D. 1969. Measurements of pressure-wave transmission in liquid-filled tubes used for intravascular blood pressure recording. *Med. Biol. Eng.* 7:143–68

123. Lee, J. S., Frasher, W. G., Fung, Y. C. 1968. Comparison of elasticity of an artery in vivo and in excision. *J. Appl. Physiol.* 25:799–801

124. Lew, H. S., Fung, Y. C. 1970. Entry flow into blood vessels at arbitrary Reynolds number. *J. Biomech.* 3:23–38

125. Lewi, P. J., Schaper, W. K. A. 1971. The estimation of coronary volume elasticity in the beating heart of the dog. *Pfluegers Arch.* 325:191–98

126. Leyton, R. A., Spotnitz, H. M., Sonnenblick, E. H. 1971. Cardiac ultrastructure and function: sarcomeres in the right ventricle. *Am. J. Physiol.* 221: 902–10

127. Lie, M., Sejersted, O. M., Kiil, F. 1970. Local regulation of vascular cross-section during changes in femoral arterial blood flow in dogs. *Circ. Res.* 27:727–37

128. Lindström, L. H. 1970. Miniaturised pressure transducer intended for intravascular work. *IEEE Trans. Bio-Med. Eng.* 17: 207–19

129. Ling, S. C., Atabek, H. B., Fry, D. L., Patel, D. J., Janicki, J. S. 1968. Application of heated-film velocity and shear probes to hemodynamic studies. *Circ. Res.* 23:789–801

130. Lowe, R. D. 1968. Use of a local indicator dilution technique for the measurement of oscillatory flow. *Circ. Res.* 22:49–56

131. Lynch, P. R., Bove, A. A. 1969. Geometry of the left ventricle as studied by a high-speed cinematographic technique. *Fed. Proc.* 28:1330–33

132. MacCanon, D. M., Bruce, D. W., Lynch, P. R., Nickerson, J. L. 1969. Mass excursion parameters of first heart sound energy. *J. Appl. Physiol.* 27:649–52

133. McDonald, D. A. 1960. *Blood Flow in Arteries.* London: Arnold. 328 pp.

134. McDonald, D. A. 1968. Regional pulse-wave velocity in the arterial tree. *J. Appl. Physiol.* 24: 73–78

135. Malindzak, G. S. 1970. Fourier analysis of cardiovascular

HEMODYNAMICS 113

events. *Math. Biosci.* 7:273–289
136. Maseri, A., Caldini, P., Permutt, S., Zierler, K. L. 1970. Frequency function of transit times through dog pulmonary circulation. *Circ. Res.* 26:527–43
137. Mason, D. T. et al 1970. Applications of the catheter-tip electromagnetic velocity probe in the study of the central circulation in man. *Am. J. Med.* 49:465–71
138. Maxwell, J. A., Anliker, M. 1968. The dissipation and dispersion of small waves in arteries and veins with viscoelastic wall properties. *Biophys. J.* 8:920–50
139. Meinecke, E. A. 1971. Dynamisches Verhalten von Elastomeren bei grossen Dehnungen überlagerten kleinen Schwingungen. *Rheol. Acta* 10:302–9
140. Melbin, J., Noordergraaf, A. 1971. Elastic deformation in orthotropic oval vessels: a mathematical model. *Bull. Math. Biophys.* 33:497–519
141. Melbin, J., Noordergraaf, A. 1971. Elastic deformation in orthotropic vessels. *Circ. Res.* 28:680–92
142. Melbin, J., Spohr, M. 1969. Evaluation and correction of manometer systems with two degrees of freedom. *J. Appl. Physiol.* 27:749–55
143. Messmer, K., Meisner, H., Pfau, B., Hagl, S. 1969. Modellanalyse eines Doppler-Ultraschallströmungsmessers. *Pfluegers Arch.* 308:80–90
144. Mills, C. J. et al 1970. Pressure-flow relationships and vascular impedance in man. *Cardiovasc. Res.* 4:405–17
145. Milnor, W. R., Conti, C. R., Lewis, K. B., O'Rourke, M. F. 1969. Pulmonary arterial pulse wave velocity and impedance in man. *Circ. Res.* 25:637–49
146. Mirsky, I. 1969. Left ventricular stresses in the intact human heart. *Biophys. J.* 9:189–208
147. Mirsky, I. 1970. Effects of anisotropy and nonhomogeneity on left ventricular stresses in the intact heart. *Bull. Math. Biophys.* 32:197–213
148. Mitchell, J. H., Wildenthal, K., Mullins, C. B. 1969. Geomet-

rical studies of the left ventricle using biplane cinefluorography. *Fed. Proc.* 28:1334–43
149. Neufeld, G. R. 1971. Computation of transit time distributions using sampled data Laplace transforms. *J. Appl. Physiol.* 31:148–53
150. Nicolosi, G. R., Pieper, H. P. 1971. Aortic smooth muscle responses to changes in venous return studied in intact dogs. *Am. J. Physiol.* 221:1209–16
151. Nippa, J. H., Alexander, R. H., Folse, R. 1971. Pulse wave velocity in human veins. *J. Appl. Physiol.* 30:558–63
152. Noordergraaf, A., Kresch, E., Eds. 1968. The venous system: characteristics and function, a biomedical engineering approach. *IEEE Trans. Bio-Med. Eng.* 16:233–338
153. Norwich, K. H., Zelin, S. 1970. Dispersion of indicator in the cardiopulmonary system. *Bull. Math. Biophys.* 32:25–43
154. Okai, O., Togawa, T., Oshima, M. 1971. Magnetorheography: nonbleeding measurement of blood flow. *J. Appl. Physiol.* 30:564–66
155. Olson, R. M. 1968. Aortic blood pressure and velocity as a function of time and position. *J. Appl. Physiol.* 24:563–69
156. O'Rourke, M. F. 1971. The arterial pulse in health and disease. *Am. Heart J.* 82:687–702
157. O'Rourke, M. F., Cartmill, T. B. 1971. Influence of aortic coarctation on pulsatile haemodynamics in the proximal aorta. *Circulation* 44:281–92
158. Päuser, H., Kenner, T. 1968. Untersuchungen zu Ph. Broemsers Abstimmungstheorie. *Z. Kreislaufforsch.* 57:1060–73
159. Paraskos, J. A., Grossman, W., Saltz, S., Dalen, J. E., Dexter, L. 1971. A noninvasive technique for the determination of velocity of circumferential fiber shortening in man. *Circ. Res.* 29:610–15
160. Patel, D. J., Fry, D. L. 1969. The elastic symmetry of arterial segments in dogs. *Circ. Res.* 24:1–8
161. Patel, D. J., Janicki, J. S. 1970. Static elastic properties of the left coronary circumflex artery and the common carotid artery

in dogs. *Circ. Res.* 27:149–158

162. Patel, D. J., Tucker, W. K., Janicki, J. S. 1970. Dynamic elastic properties of the aorta in radial direction. *J. Appl. Physiol.* 28: 578–82

163. Pech, H. J., Porstmann, W. 1968. Bestimmung des Schlagvolumens des linken Ventrikels durch Angiokardiographie. *Z. Kreislaufforsch.* 57:319–33

164. Perl, W., Chinard, F. P. 1968. A convection-diffusion model of indicator transport through an organ. *Circ. Res.* 22:273–98

165. Pieper, H. P., Paul, L. T. 1969. Responses of aortic smooth muscle studied in intact dogs. *Am. J. Physiol.* 217:154–60

166. Pollack, G. H., Reddy, R. V., Noordegraaf, A. 1968. Input impedance, wave travel, and reflections in the human pulmonary arterial tree: studies using an electrical analogue. *IEEE Trans. Bio-Med. Eng.* 15:151–64

167. Pombo, J. F., Russell, R. O., Rackley, C. E., Foster, G. L. 1971. Comparison of stroke volume and cardiac output determination by ultrasound and dye dilution in acute mycoardial infarction. *Am. J. Cardiol.* 27: 630–35

168. Pürschel, S., Reichel, H., Vonderlage, M. 1969. Vergleichende Untersuchungen zur statischen und dynamischen Wanddehnbarkeit von Vena cava und Aorta des Kaninchens. *Pfluegers Arch.* 306:232–46

169. Ramirez, A. et al 1969. Registration of intravascular pressure and sound by a fiberoptic catheter. *J. Appl. Physiol.* 26:679–83

170. Ray, G., Davids, N. 1970. Shear stress analysis of blood-endothelial surface in inlet section of artery with plugging. *J. Biomech.* 3:99–110

171. Rees, P. M. 1968. Electron microscopical observations on the architecture of the carotid arterial walls, with special reference to the sinus portion. *J. Anat.* 103: 35–47

172. Reuben, S. R. 1971. Compliance of the human pulmonary arterial system in disease. *Circ. Res.* 29:40–50

173. Reuben, S. R., Swadling, J. P., Lee, G. de J. 1970. Velocity profiles in the main pulmonary artery in dogs and man, measured with a thin-film resistance anemometer. *Circ. Res.* 27: 995–1001

174. Reuben, S. R., Gersh, B. J., Swadling, J. P., Lee, G. de J. 1970. Measurement of pulmonary arterial distensibility in the dog. *Cardiovasc. Res.* 4:473–81

175. Rittenhouse, E. A., Strandness, D. E., Jr. 1971. Oscillatory flow patterns in patients with aortic valve disease. *Am. J. Cardiol.* 28:568–74

176. Roach, M. R. 1970. Reversibility of poststenotic dilatation in the femoral arteries of dogs. *Circ. Res.* 27:985–93

177. Ross, J., Jr., Sonnenblick, E. H., Taylor, R. R., Spotnitz, H. M., Covell, J. W. 1971. Diastolic geometry and sarcomere lengths in the chronically dilated canine left ventricle. *Circ. Res.* 28:49–61

178. Rothe, C. F., Nash, F. D. 1968. Renal arterial compliance and conductance measurement using on-line self-adaptive analogue computation of model parameters. *Med. Biol. Eng.* 6:53–69

179. Sacks, A. H., Tickner, E. G., Macdonald, I. B. 1971. Criteria for the onset of vascular murmurs. *Circ. Res.* 29:249–56

180. Sallin, E. A. 1969. Fiber orientation and ejection fraction in the human left ventricle. *Biophys. J.* 9:954–64

181. Sandler, H., Dodge, H. T. 1968. The use of single plane angiocardiograms for the calculation of left ventricular volume in man. *Am. Heart J.* 75:325–34

182. Sanmarco, M. E., Philips, C. M., Marquez, L. A., Hall, C., Davila, J. C. 1971. Measurement of cardiac output by thermal dilution. *Am. J. Cardiol.* 28:54–58

183. Sato, T., Yamashiro, S. M., Grodins, F. S. 1971. Measurement of peripheral vascular properties by a frequency response method. *Am. J. Physiol.* 220: 1640–50

184. Saunders, K. B., Hoffman, J. I. E., Noble, M. I., Domenech, R. J. 1970. A source of error in measuring flow with indocyanine

green. *J. Appl. Physiol.* 28: 190–98

185. Schmid-Schönbein, H., Wells, R. E., Jr. 1971. Rheological properties of human erythrocytes and their influence upon the "anomalous" viscosity of human blood. *Ergeb. Physiol.* 63: 146–219

186. Schoenberg, M. 1968. Pulse wave propagation in elastic tubes having longitudinal changes in area and stiffness. *Biophys. J.* 8: 991–1008

187. Schultz, D. L., Tunstall-Pedoe, D. S., Lee, G. de J., Gunning, A. J., Bellhouse, B. J. 1969. Velocity distribution and transition in the arterial system. *Circulatory and Respiratory Mass Transport,* ed. G. E. W. Wolstenholme, J. Knight, 172–99. London: Churchill

188. Seed, W. A., Wood, N. B. 1970. Development and evaluation of a hot-film velocity probe for cardiovascular studies. *Cardiovasc. Res.* 4:253–63

189. Seed, W. A., Wood, N. B. 1970. Use of a hot-film velocity probe for cardiovascular studies. *J. Sci. Instrum. (Ser. 2)* 3:377–84

190. Sepibus, G. de, Fricke, G., Rutishauser, W. 1969. Wie entsteht die Primärkurve bei Indikatorverdünnung im Kreislaufsystem? *Arch. Kreislaufforsch.* 60: 240–61

191. Shapiro, G. G., Krovetz, L. J. 1970. Damped and undamped frequency responses of underdamped catheter manometer systems. *Am. Heart J.* 80:226–36

192. Shelton, C. D., Watson, B. W. 1968. A pressure generator for testing the frequency response of catheter/transducer systems used for physiological pressure measurements. *Phys. Med. Biol.* 13:523–28

193. Simmons, R., Shephard, R. J. 1971. Does indocyanine green obey Beer's Law? *J. Appl. Physiol.* 30:502–07

194. Simon, B. R., Kobayashi, A. S., Strandness, D. E., Wiederhielm, C. A. 1971. Large deformation analysis of the arterial cross section. *J. Basic Eng.* 93:138–46

195. Somlyo, A. P., Somlyo, A. V. 1968. Vascular smooth muscle. I. Normal structure, pathology, biochemistry, and biophysics. *Pharm. Rev.* 20:197–272

196. Spieckermann, J. G., Bretschneider, H. J. 1968. Vereinfachte quantitative Auswertung von Indikatorverdünnungskurven. *Arch Kreislaufforsch.* 55: 211–82

197. Starmer, C. F., Clark, D. O. 1970. Computer computations of cardiac output using the gamma function. *J. Appl. Physiol.* 28: 219–20

198. Steadham, R. E., Blackwell, L. H. 1970. A new method for the determination of the area under a cardiac output curve. *IEEE Trans. Bio-Med. Eng.* 17:335–38

199. Strandness, D. E., Kennedy, J. W., Judge, T. P., McLeod, F. D. 1969. Transcutaneous directional flow detection: a preliminary report. *Am. Heart J.* 78: 65–74

200. Streeter, D. D., Bassett, D. L. 1966. An engineering analysis of myocardial fiber orientation in pig's left ventricle in systole. *Anat. Rec.* 155:503–11

201. Streeter, D. D., Spotnitz, H. M., Patel, D. J., Ross, J., Sonnenblick, E. H. 1969. Fiber orientation in the canine left ventricle during diastole and systole. *Circ. Res.* 24:339–47

202. Streeter, D. D. et al 1970. Stress distribution in the canine left ventricle during diastole and systole. *Biophys. J.* 10:345–63

203. Takeuchi, J., et al 1970. Intrarenal distribution of blood flow in man. A new analytical method for dye-dilution curves. *Circulation* 42:347–60

204. Taylor, M. G. 1969. Arterial impedance and distensibility. *The Pulmonary Circulation and Interstitial Space,* ed. A. P. Fishman, H. H. Hecht, 341–52. Chicago: Chicago Univ. Press

205. Templeton, G. H., Mitchell, J. H., Ecker, R. R., Blomqvist, G. 1970. A method for measurement of dynamic compliance of the left ventricle in dogs. *J. Appl. Physiol.* 29:742–45

206. Tibes, U., Stegemann, J. 1969. Untersuchungen über die Dehnbarkeit der Carotissinuswand an

Hund, Katze und Kaninchen. *Pfluegers Arch.* 307:47–58

207. Vatner, S. F., Franklin, D. L., Van Citters, R. L. 1970. Simultaneous comparison and calibration of the Doppler and electromagnetic flowmeters. *J. Appl. Physiol.* 29:907–10

208. Vliers, A. C. A. P., Zijlstra, W. G. 1969. Zum Problem der Mischung von Indikator und Blut. *Z. Kreislaufforsch.* 58:79–88

209. Vonderlage, M. 1968. Untersuchungen über die mechanischen Eigenschaften von Streifenpräparaten verschiedener Schnittrichtung aus der Aorta abdominalis des Kaninchens. *Pfluegers Arch.* 301:320–28

210. Vonderlage, M. 1968. Untersuchungen über die mechanischen Eigenschaften von Streifenpräparaten verschiedener Schnittrichtung aus der Vena cava abdominalis des Kaninchens. *Pfluegers Arch.* 303:71–80

211. Voukydis, P. C. 1969. Physiological significance of the geometrical shape of the left ventricle: course and curvature of the individual myocardial fibres. *Bull. Math. Biophys.* 31:383–93

212. Voukydis, P. C. 1970. The effect of distension of the left ventricle of the heart on the length of the individual myocardial fibres. *Bull. Math. Biophys.* 32:45–58

213. Voukydis, P. C. 1970. The preload of individual myocardial fibres. *Bull. Math. Biophys.* 32: 323–35

214. Warbasse, J. R., Hellman, B. H., Gillilan, R. E., Hawley, R. R., Babitt, H. I. 1969. Physiologic evaluation of a catheter-tip electromagnetic velocity probe. *Am. J. Cardiol.* 23:424–33

215. Wessel, H. U., Paul, M. H., James, G. W., Grahn, A. R. 1971. Limitations of thermal dilution curves for cardiac output determinations. *J. Appl. Physiol.* 30:643–52

216. Wetterer, E., Kenner, T. 1968. *Grundlagen der Dynamik des Arterienpulses.* Berlin:Springer. 379 pp.

217. Wildenthal, K., Mitchell, J. H. 1969. Dimensional analysis of the left ventricle in unanaesthetised dogs. *J. Appl. Physiol.* 27: 115–19

218. Wildenthal, K., Mierzwiak, D. S., Mitchell, J. H. 1969. The influence of vagal stimulation on left ventricular end-diastolic distensibility. *Am. J. Physiol.* 217:1446–50

219. Wildenthal, K., Mullins, C. B., Harris, M. D., Mitchell, J. H. 1969. Left ventricular end-diastolic distensibility after norepinephrine and propranolol. *Am. J. Physiol.* 217:812–18

220. Wissler, R. W. 1968. The arterial medial cell, smooth muscle or multi-functional mesenchyme? *J. Atheroscler. Res.* 8:201–13

221. Womersley, J. R. 1955. Oscillatory motion of a viscous fluid in a thin-walled elastic tube. I. The linear approximation for long waves. *Phil. Mag.* 46:199–221

222. Womersley, J. R. 1957. Oscillatory flow in arteries: the constrained elastic tube as a model of arterial flow and pulse transmission. *Phys. Med. Biol.* 2: 178–87

223. Wong, A. Y. K. 1970. A concentric layer model for estimating the energy expenditure of the left ventricle. *Bull. Math. Biophys.* 32:581–98

224. Wong, A. Y. K., Rautaharju, P. M. 1968. Stress distribution within the left ventricular wall approximated as a thick ellipsoidal shell. *Am. Heart J.* 75:649–62

225. Wong, A. Y. K., Rautaharju, P. M. 1971. Relation of sarcomere lengths to filling pressures in normal and hypertrophied hearts. *Bull. Math. Biophys.* 33: 203–14

226. Wyatt, D. G. 1968. Dependence of electromagnetic flowmeter sensitivity upon encircled media. *Phys. Med. Biol.* 13:529–34

227. Yoder, R. D., Swan, E. A. 1971. Cardiac output: comparison of Stewart-Hamilton and gamma-function techniques. *J. Appl. Physiol.* 31:318–21

Ann. Rev. Physiol. 1973. 35:117–150

MICROCIRCULATION[1] 1091

B. W. ZWEIFACH

University of California, San Diego
La Jolla, California

REVIEWS

This article covers only the years 1970, 1971, and early 1972, except where for the sake of continuity a few older references are cited. A computer search provided over 500 references, of which almost 350 were clearly relevant to the physiology or pathophysiology of the blood capillary system. It is obvious that only a portion of the activities in the field can be reviewed in the space allocated for the subject; the selection and orientation of the subject matter reflects my own prejudices and preoccupation. Fortunately, during the past two years many excellent reviews of particular aspects of microcirculation have become available.

Theoretical approaches to the transport and exchange aspects of micro-iirculation have been covered in two reviews of the mechanics of blood (59, 60) and the Benzon symposium on capillary permeability (44). Likewise, there have been reviews of interstitial pressure (70), red blood cells and flow properties of blood (24), microcirculatory organization (75), physicochemical aspects of the interstitium (125), and rheologic aspects of blood flow (64, 156). Several review articles are cited later in relevant sections covering particular aspects of the problem.

METHODOLOGY

Many new techniques and instruments are now available for quantitation and analysis of small blood vessel behavior. An increased awareness of the factors which are needed to sustain exteriorized tissues has brought about a refinement of existing techniques and the development of new procedures for the observational study of the microcirculation.

Skeletal muscle has not been subjected to the same critical quantitative analysis at the microscopic level as has been possible by organ perfusion in situ. Techniques for such an approach have now been devised (26) for the tenuissimus muscle of the cat. Examples of other improvements are special

[1] The author has been supported by grants from the USPHS (HL-10881) and the National Science Foundation (GK-31160X).

117

mountings for mesentery preparations (187), newly designed ear chambers (3, 106, 138), the in situ study of the gastric microcirculation (148), and various skin preparations in man (82, 120). Perfusion of single capillaries in the frog (128) presents an approach with challenging possibilities. Online measurement of erythrocyte velocity is possible not only for single capillaries (61), but for larger arterioles and venules through the use of video and computer crosscorrelation techniques (86). Vessel dimensions can be recorded continuously be television microscopy (85). Improvements in membrane osmometers (89) permit accurate and rapid recording of shifts in plasma colloid osmotic pressures. Permeability to macromolecules has been studied by regional radioisotope levels (177), and by the transport of fluorescent tagged macromolecules (74). New types of microelectrodes for determining tissue oxygen levels (21) have been applied to brain tissue. Surface characteristics of endothelium have been studied at the ultrastructural level with the scanning electron microscope (130, 171).

The response characteristics of micropressure devices have been greatly improved (83) and measurements were made in a variety of tissues including mesentery (207), the bat wing (196), and the pial surface of the brain (162). Microangiography (181) has been found to be useful for establishing the blood supply in solid tissues. Quantitative estimations of the contributions of interstitial permeability to the exchange between blood and extravascular compartment have been made using sheets of mesentery as a permeability barrier (182). The local clearance method remains a favorite approach for studying blood flow in whole organs or tissues (101) and has been used to establish intercapillary spacing or density (68). Refinements in the Landis micro-occlusion procedure (204) have permitted repeated measurements of capillary filtration coefficients in selected capillaries.

ORGANIZATIONAL FEATURES
DESIGN OF THE CAPILLARY BED

Module.—Frasher & Wayland have proposed that the interlocking of paired arteries and veins so as to enclose discrete areas of tissue represents a modular unit which facilitates the distribution of blood in the microcirculation (55). Such an arrangement is primarily seen in flat two dimensional tissues such as the mesentery and cremaster muscle. Similar arcuate structures have not been seen in the mesentery of all laboratory species, nor in other skeletal muscles (202). A number of relevant observations make the module concept somewhat uncertain. The pressures found in paired arteriole or venous components which made up the sides of the arcade network were not uniform (207). For example, in a given five sided arcuate arrangement formed by three separate arterial vessels, the five arteries had pressures which ranged from 55 to as high as 80 mm Hg, and in their paired venous components the pressures ranged from 20 to 50 mm Hg. Vessels which formed one side of an arcuate network frequently gave off branches to other areas.

Dimensions.—A number of attempts have been made to define more rigorously the branching sequence, vessel length, vessel width, surface area, etc., in order to establish some kind of idealized microcirculatory unit, which would then serve as a framework for ancillary studies on exchange. An interesting feature of the mesenteric bed is that the branching pattern and vessel dimensions combined to provide a comparable blood volume for the successive dichotomizations (88).

Preferential channels.—Over the years different investigators have been impressed by the unique design of the capillary network in particular tissues and have attempted to relate these structural attributes to the functional needs of the system. In a recent paper, Kuprianov & Kozlov (98) distinguished between the overall needs of a microvascular bed to minimize energy requirements and the flexibility needed within the network to provide for the wide range of metabolic activity present in most tissues.

In 1938, on the basis of an analysis of the fundamental structural organization of the microcirculation in mesenteric tissues, we proposed that two features underly many of the functional attributes of the microcirculation in general—the existence of paths of least resistance (so-called thoroughfare or preferential channels) from arteriole to venule, and the unique arrangement whereby lateral branches of these channels act as sphincters regulating flow into the capillary channels. Similar features have been shown to be present in a number of tissues, but other investigators (71, 132) have been unable to demonstrate preferential channels in other tissues which have been used for in vivo studies of microcirculatory behavior. Instead they described an apparently random distribution of small vessels beyond the terminal arterioles. In a number of structures where the small blood vessels dichotomize repeatedly to form capillaries, it has been difficult to identify sphincters as a regular feature of precapillary arrangement (26, 71).

Despite the physiological importance of skeletal muscle and the extraordinary amount of effort which has been put into studies of its circulation, there is as yet no consensus on some of the most fundamental features of its structure and behavior. Direct visual studies of muscle circulation must perforce by confined to comparatively flat, thin tissues. Emphasis has thus been placed on a two dimensional disposition of the microvasculature with no clear indication of its three dimensional architecture. When different skeletal muscles were compared (69), dissimilar branching patterns were found; shunt vessels of capillary dimensions were seen in one set of muscles but not in another; precapillary sphincter arrangement was found to be common in one site whereas in others repeated arteriolar dichotomization into a nondescript capillary network was observed. Whether such differences stem from particular functional needs of certain sets of muscles remains to be determined.

The preferential channel concept deals with a number of structural features within the capillary bed proper which are, in fact, basic elements of design and which should not be discarded because in some tissues arteriolar vessels simply terminate by splaying out into a nondescript network of capillary channels. In almost every tissue examined in vivo, arterial blood is distributed into the capillary network by direct, almost linear extensions of the feeding arteriole. Along their course these vessels distribute lateral branches which then dichotomize to form the capillary network proper. In a tissue such as skeletal muscle, over 80% of the capillaries have been found to be delivered as lateral branches (26, 71). The capillary bed proper is, therefore, not simply a terminal in-series network, but in large part originates along the entire course of the arteriole. These lateral offshoots (about 15μ wide) are operationally in parallel with the main arteriole to venule pathway and since they are endowed with smooth muscle, they can serve as active controls for the distribution of blood into particular networks of capillaries. In most tissues such side branches break up into five or six separate capillary vessels (202). Many of these major side branches do not form structurally recognizable preferential pathways.

This structural alignment within the capillary bed proper represents a mechanism for bypassing varying percentages of these lateral precapillary branches. In other structures, such as the omentum, which is an important organ for fat storage, the arterioles terminate abruptly and splay out into a capillary mesh. Detailed reconstructions are needed to depict the three dimensional distribution of all of the capillary branches of a major feeding arteriole and the venular effluence of such a network in representative tissues.

Sphincters.—The term precapillary sphincter has become synonymous with a vessel which guards the entrance to one or two capillaries and determines the selective distribution of blood within the capillary network (202). Sphincters in this classical sense do exist in many tissues, but in others the major control for the distribution of blood within the capillary network appears to be the terminal arterioles or their immediate muscular branches. Recent studies on the tenuissimus muscle of the cat (26), for example, have shown that the terminal arterioles which are only 14 to 16μ wide subdivide some five to six times in rapid succession with no evidence of perivascular muscle after the second dichotomy. Thus, the vasomotor activity of such terminal arterioles controls some N^6 branches whereas in other tissues only 4–5 branches are directly affected by the activity of a single precapillary vessel. This type of arrangement is not, however, characteristic of other muscle. Honig et al (80), have examined the effects of denervation and metabolic factors on the number of open capillaries in heart muscle and concluded that capillary density is influenced on the immediate precapillary level by locally elaborated chemicals, and not by the nervous system, which affects the arterioles and larger vessels only.

Neurogenic control.—Observational studies on the distribution of blood in a skeletal muscle following nerve stimulation (51) have shown groups of stagnant capillaries without an active flow, presumably as a result of contraction of the larger arterioles upstream. In another study (71), in which the injection of colored gelatin was used to examine the distribution of blood, no evidence could be found for a uniform distribution of sphincters in relation to regularly spaced preferential channels.

The suggestion that vasomotor control of capillary flow in skeletal muscle resides in the feeding arterioles removes from the microcirculation a type of local control believed indigenous to it. In view of the many orders of branching between the arterioles and capillaries in skeletal muscle, contraction of a given arteriole will perforce affect almost one hundred capillaries by regional or group control. This may be useful for working skeletal muscle where an entire mass of muscle fibers are activated simultaneously. Such an arrangement, however, does not allow for uniform distribution of blood during periods of comparative inactivity.

SHUNTS

The concept of "shunting" at the capillary level has been developed in two contexts—a diffusive type of exchange (140) between adjacent large blood vessels so as to bypass to a considerable degree the capillary network, and short convective pathways (69, 81) between arterioles and venules. This latter type of shunt has not been regularly encountered in all tissues, although indirect evidence points to its existence even in skeletal muscle. For example, pressures recorded simultaneously with two microprobes placed in the arteriole and venule bridging a common area show that some 15–20% of these vessels have a pressure drop of only 10–12 cm H_2O whereas the majority of such vessels have a pressure drop of 35–40 cm H_2O. Clearly, low resistance paths must exist, which serve in effect as shunts (145). An even higher percentage of shunts, as evidenced by a minimal A-V pressure drop, is seen in the mesentery omentum, skin, and ear microcirculation.

Grant & Wright (69) found anatomical evidence in vivo for short vessels which can serve as nonnutritive channels in the capillary network of muscle tendons. In skeletal muscle proper such shunts are not common, although there is evidence for some type of diffusional shunting. It has been difficult to establish whether the latter is due to the presence of vessels with widely differing permeabilities, or whether some type of countercurrent exchange can occur between nearby vessels. Studies on the redistribution of blood flow in the retina of the eye show a persistance of flow in preferential pathways following blood loss (112).

ENDOTHELIUM

The question of contractility of vascular endothelium is a perennial one. By far the majority of the observations made on mammalian capillaries in many different tissues favor the view that capillary endothelium is not contractile in the same sense that smooth muscle can respond to stimuli (75). Variations in the dimensions of capillaries are thought to be brought out indirectly by changes in the connective tissue matrix and possibly by some type of endothelial swelling (60). More recently electron microscopy and histochemical staining have demonstrated the presence of what appear to be contractile filaments in the endothelium of different tissues and even in the endothelium of certain lymphatics (107). It is possible that endothelial cells may be capable of undergoing changes in shape and perhaps even separate from each other so as to create slits between cells. This form of limited contractility is one of the physiologic capabilities of vascular endothelium, as it seems to be for many other parenchymal cells.

The electron microscope has increased our ability to define the precise distribution of smooth muscle in the terminal vascular bed, but it has not identified the cells found either adhering to endothelial wall or imbedded in the basement membrane of blood capillaries which some investigators have suggested could conceivably be modified smooth muscle (94). There is no physiologic evidence that smooth muscle is present in any part of the capillary network proper. On the effluent or venular side, smooth muscle reappears when collecting venules about 20μ in diameter are formed (203).

Considerable attention has been given in the literature to the functional significance of several features: the quantitative assessment of the endothelial vesicle as a dynamic element; the so-called "fenestrae" seen in highly permeable capillaries; the nature of the intercellular attachment of endothelium; and the presence of an endocapillary layer.

Vesicles.—Earlier studies had suggested that the numerous vesicles seen on the luminal and abluminal surface, as well as in the cytoplasm of the endothelial cell, could serve as a transport vehicle for larger molecules. Because of their size (200–300 Å) it was presumed that they could not be selective, and that diffusion time from one cell surface to the other would be much too slow to account for transfer of small molecules (95).

Vesicles occupy between 25 and 35% of the nonnuclear volume of the endothelial cell; their internal volume is about 0.04 $\mu m^3/\mu m^2$ of luminal surface area; about 135 vesicles were found to be attached to each surface and membrane, and between 200 and 350 were free in the cytoplasm (33). The average free life time was calculated to be about 1.5 sec. Many investigators (9, 94) have accepted these structures as the equivalent of the so-called large pores in the capillary barrier. The presence of a thin coat of polysaccharide-protein complex on the endothelial surface is believed to contribute to the rate of formation of such vesicles and to endow them with selectivity (165).

Other investigators question whether the vesicle system actually participates in transendothelial exchange. Careful quantitative counts during periods of increased and decreased exchange do not parallel one another (121). Kobayashi (97) found that vesicles continue to be labelled with ferritin whether or not the tissue has first been treated with a fixative. The system of vesicles in endothelium may function in some as yet undefined way as a selective carrier for particular molecules, but its broad function as the mechanism for macromolecular transport between blood and tissue compartments remains largely unproven.

Fenestrae.—Another structural element believed to be involved in the blood-tissue exchange of large molecules are the thinned-out portions of endothelium which form circular-shaped structures with only a thin membraneous diaphragm (40–50 Å thick) separating the bloodstream from the extravascular compartment (34, 35, 56, 180, 198). These so-called fenestrae have been shown to permit passage of particles and macromolecules under different conditions depending upon the absence or presence of the diaphragm-like partition bridging the circular opening. For example, the sequestration of calcium by a chelating agent has been found to influence the completeness of the diaphragm (40).

Intercellular junctions.—There is increasing evidence that much of the exchange through the capillary wall occurs by way of the intercellular junctions (95). Except for very specialized areas, no continuum of tight junctions has been demonstrated. Interendothelial cell attachments are believed to involve some type of chemical bonding that is susceptible to local modification. The problem may be similar to that encountered in the attachment of tumor cells or multicellular structures to one another through the intermediary of a special protein which permits sialic acid linkages to cell surfaces.

Endocapillary surface.—The presence of a lining material on the luminal surface of the endothelium has been disputed because of its absence in conventional electron micrographs. Recent attention to fixation artifacts and extraction of water soluble components has brought to light a thin (50–60 Å) layer of what appears to be a polysaccharide complex that is heavily stained by the PAS procedure (165). The material appears to be continuous with the intercellular matrix. Although the chemical specificity of the staining procedure for polysaccharides is not clear, the consistent presence of this layer in all blood vessels reenforces the evidence originally presented by Luft on the basis of staining with ruthenium red (163).

The scanning electron microscope (171) has brought to light the presence of numerous fine surface projections on the luminal side of endothelial surfaces; these may be up to several hundred angstroms in length and could conceivably set up a buffer zone between the bloodstream and the vessel wall. Why these structures have not been seen in routine electron micrographs remains in dispute.

Basement membrane.—The endothelium proper of small blood vessels is encased in a basement membrane. Although this supporting structure appears to be attached directly to the outer surface of the endothelial cells, the two structures can become separated under conditions of abnormal leakage of protein and blood cellular elements (95). A number of studies (188, 189) have indicated that the subendothelial space represents a potential compartment for controlling the exchange of materials between the blood and interstitium proper. The basement membrane of small blood vessels is an exchange barrier only in the sense that it restricts movement of blood cells, platelets, and the largest immune complexes.

PHYSICAL PROPERTIES

Vessel wall rheology.—The concept of a critical closing pressure for small blood vessels, originally developed by Burton, was based on an instability arising when wall tension was greater than intravascular pressure. Oka & Azuma (133) have shown in a theoretical analysis that calculations of circumferential pressure should include, in addition to the vessel radius, wall thickness. Depending upon the elastic properties of the wall, arterioles under conditions of decreased pressure were shown to increase in diameter and not to collapse as proposed by Burton. They suggested that the viscoelastic properties of the smooth muscle may be the determining factor in closure of resistance vessels under conditions of reduced blood pressure.

The observation that thin-walled capillaries remain open despite reduced flow and pressure has been ascribed to the fact that the surrounding tissue provides the elastic environment for such vessels, so that in effect they behave as comparatively rigid tubes (59). This concept is supported by online velocity measurements of terminal arterioles and venules (87). Analysis of the phase shifts in the pressure wave on the venular side indicated a comparatively rigid microvasculature.

Distensibility.—Studies on small blood vessels are difficult to make because such structures cannot be isolated and simultaneous pressure-diameter studies have not been made. An approach to such an analysis has been made by Baez (11) who used an image-splitting technique to quantify changes in wall thickness and lumen size of the successive components of the microcirculation in skeletal muscle.

In a study of vessel distensibility in the alveolar membrane of the cat lung (173), it was found that the dynamics of the lung vessels are entirely different from those in connective tissue or in skeletal muscle. These workers developed a sheet flow theory in which the effects of pressure and thickness remain uniform in the alveolar sheet; the most rapid changes in thickness and pressure occur near the venous outflow. Impedance of the alveolar sheet is not purely a resistive phenomenon.

INTERSTITIUM

Although the interstitial tissue is an integral part of blood-tissue exchange processes, it remains largely unexplored in this regard (197). Recent work (104) on the physicochemical makeup of the connective tissue has focused on the interfibrillar material, which consists primarily of polysaccharides of the hyaluronate type.

The physicochemical properties of the interstitium have been modeled on the basis of in vitro studies of hyaluronic acid gels and mixtures of proteins (118, 142, 143). The connective tissue ground substance is visualized as consisting of two phases–a colloid-rich gel phase with a high content of hyaluronate (about 1%) and a fluid phase which is either in equilibrium with or in a steady state with the gel phase. The makeup and properties of these two phases will determine the transport of fluid and solutes between the blood capillaries and parenchymal cells. [For details, the reader is referred to the recent conference on hemodilution (125)]. The actual resistance to water movement depends upon the concentration of polysaccharides (124). Other contributing factors (104) are exclusion and sieving of molecules, swelling pressure, and the anamolous osmotic pressure generated by mixtures of polysaccharides and plasma protein as developed by Ogton. A disproportionate distribution of small ions because of Donnan equilibrium considerations could further exaggerate osmotic differences (96).

The peritoneal membrane has been used as a model for exchange across the interstitial compartment (7). Its properties, as in the case of a barrier such as the glomerular membrane, can be explained on the basis of a large and small pore system. It is difficult to balance all of the tissue forces in terms of transcapillary fluid movement since the various compartments need not be in simple equilibrium but are kept in a balanced steady-state condition.

TISSUE PRESSURE

The concept of a negative tissue pressure has been both contradicted and supported by recent work. The negative pressure measured by the implanted capsule procedure (70) has been explained by Stromberg & Wiederhielm (176) as an experimental artifact resulting from the presence of a capsular membrane with a high reflection coefficient for protein and a comparatively high concentration of ground substance materials outside the capsule. The colloid osmotic pressure differential would thus tend to draw fluid out of the capsular compartment, which because of its high compliance will develop a subatmospheric or negative pressure. This tendency for interstitial tissue to take up water is supported by swelling experiments in an osmometer where tissue volume is kept constant by a servo mechanism (175). It is difficult to transpose such numbers into in vivo situations dealing with blood-tissue exchange and satisfy the needs of the Starling equation.

Measurements made with the cotton wick technique pioneered by Scholander provide strong support for the existence of negative tissue pressures (99, 136, 172). The wick measurements are not based on an osmometer principle so that the Stromberg & Wiederhielm argument cannot be used against these experiments. Subcutaneous pressures of -2 to -6 mm Hg have been recorded in man and in various mammals (172). Comparison with implanted capsule measurements showed an identical trend during perturbations which led either to tissue hydration or dehydration. The precise principle by which the cotton wick acts has not been clearly demonstrated. In preliminary experiments on brain tissue, wick readings showed positive pressures and closely followed shifts in cerebrospinal fluid pressure (27). A balloon tipped catheter has also been used to measure tissue pressure (78), but such an indirect approach gives a resultant value of both physical and free fluid forces.

In related experiments (124) it has been shown that the pressure exerted by a gel across a membrane varied with its state of hydration: in the dehydrated state, highly negative pressures developed; after hydration the pressure returned to baseline values dependent on concentration. Pressure readings recorded by the insertion of microneedles into the interstitium have always been positive or near atmospheric. It is apparent that the significance of specific experimental values cannot be determined until we can identify the compartment with which hydraulic conductivity has been established.

TERMINAL LYMPHATICS

A somewhat neglected aspect of blood-tissue exchange is the mechanics of fluid return via the lymphatics at the microcirculatory level. Only sketchy outlines of the distribution of lymphatic capillaries are available. These vessels are difficult to recognize in living structures and have been described primarily under circumstances where dye or particulate materials are injected into the interstitium. Through the use of darkfield illumination, Hauck (75) has been able to identify extremely fine lymphatic networks in a contiguous relationship to the venules and in the free spaces of the mesentery. These channels fill rapidly with fluorescent labelled proteins. A more direct approach has been the filling of lymphatic capillaries with colored solutions from micropipettes so as to bypass valvular obstructions (206). The terminal lymphatics in the mesentery of the cat and rabbit are flattened endothelial sacs about $40-60\mu$ wide and only $5-6\mu$ deep. They interconnect with one another freely to form collecting channels in which valves are present.

There is good evidence that higher molecular weight materials such as dextran are selectively taken up and concentrated within the lymphatic capillary (32, 92). Courtice (43) believes that a continuous movement of protein into the lymph is essential to maintain extracellular fluid balance. Dextran was found to enter the terminal lymphatics by way of direct communication between postcapillary venules and the lymphatic capillaries (92). Similar connections have not however been reported in other tissues. When low molecular weight materials or ions are maintained at a steady state concentration in the blood stream, their concentration in the lymphatics likewise remains at a steady state, indicating a direct relationship between the diffusion of these materials into tissue and a comparable diffusion gradient into lymphatic terminals (141).

In electron microscope studies wide gaps have been described between overlapping endothelial cells in the terminal lymphatics (35, 107). The absence of a basement membrane and the presence of fibrils anchored in both the endothelial surface and the tissue matrix would appear to facilitate free exchange with the interstitium (107). Although the larger lymphatics have been shown to be contractile, the evidence for contractions of terminal lymphatic capillaries is inconsistent. The terminal lymphatics in many tissues show comparatively few endothelial vesicles, but in the intestine, for example, substantial numbers are present (48).

A number of mechanisms have been proposed for transfer of fluid and materials from the interstitium into the lymphatic capillaries. Casley-Smith (32) favors an osmotic mechanism which becomes more effective as the vessel fills and the endothelial cell overlap is closed. He has also proposed an active vesicular transport of protein into the lymph. Experimental data to support this concept is not substantial.

Most workers (43, 70) believe the major force driving fluid into the lymph capillaries is the tissue pressure, which tends to increase periodically until it exceeds that needed to open the valves guarding the earliest lymph channels. Passive movements, including skeletal muscle contraction, respiratory movements, etc., contribute to the entrance of fluid into lymphatics in different organs. The physical contributions of the interstitium in supporting the lymphatics and in the selective transport of materials between the blood and the lymphatic capillaries are critical aspects which remain to be defined.

Observational studies using fluorescent tagged materials (75, 92) describe direct contact between terminal lymphatics and venules of the capillary network. Such bulk transfer is not encountered in other tissues, e.g. skeletal muscle, where blood-lymph ratios for larger molecules clearly indicate a sieving action beyond the blood vessel wall (8).

The relative contribution of lymph drainage to the local vascular balance of hydrostatic and colloid osmotic forces appears to depend upon the concentration of protein which is present in the interstitial compartment (200). Thus, in some regions a modest hydrostatic pressure suffices, while in others a more substantial change is needed to achieve a steady state.

The existence of regional specialization in lymphatic capillary function depends upon the particular function involved (41). Hauck & Schröer (77) have placed emphasis on the lymphatic removal of fluid from the tissue compartment as an essential feature for fluid balance. In part, this need exists because of the unequal permeability (both hydrodynamic and diffusive) on the arterial and venous sides of the microcirculation.

Most data based on blood-lymph content of materials suggest that plasma proteins in the tissue compartment are returned primarily by way of the lymphatic system and not via the venular capillaries (75). There are, however, studies which show that in important tissues such as heart muscle and the kidney cortex more than 75–80% of the protein is returned to the blood stream directly. It is not clear precisely how protein is moved against a substantial concentration gradient. Possibly some type of selective vesicular transport is present in such tissues.

Casley-Smith in comparative studies (34, 35) has found an inverse relationship between the presence of fenestrated blood capillaries and terminal lymphatics. The ultrastructure of lymphatic endothelium, as in the case of blood capillaries, varies considerably in particular organs and species, with wide ranges in the number of endothelial vesicles, infoldings, and the extent of endothelial overlap (30).

Pressure measurements in accessible terminal lymphatics (bat wing, skin, mesentery) are consistently in the positive range between 0 and 3 cm H_2O (132, 206). In view of the free connection of these terminal lymph capillaries with the interstitial compartment, it is difficult to see how the prevailing pressure in the interstitium could be subatmospheric or negative without the intervention of some active process.

TRANSPORT FUNCTIONS

MICROPRESSURES

Substantial strides have been made in the analysis of blood flow in the microcirculatory bed through the continued improvement of techniques for measuring micropressures. Nicoll (132) used a hydraulic linkage to a micropipette to obtain mean pressure readings in selected vessels of the bat wing and found a considerable scatter. The Wiederhielm servo-electronic null technique (196) has made possible continuous measurement of all of the components of the pressure wave in vessels as small as 5–6 μ in diameter. He was able to calculate the driving force in consecutive segments of the capillary bed. In the bat wing it was necessary to use micropipettes with tips as fine as 1 μ, and some of the pressure instability noted may thus be a direct result of the tendency for such fine openings to become obstructed.

Continuous measurements of capillary pressure in selected regions of the mesentery or omentum, using an improved version of this servonulling system, have demonstrated that the pressure is maintained (83) in the narrow range of 25 ± 4 cm H_2O, and that this range is reestablished within 4–5 min after shifting central arterial or venous pressures (203). The pressure drop across single capillaries in this tissue is on the order of 1.0–1.5 cm H_2O for vessels 200–250 μ long. The pressure drop across an average capillary network, as measured by two microprobes in the feeding arteriole and effluent venule, ranged between 6 and 8 cm H_2O. In the cremaster muscle of the rat, the pressure drop across the capillary network averaged 10–12 cm H_2O (169). The pressure drop in paired vessels feeding a given area of the mesentery usually averages 55–60 cm H_2O. In about 15–20% of the paired vessels, evidence of shunting was clearly demonstrated (145). An interesting finding in the pial circulation of the brain (162) was the substantial reduction in pressure in the largest surface arteries relative to central arterial pressure (a 39% drop). In most tissues, pressure in the feeding artery is usually quite close (-10%) to systemic arterial levels.

Capillary pressures are significantly lower in skeletal muscle than in mesentery (169). Despite substantial shifts in central arteriolar or venous pressures, pressure in the minute capillaries is quickly readjusted to control levels (203). For example, under conditions where pressure in the feeding artery is increased by 25–30 mm Hg, capillary pressure is brought back in 1 to 2 min to within 1 mm Hg of its original level. In some capillary beds, such as that of the omentum, mean capillary pressure is significantly higher than the colloid osmotic pressure, indicating that this bed is primarily a filtration organ.

Simultaneous records of micropressures and velocity in arterioles and venules of the mesentery (144) indicated that the pulsatile characteristics of arteriolar pressure were transmitted through the capillary network into the venules. Pressure wave characteristics of microvessels have been compared with central pressure recordings (4): shifts in the amplitude were more significant than phasic delays in analyzing the wall characteristics of the smaller blood vessels.

BLOOD FLOW

Flow in microvessels has been recorded by a photometric dual slit method (61), or online by a crosscorrelation method by which the images passing across the face of two diodes placed along the length of vessel are matched continuously by a small computer (86). The fact that pressure and velocity show clearly pulsatile characteristics in both the arteriole and venule has important implications with respect to rapid transients in transcapillary fluid movement.

Although flow velocities in most of the small muscular vessels are pulsatile, mean flow velocity has been found to remain reasonably constant for several minutes (90). Capillary velocities, however, varied considerably in different vessels of a given network in the mesentery (91).

Increasing attention has been given to factors which may influence the relative distribution of red blood cells through the various subdivisions of the microcirculation. Johnson and co-workers (91) used precisely spaced diodes and computer analysis of photometric signals to obtain average hematocrit values in selected capillaries and found the level to remain reasonably stable in the cat mesentery. The hematocrit depended more on local factors at the points of branching than on the absolute flow rate through the capillary network (90). The major determinant was the relative velocity in the two branches so that the greatest percentage of red cells moved into the vessel which had the greatest pressure drop. The apparently random branching of most networks results in an uneven distribution of plasma and red cells through the various subdivisions of the microcirculation.

Attempts to define precapillary regulation by monitoring red blood cell fluxes or velocity characteristics take a somewhat oversimplified view of the many other factors affecting the capillary circulation. Included are red blood cell spacing, relative size of the tube with respect to the red cell, and velocity at bifurcation points—all of which influence the local distribution of red cells and introduce a considerable degree of variability in different capillary vessels.

Stochastical analyses of erythrocyte movements through the capillaries (36) have suggested that the fluxes recorded are reflections of vasomotor changes within the microvasculature. The existence of periodic autoregulation in skeletal muscle is supported also by analyses of high speed motion picture recordings of red cell movement in the capillary bed (31). Studies in which simultaneous measurements were made of blood pressure and flow in microvessels (84) have suggested that a property analogous to compliance is imparted to the capillary bed by a combination of hydraulic and osmotic forces and the phase shift in pressure-flow disturbances.

Red blood cells and plasma are not evenly distributed in the capillary network. During periods of maximal blood flow in muscle, as following exercise, plasma and red blood cell passage becomes more nearly equal, suggesting that the number of paths poorly perfused with red blood cells is significantly decreased (129). Another inhomogeneity may arise from the presence in skeletal muscle of paths with different exchange properties, the so-called nutritive and nonnutritive paths for blood flow. The extent of nutritional blood flow to total blood flow has been evaluated (57) in the isolated gracilis muscle by utilizing the extraction of rubidium which traverses the blood capillary barrier readily.

The mechanism by which blood flow is adjusted locally in accord with changing metabolic needs can be conveniently studied in skeletal muscle. The concept that the local vasodilation is for the most part due to hyperosmolarity per se, rather than to specific chemical mediators, has been intensively explored (123). Some workers (155, 158, 159, 168), however, believe that osmolarity alone cannot reproduce reactive or exercise hyperemia and indicate that factors such as K^+, pH, and Po_2 are also involved in the full response. Extracellular hyperosmolarity has a direct effect on the response characteristics of vascular smooth muscle (93). Vascular tone and the response to myogenic stimuli were found to be markedly reduced.

The responsiveness of the microvascular elements to endogenous mediators has been examined in a number of different contexts. In one, the physical tension or stretch to which the cremaster muscle was subjected during microscopic study was varied (12). As the mechanical tension on the tissue was increased, the response or sensitivity to standard doses of norepinephrine was decreased. Somewhat analogous conclusions were reached (66) in experiments where vessel reactivity was compared with the physical tension existing in the vessel wall as calculated from the vessel radius, pressure, and wall thickness. The higher responsiveness in most peripheral vessels appeared to be related to the lower tension present in the walls of the metarterioles and precapillaries. Analyses of this kind may hold for the arteriole side, but do not explain the reduced responsiveness in the venules, where the wall tension is much lower than that in the arteriole side.

The extent to which the smallest subdivisions of the arteriolar and venular tree are under the influence of the nervous system (54) remains uncertain. Histochemical staining of adrenergic fibers has indicated that the arterioles and some of their branches are directly innervated by adrenergic fibers. Cholinergic innervation has been demonstrated by direct stimulation with microelectrodes in the retrolingual membrane of the frog (166). There is some evidence that even structures of capillary dimensions may each be accompanied by a single adrenergic fiber in tissues such as the mesentery. Such data are suggestive but certainly not clearly indicative of a direct innervation.

When the sympathetic nerves to an exteriorized skeletal muscle are stimulated, a significant reduction in blood flow occurs. Direct observation (51) has indicated that blood flow in groups of capillary vessels comes to a stop without any direct evidence of contraction in these particular vessels, so that the stoppage of blood must be attributed to closure of the feeding terminal arteriole. Honig (80), using a different approach, came to a similar conclusion—that sympathetic control of the microcirculation in cardiac muscle is restricted to the feeding arteriole, while the more distal precapillary vessels seem to be influenced primarily by local chemical factors. A word of caution is needed here since in exteriorized structures prepared for microscopic observation, the influence of local metabolic factors may supersede neurogenic controls and the response may not be representative of that under totally physiologic conditions.

Vascular smooth muscle in the microcirculation is believed to be regulated locally be factors which antagonize adrenergic mediated responses. Histamine and a histamine analog both were shown to abolish the action of catecholamines and polypeptides on the terminal vascular beds in the mesentery (13). Histamine, however, remains an enigma—its precise involvement in physiologic adjustments of the microcirculation remain unsettled. Altura (1), in an extensive series of studies, demonstrated that control of blood flow through the microcirculation is achieved mainly by chemical agents acting on precapillary vessels. The hypothesis was advanced that the graded interaction of various combinations of chemical and humoral substances serves to control nutritive blood supply to the microcirculation in particular tissues of the body.

The influence of local dilator chemicals on centrally mediated vasomotor adjustments was investigated in an isolated dog skeletal muscle preparation (80). Local mechanisms were found to be strong enough to override central constrictor mechanisms and it has been suggested that this type of interaction may serve to modulate blood flow through the terminal vascular bed of muscle. Local variations in pH, associated particularly with elevations of P_{CO_2}, were shown to produce intense constriction of the arterioles on the surface of the brain (191), suggesting that metabolic regulation of blood flow in the brain may involve changes in periarteriolar pH. A propagated type of vasodilation, which spreads both upstream and downstream, could be demonstrated with microtechniques by the local application of acetylcholine on arterioles (50).

Among the new types of mediators which have been uncovered in recent years, the prostaglandins appear to be most significant. The mechanism of action of prostaglandin E_1 was studied on an exteriorized mesentery preparation (193); it appears to serve as a local regulator by suppressing vascular responsiveness to endogenous adrenergic materials and to vasoactive polypeptides. Prostaglandins injected into the feeding artery of a skeletal muscle bed (45) produced an extensive increase in blood flow, but capillary filtration was not affected because of a proportional change in pre- and postcapillary segments.

The role of low tissue oxygen during periods of increased metabolic activity has likewise been explored in relation to the vasodilation accompanying reactive hyperemia and autoregulation. As has been noted earlier, oxygen deficits by themselves are not the sole explanation for autoregulation (168). Many endogenous factors have been found to produce an increase in blood flow in skeletal muscle, but none of them alone can reproduce the in vivo phenomena completely (137).

TRANSCAPILLARY EXCHANGE

Single Vessels

The constitutive equation for fluid movement across the blood capillary barrier as originally derived by Starling is concerned with factors which operate across single blood vessels. Attempts to apply this same mathematical relationship to whole organs (16, 44) have encountered formidable difficulties, chiefly because the morphology of the vascular bed as a whole is not sufficiently well defined and because the arrangement of vessels in different parts of a tissue is not homogenous. In recent years the Starling relationship for single capillaries has been subjected to a more rigorous analysis. These studies in principle adopted the original Landis micro-occlusion procedure and have refined the data reduction methods (204, 205). The permeability coefficient for mammalian capillaries was found to vary in different portions of the same bed and tended to be significantly higher on the venous side. The validity of this method of approach has been supported by a number of theoretical analyses (110, 111, 116).

The hydrodynamic coefficient for the capillary wall as determined by the Landis micro-occlusion procedure is an operational term which does not indicate which parts of the barrier are involved. The existence of several pathways is suggested by the experiments of Landis & Sage (100), who determined a separate proportionality constant based on an osmotic transient which was induced by irrigating the surface of the mesentery with different concentrations of small hydrophilic substances. Osmotically generated forces were found to be less effective in producing fluid shifts then was an equivalent hydrostatic force. The study implies that hyperosmolarity of metabolic origin is not as effective as hydraulic factors in producing filtration of fluid into tissues.

In vivo measurements of capillary filtration rates for tissues such as skeletal muscle have been expressed numerically as CFC (capillary filtration coefficient), a value which necessarily must encompass the surface area involved in the exchange (53). Difficulties continue to be encountered with such techniques since it is not possible to establish unequivocally by isogravimetric or isovolumetric procedures that the changes are due not to shifts in hydrostatic pressure but to shifts in surface area (44). Friedman (58) has made an even more fundamental criticism of these methods. He has found that changes in venous blood colloidal osmotic pressure recorded continuously in a perfused muscle preparation gave more consistent CFC values when venous pressure was elevated than did the isogravimetric procedure, which gave progressively lower CFC values as the venous pressure was increased. Some form of delayed compliance appeared to be involved.

There is no well defined formula for handling the problem of the gradient of permeability in terms of both diffusive and convective exchange. A topographical gradient of permeability is readily observed in exteriorized tissues (73), using as a yardstick the escape of dye-colored or fluorescent-tagged protein. As previously indicated, venous vessels have a higher filtration coefficient. Electron microscope studies have demonstrated structural adaptations (fenestrae) for venular endothelium (34), which are the same as those found in capillaries of organs where vascular permeability to protein is high.

Wiederhielm (195) incorporated both an increased permeability and a high venular surface area into a computer simulation of the capillary bed. He then attempted to establish the range of tissue pressure needed to keep such a system in fluid balance. The computer analysis in all instances gave positive values for tissue pressure. It is interesting to note that a theoretical analysis (111) of fluid movement following micro-occlusion of single capillaries has predicted that about 10 cm H_2O out of an effective driving pressure of from 28 to 38 cm H_2O is contributed by tissue factors (a negative hydrostatic or a substantial colloid osmotic pressure, or both). Other theoretical studies (116, 134, 143) found it necessary to include changes in tissue factors as determinants of blood-tissue fluid exchange.

Levick & Michel (113, 115) analyzed the permeability properties of small blood vessels by perfusing single capillaries in the frog mesentery and found (114) that the permeability coefficient of selected capillaries could be varied by changing the concentration of protein used to perfuse these vessels.

Pathways for Exchange

A number of attempts have been made with electron microscopy using visible tracers to determine the route taken by different materials during their passage through the capillary wall. Most studies (95) with larger molecules have indicated an intercellular pathway but still leave open the possibility of vesicular transport. Shirahama & Cohen (165) concluded that a mucopolysaccharide coating of the endothelial cell wall participates in the formation of pinocytotic vesicles and may introduce a degree of selectivity for the material which is taken up. Other workers (97) have downgraded the significance of such ultrastructural evidence. They found that identical movement of material into vesicles occurs even when the material has previously been fixed.

With respect to diffusive exchange of small hydrophilic molecules, the evidence for intercellular pathways is reasonably convincing (16, 102). If one compares the transcapillary diffusion of sodium, sucrose, or glucose relative to water, the ratios are essentially the same as in aqueous solutions. This suggests that diffusion is occurring through water filled pores much larger than are believed to be present in the endothelial cell membrane. Michel (127) arrived at a similar conclusion on the basis of experiments with microelectrodes by which he traced the movement of sodium chloride across the mesothelium of the mesentery. He also noted that complexes of blue dye and albumin diffused out of perfused capillaries at intervals which corresponded to endothelial cell junctions. There is good evidence (186) that the permeability characteristics of such slits or pores can be changed under different physiologic conditions.

The experiments of Lassen & Trap-Jensen (102, 103) indicated a much smaller permeability to water in the vessels of skeletal muscle than was originally estimated by Pappenheimer. This discrepancy could be circumvented if the calculations were based on open interendothelial slits rather than pores as the passage sites for small hydrophilic substances. A similar conclusion was reached by Karnovsky (95) using electron microscope material.

A number of pathophysiological phenomena associated with fluid loss into tissues have been attributed to changes in the filtration coefficient of the vessel wall. Studies on hypothermia (179) and local hypoxia (158) failed to show a change in capillary permeability per se.

FUNCTIONAL SHUNTING

The term "functional shunting" has come into the literature primarily because changes in flow are not always associated with a proportionate shift in exchange. Such discrepancies may be explained on the basis either of sets of vessels with different permeability properties, or of a shift in the permeability of the capillary barrier associated with changes in flow (81). To accept the existence of vessels with widely different permeabilities would imply that some type of regulation exists whereby flow can be diverted selectively into or away from particular vessels (140). There is as yet no indication for any such mechanism.

The fact that such "shunting" of hydrophilic substances occurs with increased flow rates (185, 186) suggests that "restricted diffusion" becomes more prominent as flow increases. Some type of "pore" structure is usually presented as the basis for this type of effect. It should be pointed out, however, that "functional shunting" has been described in skeletal muscle even for gases such as hydrogen which presumably diffuse across the entire cell surface and do not require pores for their diffusion between the blood and tissue compartments. The only plausible alternative would then be either re-distribution of blood or a change in the permeability of the vessel wall.

Chien (38) has attempted to incorporate the possibility of shunting into a mathematical model of the microcirculation modified from that of Wieder-hielm. The term "shunting" as indicated encompasses both diffusion and con-vective flow so that a much more detailed analysis of geometrical factors is needed before proper physiologic controls can be introduced.

Despite the widespread acceptance and use of indicator dilution techni-ques as a measure of flow, reports continue to show that tracer disappearance and flow are not necessarily parallel phenomena (22, 67). The extravascular movement of materials which penetrate into cells (K, Rb) is especially diffi-cult to analyze by such techniques (164).

Gas Exchange

All segments of the microcirculation are highly permeable to gases (160) and recent studies have indicated that a substantial portion of the oxygen in the blood may have diffused into the tissue before the immediate precapillary vessels are reached.

Duling (49), in studies on the hamster cheek pouch, used microelec-trodes to map the perivascular oxygen tension adjacent to successive branches of the capillary bed. Oxygen tension was observed to fall off pro-gressively until, at the level of the precapillary vessels, the tension was about 16% of the arteriole levels. He postulated that the regulation of tissue oxygen tension must therefore be manifest chiefly between the arteriole and precapil-lary sphincter. Substantial changes in oxygen supply were needed to produce a significant increase in pericapillary oxygen tension. Similar conclusions were reached in studies of other tissues (126), where hypercapnia vasodila-tion was found to be much more effective in elevating tissue PO_2 than was hyperoxia.

Mathematical models of oxygen exchange have been applied to various tissues, using the Krogh cylinder for oxygen diffusion as their basis (183). The model of Reneau and co-workers (139) for brain tissue is applicable only if the suggested idealized arrangement of capillary tissue cylinders does in fact represent the actual in vivo situation. Obviously this is not correct, and even in other tissues such as the heart (79) or skeletal muscle (105) where capil-lary alignment is highly regular, models of this type are not accurate. The fall in oxygen in most tissues is nonlinear (105, 190, 194). Bicher et al (20) used metal microelectrodes to follow brain oxygen tension and found reoxygena-tion time after periods of hypoxia to be a more appropriate measure of gas exchange than PO_2 levels alone.

Exchange of Macromolecules

Visual evidence of vascular permeability is difficult to quantitate. The mechanism of protein leakage has not been satisfactorily explained (8, 63).

Intravenous injection of fluorescent-tagged plasma proteins or dextrans of graded molecular weight colored the perivenular tissue diffusely, and then spread into the interstitium until after some 20–35 min it was no longer evident, depending upon the amount of macromolecule which was injected (76). If the blood flow to the vascular bed was temporarily interrupted, the dye-colored albumin, or fluorescent-tagged protein did not appear in the perivenular tissue in sufficient concentrations to be detectable (199).

The experiments of Arturson and colleagues (9) and of Renkin & Garlick (141) were based on a comparison of blood and lymph concentrations of labelled macromolecules injected into the bloodstream. The distribution spaces involved are not known so that concentration gradients between the interstitium and the lymphatics, for example, cannot be set up with any degree of certainty. Depending upon whether one uses lymph values or total distribution within a tissue, completely different values will be obtained for the resistance to diffusion of macromolecules through the tissue compartment.

BLOOD RHEOLOGY

In Vivo Studies

In vivo recording of the microcirculation, with exposures of 10^{-4} sec or less, has shown the highly deformable nature of the red blood cell (167), but without factual data on red blood cell deformability, pressures, and flow, it will not be possible to determine the stresses (25) which are responsible for the shapes assumed in the flowing blood stream. Model experiments using flexible simulated red cells are suggestive (161, 178), but the data are not directly applicable until precise figures for the elasticity of the red cell have been established. Several groups of workers in Folkow's laboratory (10, 47) have compared pressure-flow relationships for solutions in which viscosity and hematocrit were varied, using the partially isolated hind limb preparations as a viscometer. They found a poor relationship between viscosity as measured in conventional viscometers and the flow properties of particular solutions with different amounts of protein or hematocrits. Blood viscosity is a complex property determined by many factors other than shear rate or hematocrit (64, 184). Geometry is an especially important factor and unless a comparison can be made under identical conditions, flow values for material of different macroscopic viscosity cannot be adequately evaluated. The plate spacing in viscometers is macroscopic when compared to the flow through the microcirculation, and in that context the broad implications of these in vivo studies are well taken. In the microcirculation, viscosity is determined primarily by the interaction between the deformed red cells and the capillary wall and not by the bulk flow properties of blood.

In considering pressure-flow relationships through the isolated paw of the dog, Benis et al (17, 18) distinguished between viscous and inertial factors and set up a power series expansion $\Delta P = A\eta Q + BQ^2$, which includes two constants A and B representing geometrical parameters, and η the apparent viscosity of blood. It will be necessary, however, to determine the extent to which the inertial term enters into calculations for the smallest blood vessels.

IN VITRO STUDIES

Red blood cell aggregation strongly influences the apparent viscosity of blood during its flow through microscopically small blood vessels (167). Such calculations should take into account not only the properties of single red cells, but also what might be called the effective volume of red cell masses or aggregates in the blood stream (37). Factors such as a high fibrinogen content (122) or the addition of macromolecules such as dextran (2) can affect the blood viscosity and introduce a departure from Newtonian behavior by the formation of cell aggregates (28). Under physiological conditions red cell aggregates are readily dissipated by the shear stress which is encountered in the small blood vessels (156). Under pathological conditions, however, the blood cell aggregates are more permanent (65), indicating important differences in the factors responsible for cell-cell adhesion under normal and pathological conditions. There has been a tendency to consider red blood cell aggregation as a phenomena with a unique chronology, but a variety of factors including changes in red cell size, red cell shape, plasma proteins, as well as the shear rates which are developed, all have been found to contribute to the development of such aggregates and their dissolution (46, 62, 119, 122, 194). Blood viscosity rose significantly in experiments where fibrinogen content was increased (122). There is no consensus on a yield stress value for blood under physiological conditions.

The ability of the red cell to undergo deformation (24) is perhaps the single most important feature influencing the passage of blood through the narrow capillaries. Studies on cells whose deformability has been altered by fixatives show that altered red cells are unable to be perfused through tubes or vessels whose diameter is smaller than that of the red blood cell (24). In contrast to normal red cells, such deformed cells are difficult to pass through 1–2 μ pores in synthetic membranes (39). When the driving pressure is raised so as to force these cells through small openings, the red cells undergo hemolysis. An obvious parallel exists under abnormal conditions involving hemolysis in vivo in which red cells may show signs of crenation or other shape changes (19).

The range of changes of red cell shape, from crenation to sphering, is believed to be directly related to effects on the cell surface by different materials. Sphered red blood cells require a longer period of time to pass through 4 μ pores in glass capillary (23), a phenomenon which can be reversed by a metabolic antagonist such as chlorpromazine. Model experiments with flexible red cells (161, 178) may offer some insight into the elastic properties of red cells subjected to deformation under different shear rates.

Red blood cell deformability probably is an important determinant of red cell life span in vivo, as well as of the hemolysis associated with certain hemolytic anemias (192). In a similar context, red cell deformability is believed to regulate the normal release of maturing cells from the bone marrow (108).

Normally, hemoglobin is confined to the interior of the red cell but under some circumstances it can become free in plasma. Recrystallized hemoglobin solutions have also been used as blood replacement measures. Hemoglobin solutions were found to have a viscosity which is lower than the apparent viscosity of red blood cells suspensions with equal oxygen carrying capacity (42). Inasmuch as the apparent viscosity of blood is increased at low shear rates, the place where such effects would most likely occur would be on the venular side of the microcirculation (46). Such factors are believed to contribute to the complete stasis which occurs in such venules (157).

The velocity profile which is developed under different pressure differentials under normal circumstances is influenced by particle-to-particle interactions (62). The smaller the tube in which the blood is flowing and the higher the hematocrit, the more the velocity profile will be deformed. The flow of blood through tubes as small as 29 μ is associated with a lower hematocrit than is presented in the inflow chamber, and, when correction is made for this fact, accurate calculation of pressure-flow relations can be made (14). Such an effect may explain the presumed nonlinearities of the so-called Fåhraeus-Lindquist phenomenon (15).

Dintenfass (46) and Wells (194) discussed the clinical implications of the so-called "hyper-viscosity syndrome" and its recognition by appropriate in vitro viscometry tests. Emphasis was placed on an increased internal rigidity of the red blood cell, and the multifactoral character of such abnormal states.

A series of papers (149–153) on the cerebral microcirculation dealt with a comparison in situ of changes in red blood cell velocity and plasma transit times (fluorescein) under conditions where blood viscosity differed significantly. With a decrease in viscosity (e.g. anemia), the rate of blood flow increased, and conversely, with an increased visosity—for example, following IV injection of high molecular weight dextran, or in macroglobulinemia—there was a marked retardation of the flow of plasma. The data suggest an in vivo relationship between blood viscosity and the shape of the velocity profile in the cerebral microvessels.

THEORETICAL ANALYSES
SINGLE CAPILLARY MODELS

Mathematical analyses of capillary flow have treated the vessel as an idealized structure with fixed properties. A number of studies have modified the classical Starling relationships for fluid exchange to include the tissue contribution (116, 134). Others have used computer simulation to take into account the effect of increases in the perviousness of the wall for water and water soluble substances on the osmotic and hydrostatic relationships in the blood and tissue compartments (72). The discontinuities which develop as the blood separates into plasma and red blood cells in the capillaries have focused attention on theoretical solutions for such features as the axial plasmatic gaps (29) and the so-called plug flow, in terms of the relative transport of plasma and red cells and the apparent hematocrit in capillaries (117). Aroesty & Gross (5, 6) have analyzed the pulsatile characteristics of the blood in the capillary vessels by solving the problem as a Casson fluid under conditions where time acts as a parameter and not as an independent variable. Since the inertial terms are negligible, flow behavior in arterioles and venules can be approximated accurately. The model of Stoltz & Larcan (174) has attempted to characterize the interaction of viscous and inertial forces for plasma with blood cell rheological features.

In their analysis of the pressure-flow relationships in capillary vessels, Aroesty et al (4) discussed the lubricant action of a layer of plasma at the periphery to increase flow rate. In somewhat analogous calculations of flow through small tubes, Charm originally had claimed that the finite layer of plasma at the periphery of the tube could not be adequately accounted for by the classical formulations for flow-viscosity interactions. In contrast, Cokelet (14) has shown that the Hagen-Poiseuillian relationship holds even for blood flow through tubes as small as 29 μ.

The mathematical details of the red blood cell-vessel lubrication layer, originally developed by Lighthill and expanded by Fitz-Gerald (52) to include details of red blood cell flow, led the latter to postulate that "seizure" would occur when the lubrication layer became too thin. Rowlands & Skibo (154) could find no experimental evidence for such a binding of red cells in glass capillaries 4 to 6 μ wide.

Exchange across single capillaries has been modeled both on the existence of idealized pores and on the intercellular clefts demonstrated by the electron microscope. Perl (135) was able to reconcile discrepancies in such models for existing transcapillary permeability and reflection coefficients by assuming clefts 40 Å wide as the pathways for exchange.

Capillary Bed Models

Intaglietta & Zweifach (88) constructed idealized models of the microvasculature in the omentum as an initial step in circumventing the difficulties of arbitrarily assembling data on a single capillary into completed microcirculatory units. A striking feature was the uniform distribution of surface area and volume throughout the capillary bed from arteriole to venule. Lee & Fronek (109) utilized such idealized beds as a frame of reference for a theoretical analysis of exchange of small molecular weight solutes and were able to show that back diffusion comes into play very early so that a concentration buildup adjacent to exchange vessels reduces overall exchange.

Rodbard and colleagues (146, 147) have presented additional calculations to support their "capillaron" concept. The compartmentalization of the tissue into encapsulated structures is offered as a major feature of microcirculation control, operating through periodic changes in tissue pressure. Such substantial periodic increases in tissue pressure have not yet been demonstrated by direct measurements.

WHOLE ORGANS OR TISSUES

The literature contains a whole array of models based on some modification of the Krogh tissue cylinder concept. The reader is referred to the Benzon symposium on capillary permeability held in Copenhagen in 1970 (44) for a thorough discussion of the values and shortcomings of particular approaches to blood flow and exchange at the organ level. An especially incisive examination of the indicator dilution approach used to provide data for such analyses has been made by Bassingthwaighte (16). He has modified the computer models of Wiener to take into account bolus flow, longitudinal diffusion in the capillary permeability of the vessel walls, geometrical factors, etc. Difficulties persist, however, in establishing a linear relationship between blood flow and the tissue extraction of different sized solutes. Lassen & Trap-Jensen (103) found small molecules (EDTA) to follow reasonably well the predicted tissue distribution from the blood stream. Ziegler & Goresky (201), on the other hand, concluded that current models based on multiple indicator dilution curves do not provide an appropriate description of flow and volume of distribution relationships.

Neufeld & Smith (131, 170) suggested the use of La Place transform numerical convolution to avoid many of the constraints and assumptions required for Fourier analysis of indicator dilution data. These workers were able to apply the method to the study of multiple tracers as a measure of capillary permeability in the lung and brain.

LITERATURE CITED

1. Altura, B. M. 1971. Chemical and humoral regulation of blood flow through the precapillary sphincter. *Microvasc. Res.* 3: 361–84
2. Appelgren, K. C., Lewis, D. H. 1970. Capillary flow and transcapillary transport in dog skeletal muscle after induced RBC aggregation and disaggregation. *Eur. Surg. Res.* 2:161–70
3. Arfors, K. E., Jonsson, J. A., McKenzie, F. N. 1970. A titanium rabbit ear chamber: assembly, insertion, and results. *Microvasc. Res.* 2:516–19
4. Aroesty, J., Gazley, C., Jr., Gross, J. F. 1970. On pulsatile, non-Newtonian flow in the microcirculation. In *6th Eur. Conf. Microcirc.*, ed. J. Ditzel, D. H. Lewis, 234–37. Basel, Switzerland: Karger, 451 pp.
5. Aroesty, J., Gross, J. F. 1970. Convection and diffusion in the microcirculation. *Microvasc. Res.* 2:247–67
6. Aroesty, J., Gross, J. F. 1972. The mathematics of pulsatile flow in small vessels I. Casson theory. *Microvasc. Res.* 4:1–12
7. Arturson, G. 1971. Permeability of the peritoneal membrane. In *6th Eur. Conf. Microcirc.*, ed. J. Ditzel, D. H. Lewis, 197–202. Basel, Switzerland: Karger. 451 pp.
8. Arturson, G. 1972. Effect of colloids on transcapillary exchange. In *Hemodilution,* ed. K. Messmer, H. Schmid-Schönbein, 84–104. Basel, Switzerland: Karger. 322 pp.
9. Arturson, G., Groth, F., Grotte, G. 1972. The functional ultrastructure of the blood-lymph barrier. Computer analysis of data from dog heart-lymph experiments using theoretical models. *Acta Physiol. Scand. Suppl.* 374:1–30
10. Baeckstrom, P., Folkow, B., Kendrick, E., Löfving, B., Öberg, B. 1971. Effects of vasoconstriction on blood viscosity in vivo. *Acta Physiol. Scand.* 81:376–84
11. Baez, S. 1969. Simultaneous measurements of radii and wall thickness of microvessels in the anesthetized rat. *Circ. Res.* 25: 315–29
12. Baez, S. 1971. Supporting tissue tension and microvascular reactions. *Microvasc Res.* 3:95–103
13. Baez, S., Orkin, L. R., Lagisquet, J. A. L. 1971. Antagonism of some vascular smooth muscle agonists by histamine and betahistine. *Microvasc. Res.* 3: 170–82
14. Barbee, J. H., Cokelet, G. R. 1971. Prediction of blood flow in tubes with diameters as small as 29μ. *Microvasc. Res.* 3: 17–21
15. Barbee, J. H., Cokelet, G. R. 1971. The Fahraeus effect. *Microvasc. Res.* 3:6–16
16. Bassingthwaighte, J. B. 1970. Blood flow and diffusion through mammalian organs. *Science.* 167:1347–53
17. Benis, A. M., Usami, S., Chien, S. 1970. Effect of hematocrit and inertial losses on pressure flow relations in the isolated hind paw of dog. *Circ. Res.* 27: 1047–68
18. Benis, A. M., Usami, S., Chien, S. 1972. Evaluation of viscous and inertial pressure losses in isolated tissue with a simple mathematical model. *Microvasc. Res.* 4:81–93
19. Bessis, M., Döbler, J. 1970. Discocytes et échinocytes dans l'anemie à cellules falciformes. II. Disposition des polymèrs d'hémaglobine. *Nouv. Rev. Fr. Hématol.* 10:793–800
20. Bicher, H. I. et al 1971. Effect of microcirculation changes on brain tissue oxygenation. *J. Physiol. London.* 217:689–707
21. Bicher, H. I., Knisely, M. H. 1970. Brain tissue re-oxygenation time, demonstrated with a new ultramicro oxygen electrode. *J. Appl. Physiol.* 28: 387–90
22. Bolme, P., Edwall, L. 1970. Dissociation of tracer disappearance rate and blood flow in isolated

skeletal muscle during various vascular reactions. *Acta Physiol. Scand.* 82:17–27

23. Braasch, D. 1970. Deformability and traversing time of shape-transformed single red cells passing through a 4μ glass-capillary. *Pfluegers Arch.* 329:167–71

24. Braasch, D. 1971. Red cell deformability and capillary blood flow. *Physiol. Rev.* 51:679–701

25. Braasch, D., Rogausch, H. 1970. Decreased red-cell deformability after severe burns, determined with the chlorpromazine test. *Pfluegers Arch.* 323:41–49

26. Brånemark, P.-I., Eriksson, E. 1971. Method for studying qualitative and quantitative changes of blood flow in skeletal muscle. *Acta. Physiol. Scand.* 84:284–88

27. Brock, M., Winkelmüller, W., Pöll, W., Markakis, E., Dietz, H. 1972. Measurement of brain-tissue pressure. *Lancet:* 595–96

28. Brooks, D. E., Goodwin, J. W., Seaman, G. V. 1970. Interactions among erythrocytes under shear. *J. Appl. Physiol.* 28:172–77

29. Bugliarello, G., Hsiao, G. C. 1970. A mathematical model of the flow in the axial plasmatic gaps of the smaller vessels. *Biorheology* 7:5–36

30. Bullon, A., Huth, F. 1972. Fine structure of lymphatics in the mycocardium. *Lymphology* 5:42–48

31. Cardon, S. F., Oestermeyer, C. F., Bloch, E. H. 1970. Effect of oxygen on cyclic red blood cell flow in unanesthetized mammalian striated muscle as determined by microscopy. *Microvasc. Res.* 2:67–76

32. Casley-Smith, J. R. 1968. How the lymphatic system works. *Lymphology* 1:77

33. Casley-Smith, J. R. 1969. The dimensions and numbers of small vesicles in cells, endothelial and mesothelial and the significance of these for endothelial permeability. *J. Micros.* 90:251–68

34. Casley-Smith, J. R. 1971. Endothelial fenestrae in intestinal villi, differences between the arterial and venous ends of the capillaries. *Microvasc. Res.* 3:49–68

35. Casley-Smith, J. R. 1971. The fine structure of the vascular system of amphioxus, implications in the development of lymphatics and fenestrated blood capillaries. *Lymphology* 3:79–94

36. Cerimele, B. J., Greenwald, E. K. 1970. Stochastic aspects of erythrocyte transit in capillaries. *Microvasc. Res.* 2:139–150

37. Chien, S. 1970. Shear dependence of effective cell volume as a determinant of blood viscosity. *Science* 168:977–79

38. Chien, S. 1971. A thoery for quantitation of transcapillary exchange in the presence of shunt flow. *Circ. Res.* 29:173–80

39. Chien, S., Luse, S. A., Bryant, C. A. 1971. Hemolysis during filtration through micropores: A scanning electron microscopic and hemorheologic correlation. *Microvasc. Res.* 3:183–203

40. Clementi, F., Palade, G. E. 1969. Intestinal capillaries II. Structural effects of EDTA and histamine. *J. Cell Biol.* 42:706–14

41. Cliff, W. J., Nicoll, P. A. 1970. Structure and function of lymphatic vessels of the bat's wing. *Quart. J. Exp. Physiol.* 55:112–21

42. Cokelet, G. R., Meiselman, H. J. 1968. Rheological comparison of hemoglobin solutions and erythrocyte suspensions. *Science* 162:275–77

43. Courtice, F. C. 1971. Lymph and plasma proteins: Barriers to their movement throughout the extracellular fluid. *Lymphology* 1:9–17

44. Crone, C., Lassen, N. A., Eds. 1970. Alfred Benzon Symposium II. *Capillary Permeability* New York: Academic. 681 pp.

45. Daugherty, R. M., Jr. 1971. Effects of iv and ia prostaglandin E_1 on dog forelimb skin and muscle blood flow. *Am. J. Physiol.* 220:392–96

46. Dintenfass, L. 1969. Blood rheology in pathogenesis of the coronary heart diseases. *Am. Heart J.* 77:139–47

47. Djojosugito, A. M., Folkow, B.,

Öberg, B., White, S. W. 1970. A comparison of blood viscosity measured in vitro and in a vascular bed. *Acta Physiol. Scand.* 78:70–84

48. Dobbins, W. O., Rollins, E. L. 1970. Intestinal mucosal lymphatic permeability. An electron microscopic study of endothelial vesicles and cell junctions. *J. Ultrastruct. Res.* 33:29–59

49. Duling, B. R., Berne, R. M. 1970. Longitudinal gradients in periarterial oxygen tension in the hamster cheek pouch. *Fed. Proc.* 29:320

50. Duling, B. R., Berne, R. M. 1970. Propagated vasodilation in the microcirculation of the hamster cheek pouch. *Circ. Res.* 26:163–70

51. Eriksson, E., Lisander, B. 1972. Changes in precapillary resistance in sketetal muscle vessels studied by intravital microscopy. *Acta Physiol. Scand.* 84:295–305

52. Fitz-Gerald, J. M. 1969. Implications of a theory of erythrocyte motion in narrow capillaries. *J. Appl. Physiol.* 27:912–918

53. Folkow, B., Mellander, S. 1970. Measurements of capillary filtration coefficient and its use in studies of the control of capillary exchange. In *Capillary Permeability*, ed. C. Crone, N. A. Lassen, 614–23. New York: Academic. 681 pp.

54. Folkow, B., Sonnenschein, R. R., Wright, D. L. 1971. Loci of neurogenic and metabolic effects on precapillary vessels of skeletal muscle. *Acta Physiol. Scand.* 81:459–71

55. Frasher, W. G., Jr., Wayland, H. 1972. A repeating modular organization of the microcirculation of cat mesentery. *Microvasc. Res.* 4:62–76

56. Friederici, H. H. 1969. On the diaphragm across fenestrae of capillary endothelium. *J. Ultrastruct. Res.* 27:373–75

57. Friedman, J. J. 1971. [86]RB extraction as an indicator of capillary flow. *Circ. Res.* 28: Suppl. 1, 15–20

58. Friedman, J. J. 1972. Comparison of the volumetric and osmometric methods for estimating transcapillary fluid movement. *Fed. Proc.* 31:365

59. Fung, Y. C., Perrone, N., Anliker, M. 1972. *Biomechanics—Its Foundation and Objectives*. Englewood Cliffs, New Jersey: Prentice-Hall. 641 pp.

60. Fung, Y. C., Zweifach, B. W. 1971. Microcirculation: Mechanics of blood flow in capillaries. *Ann. Rev. Fluid Mech.* 3:189–210

61. Gaehtgens, P., Meiselman, H. J., Wayland, H. 1970. Erythrocyte flow velocities in mesenteric microvessels of the cat. *Microvasc. Res.* 2:151–62

62. Gaehtgens, P., Meiselman, H. J., Wayland, H. 1970. Velocity profiles of human blood at normal and reduced hematocrit in glass tubes up to 130μ diameter. *Microvasc. Res.* 2:13–23

63. Garlick, D. G., Renkin, E. M. 1970. Transport of large molecules from plasma to interstitial fluid and lymph in dogs. *Am. J. Physiol.* 219:1595–1605

64. Goldsmith, H. C. 1971. Deformation of human red cells in tube flow. *Biorheology* 7:235–42

65. Goldstone, J., Schmid-Schönbein, H., Wells, R. E., Jr. 1970. The rheology of red blood cell aggregates. *Microvasc. Res.* 2:273–86

66. Gore, R. W. 1972. Wall stress: A determinant of regional differences in response of frog microvessels to norepinephrine. *Am. J. Physiol.* 222:82–91

67. Goresky, C. A., Ziegler, W. H., Bach, G. G. 1970. Barrier-limited distribution of diffusible substances from the capillaries in a well-perfused organ. In *Capillary Permeability*, ed. C. Crone, N. A. Lassen, 171–84. New York: Academic. 681 pp.

68. Gosselin, R. E., Audino, L. F. 1971. Muscle blood flow and functional capillary density evaluated by isotope clearance. *Pfluegers Arch.* 322:197–216

69. Grant, R. T., Wright, H. P. 1970. Anatomical basis for non-nutritive circulation in sketetal muscle exemplified by blood vessels of rat biceps femoris

tendon. *J. Anat.* 106:125–33

70. Guyton, A. C., Granger, H. J., Taylor, A. 1971. Interstitial fluid pressure. *Physiol. Rev.* 51: 527–63

71. Hammersen, F. 1970. The terminal vascular bed in skeletal muscle with special regard to the problem of shunts. In *Capillary Permeability*, ed. C. Crone, N. A. Lassen, 351–65. New York: Academic. 681 pp.

72. Hantos, Z., Lazar, Z. 1970. The flow of fluid through the wall of capillary systems studied by a mathematical model. *Acta Physiol. Budapest* 38:265–80

73. Hauck, G. 1969. Zur Frage der Existenz eines "gradient of vascular permeability" an der Endstrombahn. *Arch. Kreislaufforsch.* 59:197–227

74. Hauck, G. 1970. Modern fluorescent technic for cutaneous microcirculatory studies. *Arch. Klin. Exp. Dermatol.* 237:371–77

75. Hauck, G. 1971. Physiology of blood and lymph. *Angiologica* 8:129–275

76. Hauck, G. 1971. Physiology of the microvascular system. *Angiologica* 8:236–60

77. Hauck, G., Schröer, H. 1971. Importance of lymph drainage for the fluid balance of the tissue spaces. *6th Eur. Conf. Microcirc.*, ed. J. Ditzel, D. H. Lewis, 203–6. Basel, Switzerland: Karger. 451 pp.

78. Hesse, B. 1971. Tissue pressure variations measured by a miniature balloon technique. *Scand. J. Clin. Lab. Invest.* 27:139–44

79. Honig, C. R., Frierson, J. L., Nelson, C. N. 1972. O_2 transport and VO_2 in resting muscle: Significance for tissue-capillary exchange. *Am. J. Physiol.* 220: 357–63

80. Honig, C. R., Frierson, J. L., Patterson, J. L. 1970. Comparison of neural controls of resistance and capillary density in resting muscle. *Am. J. Physiol.* 218: 937–42

81. Hyman, C. 1971. Independent control of nutritional and shunt circulation. *Microvasc. Res.* 3; 89–94

82. Illig, L. 1970. Development of microcirculatory research in general and in dermatology. *Arch. Klin. Exp. Dermatol.* 237:350–56

83. Intaglietta, M., Pawula, R. F., Tompkins, W. R. 1970. Pressure measurements in the mammalian microvasculature. *Microvasc. Res.* 2:212–20

84. Intaglietta, M., Richardson, D. R., Tompkins, W. R. 1971. Blood pressure, flow, and elastic properties in microvessels of cat omentum. *Am. J. Physiol.* 221: 922–28

85. Intaglietta, M., Tompkins, W. R. 1972. On-line measurement of microvascular dimensions by television microscopy. *J. Appl. Physiol.* 32:546–51

86. Intaglietta, M., Tompkins, W. R. 1972. On-line microvascular blood cell flow velosity measurement by simplified correlation technique. *Circ. Res.* 4: 217–20

87. Intaglietta, M., Tompkins, W. R., Richardson, D. R. 1970. Velocity measurements in the microvasculature of the cat omentum by on-line method. *Microvasc. Res.* 2:462–73

88. Intaglietta, M., Zweifach, B. W. 1971. Geometrical model of the microvasculature of rabbit omentum from in vivo measurements. *Circ. Res.* 28:593–600

89. Intaglietta, M., Zweifach, B. W. 1971. Measurement of blood plasma colloid osmotic pressure I. Technical aspects. *Microvasc. Res.* 3:72–82

90. Johnson, P. C. 1971. Red cell separation in the mesenteric capillary network. *Am. J. Physiol.* 221:99–104

91. Johnson, P. C., Blaschke, J., Burton, K. S., Dial, J. H. 1971. Influence of flow variations on capillary hematocrit in mesentery. *Am. J. Physiol.* 221:105–112

92. Jonsson, J. A., Arfors, K. E., Hint, H. C. 1971. Studies on relationship between the blood and lymphatic systems within the microcirculation. In *6th Eur. Conf. Microcirc.*, ed. J. Ditzel,

D. H. Lewis, 214–18. Basel, Switzerland: Karger, 451 pp.

93. Jonsson, O. 1970. Extracellular osmolality and vascular smooth muscle activity. *Acta Physiol. Scand., Suppl.* 359:5–48

94. Karnovsky, M. J. 1970. Morphology of capillaries with special reference to muscle capillaries. *Capillary Permeability*, ed. C. Crone, N. A. Lassen. New York: Academic. 681 pp.

95. Karnovsky, M. J., Shea, S. M. 1970. Transcapillary transport by pinocytosis. *Microvasc. Res.* 2:353–60

96. Kirsch, K., Rafflenbeul, W., Roedel, H. 1971. Untersuchungen zur Ursache des negativen interstitiellen Gewebsdruckes (Guyton-Kapsel). *Pfluegers Arch.* 328:193–204

97. Kobayashi, S. 1970. Ferritin labeling in the fixed muscle capillary. A doubt on the tracer-experiments as the basis for the vesicular transport theory. *Arch. Histol. Jap.* 32:81–86

98. Kuprianov, V. V., Kozlov, V. I. 1971. Dynamic structures of the microvascular bed. *Microvasc. Res.* 3:22–34

99. Lagegaard-Pedersen, H. J. 1970. Measurement of the interstitial pressure in subcutaneous tissue in dogs. *Circ. Res.* 26:765–70

100. Landis, E. M., Sage, L. E. 1971. Fluid movement rates through walls of single capillaries exposed to hypertonic solutions. *Am. J. Physiol.* 221:520–34

101. Lassen, N. A. 1967. On the theory of the local clearance method for measurement of blood flow including a discussion of its application to various tissues. *Acta Med. Scand., Suppl.* 472:136–45

102. Lassen, N. A., Trap-Jensen, J. 1970. Estimation of the fraction of the inter-endothelial slit which must be open in order to account for the observed transcapillary exchange of small hydrophilic molecules in skeletal muscle in man. In *Capillary Permeability*, ed. C. Crone, N. A. Lassen, 647–53. New York: Academic. 681 pp.

103. Lassen, N. A., Trap-Jensen, J. 1970. On the validity of the indicator dilution method for measuring capillary diffusion capacity for ^{51}Cr-EDTA in hyperemic skeletal muscle. *Eur. J. Clin. Invest.* 1:118–23

104. Laurent, T. C., 1970. The structure and function of the intercellular polysaccharides in connective tissue. In *Capillary Permeability*, ed. C. Crone, N. A. Lassen, 261–77. New York: Academic. 681 pp.

105. Lawson, W. H., Jr., Forster, R. E. 1967. Oxygen tension gradients in peripheral capillary blood. *J. Appl. Physiol.* 22:970–73

106. Leaf, N., Zarem, H. A. 1970. Construction and use of a miniaturized rabbit ear chamber. *Microvasc. Res.* 2:72–85

107. Leak, L. V. 1970. Electron microscopic observations on lymphatic capillaries and the structural components of the connective tissue-lymph interface. *Microvasc. Res.* 2:361–91

108. Leblond, P. F., Lacelle, P. L., Weed, R. I. 1971. Cellular deformability: A possible determinant of the normal release of maturing erythrocytes from the bone marrow. *Blood* 37:40–46

109. Lee, J. S., Fronek, A. 1970. An analysis on the exchange of indicators in single capillaries. *Microvasc. Res.* 2:302–18

110. Lee, J. S., Fung, Y. C. 1969. Modeling experiments of a single red blood cell moving in a capillary blood vessel. *Microvasc. Res.* 1:221–43

111. Lee, J. S., Smaje, L. H., Zweifach, B. W. 1971. Fluid movement in occluded single capillaries of rabbit omentum. *Circ. Res.* 28:358–70

112. Lemmingson, W. 1971. Distribution of blood flow in the retina during hemorrhagic shock. In *6th Eur. Conf. on Microcirc.*, ed. J. Ditzel, D. H. Lewis, 106–9. Basel, Switzerland: Karger. 451 pp.

113. Levick, J. R., Michel, C. C. 1969. The passage of T1824-albumin out of individually perfused capillaries of the frog mesen-

tery. *J. Physiol. London* 202: 114–15P

114. Levick, J. R., Michel, C. C. 1970. The effect of bovine albumin on the permeability of frog mesenteric capillaries. *J. Physiol. London* 210:36–37P

115. Levick, J. R., Michel, C. C. 1971. A densitometric method for estimating the filtration coefficient of frog mesenteric capillaries. *J. Physiol. London* 218:25–26P

116. Lew, H. S., Fung, Y. C. 1969. Flow in an occluded circular cylindrical tube with permeable wall. *Z. angew. Math. Phy.* 20:750–66

117. Lew, H. S., Fung, Y. C. 1970. Plug effect of erythrocytes in capillary blood vessels. *Biophys. J.* 10:80–99.

118. McCabe, M. 1972. The diffusion coefficient of caffeine through agar gels containing a hyaluronic acid-protein complex. A model system for the study of the permeability of connective tissues. *Biochem. J.* 127:249–53

119. Malcolm, R., Bicher, H. I., Duncan, R. C., Knisely, M. H. 1972. Behavioral effects of erythrocyte aggregation. *Microvasc. Res.* 4:94–97

120. Maricq, H. R. 1970. "Wide-Field" photography of nailfold capillary bed and a scale of plexus visualization scores. *Microvasc. Res.* 2:335–340

121. Marquart, K.-H., Caesar, R. 1970. Quantitative study of the so-called pinocytic vesicles in the capillary endothelium. *Virchows Arch. B* 6:220–33

122. Meiselman, H. J., Frasher, W. G., Jr., Wayland, H. 1972. The effects of fibrination on the in vivo rheology of dog blood. *Microvasc. Res.* 4:26–44

123. Mellander, S., Lundvall, J. 1971. Role of tissue hyperosmolality in exercise hyperemia. *Circ. Res.* 28: Suppl. 1, 39–45

124. Mendler, N., Schröck, R. 1972. Osmotic properties of macromolecular solutions and gels—Physical aspects and physiological relevance. In *Hemodilution*, ed. K. Messmer, H. Schmid-Schönbein, 105–17. Basel, Switzerland: Karger. 322 pp.

125. Messmer, K., Schmid-Schönbein, H. 1972. *Hemodilution*. Basel, Switzerland: Karger. 322 pp.

126. Metzger, H., Erdmann, W., Thews, G. 1971. Effect of short periods of hypoxia, hyperoxia, and hypercapnia on brain O_2 supply. *J. Appl. Physiol.* 31: 751–59

127. Michel, C. C. 1970. Direct observations of sites of permeability to ions and small molecules in mesothelium. In *Capillary Permeability*, ed. C. Crone, N. A. Lassen, 628–42. New York: Academic. 681 pp.

128. Michel, C. C., Baldwin, R., Levick, J. R. 1969. Cannulation, perfusion and pressure measurements in single capillaries in the frog mesentery. *Proc. Brit. Microcirc. Soc.* 28–32

129. Moore, J. C., Baker, C. H. 1971. Red cell and albumin flow circuits during skeletal muscle reactive hyperemia. *Am. J. Physiol.* 220:1213–19

130. Murakami, T. 1971. Application of the scanning electron microscope to the study of the fine distribution of the blood vessels. *Arch. Histol. Jap.* 32:445–54

131. Neufeld, G. R., Marshall, B. 1970. Application of Z transform method in the analysis of indicator dilution data. *Proc. Eng. Med. Biol.* 12:3

132. Nicoll, P. A. 1969. Intrinsic regulation in the microcirculation based on direct pressure measurements. In *The Microcirculation*, ed. W. L. Winters, A. N. Brest, 89–101. Springfield, Ill: C. C. Thomas. 195 pp.

133. Oka, S., Azuma, T. 1970. Physical theory of tension in thick-walled blood vessels in equilibrium. *Biorheology* 7:109–17

134. Oka, S., Murata, T. 1970. A theoretical study of the flow of blood in a capillary with permeable wall. *Jap. J. Appl. Phys.* 9: 345–52

135. Perl, W. 1971. Modified filtration permeability model of transcapillary transport—a solution of the Pappenheimer pore puzzler? *Microvasc. Res.* 3:233–251

136. Prather, J. W., Bowes, D. N., Warrell, D. A., Zweifach, B. W. 1971. Comparison of capsule

and wick techniques for measurement of interstitial fluid pressure. *J. Appl. Physiol.* 31: 942–45

137. Radawski, D., Dabney, J. M., Daugherty, R. M., Jr., Haddy, F. J., Scott, J. B. 1972. Local effects of CO_2 on vascular resistances and weight of the dog forelimb. *Am. J. Physiol.* 222: 439–443

138. Rand, P. W., Wilkinson, A. F., Lacombe, E., Barker, N. 1970. An electrode-containing rabbit ear chamber for microvascular measurements. *Microvasc. Res.* 2:508–19

139. Reneau, D. D., Bruley, D. F., Knisely, M. H. 1969. A digital simulation of transient oxygen transport in capillary-tissue systems. *Am. Inst. Chem. Eng.* 15: 916–25

140. Renkin, E. M. 1971. The nutritional-shunt-flow hypothesis in skeletal muscle circulation. *Circ. Res.* 28: Suppl. 1, 21–25

141. Renkin, E. M., Garlick, D. G. 1970. Blood-lymph transport of macramolecules. *Microvasc. Res.* 2:392–98

142. Reichel, A. 1970. Comparative investigations of plasma and lymph in the frog—a qualitative approach to the blood-lymph transfer of proteins. *Acta Physiol. Budapest* 37:1–17

143. Reichel, A. 1971. Vergleichende Untersuchung zwischen der Migration von Plasmaprotein-Fraktionen in kunstlichen molekulariebenden Gelen und ihrem Transfer durch die Blut-Lymph-Schranke. *Pfluegers Arch.* 323:310–14

144. Richardson, D. R., Intaglietta, M., Zweifach, B. W. 1971. Simultaneous pressure and flow velocity measurements in the microcirculation. *Microvasc. Res.* 3:69–71

145. Richardson, D. R., Zweifach, B. W. 1970. Pressure relationships in the macro- and microcirculation of the mesentery. *Microvasc. Res.* 2:474–88

146. Rodbard, S. 1971. Capillary control of blood flow and fluid exchange. *Circ. Res.* 28: Suppl. 1, 51–58

147. Rodbard, S., Handel, N., Sadja, L.

148. Rosenberg, A., Guth, P. H. 1970. A method for the in vivo study of the gastric microcirculation. *Microvasc. Res.* 2:111–12

149. Rosenblum, W. I. 1970. Effects of blood pressure and blood viscosity on fluorescein transit time in the cerebral microcirculation in the mouse. *Circ. Res.* 27:825–33

150. Rosenblum, W. I. 1970. The differential effect of elevated blood viscosity on plasma and erythrocyte flow in the cerebral microcirculation of the mouse. *Microvasc. Res.* 2:399–408

151. Rosenblum, W. I. 1971. Effects of reduced hematocrit on erythrocyte velocity and fluorescein transit time in the cerebral microcirculation of the mouse. *Circ. Res.* 29:96–103

152. Rosenblum, W. I. 1971. Erythrocyte velocity and fluorescein transit time in the cerebral microcirculation of macroglobinemic mice: differential effect of a hyperviscosity syndrome on the passage of erythrocytes and plasma. *Microvasc. Res.* 3:288–96

153. Rosenblum, W. I. 1972. Ratio of red cell velocities near the vessel wall to velocities at the vessel center in cerebral microcirculation, and an apparent effect of blood viscosity on this ratio. *Microvasc. Res.* 4:98–107

154. Rowlands, S., Skibo, L. 1971. Erythrocyte flow in capillary tubes. *Can. J. Physiol. Pharmacol.* 49:373–74

155. Sachs, R. G., Hanley, H. G., Skinner, N. S., Jr. 1971. K⁺ osmolality and subcutaneous adipose tissue blood flow. *Pfluegers Arch.* 327:337–48

156. Schmid-Schönbein, H., Wells, R. E., Jr. 1971. Rheological properties of human erythrocytes and their influence upon the "anomalous" viscosity of blood. *Ergeb. Physiol., Biol. Chem. Exp. Pharmakol.* 63: 146–74

157. Scott, J. B., Daugherty, R. M., Jr., Haddy, F. J. 1967. Effect of severe local hypoxemia on trans-

capillary water movement in dog forelimb. *Am. J. Physiol.* 212:847–51

158. Scott, J. B., Radawski, D. 1971. Role of hyperosmolarity in the genesis of active and reactive hyperemia. *Circ. Res.* 28: Suppl. 1, 26–32

159. Scott, J. B. et al 1970. Role of osmolarity, K^+, H^+, Mg^{++}, and O_2 in local blood flow regulation. *Am. J. Physiol.* 218: 338–45

160. Sejrsen, P. 1970. Convection and diffusion of inert gases in cutaneous, subcutaneous, and skeletal muscle tissue. In *Capillary Permeability*, ed. C. Crone, N. A. Lassen, 586–596. New York: Academic. 681 pp.

161. Seshadri, V., Hockmuth, R. M., Croce, P. A., Sutera, S. P. 1970. Capillary blood flow III. Deformable model cells compared to erythrocytes in vitro. *Microvasc. Res.* 2:434–42

162. Shapiro, H. M., Stromberg, D. D., Lee, D. R., Wiederhielm, C. A. 1971. Dynamic pressures in the pial arterial microcirculation. *Am. J. Physiol.* 221:279–83

163. Shea, S. M. 1971. Lanthanum staining of the surface coat of cells. *J. Cell Biol.* 51:611–20

164. Sheehan, R. M., Renkin, E. M. 1972. Capillary, interstitial and cell membrane barriers to blood-tissue transport of potassium and rubidium in mammalian skeletal muscle. *Circ. Res.* 30:588–607

165. Shirahama, T., Cohen, A. S. 1972. The role of mucopolysaccharides in vesicle architecture and endothelial transport. An electron microscope study of myocardial blood vessels. *J. Cell Biol.* 52:198–206

166. Siggins, G. R., Weitsen, H. A. 1971. Cytochemical and physiological evidence for cholinergic, neurogenic vasodilation of amphibian arterioles and precapillary sphincters. *Microvasc. Res.* 3:308–22

167. Skalak, R., Brånemark, P.-I. 1969. Deformation of red blood cells in capillaries. *Science* 164: 717–19

168. Skinner, N. S., Jr., Costin, J. C. 1971. Interactions between oxygen, potassium, and osmolality in regulation of skeletal muscle blood flow. *Circ. Res.* 28: Suppl. 1, 73–85

169. Smaje, L. H., Zweifach, B. W., Intaglietta, M. 1970. Micropressures and capillary filtration coefficients in single vessels of the cremaster muscle of the rat. *Microvasc. Res.* 2:96–110

170. Smith, A. L., Neufeld, G. R., Ominsky, A. J., Wollman, H. 1972. Effect of arterial CO_2 tension on cerebral blood flow, mean transit time and vascular volume. *J. Appl. Physiol.* 31: 701–07

171. Smith, V., Ryan, J. W., Michie, D. D., Smith, D. S. 1971. Endothelial projections as revealed by scanning electron microscopy. *Science* 173:925–27

172. Snashall, P. D., Lucas, J., Guz, A., Floyer, M. A. 1971. Measurement of interstitial 'fluid' pressure by means of a cotton wick in man and animals: An analysis of the origin of the pressure. *Clin. Sci.* 41:35–53

173. Sobin, S. S., Tremer, H. M., Fung, Y. C. 1970. Morphometric basis of the sheet-flow concept of the pulmonary alveolar microcirculation in the cat. *Circ. Res.* 26:397–414

174. Stoltz, J. F., Larcan, A. 1970. Theoretical aspects concerning microcirculation rheology apropos of a capillary model. *Agressologie* 11:111–18

175. Stromberg, D. D., Lee, D. R., Wiederhielm, C. A. 1972. Interstitial oncotic pressures measured by implanted membrane osmometers. *Fed. Proc.* 31:365

176. Stromberg, D. D., Wiederhielm, C. A. 1970. Effects of oncotic gradients and enzymes on negative pressures in implanted capsules. *Am. J. Physiol.* 219:928–32

177. Studer, R., Potchen, J. 1971. The radioisotopic assessment of regional microvascular permeability to macromolecules. *Microvasc. Res.* 3:35–48

178. Sutera, S. P., Seshadri, V., Croce, P. A., Hochmuth, R. M. 1970. Capillary blood flow II. Deformable model cells in tube flow. *Microvasc. Res.* 2:420–33

179. Svanes, K., Zweifach, B. W., Inta-glietta, M. 1970. Effect of hypo-thermia on transcapillary fluid exchange. *Am. J. Physiol.* 218: 981–89

180. Takeda, M. 1969. Fenestrated capillaries seen in most organs of the digestive system. *Nagoya Med. J.* 15:29–32

181. Tashiro, K. 1970. Microangio-graphic study of the microcircu-latory system of the lingual mu-cosa, especially of the lingual papillae in the dog. *J. Otolaryn-gol. Jap.* 73:800–10

182. Tesi, D., Forssmann, W. G. 1971. Permeability studies with the interstitial tissues of the rat mesentery. *Pfluegers Arch.* 322: 188–91

183. Thuning, C. A., Buerk, D. G. 1972. Some factors affecting the transient cylindrical diffusion of oxygen in an artificial capillary model and comparisons with in vivo data. *Microvasc. Res.* 4: 13–25

184. Tickner, E. G. 1972. Concentra-tion effects on viscosity in mod-els of blood flow through capil-laries. *Microvasc. Res.* 4:102–4

185. Trap-Jensen, J., Korsgaard, O., Lassen, N. A. 1970. Capillary permeability to human skeletal muscle measured by local in-jection of ^{51}Cr-EDTA and ^{133}XE. *Scand. J. Clin. Lab. In-vest.* 25:93–99

186. Trap-Jensen, J., Lassen, N. A. 1971. Restricted diffusion in skeletal muscle capillaries in man. *Am. J. Physiol.* 220:371–76

187. Vacek, L. et al 1970. Mesenteric microcirculation in the rat, the P-phenomenon. *Sb. Ved. Pr. Lek. Fak. Karlovy Univ.* 13: 293–294

188. Voitkevich, A. A. Dedov, I. I. 1969. Pericapillary space—a zone of functional mediation between blood and tissue cells. *Arkh. Anat. Gistol. Embriol.* 57:3–15

189. Voitkevich, A. A., Dedov, I. I. 1969. Subendothelial spaces of capillary blood vessels. *Dokl. Akad. Nauk. SSSR.* 186:697–700

190. Wagner, E. P., Jr., Goldstick, T. K. 1971. Oxygen pathways in skeletal muscle: Nonlinear re-sponse to hyperoxia. *Proc. Ann. Conf. Eng. Med. Biol.* 13:16

191. Wahl, M., Deetjen, P., Thurau, K., Ingvar, D. H., Lassen, N. A. 1970. Micropuncture evaluation of the importance of perivascu-lar pH for the arteriolar di-ameter on the brain surface. *Pfluegers Arch.* 316:152-63

192. Weed, R. I. 1970. The importance of erythrocyte deformability. *Am. J. Med.* 49:147–50

193. Weiner, R., Kaley, G. 1969. Influ-ence of prostaglandin E_1 on the terminal vascular bed. *Am. J. Physiol.* 217:563–66

194. Wells, R. E., Jr. 1970. Syndromes of hyperviscosity. *N. Engl. J. Med.* 283:183–86

195. Wiederhielm, C. A. 1968. Dynam-ics of transcapillary fluid ex-change. *J. Gen. Physiol.* 52:29–63

196. Wiederhielm, C. A. 1969. Physio-logic characteristics of small vessels. In *The Microcircula-tion,* ed. W. L. Winters, A. N. Brest, 75–88. Springfield, Ill.: Thomas. 195 pp.

197. Wiederhielm, C. A. 1972. The in-terstitial space. In *Biomechanics Its Foundations and Objectives,* ed. Y. C. Fung, N. Perrone, M. Anliker, 273–86. Englewood Cliffs, New Jersey: Prentice-Hall. 641 pp.

198. Wisse, E. 1970. An electron micro-scopic study of the fenestrated endothelial lining of rat liver si-nusoids. *J. Ultrastruct. Res.* 31: 125–50

199. Witte, S., Goldenberg, D. M., Schricker, K. T. 1968. The propagation of fluorescent dyes in the hamster cheek pouch. *Z. Gesamte Exp. Med.* 148:72–80

200. Witte, C. L., Witte, M. H., Du-mont, A. E. 1971. Significance of protein in edema fluids. *Lymphology* 4:29–31

201. Ziegler, W. H., Goresky, C. A. 1971. Transcapillary exchange in the working left ventricle of the dog. *Circ. Res.* 29:181–207

202. Zweifach, B. W. 1969. Small blood vessel dynamics. In *Dy-namics of Thrombus Formation and Dissolution,* ed. S. A. John-son, M. M. Guest, 45. Philadel-phia: Lippincott, 376 pp.

203. Zweifach, B. W. 1971. Local regulation of capillary pressure. *Circ. Res.* 28, 29: Suppl. 1, 129–34
204. Zweifach, B. W., Intaglietta, M. 1969. Mechanics of fluid movement across single capillaries in the rabbit. *Microvasc. Res.* 1: 83–101
205. Zweifach, B. W., Intaglietta, M. 1971. Measurement of blood plasma colloid osmotic pressure II. Comparative study of different species. *Microvasc. Res.* 3: 83–88
206. Zweifach, B. W., Prather, J. W. 1971. Pressures in the terminal lymphatics of mesentery. *Fed. Proc.* 30:M20
207. Zweifach, B. W., Richardson, D. R. 1971. Microcirculatory adjustments of pressure in the mesentery. In *6th Eur. Conf. Microcirc.*, ed. J. Ditzel, D. H. Lewis, 248–53. Basel, Switzerland: Karger. 451 pp.

Ann. Rev. Physiol. 1973. 35:151–168

LOCAL CONTROL OF REGIONAL BLOOD FLOW 1092

WENDELL N. STAINSBY[1]

Department of Physiology, College of Medicine
University of Florida, Gainesville, Florida

Preliminary examination of the literature during the current year showed a large number of reports dealing with nervous control of many vascular regions. These reports appeared to be mainly descriptive: an anatomy lesson. Making an arbitrary decision to cover a different aspect of the circulation, I began a search for information about local control mechanisms—an area which seemed controversial and in need of critical review. The search was frustrating. Rather little research into local control mechanisms has been very probing, and new ideas seem to be few relative to the amount of experimentation. My intent is to review recent research on these mechanisms, and to suggest some problems for future investigation. This review is far from exhaustive and I apologize for omission of important reports. Further, I am sure my views are biased because of long experience with mammalian skeletal muscle. If this bias shows, it is unintentional.

SKELETAL AND CARDIAC MUSCLE

Comparisons of circulatory control in "red" and "white" skeletal muscle have not been made recently. The reports reviewed seem to apply equally for circulations in both skeletal and cardiac muscle and are, therefore, lumped together.

There have been some interesting studies of coronary flow in intact conscious baboons and dogs (94, 95). One study showed that in the resting animal coronary flow seemed to vary with the metabolic rate (94); it followed heart rate, blood pressure, and other variables, which have previously been associated with changes in myocardial oxygen uptake. In addition, there were periods of spontaneous coronary dilatation not associated with visible changes that would alter oxygen uptake. These responses were thought to be due to neural control. When the animal was running, coronary flow again varied with factors affecting oxygen uptake, with heart rate most important, and blood pressure and changes in myocardial contractility less so (95).

In a recent study of the effects of changes in venous blood Pco_2 and pH

[1] Supported in part by Grant GM 6264-13 from the National Institutes of Health.

151

on blood flow in dog skeletal muscle, a linear decrease in resistance occurred when pH decreased from 7.4–6.7 (62). The authors reported a similar decrease to increasing Pco_2 in the range of 30–100 mm Hg and noted that the response was similar to but smaller than that observed in man. In view of the small dose of heparin used in these pump-perfusion experiments (3000–4000 units[2] or about 2 mg/kg), and from my own experience with perfusions using dog blood, this dose is about a tenth the dose needed to keep blood even reasonably free of microemboli. Since the effect of such embolization has never been considered experimentally by anyone, I wonder what effect it must have had on the results. Another study on foreleg suggested that change in pH and Pco_2 had only a small effect in this preparation (76), with the response somewhat greater in skin than in muscle. No mention was made of how these effects were mediated.

Studies on the role of adenosine in control of coronary flow have continued and have been extended into skeletal muscle (14, 26). Vessels in skeletal muscle respond similarly to those in cardiac muscle, except that the former dilate with lower concentrations of adenosine (26). This study also suggests that ATP, ADP, AMP, and Pi have little function in reactive hyperemia or active hyperemia. The same has been suggested for Pi in the human forearm (8). An interesting aspect of the study on dog muscle (26) is that the adenosine concentration in the sartorius muscle was measured only during ischemia and when muscle was not contracting.[3]

The role of adenosine in the regulation of coronary flow has been questioned by Bittar & Pauly because in their experiments lidoflazine increased the response to infused adenosine but did not alter the response to reactive hyperemia (15). These authors also reported that aminophyllin decreased the response to infused adenosine but did not decrease the response to reactive hyperemia. It is still necessary to prove that these drugs reach the active sites, but the question is clear. The role of adenosine in active hyperemia is also questionable. The adenosine system proposed (14, 26) assumes that ATP concentration decreases during contractions creating an increase in ADP, AMP, and, therefore, adenosine in the muscles. There is no evidence to support this assumption since it seems that ATP concentration is constant under most conditions of contraction [for example, see (75)]. There is need for further critical research in this area.

Blood oxygen tension has again been reported to act directly on blood vessels in dogs (5). This report is of complex, straight and crossed, perfusion experiments with only 3 mg/kg heparin and vascular beds which seem passive to changes in flow. The presence of responses to hyperoxia and hypoxia at a time when autoregulation to flow change was absent is the first example I have seen reported of separation of two sorts of local control, although I

---

[2] H. A. Kontos, personal communication. The values are not given in the report.

[3] R. M. Berne, personal communication.

have heard such separation reported at meetings. The possible effect of micro-embolization must again be considered. The relationship between the presence of autoregulation to a change in perfusion pressure and the presence of responses to change in oxygen concentration has not been examined; it was not mentioned in a discussion of flow control mechanisms in skeletal muscle during exercise which favors direct control by oxygen (9).

In a recent investigation of the interaction of constrictor and dilator mechanisms in muscle vasculature (21) a basic resemblance can be seen to the autoregulatory escape seen in the intestinal vascular bed. A study of the loci of action of some neurogenic and metabolic effects on precapillary vessels (31) has shown that the local metabolic effects are apparently on vessels closest to the capillaries, being largely in the precapillary sphincter areas, while the neurogenic effects are further upstream, in the arterioles. This is not the first report of such an arrangement but it is presented more definitively here. In another interesting study of this sort, it was found that the largest change of vessel diameter with constriction and dilatation occurred in vessels about 30 μ in diameter; the relative size of the diameter change decreased as the vessels become larger or smaller (28).

Perfusion heterogeneity (74), arteriovenous anastomoses (89), and functional capillary density (42) have been examined; although these all seem to be problems related to control of metabolism-perfusion ratios, their names sound as if they were quite different. Heterogeneity measured using tritiated water was worsened by pump perfusion (74). Arteriovenous anastomoses were reported to be under extrinsic control (89). And it was suggested that perhaps the permeability P of PS (permeability $\times$ surface area) can be estimated by using ^{133}Xe and ^{131}I simultaneously (42). None of these reports has suggested that the matching of metabolism and perfusion in individual capillaries is associated with the broader picture of local control responses. Muscle is a risky tissue to study by indicator washin or washout. Simple passive stretch has been shown to destroy the relationship between flow calculated from ^{133}Xe clearance and measured flow (40). I can only imagine what contractions or other procedures might do to "stir" the contents of the muscle, and thereby invalidate some of the assumptions necessary for the clearance methods. Such methods are very popular but they have not been critically tested in muscle.

The distribution of flow in the coronary circulation has been assessed by ^{133}Xe washin (7). The left ventricle received more flow per gram of tissue than the right, and the endocardial half of the left ventricle wall was at least as well perfused as the epicardial portion. A similar study using microspheres gave generally similar results (12). In this study an effect of size of the spheres was noted, but I could not understand their explanation of this observation. They also reported the effects of nitroglycerine and propranolol on distribution of flow during ischemia. These drugs improved endocardial perfusion relative to epicardial perfusion. Usually endocardial perfusion decreased more during relative ischemia than did epicardial flow. The role of extravascular compression by the muscle of the heart was not discussed as a factor that might influence the effects of the drugs on flow distribution.

Radially applied tension was found to have little effect on microvessels until it became large (6). Externally applied hyperosmotic solutions produced relaxation of vascular smooth muscle, more in arterioles than venules (44). One interesting aspect of this study was the observation that the responses could not be clearly ascribed to changes in intracellular volume and intracellular-extracellular ion concentration. This in effect disagrees with a current suggestion (71) that the osmotic effects are the result of changes in intracellular K^+ concentration and the resulting membrane potential changes.

Active hyperemia has been reported to be greater in human legs when they are dependent than when they are horizontal (30) probably because of the changes in arterial pressure due to gravity. However, post contraction hyperemia was not changed by altering the position of the leg, probably because the muscle pump is equally effective during exercise whether the legs are dependent or horizontal. Post contraction, venous pressure is affected by gravity the same as is the arterial pressure. These explanations of these observations emphasize the importance of the venous pump.

There were a number of miscellaneous observations. Rabbit coronary vascular strips in vitro contracted when acetylcholine was added to the bath and when external potassium was increased (71). The results of such in vitro studies are often treated as though they indicated functions which are normal and relevant to local control of blood flow in vivo. Unfortunately, the unexpected response to acetylcholine is just one of the observations that suggests that studies of this nature should be considered with great care before the results are extrapolated to intact animals.

The resistance changes in flow through the gracilis muscle in responses to square pressure pulses suggest that the vessels respond only to increased pressure transients, and do so with a larger dilatation than can be accounted for on a passive mechanical basis (87). The author, therefore, proposes an active dilatation to sudden distension and he suggests that this response is separate from the steady-state response to pressure reported by Bayliss. The structure and dilator activity of prostaglandins (68) and the interaction of a few of the prostaglandins with other extrinsic vascular control systems (23, 53) have been assessed.

Harris & Longnecker have suggested that the local control responses of the precapillary vessels have a dual function (50): first, these vessels respond to regulate downstream capillary pressure to control capillary-tissue fluid exchange, and second, these vessels respond to regulate the delivery or removal of one or more tissue metabolites.

THE KIDNEY

Local control of blood flow in the dog kidney relative to changes in arterial and venous pressure has been examined carefully, and the results have been treated statistically (80). Such studies provide a solid background for other research in control of renal blood flow. A pulse pressure was found to be unnecessary in the kidney (85); pulseless perfusion lengthened urine transit time slightly, but did little else compared to normal pulsatile perfusion. Sinusoidal pressure perfusion at different frequencies has been reported to indicate a slow pressure regulating response with a cycle length of 1000 sec, in addition to flow autoregulation (61). The significance of this observation was not clear.

Although the past literature contains a few reports that autoregulation does not occur normally when artificial, non-plasma-containing perfusates are used, most of the knowledge in this area has only been passed around in the halls at meetings; such negative data too often end in a drawer and not in print. However, this negative suggestion has recently been repeated in print by Hysell & Bohr (57). These authors found long lasting increased resistance when plasma was added to artificial perfusate. Also interesting was the observation that essentially normal resistance was found when a Sephadex-separated protein-free fraction of plasma was added to the perfusate. Several familiar constrictor agents added to the perfusate instead of the protein-free fraction did not restore tone nearly as well. However, it has also been reported that pressure-induced changes in resistance to renal blood flow were the same as the responses reported previously for isolated kidneys perfused with a non-plasma-containing perfusate (54). The necessity for a substance or substances in plasma to be present in the perfusate before normal autoregulation will occur ought to have been clarified long ago in other tissues as well as the kidney.

Another problem is evident in the search for substances in renal venous effluent that might mediate postischemic hyperemia (47). When a leg was used as an assay organ, the postischemic venous effluent caused dilatation, but when a second kidney was used as the assay organ, constriction occurred. The authors suggested that adenosine may have been the effluent substance because it is one of few substances which cause constriction in the kidney and dilatation in legs. This may well be correct, but I suggest that the presence of a constrictor substance in the venous blood coming from a postischemic vaso-dilated kidney is quite remarkable. The question to be tested is whether anything in the venous blood is relevant to flow control in the organ that the venous blood came from.

Still another controversy concerns changes in distribution of blood flow within a kidney. The authors described a microsphere technique and reported that skimming of the spheres did not occur (86). But a comparison of microspheres and antiglomerular basement membrane antibody suggested clearly that microspheres were skimmed (97). A careful analysis of microsphere technique as well as indicator clearance methods has suggested that they need to be applied with great care (60). With these problems sometimes in mind, it has been reported that outer cortical flow decreases with decreased renal flow and perfusion pressure (64, 65, 86). Drug-induced dilatation also decreased outer cortical relative flow, but increased flow in deeper areas (90).

Increased venous pressure or ureteral pressure also shifted flow from outer to inner cortical areas (67). Dye curves from bolus injections directly into the renal artery have suggested that outer cortex has the greater flow (19). Acute denervation increased medullary flow most (13). Some of the distribution changes were not related to Na^+ excretion; this suggests that the two are not related (13, 97). Prostaglandin PGE_1 and acetylcholine increased inner and outer cortical flow, but not outer medullary flow which was constant (18). The unique circulation in the cat kidney allowed separate direct measurement of cortical and deep area flows (36); both were reported uniformly regulated.

In one study a "hyperoncotic" infusion upset the kidney's capacity to autoregulate (70) but the methods and data presented in this paper do not permit one to determine if the loss of autoregulation was more than might be expected simply because flow was elevated closer to maximal levels. In another study, the induction of hemorrhagic shock reduced intrarenal Po_2 severely (91), with much variation with time, place, and recovery. The authors suggested considerable vasomotion was occuring.

Falchuk & Berliner (29) have measured intrarenal pressures by careful micropuncture technique. The interstitial pressure was 5 mm Hg or less, lower than previously reported. Pressures in proximal tubule, peritubular capillaries, distal tubules, and star vessels changed with various experimental procedures, but the relative differences between different sites remained. Interstitial pressure was also measured using small porous capsules (73). The mean pressure found was 6 mm Hg, which is about the same as that in the micropuncture study mentioned above. These authors observed that interstitial pressure was only slightly affected by changes in arterial pressure, but a tenfold greater change was observed when venous pressure or ureteral pressures were altered. They suggested that interstitial pressure is "autoregulated" when arterial pressure is changed. It has been reported that renal size is autoregulated (20), and it seems appropriate that interstitial pressure and size go together.

Renin secretion was found to vary inversely with blood pressure, but was unrelated to [Na^+] in the macula densa (16). A new pressor agent of renal origin called nephrotensin was found in human kidneys when the renal artery was constricted or the kidney infarcted (46). It will be interesting to learn the significance of this substance.

The Brain

That autoregulation in the brain is indeed locally controlled has been reaffirmed. It is clearly present following acute sympathectomy and sympathetic blockers (98), and following chronic sympathectomy (27). Reactive hyperemia is brisk following ischemia, overpaying the flow debt maximally after 15 min of occlusion (99). Lesser overpayments were associated with shorter or longer occlusion periods. Examination of localized cerebral ischemia by direct observation and ^{85}Kr washout showed that flow decreased to

20–50% of control values in the core area for the occluded artery (92). During occlusion, flow was pressure-dependent in the core area. Correlation between flow and the visual dilatation was poor. "Luxury hyperemia" was seen and interpreted as the result of reactive hyperemia occurring simultaneously with reduced metabolism. Correlation between the hyperemia and the degree of preceding ischemia was poor. No failure of collateral circulation with time was observed. Cerebral edema was a chief cause of death during the experiments. It began during ischemia, was progressive and unrelated to the degree of ischemia, and continued during the hyperemia.

It has been reaffirmed that hypoxia produces dilatation of cerebral vessels (43). Light anesthesia with several agents allowed good responses to hypoxia, but deeper anesthesia with some agents reduced the response. Hypercapnia continues as it has for many years to produce good dilatation in the brain. The dilation during hypercapnia is faster and greater than the constriction during hypocapnia, and both responses are reported to be a direct effect of CO_2 on vascular smooth muscle (77). The response to CO_2 has also been reported to be indirect; the flow seemed to be better correlated with CSF pH than with blood pH (32, 33). Hypothalamic flow was also responsive to P_{CO_2} and seemed little affected by "baritone" anesthesia (22).

Renin has been found in the brains of nephrectomized dogs kept alive by hemodialysis (37). The authors suggested that the renin was synthesized in the brain.

THE GUT

When portions of the small intestine were tested with a sharp, sustained drop in perfusion pressure, resistance to blood flow fell immediately, then for 2–5 min decreased slowly and finally after a period of 10–30 min decreased further before becoming steady (48). The first drop in resistance was ascribed to a myogenic response related to the decrease in transmural pressure, the second drop was considered to be a metabolically linked mechanism, while the last phase, in view of measured changes in capillary filtration coefficient and water exchange, was thought to be the effect of a mechanism to regulate capillary pressure and hence transcapillary water exchange.

Measurement of gastric mucosal blood flow by an amidopyrine technique suggests that mucosal flow is dependent more upon acid secretion than on pepsin secretion (78). However, the flow was greater relative to H^+ output when there was pepsin secretion. Splanchnic nerve stimulation reduced motility, acid secretion, and blood flow, but not pepsin secretion. Later studies using a wide dose range of gastrin extracts, pentapeptide and histamine, further affirmed the relationship between blood flow and acid secretion (79). Deviations from this strong relationship appeared to be only transient. It is unfortunate that metabolic rate was not measured in these studies to see if it was an important determinant of flow in this tissue. Prostaglandins PGE_1 and PGA_1 have been shown to be potent vasodilators of gastric vessels in dogs (69).

When the upper gastrointestinal tract of the rat was isolated and perfused with an artificial perfusate, a large fraction of the flow passed through arteriovenous anastomoses (59). These observations are not in accord with earlier reports, and I suppose this is to be expected considering the methods used. Local control of flow distribution probably was disturbed, as were other aspects of local control of blood flow, when artificial perfusates were used. When such controls were absent loss of tone of all vessels apparently occurred. Under these conditions, a few large bore short vessels—arteriovenous anastomoses—could carry a large fraction of the flow. I question the significance of such studies beyond their showing the maximal capacity of the arteriovenous anastomoses and the increase in shunt flow when local control of flow is disturbed.

THE LUNG

The pulmonary circulation was studied in complex experiments on adult, newborn, and fetal lungs (45). The results in newborn and adult lungs did not present any new data. However, in contrast to earlier reports, the fetal lungs showed neither autoregulation when perfusion pressure was changed nor reactive hyperemia. It is possible that perfusion of the lungs with maternal rather than the fetus' own blood created this difference. If correct, this would seem to be an important observation. The effects of perfusion with the fetus' own blood and maternal blood should be compared directly.

Blood flow in the lungs of cats responded in a manner similar to that in muscle when blood osmolality was altered (52). A simple osmolar-related dilatation occurred with graded hyperosmolality except with glycerol, which penetrates cells rapidly. Hyperosmolality of the blood perfusing the lung decreased lung blood volume (17). The authors concluded that the capacitance vessels were constricted even though the resistance vessels were dilated.

Comparison of rat and cat lung responses to CO_2 breathing showed dilatation in rat lung blood vessels if the vascular tone was already high due to hypoxia (10). When tone was normal, breathing gas high in CO_2 produced weak constriction. The authors proposed a rather complex interaction of a direct vasodilator action of CO_2 itself with a vasoconstrictor action of carbonic acid. In the same report cat lungs showed consistent vasoconstriction in response to inhalation of CO_2 although the authors discussed the direct action of CO_2 as a dilator. The vessels of dog lungs have been reported to constrict with decreased pH, but the response was not believed to be due to pH changes alone (55).

Isolated pulmonary artery smooth muscle constricted in response to hypoxia and relaxed in response to increased O_2 (24). These responses to oxygen are the opposite of those seen for ductus arteriosus (66) and of those seen for systemic arterial smooth muscle. The meaning of studies of isolated vessels has already been discussed.

Perfusing the circulation of rat and guinea pig lungs with Krebs' solution containing angiotensin I or II resulted in the release of an unidentified myotropic substance (93). In addition, it was suggested that an inhibitory substance had been released.

The sites of vasomotor activity due to hypoxia, serotonin, and histamine were investigated using red cells as an indicator of capillary volume (41). For example, hypoxia decreased capillary volume; this was interpreted as indicating precapillary constriction which in turn reduced capillary pressure, and hence volume. Segmental resistances have been calculated for fetal lung (31). But the reasoning in these reports is oversimplified. Part of the problem, I think, lies in the inadvertent use of two very different models of the pulmonary circulation, the waterfall and the Starling resistor, as if they were essentially the same. They are not.

Confusion in using these models seems to be based on the fact that both show a range of operation over which changes in downstream pressure do not alter flow through the system. For example, raising the lower Niagara river fifty feet would not alter flow over Niagara Falls. Likewise, in a Starling resistor system, raising outflow pressure up to the level of pressure surrounding the collapsible part of the system does not alter flow through the system. This is the extent of the similarity. In a waterfall there is a break in the system. What occurs below the fall is irrelevant to what happens above the fall. As most waterfalls exist, flow is determined only by the pressure head at some point upstream, and the resistance to flow only to the edge of the fall. The relationship in a given waterfall between flow rate and pressure head is approximately linear and no minimal pressure is required to initiate flow; i.e., there is no minimal or critical pressure head (assuming the upper river bed is perfectly horizontal). Any difference in water level between upstream and the lip of its falls will produce flow. However, there is a minimal or critical pressure in a Starling resistor. Inflow pressure must exceed the surrounding pressure of the collapsible part of the system to open it partially before any flow can occur. The lung seems to work this way (39).

Visual inspection of a Starling resistor model in operation revealed that the partially collapsed portion does not always remain at the extreme distal end of the collapsible portion, and pressures measured within the collapsible portion were not always equal to or above the surrounding pressure [personal observation with S. Cassin of the model in (39)]. The intent here is not to tell how a Starling resistor changes its resistance, but to plead for the use of the correct model for flow in the lung and, since the Starling resistor seems more correct than a waterfall, for careful analysis of how a Starling resistor functions. I do not think the operation of a Starling resistor is well understood.

Sobin and associates have described in detail a modification of the basic Starling resistor to a "sheet" form as it applies to the cat lung (34, 35, 88). Their series of papers is very detailed and complex. The basic model appears to fit the lung better than a simple Starling resistor model. Smooth muscle activity seems to be missing from the model. I am not sure that all of the questions raised for the simple Starling resistor are answered by the sheet model, but more about this model will surely come in the future.

SOME OTHER VASCULAR AREAS

The spleen seems able to dump red cells in response to stimulation of alpha receptors but can increase its flow without dumping its red cells with stimulation of beta receptors (72). Splenic blood flow oscillated frequently during the period after release of occlusion of the blood flow (51). If the oscillations were weak, infused adenosine enhanced the oscillations. Several other substances—tetrodotoxin, guanethidine, ATP, ADP, and AMP—had no effect. The authors imply that adenosine played a role in local flow control. This is possible. In the pancreas, electrical conductance through the tissue and secretion seemed to be correlated with an increase in blood flow (11). Again, metabolism was not measured, and it is difficult to establish the flow control mechanisms. The same may be said for the salt gland of the goose (49). In this gland, secretion stopped following acute denervation, but blood flow could still be increased pharmacologically without causing secretion. It seems fair to conclude that increase in flow alone does not cause secretion. In adipose tissue blood flow is related to the number of fat cells and not to cell size (25); cell size is determined by the fat content but the cell tissue determines the blood flow. Blood flow to adipose tissue increases irregularly to increased osmolality and weakly to increased K^+, but when both are increased together a large increase always occurs (82). From measurements of Po_2 in the vitreous body of the eye, it has been shown that flow is locally regulated in response to changes in intraocular pressure, arterial pressure, changes in blood Po_2, and changes in blood Pco_2 (1).

SOME MISCELLANEOUS OBSERVATIONS

The responses to changes in plasma osmolality have been compared in three different vascular areas of dogs—the forelimb, the kidney, and the coronary circulation of the heart (38). All three areas showed dilatation when osmolality was increased by NaCl, dextrose, or urea. The responses to NaCl and dextrose waned slowly with time, except in the heart. The response to hyperosmolality due to urea diminished more rapidly in all areas. With urea, all vascular beds showed a reverse response, constriction, when the hyperosmolal infusion fluid was stopped. The kidney showed this reverse response to NaCl and dextrose; this suggests that in the kidney NaCl and dextrose are doing what urea does in all tissues. Urea has generally been considered to be different from most other substances used to raise plasma osmolality because of its ability to enter cells. Perhaps in the kidney, dextrose and NaCl can do this also. It is also possible that the answer lies elsewhere. If it does, then the simple concentration effect of infusion of hypertonic solutions on vascular smooth muscle K^+, and hence on membrane potential and tone as was proposed earlier (71), is questioned again. The heparin dose was not given in this paper—I wonder if it was adequate.

An interesting conflict appeared in two papers from Altura's laboratory. In one, all-or-none behavior of precapillary sphincters was assumed for a detailed analysis of the pharmacology of these structures (2). In the other, it was reported that precapillary sphincters operate in a graded dose-dependent fashion in response to catecholamines in low doses that were suggested to be more physiological than pharmacological (3). It would be nice to know more clearly how precapillary sphincters operate: do they operate in an all-or-none fashion under some conditions, and in a graded fashion under other conditions? The answers are not yet clear.

A disturbing paper on mechanical equilibria of blood vessels has suggested that circumferential wall tension must be negative; therefore, physical stability is determined by vasomotor tone, not by transmural pressure (4). It is not clear to me from this report how tone and transmural pressure interact, but the paper certainly raises some new and interesting questions. In a different type of analysis, peripheral vascular properties have been examined using a frequency response method (83). My intuitive response is that such studies will not elucidate the mechanisms of local control. Nevertheless, it is likely that understanding the physical properties may aid in unravelling the mysteries of local control. The presence of autoregulation was not mentioned.

Control of "nutritional and shunt" circulations has been discussed (56) in a treatise which every student of the circulatory system should read. In addition, there has been an elegant discourse on capillary exchange (63) and a detailed study of the pathways of the sympathetic nervous system relative to flow control in the cat (84).

Last, but not least, is a brief paper on the tone-inducing effect of Evans blue dye on isolated, artificially perfused resistance vessels (96). If this information means nothing more than that some part of the dye molecule fits into some receptor, then a small step forward has been achieved. The fact that the dye altered the response to bolus injections of Ca^{2+} raises another possibility. The authors have suggested the dye might have altered the affinity for Ca^{2+} of some of the membranes of the resistance vessel. Perhaps that is a mechanism used by the local control system. If this possibility could be tested, there might be a larger step forward.

CONCLUSIONS

The mechanisms of local control of blood flow remain essentially unknown. Even whether adenosine is a normal part of the mechanisms has been challenged. The fact of the matter is that except for an almost all-inclusive multiple factor theory and the notion that low-oxygen tension may act directly on precapillary smooth muscles, we really have no idea how the system operates. Some of the earliest and most basic questions still lack clear answers. Why does local control of blood flow spontaneously disappear if a preparation is not perfectly prepared and cared for? That a phenomenon which seems so essential should be so easily upset seems odd. What are the real functions of local control of blood flow? It does not seem to be clear since the observations of Roy & Brown (81) nearly 100 years ago, what it is that local control is regulating. It has been proposed that vessel circumference is regulated: the myogenic theory. It has been suggested that flow is regulated to maintain the concentration of some metabolite, or metabolites: the metabolic theory. It has been suggested that the system serves to regulate transcapillary water exchange. As an active system utilizing smooth muscle, this theory is unnamed; it might be called the hydrometer theory. And, as a passive system, it has been explained by the tissue pressure theory. What is there about plasma that is important for normal autoregulation? Does the labile aspect lie here? Indeed, it is not yet certain whether local control requires plasma.

Excluding the lung and portal circulation of the liver, it seems to me that, based on the data to date, the physiological functions served by local control of blood flow are transcapillary water exchange, as an active system, and metabolite control.

I suggest that water-exchange regulation operates as a vasoconstrictor system; that water movement toward the interstitial space or too much water in the interstitial space causes precapillary constriction. Therefore, increased venous pressure and hypoosmolality of the plasma can result in an increase in resistance to flow, even though there may be a simultaneous decrease in postcapillary resistance to flow. This system might also explain the very low flows that follow relatively long and fairly intense muscular activity. The muscles are edematous and the system acts to hasten water removal. This is the system that responds to increased perfusion pressure or pump-forced increases in blood flow. Both procedures raise capillary pressures and blood-to-interstitial-space water movement. The system turns off constriction for the reverse of the above situations. The mechanism is unknown and is somehow labile. Perhaps plasma factors are necessary.

I suggest that the metabolic system uses a dilator mechanism. The dilator principle is produced in response to the relative availability of some metabolite. Oxygen is a good candidate. This does not imply a direct action of oxygen. Instead, the system senses the availability of oxygen relative to metabolic rate. If the blood flow is high, dilatation does not occur with an increase in metabolic rate until extraction is increased to some value. Then flow increases. If flow is low, dilatation will occur with small increases in metabolic rate. These response patterns are very easily observed in red muscles of dog. White muscles presumably would respond to smaller changes in metabolic rate. This system must work best on the vascular smooth muscle closest to the capillaries, and thereby controls metabolism to flow ratios. But the system must also be able to operate further upstream. Being a ratio detector, the system can produce maximal dilatation without an increase in metabolic rate. Severe hypoxia produces maximal dilatation in resting skeletal muscle.

The mechanism for this metabolically linked system is unknown. I suggest that it must sense the oxidation-reduction state of the cytoplasm, because mitochondrial components are more oxidized during contractions than at rest (58). The system cannot operate through gain or loss of an ion or other non-metabolized substances, because the system must be capable of operating indefinitely under steady-state conditions—the heart remains in active hyperemia for a lifetime. Much effort has already come to naught, because of all the substances that come out of skeletal muscle during the first ten to twenty minutes of transition from rest to steady activity. Although many of these substances may aid in getting active hyperemia started, the basic system operates using a mechanism or mechanisms yet to be discovered.

ACKNOWLEDGEMENT

The author gratefully acknowledges the assistance of Mrs. C. Mc. Marshall and of his MED 620 class: R. A. Ackerman, P. D. Allen, C. A. Ellis, R. D. Hunt, E. L. Nelson, Jr., D. G. Newsome, and S. I. Noel.

LITERATURE CITED

1. Alm, A., Bill, A. 1972. The oxygen supply to the retina, I. Effects of changes in intraocular pressures and arterial blood pressures, and in arterial Po_2 and Pco_2 on oxygen tension in the vitreous body of the cat. *Acta Physiol. Scand.* 84:261–74

2. Altura, B. M. 1971. Chemical and humoral regulation of blood flow through the precapillary sphincter. *Microvasc. Res.* 3:361–384.

3. Altura, B. M. 1971. Do precapillary sphincters respond to vasoactive substances in an all-or-none manner? *Proc. Soc. Exp. Biol. Med.* 138:273–76

4. Azuma, T., Oka, S. 1971. Mechanical equilibrium of blood vessel walls. *Am. J. Physiol.* 221:1310–18

5. Bachofen, M., Gage, A., Bachofen, H. 1971. Vascular response to changes in blood oxygen tension under various flow rates. *Am. J. Physiol.* 220:1786–92

6. Baez, S. 1971. Supporting tissue tension and microvascular reactions. *Microvasc. Res.* 3:95–103

7. Bagger, H. 1972. The distribution of Xe-133 in the left and right ventricular walls of dog hearts after left ventricular bolus infection. *Acta Physiol. Scand.* 84:275–83

8. Barcroft, H., Foley, T. H., McSwiney, R. R. 1971. Experiments on liberation of phosphate from the muscles of the human forearm during vigorous exercise, and the action of sodium phosphate on forearm muscle blood vessels. *J. Physiol London* 213:411–20

9. Barcroft, H. 1972. An enquiry into the nature of the mediator of the vasodilatation in skeletal muscle in exercise. *J. Physiol. London* 222:99P–118P

10. Barer, G. R., Shaw, J. W. 1971. Pulmonary vasodilator and vasoconstrictor actions of carbon dioxide. *J. Physiol. London* 213:633–45

11. Barlow, T. E., Greenwell, J. R., Harper, A. A., Scratcherd, T. 1971. The effect of adrenaline and noradrenaline on the blood flow, electrical conductance and external secretion of the pancreas. *J. Physiol. London* 217:665–678

12. Becker, L. C., Fortuin, N. J., Pitt, B. 1971. Effect of ischemia and antianginal drugs on the distribution of radioactive microspheres in the canine left ventricle. *Circ. Res.* 28:263–69

13. Bencsáth, P., Takács, L. 1971. Intrarenal distribution of blood flow and cortico-medullary sodium gradient after unilateral spanchnicotomy in the dog. *J. Physiol. London* 212:629–640

14. Berne, R. M., Rubio, R., Dobson, J. G., Jr., Curnish, R. R. 1971. Adenosine and adenosine nucleotides as possible mediators of cardiac and skeletal muscle blood flow regulation. *Circ. Res.* 28: Suppl. I, 115–19

15. Bittar, N., Pauly, T. J. 1971. Myocardial reactive hyperemia responses in the dog after aminophyllin and lidoflazine. *Am. J. Physiol.* 220:812–15

16. Blaine, E. H., Davis, J. O., Prewitt, R. L. 1971. Evidence for a renal vascular receptor in control of renin secretion. *Am. J. Physiol.* 220:1593–97

17. Bø, G., Hauge, A., Nicolaysen, G. 1971. Hyperosmolarity and pulmonary vascular capacitance. *Acta Physiol. Scand.* 82:375–81

18. Carrière, S., Friborg, J., Guay, J. P. 1971. Vasodilators, intrarenal blood flow, and natriuresis in the dog. *Am. J. Physiol.* 221:92–98

19. Cohn, J. N., Velasquez, M. T., Notargiacomo, A., Khatri, I. M. 1971. Cortical blood flow, cortical fraction and cortical blood volume in the dog kidney. *Am. J. Physiol.* 221:877–82

20. Collier, R. O., Swann, H. S. 1971. Relationship of kidney size to blood pressure. *Am. J. Physiol.* 220:488–91

21. Costin, J. C., Skinner, N. S., Jr. 1971. Competition between vasoconstrictor and vasodilator mechanisms in skeletal muscle. *Am. J. Physiol.* 220:462–66

22. Cranston, W. I., Rosendorff, C.

1971. Local blood flow, cerebrovascular autoregulation and CO_2 responsiveness in the rabbit hypothalamus. *J. Physiol. London* 215:577–90

23. Daugherty, R. M., Jr. 1971. Effects of IV and IA prostaglandin E_1 on dog forelimb skin and muscle blood flow. *Am. J. Physiol.* 220: 392–96

24. Detar, R., Gellai, M. 1971. Oxygen and isolated vascular smooth muscle from the main pulmonary artery of the rabbit. *Am. J. Physiol.* 221:1791–94

25. Di Girolamo, M., Skinner, N. S., Jr., Hanley, H. G., Sachs, R. G. 1971. Relationship of adipose tissue blood flow to fat cell size and number. *Am. J. Physiol.* 220: 932–37

26. Dobson, J. G., Jr., Rubio, R., Berne, R. M. 1971. Role of adenosine nucleotides, adenosine, and inorganic phosphate in the regulation of skeletal muscle blood flow. *Circ. Res.* 29:375–84

27. Eklöf, B., Ingvar, D. H., Kågstrom, E., Olin, T. 1971. Persistence of cerebral blood flow autoregulation following chronic bilateral cervical sympathecomy in the monkey. *Acta Physiol. Scand.* 82:172–76

28. Ericksson, E., Lisander, B. 1972. Changes in precapillary resistance in skeletal muscle vessels studies by intravital microscopy. *Acta Physiol. Scand.* 84:295–305.

29. Falchuk, K. H., Berliner, R. W. 1971. Hydrostatic pressures in peritubular capillaries and tubules in rat kidney. *Am. J. Physiol.* 220:1422–26

30. Folkow, B., Haglund, U., Jodal, M., Lundgren, O. 1971. Blood flow in the calf muscle of man during heavy rhythmic exercise. *Acta Physiol. Scand.* 81:157–63

31. Folkow, B., Sonnenschein, R. R., Wright, D. L. 1971. Loci of neurogenic and metabolic effects on precapillary vessels of skeletal muscle. *Acta Physiol. Scand.* 81: 459–71

32. Fujishima, M. 1971. The metabolic mechanism of cerebral blood flow autoregulation in dogs. *Jap. Heart J.* 12:376–382.

33. Fujishima, M. 1971. Effect of constricting carotid arteries on cerebral blood flow and on cerebrospinal fluid pH, lactate, and pyruvate in dogs. *Jap. Heart J.* 12: 467–73

34. Fung, Y. C., Sobin, S. S. 1972. Elasticity of the pulmonary alveolar sheet. *Circ. Res.* 30:451–69

35. Fung, Y. C., Sobin, S. S. 1972. Pulmonary alveolar blood flow. *Circ. Res.* 30:470–90

36. Galskov, Å., Nissen, O. 1972. Autoregulation of directly measured blood flows in the superficial and deep venous drainage areas of the cat kidney. *Circ. Res.* 30: 97–103

37. Ganten, D. et al 1971. Renin in dog brain. *Am. J. Physiol.* 221: 1733–37

38. Gazitùa, S., Scott, J. B., Swindall, B., Haddy, F. J. 1971. Resistance responses to local changes in plasma osmolality in three vascular beds. *Am. J. Physiol.* 220: 384–91

39. Gilbert, R. D., Hessler, J. R., Eitzman, D. V., Cassin, S. 1972. Site of pulmonary vascular resistance in fetal goats. *J. Appl. Physiol.* 32:47–53

40. Gimlette, T. M. D., Nasrallah, A. 1969. Effect of stretch on blood flow in dog skeletal muscle evaluated by simultaneous [133]Xenon clearance and direct recording methods. *Cardiovasc. Res.* 3:88–91

41. Glazier, J. B., Murray, J. F. 1971. Sites of pulmonary vasomotor reactivity in the dog during alveolar hypoxia and serotonin and histamine infusion. *J. Clin. Invest.* 50:2550–58

42. Gosselin, R. E., Audino, L. F. 1971. Muscle blood flow and functional capillary density evaluated by isotope clearance. *Pfluegers Arch.* 322:197–216

43. Gray, I. G., Mitra, S. K., Nisbet, H. I. A., Aspin, N., Creighton, R. E. 1971. Cerebral blood flow in hypoxemic anesthetized dogs. *Anesth. Analg.* 50:594–608

44. Gray, S. D. 1971. Effect of hypertonicity on vascular dimensions in skeletal muscle. *Microvasc. Res.* 3:117–24

45. Grega, G. F., Daugherty, R. M., Jr., Scott, J. B., Radawski, D. P.,

Haddy, F. J. 1971. Effect of pressure, flow and vasoactive agents on vascular resistance and capillary filtration in canine fetal, newborn, and adult lung. *Microvasc. Res.* 3:297–307

46. Grollman, A., Krishnamurty, V. S. R. 1971. A new pressor agent of renal origin: its differentiation from renin and angiotensin. *Am. J. Physiol.* 221:1499–1506

47. Haddy, F. J., Scott, J. B. 1971. Bioassay and other evidence for participation of chemical factors in local regulation of blood flow. *Circ. Res.* 28:Suppl. I, 86–92

48. Haglund, U., Lundgren, O. 1972. Reactions within consecutive vascular sections of the small intestine of the cat during prolonged hypotension. *Acta Physiol. Scand.* 84:151–63

49. Hanwell, A., Linzel, J. L., Peaker, M. 1971. Salt-gland secretion and blood flow in the goose. *J. Physiol. London* 213:373–87

50. Harris, P. D., Longnecker, D. E. 1971. Significance of precapillary activity for microcirculatory function. *Microvasc. Res.* 3:385–95

51. Hashimoto, K., Satoh, S. 1971. Enhancement of the post-occlusive oscillation in the splenic circulation by adenosine. *J. Physiol. London* 218:295–304

52. Hauge, A., Bø, G. 1971. Blood hyperosmolality and pulmonary vascular resistance in the cat. *Circ. Res.* 28:371–76

53. Hedwall, P. R., Abdel-Sayed, W. A., Schmid, P. G., Mark, A. L., Abboud, F. M. 1971. Vascular responses to prostaglandin E_1 in gracilis muscle and hindpaw of the dog. *Am. J. Physiol.* 221:42–47

54. Held, K., Niedermayer, W., Schaefer, J., Schwartzkopf, H. J., Weiss, Ch. 1971. Pressure induced changes of renal blood flow resistance in the dog kidney in situ. *Pfluegers Arch.* 325:95–102

55. Hyman, A. L., Woolverton, W. C., Guth, P. S., Ichinose, H. 1971. The pulmonary vasopressor response to decreases in blood pH in intact dogs. *J. Clin. Invest.* 50:1028–43

56. Hyman, C. 1971. Independent control of nutritional and shunt circulations. *Microvasc. Res.* 3:89–94

57. Hysell, J. W., Bohr, D. F. 1970. Renal vascular response to plasma and to known vasoactive substances. *Proc. Soc. Exp. Biol. Med.* 135:930–33

58. Jöbsis, F. F., Stainsby, W. N. 1968. Oxidation of NADH during contrations of circulated mammalian skeletal muscle. *Resp. Physiol.* 4:292–300

59. Johnson, R. C. 1970. Arteriovenous shunting in isolated perfused rat upper gastrointestingal tract. *Am. J. Physiol.* 219:17–22

60. Katz, M. A., Blantz, R. C., Rector, F. L., Jr., Seldin, D. W. 1971. Measurement of intrarenal blood flow. I. Analysis of microsphere method. *Am. J. Physiol.* 220:1903–13

61. Kenner, T., Ono, K. 1971. The low frequency input impedance of the renal artery. *Pfluegers Arch.* 324:155–64

62. Kontos, H. A., Thames, M. D., Lombana, A., Watlington, C. O., Jessee, F., Jr. 1971. Vasodilator effects of local hypercapnic acidosis in dog skeletal muscle. *Am. J. Physiol.* 220:1569–72

63. Landis, E. M., Sage, L. E. 1971. Fluid movement rates through walls of single capillaries exposed to hypertonic solutions. *Am. J. Physiol.* 221:520–34

64. Logan, A., Jose, P., Eisner, G. M., Lilinfield, L., Slotkoff, L. 1971. Intracortical distribution of renal blood flow in hemorrhagic shock in dogs. *Circ. Res.* 29:257–66

65. Løyning, E. W. 1971. Effect of reduced perfusion pressure on intrarenal distribution of blood flow in dogs. *Acta Physiol. Scand.* 83:191–202

66. McMurphy, D., Heymann, M. A., Rudolph, A. M., Melmon, K. L. 1972. Developmental changes in constriction of the ductus arteriosus: responses to oxygen and vasoactive agents in the isolated ductus arteriosus of the fetal lamb. *Pediat. Res.* 6:231–38

67. Miyazaki, M., McNay, J. 1971. Redistribution of renal cortical blood flow during ureteral occlusion and renal venous constric-

tion. *Proc. Soc. Exp. Biol. Med.*
138:454–61
68. Nakano, J. 1972. Relationship between the chemical structure of prostaglandins and their vasoactivities in dogs. *Brit. J. Pharmacol.* 44:63–70
69. Nakano, J., Prancan,, A. V. 1972. Effect of prostaglandins E_1 and A_1 on the gastric circulation in dogs. *Proc. Soc. Exp. Biol. Med.* 139:1151–54
70. Navar, L. G., Baer, P. G., Wallace, S. L., McDaniel, J. K. 1971. Reduced intrarenal resistance and autoregulatory capacity after hyperoncotic dextran. *Am. J. Physiol.* 221:329–34
71. Norton, J. M., Detar, R. 1972. Potassium and isolated coronary vascular smooth muscle. *Am. J. Physiol.* 222:474–79
72. Opdyke, D. F. 1970. Hemodynamics of blood flow through the spleen. *Am. J. Physiol.* 219:102–6
73. Ott, C. E., Navar, L. G., Guyton, A. C. 1971. Pressures in static and dynamic status from capsules implanted in the kidney. *Am. J. Physiol.* 221:394–400
74. Paradise, N. F., Swayze, C. R., Shin, D. H., Fox, I. J. 1971. Perfusion heterogeneity in skeletal muscle using tritiated water. *Am. J. Physiol.* 220:1107–14
75. Piiper, J., Spiller, P. 1970. Repayment of O_2 debt and resynthesis of high-energy phosphates in gastrocnemius muscle of the dog. *J. Appl. Physiol.* 28:657–62
76. Radawski, D., Dabney, J. M., Daugherty, R. M., Jr., Haddy, F. J., Scott, J. B. 1972. Local effects of CO_2 on vascular resistances and weight of the dog forelimb. *Am. J. Physiol.* 222:439–43
77. Raper, A. J., Kontos, H. A., Patterson, J. L., Jr. 1971. Response of pial precapillary vessels to changes in arterial carbon dioxide tension. *Circ. Res.* 28:518–23
78. Reed, J. D., Sanders, D. J. 1971. Pepsin secretion, gastric motility and mucosal blood flow in the anesthetized cat. *J. Physiol. London* 216:159–70
79. Reed, J. D., Smy, J. R. 1971. Mechanisms relating gastric acid

secretion and mucosal blood flow during gastrin and histamine stimulation. *J. Physiol. London* 219:571–85
80. Rothe, C. F., Nash, F. D., Thompson, D. E. 1971. Patterns in autoregulation of renal blood flow in the dog. *Am. J. Physiol.* 220:1621–26
81. Roy, C. S., Brown, J. G. 1880. The blood pressure and its variations in the arterioles, capillaries and smaller veins. *J. Physiol. London* 2:323–59
82. Sachs, R. G., Hanley, H. G., Skinner, N. S., Jr. 1971. K^+, osmolality and subcutaneous adipose tissue blood flow. *Pfluegers Arch.* 327:337–48
83. Sato, T., Yamashiro, S. M., Grodins, F. S. 1971. Measurement of peripheral vascular properties by a frequency response method. *Am. J. Physiol.* 220:1640–50
84. Schramm, L. P., Bignall, K. E. 1971. Central neural pathways mediating active sympathetic muscle vasodilatation in cats. *Am. J. Physiol.* 221:754–67
85. Seely, J. F., Boulpaep, E. L. 1971. Renal function studies on the isobaric autoperfused kidney. *Am. J. Physiol.* 221:1075–83
86. Slotkoff, L., Logan, A., Jose, P., Avella, J. D., Eisner, G. M. 1971. Microsphere measurement of intrarenal circulation of the dog. *Circ. Res.* 28:158–65
87. Smieško, V. 1971. Unidirectional rate sensitivity component in local control of vascular tone. *Pfluegers Arch.* 327:324–36
88. Sobin, S. S., Fung, Y. C., Tremer, H. M., Rosenquist, T. H. 1972. Elasticity of the pulmonary alveolar microvascular sheet in the cat. *Circ. Res.* 30:440–50
89. Spence, R. J., Rhodes, B. A., Wagner, H. N., Jr. 1972. Regulation of arteriovenous anastomotic and capillary blood flow in the dog leg. *Am. J. Physiol.* 222:326–32
90. Stein, J. H., Ferris, T. F., Huprich, J. E., Smith, T. C., Osgood, R. W. 1971. Effect of renal vasodilatation on the distribution of cortical blood flow in the kidney of the dog. *J. Clin. Invest.* 50:1429–38
91. Strauss, J., Beran, A. V., Baker, R., Boydston, L., Reyes-Sanchez,

J. L. 1971. Effect of hemorrhagic shock on renal oxygenation. *Am. J. Physiol.* 221:1545–50

92. Sundt, T. M., Jr., Waltz, A. G. 1971. Cerebral ischemia and reactive hyperemia. Studies of cortical blood flow and microcirculation before, during, and after temporary occlusion of middle cerebral artery of squirrel monkeys. *Circ. Res.* 28:426–33

93. Türker, R. K., Yamamoto, M., Bumpus, F. M., Khairallah, P. A. 1971. Lung perfusion with angiotensins I and II: Evidence of release of myotropic and inhibitory substances. *Circ. Res.* 28: 559–67

94. Vatner, S. F. et al 1971. Coronary dynamics in unrestrained conscious baboons. *Am. J. Physiol.* 221:1396–1401

95. Vatner, S. F., Higgins, C. B., Franklin, D., Braunwald, E.

1972. Role of tachycardia in mediating the coronary hemodynamic response to severe exercise. *J. Appl. Physiol.* 32:380–85

96. Verrier, R. L., Bohr, D. F. 1971. Evans Blue dye and the development of "myogenic tone" in perfused resistance vessels. *Proc. Soc. Exp. Biol. Med.* 137:1013–15

97. Wallin, J. D. et al 1971. Effect of saline diuresis on intrarenal blood flow in the rat. *Am. J. Physiol.* 221:1297–1304

98. Waltz, A. G., Yamaguchi, T., Regli, F. 1971. Regulatory responses of cerebral vasculature after sympathetic denervation. *Am. J. Physiol.* 221:298–302

99. Zimmer, R., Lang, R., Oberdorster, G. 1971. Post-ischemic reactive hyperemia of the isolated perfused brain of the dog. *Pfluegers Arch.* 328:332–43

Ann. Rev. Physiol. 1973. 35:169–192

RESPIRATION: PULMONARY MECHANICS $\qquad$ 1093

JERE MEAD

*Department of Physiology, Harvard School of Public Health
Boston, Massachusetts*

In preparing this review I read and scanned some 200 articles dealing mainly with respiratory mechanics and then arranged them alphabetically according to topics—airways, anatomy, etc.—my plan being to attempt an overall summary. By the time I got through letter *A* it was clear that I would never make it to the chest wall and I found myself in the same difficulty I had experienced some years ago writing a review article on respiratory mechanics: I ran out of time and space then, and it's happened again. So this review is limited to the lungs, and is mainly concerned with anatomy, the airways, and lung elasticity. Nor is it at all exhaustive in these areas. I have tried to seek out articles that complement one another and I have gone into some detail—perhaps too much.

MORPHOMETRY, MORPHOGENESIS AND MORPHOSTASIS

As physiologists' models develop, so does the need for anatomic detail. Thus Weibel's monograph *Morphometry of the Human Lung* published in 1963 (58) was eagerly received. During the period under review several papers have contributed useful new knowledge in this area. Cumming, Horsfield, and their colleagues have continued their quest for a more adequate model of the bronchial tree (14, 25). To deal with the crucial problem of describing the asymmetry of branching, they developed a system for ordering dichotomously branched systems by expressing the degree of asymmetry in numbers (24). If all terminal elements are labeled order 1, and the penultimate elements order 2 etc., in the symmetrical system all branches which join are of the same order. But in asymmetrical systems the joining branches may be of a different order. Horsfield & Cumming (24) used the following convention for counting: the order of a branch is one higher than that of the two branches joining to form it. A given order, then, has a number that corresponds to the maximum number of branches between that point and the terminal unit, and the difference in order between two joining branches gives an idea of the degree of asymmetry. For example, a difference of three indicates that the higher order branch has three more generations of branching to the terminal unit than its fellow branch. The authors showed that regularly

169

irregular branching systems, whose branches differ in order by fixed amounts, have fixed ratios of the number of branches of a given order to the number of branches of the order one lower. The branching ratio for the example given would be 1.38, which, incidentally, is the ratio they observed in lobar airways of human lungs. Since this ratio appears to be fairly stable for airways 0.7 mm i.d. and larger, up to lobar bronchi, they modeled lobar branching with this particular regular irregularity—namely, joining branches differing in order by three. For the central airways they did not attempt any average representation, but merely gave the direct measurements. For airways smaller than 0.7 mm i.d. they relied on measurements recorded in a separate study; namely, of six to seven orders of symmetrical dichotomy down to and including the most distal respiratory bronchiole (46).

Here they appear to be in disagreement with Gamsu et al (18), who concluded from microbronchographic measurements that there is considerable irregularity of branching at the bronchiolar level. They claimed to be able to visualize all branches distal to 1 mm i.d. bronchioles in eight different areas within one lung. They found six generations of branching down to terminal bronchioles but the total number of terminal bronchioles was less than half the number expected for symmetrical dichotomy. It is important to note that the airways described by Parker et al (46) were more peripheral. They found an average of six generations from 0.7 mm i.d. bronchioles down to and including three generations of respiratory bronchioles. Thus Gamsu et al, beginning with bronchioles 1 mm i.d., were some three generations further down the tree (i.e. mouthward), and this probably explains the irregularity they observed.

The confusion that "down the tree" creates makes this a good spot to point out that Horsfield & Cumming, following the lead of geologists who studied branching of river systems, have got us usefully turned around on this point (24). We tend to think of the alveoli as being at the end of this system, rather than at its beginning. As far as branching is concerned it wouldn't matter which way we thought if the branching were symmetrical, but in asymmetrical systems it does matter. As Horsfield & Cumming point out, in systems asymmetrical in the sense of having variations in the number of divisions between the stem (trachea) and end branches (e.g. respiratory bronchioles), as one proceeds from the stem and counts generations one soon arrives at generations containing branches moderately different in size and performing quite different functions. If one begins at the other end, successive orders have similar sizes and similar functions. Irregularity of branching is reasonable for a wide and fairly homogeneous dispersion of similar terminals; there are great differences in distance from carina to respiratory bronchiole, for example, as between lung near hilum compared to that at the apex, and it is not at all surprising that there should be far fewer branchings to reach near than to reach distant structures. In a sense, then, the average order difference of three (implied by a branching ratio of 1.38) between joining branches reflects this matter of nearness and farness—the higher order branch coming from more distant units—that is implied by a branching system which must have its stem at a point (near the center) and serve a space with similar end units.

If irregularity relates to space filling, it is intriguing that the branching system appears to accomplish this in three or possibly four steps. Near the stem—i.e., between the trachea and the segments—the asymmetry is the greatest, and this is to be expected since the first branches define the outlines of a fairly irregular structure: the lobated lung. Between the segmental branches and the smallest bronchi the irregularity is somewhat regular, as we have seen. Between the smallest bronchi (0.7 mm i.d.) and the distal respiratory bronchioles, branching is nearly symmetrical (branching ratio 2.0), and finally the branching system of the 3–9 generations of alveolar ducts and sacs is again highly asymmetrical. Parker et al (46) suggest that the regularity of bronchiolar branching may reflect an increasing importance of diffusion of gas movement at this level. "A more rapid increase in total cross-sectional area occurs as a combined result of the more rapid increase in the number of branches and their less rapid decrease in diameter, and this facilitates gas movement by molecular diffusion." Within the ducts, sacs, and alveoli, diffusion is presumably so rapid that the asymmetry required for space filling can once more be indulged.

As these contributions have given a better grasp of the problems of asymmetry, the measurements of Angus & Thurlbeck (1) have provided an improved perspective on the matter of total number of alveoli. Based on measurements on a comparatively small number of lungs, there is a generally held belief that the number is about the same in all adults. This implies that individuals with large lungs have larger alveoli than individuals with small lungs. Angus & Thurlbeck, using carefully controlled techniques, counted alveoli in the lungs of 32 adults. They obtained a threefold range in the number of alveoli ($212-605 \times 10^6$) and found this number to be significantly correlated with body height. Indeed, the alveolar density at a fixed distending pressure was unrelated to height, indicating that alveoli have similar dimensions in large and small adult human lungs. One of the implications of the relatively wide dispersion of the number of alveoli in adult lungs is that deciding the age at which the adult number is reached cannot be as exact as has been supposed. It is certainly not possible to say that alveolar partitioning is complete at age 8, as has been maintained (17). In a separate study, Matsubu & Thurlbeck (35) found that the number of conducting airways (nonalveolated; less 2 mm i.d.) per unit area showed a striking negative correlation with body length. They interpret this as showing that the total number of these airways does not vary with body size. "Thus structurally the lungs of short subjects differ from those of tall subjects in that the former are made up of a similar number of units which contain fewer alveoli."

The functional penalty for largeness along these lines would be greater energy required for mass movement of gas; and for smallness, reduced efficiency of gas exchange per breath. The likelihood is that these differences, if they exist, vanish within the reserve of the respiratory system. Might they emerge in disease? Is there a significant correlation between body size and respiratory morbidity and mortality? Certainly if it were striking we would already know about it. But, is it possible that racial differences in the incidence of respiratory disease relate to what I will very loosely refer to as broncho-parenchymal dystrophy? Da Costa has recently summarized his own and others' comparisons of lung volumes in different races (15). Asians and Africans tend to have lung volumes which are smaller than those of Caucasians after standardization for age, size, and weight. Do Asians and Africans possibly have less parenchyma per airway? The greater incidence of chronic lung disease in north Europeans may not relate solely to environmental factors (including smoking habits) and genetic differences in the tendency of the lung to digest itself.

The morphology of carefully inflated but fixed lungs leads logically to the two problems of morphometry of living lungs and of morphogenesis. Taking up the second problem first: how does the lung grow and under what influences? The proliferation of branching is apparently complete in utero and growth of airways after birth is entirely by increase in size. Alveoli continue to proliferate through the first decade, but probably not for as long as body growth continues, so that part of alveolar growth is by increase in size. Brody et al (5) found that lung growth may resume in adults under the influence of excessive pituitary growth hormone. Six acromegalic men had abnormally large lung gas and tissue volumes but no increase in diffusion capacity. This was in contrast to a patient with pituitary gigantism who had both larger lungs and an increased diffusion capacity. The authors inferred that in the latter instance lung growth had been associated with alveolar proliferation but that growth in the acromegalic patients had been chiefly by enlargement of existing structures. These observations stimulated Bartlett to study the influence of growth hormone on lung growth in rats (2). He found that "lung weight, lung volume, alveolar surface area and alveolar number increased in concert with body weight, much as they did over a longer time course in untreated animals." This was in good agreement with the changes in pituitary gigantism which the treated rat simulates, since epiphyseal closure never takes place in rats. As Bartlett pointed out, whether or not growth hormones stimulate alveolar proliferation in the acromegalic state could be modeled on species such as the dog which undergo epiphyseal closure.

In a separate study, Bartlett & Remmers (3) confirmed earlier work of Burri & Weibel, (6) that rats exposed to fairly long periods of hypoxia (10% O_2 for some 20 days) exhibited increased lung growth and that, since alveolar size did not change, this must have been by proliferation. They reasoned that mechanical stimulation by the associated increase in ventilation could not have been responsible, since rats kept in 5% CO_2 for 20 days showed "no abnormalities of lung development." Amphibian larvae undergo excessive gill development in hypoxic environments, and the authors have suggested that it is likely that increase in respiratory surface area is a general response not limited to the lungs, and hence not likely to be determined by thoracic mechanics.

These pioneering studies combined the morphometric methods developed by Weibel with animal experiments; this approach promises definitive answers to questions which have long been unanswered. For example, how do tissue stresses influence pulmonary morphogenesis? Davies & Reid (16) have studied alveolar growth in postmortem lungs of four scoliotic patients. Here lung growth appeared to be greatly influenced by thoracic mechanics: "None of the lungs was of normal shape, and some were grossly distorted. Even after inflation and fixation the lung maintained the shape of the thorax." If the structures surrounding the lung influence lung growth certainly it must be by way of changes in distending pressure. But this presents a paradox: If transpulmonary pressure influences morphogenesis, why aren't there greater regional differences in lung growth? Certainly the upper and more anterior parts of the lung are subjected through the agency of gravity to greater average stresses in man than are the lower lobes. But the ratio of alveoli to airways is not greater in upper lobes, as would be expected if alveoli proliferate in response to stress. (The number of airways serves as a control since it is set in utero.) Nor is alveolar size at a given distending pressure larger in upper lobes, which would be the case if existing alveoli grew in response to stress. Indeed, the fact that the lungs, through the agency of gravity, grow in a systematic stress gradient (unless growth is restricted to periods of sleep!) but, nevertheless, expand nearly homogeneously when excised, strongly suggests that lung growth must be largely uninfluenced by stress between quite broad limits. So we are left with a paradox. Clearly, Davies & Reid (16) showed that the lungs of patients with severe deforming scoliosis are smaller and have fewer alveoli, and the only apparent agency is the mechanical influence of the surrounding chest wall. Perhaps the answer is in the width of the limits within which stresses do not influence growth. Conceivably, as the lung is compressed slowly, it exhibits nonuniform closure in the same manner that it does acutely, and perhaps closed units tend to atrophy in response to local failure of nutrition. If this is true, lung growth could be shaped by restraints on the container but less, or perhaps not at all, by traction; the controlling factor might be blood supply.

STUDIES IN EXCISED PREPARATIONS

Turning now to the matter of what lungs look like in the unfixed state, two studies done on excised dog lungs are complementary (26, 41). Murtagh et al (41) were interested in the role of airway smooth muscle, the effect of lung parenchyma surrounding bronchi, and the influence of volume-pressure history on bronchial caliber. By first freeing dog lobes of gas and then carefully introducing gas, the authors were able to fill the bronchial tree before expanding the parenchyma, and could thereby compare the caliber of bronchi at given distending pressures with ones measured at the same pressure after parenchymal expansion, and then after dissecting away the surrounding lungs [note: parenchyma refers to the tissues making up the alveoli, alveolar ducts, and respiratory bronchioles; this is essentially the use of Hayek (19)]. They did their best to achieve closely similar pressure-volume histories for all measurements and were most successful in the latter two instances. Comparing bronchial filling in intact lungs with and without atelectasis, they were unable to avoid the paradox that very different volume histories were required for the measurements; the bronchial filling in atelectatic lobes proved to be most useful in a separate study on the effects of mecholyl (42). They measured airway caliber from air bronchograms, thus avoiding any specific effects of contrast medium on airways.

Hughes et al (26) outlined the airways of excised dog lung with tantalum dust as described by Nadel et al (43). They used paired stereo-roentgenograms and thereby achieved a fairly high degree of accuracy, particularly in measurements of airway lengths. They confirmed the earlier finding of Hyatt et al (28) that airway length varies approximately with the cube root of lung volume. Hyatt et al had pointed out that the measurements of airway length in situ might be used to study the distribution of volume changes in lungs. Possibly the stereo techniques of Hughes et al will afford the accuracy needed to make such an approach feasible (a 20% change in lung volume means only about a 6% change in airway length). As for the relationship between airway diameter and transpulmonary pressure, Hughes et al found somewhat different results. Hyatt et al (27) found that most of the change in airway diameter with change in transpulmonary pressure occurred at pressures less than 5 cm H_2O, whereas Hughes et al found substantial changes at higher pressures. Hyatt et al (27) further found different behavior of bronchi of different sizes —small airways undergoing greater relative change than large airways; whereas Hughes et al found similar percent changes for small and large airways.

The findings of Murtagh et al (41) helped resolve this controversy: In control lungs the curvature of pressure-diameter plots is somewhat more gentle [approximately 15% of the change occurs above 5 cm H_2O in Figure 2 of (41)] than is that for lungs pretreated with atropine [10% or less of the total change occurs above 5 cm H_2O in Figure 3 of (41)]. (In Hughes et al's measurements 20–30% of the change occurred above 5 cm H_2O, and they mentioned unpublished observations to the effect that atropinized lungs gave curves more like those of Hyatt.) As for systematic differences in airways of different size, the very pretty curves of Murtagh et al qualitatively confirm the observations of Hyatt that small airways undergo larger change than large airways, both in atropinized and nonatropinized lungs. The apparently somewhat more constricted state of smooth muscle in the preparations of Hughes et al may obscure this—or put in a different way, perhaps smooth muscle activity makes the airways behave more like parenchyma and more like each other, thus improving the homogeneity of expansion.

This conjecture rises from the following further comparison of the two studies. Murtagh et al (41) made the striking observation that in atropinized lungs with similar inflation histories, airway calibers during inflation were much smaller in intact lobes than in the dissected bronchial tree, but increased to similar sizes at peak pressures and were similar on deflation. They found it "hard to believe that this could be attributed to compressive effects of lung tissue already well inflated at pressures of 15 to 20 cm H_2O when this difference is still clearly apparent. It may be that in the intact lobe effective transmural pressure is less than transpulmonary pressure during inflation; but this is hard to believe when the same effect is not noted at comparable inflation pressures during deflation and when so many studies point to the likelihood that inflated lung tissue can only result in dilation of intrapulmonary vessels and airways." They concluded "The key question of why calibers are smaller during inflation in the intact lobe than in the dissected bronchi remains to be answered. Its answer should lead to a better understanding of the changes of bronchial caliber in all other conditions." The results and discussion of Hughes et al (26) appear to supply a possible answer, as I will attempt to show.

Homogeneous expansion is one in which all regions expand in the same way. Isotropic homogeneous expansion is one in which all regions expand in the same way and equally in all directions, so that all linear dimensions change as the cube root of lung volume. The lung, a highly inhomogeneous structure in composition, could hypothetically undergo isotropic homogeneous expansion. Hughes et al found that excised lobes of their dogs did inflate and deflate roughly in this way, in that both lengths and diameters of airways changed approximately as the cube root of volume. Since the lung parenchyma exhibited substantial static hysteresis (i.e. transpulmonary pressure at a given inflation was considerably greater than at the same volume during deflation), this meant that the airways also exhibited substantial hysteresis—indeed, that they exhibited the same degree of hysteresis. But airways and parenchyma differ strikingly in size, shape, and composition, and it seemed remarkable that they should behave so similarly. This led the authors to consider the possibility that the "lung tissue exerts an influence on airways tending to make them conform to the surrounding parenchyma." In other words, the relatively high degree of homogeneity of lung and airway expansion might be accounted for by mechanical interactions between the airways and parenchyma rather than solely by the intrinsic elastic properties of the structures separately. Certainly forces expanding airways within lungs are different from the ones expanding dissected airways. In dissected airways they arise directly from the applied pressure. In the lung they arise indirectly from transpulmonary pressure by way of the tissue attachments of the intervening parenchyma. In both cases distension is caused by outwardly acting stress (force per unit area), but there is a fundamental difference: in the airway with the parenchyma dissected away the applied pressure follows Pascal's law and is thus independent of the geometry of the system. But the stresses expanding airways within lungs are highly dependent on geometry. If one maintained the pressure distending dissected airways constant and then by some magical means indefinitely increased the compliance of the airways, they would increase indefinitely in volume. But if one were to imagine the same intervention with the airways in situ in lungs exposed to a fixed transpulmonary pressure, the airways would not increase in volume indefinitely. They would increase only as long as surrounding parenchyma continued to exert a distending stress on them. And this would not continue indefinitely because as the airways expanded, circumferential elements in the surrounding parenchyma would come under increasing tension and ultimately would completely counterbalance the tendency of the parenchyma to pull outward on the airways.

I now make a sudden jump back to Murtagh et al (41). How is it possible for airways to be much smaller in lungs at a given transpulmonary pressure than in the dissected state at the same distending pressure? Since this observation was made in atropinized preparations, relaxation of airway smooth muscle would be expected to increase airway distensibility, particularly during expansion, and this circumstance is similar to the example just considered. As smooth muscle relaxes, airway volume in the dissected state would be expected to increase more than in situ. Murtagh et al found it difficult to picture a compressive effect of surrounding lung tissue. Hughes et al would picture it as a diminished expanding effect along the lines just developed. That the discrepancy would be expected to be more marked during inflation fits the influence of atropine on smooth muscle contraction, which should be greater during lengthening from a shortened state than during shortening from a lengthened state.

Mechanical interdependence and the state of smooth muscle may explain some of the other discrepancies between the observations of Hyatt et al (27) on the one hand and of Hughes et al (26) on the other. The effect of mechanical interdependence is to favor homogeneous expansion: inhomogeneities result in changes in tissue stress which tend to reduce the inhomogeneity. Thus, the stress tending to expand a region that is inherently less compliant than surrounding regions is greater than the overall stress—i.e. transpulmonary pressure, while that on a region more compliant than its surroundings (the example just considered) is less than the overall stress. Thus mechanical interdependence is homeostatic in the sense that it tends to preserve homogeneity of expansion (36). The observations that airway diameters change little at pressures greater than 5 cm H_2O when lung volume (and its linear dimensions) are changing substantially, and that small airways undergo larger relative changes in diameter, indicate that under the conditions of these experiments, lungs and airways did not expand isotropically and homogeneously. The condition common to these observations may have been a greater degree of smooth muscle relaxation than the mechanical homeostasis could cope with. Perhaps homogeneous expansion in living lungs—to the extent that it exists—depends on the action of mechanical interdependence operating on a background of smooth muscle activity. The latter might be thought of as creating a reasonable facsimile of parenchymal hysteresis—one with which mechanical interdependence is able to cope.

These considerations of the possible importance of smooth muscle have been derived from studies on "dead lung." The importance of the living state of smooth muscle has been emphasized by Colebatch & Mitchell (13). They have convincingly demonstrated in excised cat and dog lungs that smooth muscle can directly and markedly influence parenchymal distensibility without intermediation of surface forces. They immersed excised and gas-free lungs in oxygenated Krebs solution at 37°C and demonstrated that they could maintain metabolic activity during filling and emptying of the lungs, also with oxygenated Krebs solution. They showed that excised cat lungs were partially constricted by demonstrating shifts in volume-pressure curves following isoproterenol. Histamine produced increased transpulmonary pressures at a given volume, decreased liquid volume at 0 pressure, and increased hysteresis. The two cats with the greatest degree of pneumoconstriction had a relatively greater abundance of smooth muscle in alveolar ducts. The authors pointed out that the extent of constriction was larger than could be accounted for by the alveolar duct system alone—i.e. that the alveoli themselves must have changed volume.

How can smooth muscle confined to part of the respiratory unit influence its distension? The authors have suggested that if the muscle were connected by a series of nonelastic elements, it could effectively act as a continuous system. They estimated that under conditions of maximal shortening, isotropic constriction would require the muscle elements to occupy from ¼ to ⅓ of the length of the elements in the network, which is not unreasonable, but they considered the possibility that the constriction may be anisotropic—that the smooth muscle contraction may produce disproportionate shortening of ducts. That change in shape may be important was suggested by an incidental observation that "whether constricted spontaneously or by histamine, the lung lobes appeared tense and showed a slightly irregular surface, whereas after isoproterenol the lobes were flacid and the surface smooth." The authors suggested that histamine through its action on alveolar duct smooth muscle may regulate the distensibility of lung units. Since at ordinary respiratory frequencies the distribution of volume change is thought to depend almost entirely on distensibility rather than on the distribution of airway resistance, this would be a logical means for controlling distribution. But this needs to be faced with the frequent observation that smooth muscle relaxation induced in human subjects does not cause any increase in total lung capacity, nor does it cause reduction, or at most only slight reduction (4, 57), in static recoil pressures at a given lung volume in normal subjects. This suggests that at least, in man at rest, the distensibility of lung is not influenced by smooth muscle activity.

In two papers Menkes and co-workers (38, 39) reported the degree of mechanical interdependence in dog lungs. Dog lungs are essentially nonlobated and the implications of inhomogeneities might be quite different than in lobulated lungs. Hayek noted (19) that interlobular slippage might confer a degree of independence. So in effect Menkes et al were seeking to examine the interdependence of pulmonary parenchyma per se. But a price of nonlobulation is extensive collateral ventilation, and this poses two problems—the production of inhomogeneities and measurement of the pressures giving rise to them. The authors developed two ingenious approaches, one for excised lungs and one for lungs in the chest. In the first they produced steady-state inhomogeneities by sucking air out through catheters wedged into small bronchi. They measured the degree of inhomogeneity beyond from bronchograms, and the pressures producing the inhomogeneity from separate catheters that sampled alveolar pressure within the inhomogeneous region. The degree of interdependence in excised lungs was less when the segments extended to the pleural surface than when the surface was obliterated by gluing lobes together. They postulated that when the lungs were in the chest the reduced mobility of the pleural surface conferred by the surrounding chest wall might also enhance interdependence, and this led them to attempt measurements in intact animals using their second method. They showed theoretically that the degree of interdependence could be estimated from measurements of the pressures within obstructed segments and from changes in lung volume without measuring segmental volume, as long as segmental volume did not change. The problem was how to produce changes in lung volume without changing segmental volume. This they approximated by using rapid cycling. They reasoned that when further increases in cycling frequency produced no further change in the volume-pressure relationship, the segmental volume change by way of collateral pathways must be negligible. As they had anticipated, the degree of interdependence was greater in lungs within the chest than in the excised state. And in both instances it was substantially greater than would have been predicted from changes in the relative density of attachments alone (36). They defined the effective compliance of a region as the ratio of the change in volume of the segment to the change in pressure difference between the alveoli of the segment and the pleural surface. The effective compliance of a region in inhomogeneous conditions, (i.e. a region changing volume relative to its surroundings) in intact dog lungs in the chest was about ⅓ that under homogeneous conditions, (i.e. a region expanding equally with surrounding regions). A functional consequence is that collateral volume equilibration should be about three times more rapid than it otherwise would be.

Menkes et al (37) also studied the influence of surface forces on collateral ventilation. They used kerosene to partially inactivate surfactant and thereby increase surface tension at the internal surface of the lungs during inflation, and they found that collateral flow resistance at a given lung volume was reduced. They noted that the influence of a change in surface tension on the size of alveolar pores would depend on the relative size of two radii curvature: that of the pore opening, and that of the opposing curvature of the pore wall. (The two curvatures are at right angles and are opposite in sign.) If the former is the larger, which presumably is the case, increased tension should increase the pore size. On the other hand, the authors argued that tubular channels such as anastamosing respiratory bronchioles or Lambert's canals (accessory, bronchiolar alveolar communications) would, if anything, be expected to decrease in size with increases in surface tension. But they failed to consider an argument which is similar to the one which they applied to the pores. The influence of a change of surface tension on the size of a structure lined by a surface and held under traction by surrounding structures similarly lined would also depend on the relative radii of these surfaces, and on the nature of their curvatures. Tubular structures with cylindrical curvature are, if anything, probably as large or somewhat larger than the airspaces surrounding and attached to them, and these would be curved in two dimensions—i.e. more nearly spherical. For a given increase in surface tension the change in outward-acting stress would exceed that in inward-acting stress approximately in a ratio of twice the radius of the tube divided by the radius of the surrounding structures. Accordingly, tubular structures should also tend to grow larger with increases in surface tension. But this argument could not account for the decrease in collateral resistance found at the same transpulmonary pressure. For the stress distending airways is not dependent on surface forces alone; ultimately it arises, via tissue and surface forces, from transpulmonary pressure, and, indeed, in a homogeneously expanded lung it equals transpulmonary pressure. Thus if expansion remained homogeneous following kerosene, the stress distending collateral airways would remain unchanged, and for it to be increased, they would have to be decreased, not increased, in size. The authors developed this line of reasoning and thereby answered the question I've raised, although they appear not to have been aware of the similar action of surface tension per se on pores and on airways surrounded by smaller structures.

The authors also estimated the effective collateral compliance and found that it increased after kerosene. As a possible explanation they offered the influence of surface tension on mechanical interdependence and noted that a fall in surface tension resulting from compression of surfaces in regions surrounding those undergoing expansion, would tend to decrease outward-acting stress and vice versa, and that surface hysteresis would thereby increase mechanical interdependence. Inactivation of surfactant would thus be expected to decrease interdependence and increase collateral compliance. This implies that interdependence should exhibit hysteresis. It is interesting that Menkes et al (38) observed hysteresis in their studies of interdependence in living dogs.

Coburn et al (12) studied the effects of contraction of the trachealis muscle on the flow-resistance of canine tracheal segments, following up the work of Olsen et al (44) who earlier demonstrated that the trachealis smooth muscle increases the rigidity of the trachea. They were interested in observing the minimal compressive pressure at which trachealis contraction causes a fall in resistance to air flow. Contraction resulted in increases in resistance of the noncompressed trachea, but in every instance, as collapsing pressure was increased, levels were reached beyond which contraction reduced resistance. The threshold for resistance decrease during contraction ranged from 8 to 45 cm H_2O. They noted that increased tracheal resistance per se would tend to move equal pressure points (points where side pressures equal pleural pressure) at maximal flow downstream (i.e. "mouthward"), but since under conditions of maximal flow the compressing pressures are probably above the threshold levels, contraction of the trachealis muscle should reduce resistance and hence allow equal pressure points to move further upstream (i.e. toward alveoli) than they would otherwise. It has been suggested that bronchoconstriction of small airways during coughing would allow upstream migration of equal pressure points and hence lengthening of the segment of the compression. Tracheal "constriction" perhaps somewhat paradoxically would have the same effect.

Horie & Hildebrandt (23) wanted to distinguish the relative contributions of tissues and surface forces from those of airway closure, to time-dependent changes in lung compliance and stress adaptation. They carried out identical sequences of filling and emptying and volume cycling with air and saline in excised lungs, primarily from cats. Their careful experiments beautifully exemplified the high degree of consistency possible with excised lungs, even for extended measurements. Qualitatively, they found that saline-filled lungs, freed from the influence of surface tension, showed similar stress adaptation during deflation and similar time-dependence of compliance to that observed in air-filled lungs, but the changes were only about ⅛ as large. Thus most of the changes in air-filled lungs could be attributed to the surface. There were important differences in behavior at different lung volumes, however. At high lung volumes, static pressures decreased and compliance increased, whereas at lower volume static pressures increased and compliance decreased, with time. Below about ½ TLC there was some evidence of airway closure, but this was not marked until transpulmonary pressures as low as 1 cm H_2O were reached. Alveolar surface tension, estimated from differences between the saline and air curves, was also volume-dependent. At high volumes it tended toward values similar to equilibrium values for surface tension obtained on lung extracts—in the neighborhood of 20 dynes/cm. But at low volumes it remained well below these tensions, suggesting that low lung volumes can be "maintained for long periods without rapid surface stiffening and alveolar instability." Apparently within lungs a single equilibrium pressure does not exist. This implies that the in situ surface film exhibits some attributes of an elastic solid. And this in turn may reflect the thinness of the subphase which prevents extensive exchange.

Horie & Hildebrandt's studies were carried out on excised lungs at room temperature. Lempert & Macklem (34) were interested in the influence of temperature on the area-tension behavior of surfaces derived from lung extracts and on the volume-pressure behavior of excised lungs. They confirmed

Horie & Hildebrandt's conclusion that surfaces within the lung and surfaces of lung extracts behave differently, and they demonstrated substantial temperature dependence. All of their volume cycles were from complete collapse to full expansion and back, so that compared to the changes in volume seen by Horie & Hildebrandt, (23) their studies are complicated. For example, a substantial amount of hysteresis observed probably reflected airway closure. One would like to see the two approaches combined to distinguish the relative contribution of tissue and surface forces and of airway closure to the thermal effects. Lempert & Macklem revived an earlier observation by Setnikar (50), which has been hinted at in enough different experiments that it appears to be real and needs to be dealt with. They found, particularly at the lower temperature, that volume-pressure hysteresis instead of remaining constant at low frequencies as has been observed by others, actually decreased as the rate of volume change was increased. Perhaps this also relates to airway closure. If closure is time-dependent, then less time at a low volume implies less closure and hence less hysteresis during rapid than during slow cycles. Certainly the time-dependent aspects of parenchymal hysteresis during rapid cycling remain controversial.

Another study of the nature of static hysteresis is also complicated by the extent of the volume cycle. Hills (21) convincingly demonstrated that human lungs, when expanded from the collapsed state to full inflation and then allowed to deflate, have a different shape at a given volume during expansion than during deflation, and he concluded that a substantial part of the lung's static hysteresis must depend on geometric factors and not on surface hysteresis per se. But he made all of his observations under conditions which, again, favor airway closure. Lungs put through a volume cycle including collapse certainly exhibit geometric irreversibility to the naked eye. It would certainly be of interest to know whether they are geometrically reversible in the volume range where the substantial hysteresis of lungs is demonstrable with little evidence of airway closure.

With regard to hysteresis, and recalling the earlier discussion of the possible significance of a balance between airway and parenchymal hysteresis, it is interesting to note that Kahana & Thurlbeck (31) reported that patients with chronic obstructive lung disease exhibited less static volume-pressure hysteresis than healthy adults—indeed, on the average they showed very little static hysteresis at all. The authors concluded that "the surface component of hysteresis might have been minimized by structural changes such as a decrease in internal surface area of the lung or enlargement of airspaces," and that the tissue component might be reduced as a result of "permanent overstretching of fibrous elements." I find myself wondering whether such patients have normal airway hysteresis. If they do, in the face of reduced parenchymal hysteresis they should tend to have small airways at a given lung volume after a deep expiration, and vice versa. Possibly the aggravation of symptoms observed after forced expirations in many of these patients reflects in part such a mismatch.

The discovery that chronic lung disease can be produced by genetically related enzyme deficiencies (33), which presumably allow abnormal rates of proteolysis in lungs, and indeed that relative deficiencies of this sort may be a predisposing factor for chronic lung disease on a much wider basis (40), gives new significance to studies on the effects of proteolytic enzymes on lungs. Caldwell (9) injected papain into the trachea of living rabbits and later measured isovolume pressure-flow curves and related these to histologic changes. He found no significant change in static lung volume or compliance, but maximal expiratory flows at a given lung volume were decreased. Histologically he found a small but highly significant reduction in the number of alveolar attachments to noncartilagenous airways, and he suggested that the reduced expiratory flows reflected the loss of "tethering properties of alveolar walls to airways, rendering them unstable at normal maximal expiratory flow levels." Since the contribution of noncartilagenous airways to total airway resistance is probably negligible at the volumes at which maximum flows were observed to be diminished, and since dynamic compression probably does not extend to such airways, this explanation seems unlikely. The finding nevertheless emphasized that in disease mechanical coupling between parenchyma and airways is influenced not only by changes in tissue properties (i.e. force per fiber) but by changes in fiber density. The number of attachments—fixed in normal lungs—is an important variable in diseased lungs.

In a separate study Caldwell & Bland (10) administered D-penicillamine to rabbits. This agent specifically blocks collagen synthesis and increases collagen breakdown. They found small but significant increases in vital capacity and total respiratory compliance, but no significant change in maximal expiratory flow rates. It is difficult to interpret the mechanical findings without more information about absolute lung volume and static transpulmonary pressure. A promising feature of this study, however, is the observation that real changes in the living lung can be produced in comparatively short periods with an agent that acts specifically on collagen.

Johanson & Pierce (29) incubated excised rat lungs with various proteolytic enzymes: chlostridial collagenase, pancreatic elastase, and papain. The collagenase had no dramatic effect either on the volume-pressure characteristics of these lungs or on their structure as observed histologically. The elastase and papain, on the other hand, produced marked distortions including enlargement of central lobular air spaces, and abnormal staining of elastin fibers, but they also resulted in substantial increases in the slope of the static deflation curves at low lung volumes. All of the agents appeared to break down reticulin fibers. None produced demonstrable changes in the larger collagen fibers. Their findings are consistant with the supposition of Setnikar (51) that elastin contributes importantly to lung elasticity at low lung volumes, and collagen at high levels of distention. The authors put it differently and I think somewhat misleadingly: "The results suggest that elastin is the major connective tissue determinant of lung structure and elastic behavior." Although the results do suggest that reticulin probably does not greatly influence mechanical behavior (all the agents disrupted reticulin but not all produced mechanical changes), it certainly cannot be concluded that collagen is not an important determinant of lung structure and elastic behavior from these observations since the larger collagen fibers were apparently not attacked by any of the agents. Indeed after elastin digestion the volume-pressure relationship at high distending pressures was not changed appreciably, and collagen presumably must have contributed very importantly to the elastic properties of these lungs at high volumes.

STUDIES IN LIVE ANIMALS

Nadel and his co-workers, who introduced the tantalum dusting technique (43), have made excellent use of it in studies of responses of airways to nervous stimulation (8). They confirmed their earlier finding that vagal stimulation produces diffuse constriction of airways from trachea to bronchi 0.5 mm i.d. and they demonstrated that sympathetic stimulation moderated but never abolished the effect of vagal stimulation. Since sympathetic stimulation or injection of isoproterenol did not produce significant bronchodilitation in vagotomized dogs, they concluded that there is no resting tone in airways of vagotomized dogs. Sympathetic stimulation after pharmacologic β-adrenergic blockade did not produce bronchoconstriction, suggesting that no significant number of α-receptors exist in airways of dogs. Beta-receptor blockade is known to constrict airways in asthmatic subjects, and this has been thought to reflect unmasking of α-receptors. Cabezas et al (8) suggested instead that since atropine prevents this response, β-receptor blockade produces bronchoconstriction in man by increasing the effect of cholinergic parasympathetic tone.

In a separate study from the same laboratory, Sterling et al (54) examined the old question of the effects of CO_2 on airways. They vagotomized dogs so as to avoid reflex bronchoconstriction and showed that the increase in pulmonary flow resistance induced by serotonin infusion could be reversed by CO_2 inhalation, but that similar increase induced either by vagal stimulation or acetylcholine could not. They obtained similar results in isolated canine bronchial rings. Isocapnic and hypercapnic acidosis had similar effects. Three possible actions of the acidosis are suggested: it may interfere with the action of serotonin on smooth muscle receptor sites; it may redistribute serotonin into cells and hence away from receptor sites; and it may interfere with some metabolic pathway involved in serotonin-induced contraction.

Johnson & Lindskog (30), using essentially the same methods originally described by van Allen & Lindskog and co-workers some 40 years ago (56), studied the influence of isoproterenol and CO_2 on collateral overflow. In this preparation the anesthetized dog with left thoracotomy was ventilated with a piston pump. An anterior segmental bronchus of the left lower lobe was cannulated and connected to a Krogh spirometer and the rate of collection therein measured. This flow rate depends ultimately on the pressure developed by the pump and all intervening resistances, which include not only that of the collateral pathways but also that upstream from the collateral pathways—i.e. between the pump and the collateral pathways—and those downstream from the collateral pathways—i.e. that between the collateral pathways and the collecting spirometer. Since the spirometer was carefully balanced, the pressure distending the airway downstream from the collateral pathways must have been low, and it is possible that these downstream pathways contributed substantially to the overall resistance. Accordingly, the change in flow cannot clearly distinguish changes in resistance in the collateral pathways. Thus the increase in flow following isoproterenol could possibly reflect decreased resistance up and down stream from the collateral pathways. But one result in particular is of interest. Five percent (5%) CO_2, which is known to produce bronchoconstriction in anesthetized dogs with intact vagi and which in the present instance increased somewhat the "tracheal resistance pressure"—the peak pressure during inspiration, was associated with a striking increase in collateral flow (range for four animals; +31% to +198%). This is a remarkable result. Might it possibly relate to the observations of Sterling et al (54)? Is there possibly a local state of serotonin-induced bronchoconstriction which the CO_2 reverses? Or is there specific action of CO_2 (or pH) on collateral pathways as is suggested by the authors?

The two studies from Nadel's group typify the two ways in which airway responses are measured: direct estimates from dimensions and indirect inferences of dimensional changes from measurements of flow resistance. The papers of Stănescu et al (53) and of Spann & Hyatt (52) on the human upper airway are complementary in the same sense. Stănescu et al estimated transverse diameters of the glottis opening by indirect laryngoscopy. Spann & Hyatt measured laryngeal resistance during breathing by relating flow to the pressure difference between a needle passed just below the cricoid cartilage and a pharyngeal catheter. Both groups studied the effects of changing lung volume and of voluntary panting compared to quiet breathing, and their results agree with each other and with previous observations: The glottis opening is variable in and between individuals, it increases in size as lung volume is increased from resting levels, and it increases in size during panting. Spann & Hyatt also measured resistance between the pharynx and the mouthpiece and in general this resistance was equal to or slightly greater than laryngeal resistance, and changed with it. They found that upper airway resistance increased significantly both with flexion and extension of the neck but noted that the changes in head position were rather marked. It is of practical interest that change from a neutral position to 29° of extension was associated with the mean increase of resistance of about 0.4 cm H_2O liter^{-1} sec^{-1}, which suggests that variability due to head position should be fairly easy to control.

The variability of the glottic aperture during quiet breathing is of much greater practical significance. For those interested in interpreting measurements of total airway, or total pulmonary, or total respiratory resistance made during quiet breathing in terms of pulmonary changes, the nonphonating larynx remains an important source of "noise." This is clearly demonstrated in the results of Peslin et al (47), who used the method of forced oscillation and studied the variation in resistance of the total respiratory system during the respiratory cycle. With their method they were able to estimate Rohrer's constants in the expression $\Delta P = K_1 \dot{V} = K_2 \dot{V}^2$. K_2 represents the flow-dependent component of resistance, which is known to be substantial in the upper airway. In the past this component has been estimated only during voluntary hyperventilation, when the glottis tends to be fairly well open. It is not at all surprising that the values for K_2 observed by Peslin et al during quiet breathing are considerably higher (roughly three times) than previous values or that the values during expiration are significantly higher (roughly 1.4 times) than those during inspiration. In several subjects resistance increased abruptly during the cycle, most commonly toward the end of expiration. In one of these, simultaneous measurements of intratracheal pressure localized the change to the upper airway.

Combining this experience and that of previous studies, it would appear that upper airways resistance is greater during quiet breathing than during hyperventilation and that it also is more variable from breath to breath and within the breathing cycle. As yet no one has discovered how to reduce this variability except by voluntary panting and this remains the "maneuver of choice" for estimating changes in the resistance of intrathoracic airways.

Spann & Hyatt (52) made two additional observations which are relevant to their earlier studies. The breathing of increased concentrations of CO_2 (5% CO_2, 55% O_2, 40% N_2) produced fairly consistent but very small decreases in laryngeal resistance, indicating that changes in total airways resistance during CO_2 exposure do not include appreciable contribution from the upper airway in conscious man, which has previously been suggested. They also reexamined Rattenborg's conclusion that laryngeal resistance adjusts to compensate for changes in external resistance (48) and failed to find any evidence for this.

Lacourt & Polgar (32) have also described compensating changes in resistance in one part of the airway for changes in another. They have found that the substantial oscillations of nasal resistance in infants is accompanied by compensating oscillations in pulmonary resistance. They used an ingenious approach to partitioning nasal and non-nasal resistance. They measured total airway resistance in three conditions: breathing through both nostrils, through just one nostril, and through just the other nostril. They considered the total airway as three fixed resistances; two being the two nasal passages in parallel, and the third being the remainder of the airway in series. With three unknowns and three equations they solved for the individual resistances. But to the extent that the resistances are flow-dependent, the assumption of constant resistance is incorrect. With one nostril obstructed the flow through the other nostril would increase, thereby increasing its resistance, while total flow would if anything decrease, thereby decreasing non-nasal resistance. The authors state that the flow-pressure plots were only "minimally alinear." It seems unlikely that upper airway resistance in infants, however, is strikingly more linear than in adults. It might well be that the real nonlinearities lead to overestimation of nasal resistance by the method used, which in turn are greater when nasal resistance is increased, and that the compensating reduction in non-nasal resistance is the consequence of this error. This possibility can certainly be tested since the degree of linearity of nasal resistance in infants can be measured relatively simply.

Hogg et al (22) used the retrograde catheter technique to partition airway resistance in dog lungs during induced pulmonary congestion and edema. The resistance of peripheral airways (less than 2 mm i.d.) increased markedly as left atrial pressure was raised, while central airway resistance (airways greater than 2 mm i.d.) changed little. When the increase in pressure was less than about 15 mm Hg, the resistance increase was immediately reversed on lowering left atrial pressure. When the increase was greater than 15 mm Hg and prolonged, the further increase in resistance was not immediately reversible. The authors noted that total pulmonary resistance showed little change until gross edema was present. This statement is consistent with other observations of total pulmonary resistance during pulmonary congestion, but seemed not to be consistent with their own results. In their preparation peripheral resistance was about equal to central resistance under control conditions, and at a left atrial pressure of 15 mm Hg, which would not be expected to be associated with lung edema, it was very nearly doubled on the average at low transpulmonary pressure. This means that total pulmonary resistance should have increased by 50% since central airway resistance meanwhile if anything also increased slightly. This seems more than "a little change." Indeed the increase in total resistance inferred in this way is greater than has previously been reported in pulmonary congestion. The authors suggest that the immediately reversible component of the increase in pulmonary resistance may relate to compression of small airways by engorged vessels within the confinements of the bronchovascular sheath, and the less immediately reversible increase at left atrial pressures above 15 mm Hg may reflect the collection of edema in this space. It should be noted that although edema was seen to be mainly perivascular rather than peribronchial, to the extent that the structures share a common sheath, perivascular edema would be expected to result in airway compression. In addition, it is worth noting that in absolute terms all of the changes were small compared to ones that might be expected to produce symptoms. If responses are similar in humans it would be safe to say that so-called cardiac asthma could not have a purely congestive basis.

Bouhuys & van de Woestijne (4) measured airway conductance and maximum expiratory flow in normal subjects before and after bronchodilatation. Total lung capacity and static recoil pressures remained unchanged. Airway conductance increased significantly more (average increase 35%) than maximum expiratory flow at 50% vital capacity (average increase 9%). Since recoil pressures did not change, the conductance of the airways upstream from equal pressure points (the points at which intrabronchial side pressures equal pleural pressure) increased less than the conductance of the total airway. They hypothesize that bronchodilatation renders large airways more compressible and that this limits flow increase during forced expiration by limiting upstream migration of equal pressure points, thereby lengthening the upstream segment. In two instances maximum flow actually decreased—suggesting that lengthening of the upstream segment has a predominating influence on its resistance despite bronchodilatation.

It is interesting to relate their hypothesis to mechanical interdependence. Bronchodilatation would tend to diminish the local expanding stress on intrapulmonary airways. In effect, static peribronchial pressure, or its equivalent, would be less negative than pleural pressure. As a result, equal pressure points would not be where transmural pressures are zero or positive, as is the case in the normal lung, but rather at points where transmural pressures are negative and where airways are therefore somewhat compressed. Thus the resistance of the upstream segment could be increased on the basis of changes in cross-section, and changes in length need not be involved. But there is an additional possibility that needs to be considered. The state of the airway smooth muscle at the instant of maximum flow, which by definition has an immediate previous history of having been stretched, may differ from its state during the airway conductance measurement, when any previous stretch is further in the past. Might it not be possible that airways during forced vital capacities are in a relative state of dilatation on a purely mechanical basis and that they have a shorter distance to go, as it were, to the dilated state? This possibility could be tested by examining partial flow-volume curves initiated at intermediate lung volumes at various time intervals after maximal inhalation, before and after bronchodilators.

Stubbs & Hyatt (55) repeated the chest-strapping experiments of Butler et al (7, 11) and included measurements of forced expirations and isovolume pressure-flow curves. They applied thoraco-abdominal strapping with sufficient vigor to eight normal subjects to reduce vital capacity by 40% and residual volume by 11%, on the average. Measurements made as soon as two to three minutes after strapping did not change further during the next 45 min or so. As in the earlier results, static transpulmonary pressure increased at a given volume, and the associated increase in conductance was what would be expected from the relationship between static recoil pressure and conductance seen before strapping. To this Stubbs & Hyatt added the result that maximum expiratory flow also falls along the control relationship between static-recoil pressure and maximum flow. The authors were chiefly interested in the mechanism responsible for the increase in static recoil pressures, and they offered a carefully reasoned argument to the effect that the change relates mainly to changes in alveolar surface tension rather than in airway closure and atelectasis. In their observation of a fixed relationship between static recoil pressure, conductance, and maximum expiratory flow, I see a paradox: This relationship implies that airways do not exhibit pressure-volume hysteresis; but we already know that they do. Airway hysteresis means that airways are narrower at a given transpulmonary pressure during inflation from low volumes than during deflation from high volumes. And, indeed this is what may be inferred from measurements of resistance in human subjects (57). Now, although Stubbs & Hyatt's measurements were all made during expirations, they certainly were made with very different volume histories; the measurements during strapping followed inspirations from relatively low volumes, i.e. reduced FRCs which had been maintained for some time, to maximum transpulmonary pressures at peak inspiration which were comparatively modest (10 to 20 cm H_2O), whereas the control measurements followed maximal inspirations to substantially higher volumes and peak inspiratory transpulmonary pressures of from 20 to 40 plus cm H_2O. Certainly one would expect that airways should have been smaller at a given static transpulmonary pressure during strapping than before on the basis of these differences in volume history. I don't know how to explain this paradox without bringing in changes in bronchomotor tone. The authors considered the possible advantages in having lung compliance decrease when breathing occurs at low lung volumes, and they noted that if transpulmonary pressure remained low at low lung volumes airways would tend to close, and that increases in static-transpulmonary pressures would tend to prevent this. Of course, bronchodilatation would be useful in this respect as well. Is it possible that changes in smooth muscle tone in the case of airways, and of surface tension in the case of airspaces, tend to be homeostatic? When, because of force of gravity and change in posture, a given region is reduced in volume, does its smooth muscle relax and its surface tension increase so as to stabilize it and keep its airways open?

MODELING

A symposium, "Models in Ventilatory Mechanics" was held in Paris as a satellite to the International Congress of Physiological Sciences in Munich, and papers presented there have been collected in a single volume of the *Bulletin de Physio-Pathologie Respiratoire* (Vol. 8, 1972). The general impression given is that a more or less common level of sophistication exists in a number of laboratories interested in lung models, and that in the future more adequate models will surely be developed to enhance our knowledge of what we are measuring. In an introductory paper Otis (45) gave a delightful historical account with a unique collection of illustrations of famous models of the past. Many of the presentations include general comments about modeling. I found those of Schroter et al (49) particularly instructive. They distinguished three major categories: scale models, e.g., physical models of airways; analog models, i.e., electrical and mechanical equivalents; and mathematical models. They warn us that although analog models are frequently convenient they usually bear no fundamental similarity to the physical elements underlying the real process. They divide mathematical models into three groups: transport models, based on the laws of transport processes and involving the application of physical-chemical principles; statistical models, and empirical models—Hildebrandt refers to the last as "equivalent models" (20).

In empirical models experimental data are fitted to arbitrary curves and the resulting equations used to describe the real process. (An example would be Rohrer's expression for the airway pressure-flow relationship, which was developed as a transport model, and has been discarded in this capacity but remains in use as an empirical model.) Empirical models are liable to the shortcomings of analog models and indeed in essence are a form of analog model, the curve-fitting expression being the analog. Several of the presentations pointed to the limitations of linear models, typified by the electrical circuit analogies. It is somewhat paradoxical that the transport and scale models that have been developed for airways indicate nonlinearities which if anything appear to be greater than those observed in real lungs. Clearly the model makers have created the need for better and more carefully controlled measurements on lungs.

LITERATURE CITED

1. Angus, G. E., Thurlbeck, W. M. 1972. Number of alveoli in the human lung. *J. Appl. Physiol.* 32:483–85
2. Bartlett, D., Jr. 1971. Postnatal growth of the mammalian lung: influence of excess growth hormone. *Resp. Physiol.* 12:297–304
3. Bartlett, D., Jr., Remmers, J. E. 1971. Effects of high altitude exposure on the lungs of young rats. *Resp. Physiol.* 13:116–25
4. Bouhuys, A., van de Woestijne, K. P. 1971. Mechanical consequences of airway smooth muscle relaxation. *J. Appl. Physiol.* 30:670–76
5. Brody, J. S., Fisher, A. B., Gocmen, A., Dubois, A. B. 1970. Acromegalic pneumonomegaly: lung growth in the adult. *J. Clin. Invest.* 49:1051–60
6. Burri, P. H., Weibel, E. R. 1971. Morphometric estimation of pulmonary diffusion capacity. II. Effect of P_{O_2} on the growing lung. Adaptation of the growing rat lung to hypoxia and hyperoxia. *Resp. Physiol.* 11:247–64
7. Butler, J., Caro, C. G., Alcala, R., Dubois, A. B. 1960. Physiological factors affecting airway resistance in normal subjects and in patients with obstructive respiratory disease. *J. Clin. Invest.* 39:584–91
8. Cabezas, G. A., Graf, P. D., Nadel, J. A. 1971. Sympathetic versus parasympathetic nervous regulation of airways in dogs. *J. Appl. Physiol.* 31:651–55
9. Caldwell, E. J. 1971. Physiologic and anatomic effects of papain on the rabbit lung. *J. Appl. Physiol.* 31:458–65
10. Caldwell, E. J., Bland, J. H. 1972. The effect of penicillamine on the rabbit lung. *Am. Rev. Resp. Dis.* 105:75–84
11. Caro, C. G., Butler, J., Dubois, A. B. 1960. Some effects of restriction of chest cage expansion on pulmonary function in man: an experimental study. *J. Clin. Invest.* 39:573–83
12. Coburn, R. F., Thornton, D., Arts, R. 1972. Effect of trachealis muscle contraction on tracheal resistance to airflow. *J. Appl. Physiol.* 32:397–403
13. Colebatch, H. J. H., Mitchell, C. A. 1971. Constriction of isolated living liquid-filled dog and cat lungs with histamine. *J. Appl. Physiol.* 30:691–702
14. Cumming, G., Horsfield, K., Harding, L. K., Prowse, K. 1971. Biological branching systems, with special reference to the lung airways. *Bull. Physio-path. Resp.* 7:31–38
15. Da Costa, J. L. 1971. Pulmonary function studies in healthy Chinese adults in Singapore. *Am. Rev. Resp. Dis.* 104:128–31
16. Davies, G., Reid, L. 1971. Effect of scoliosis on growth of alveoli and pulmonary arteries and on right ventricle. *Arch. Dis. Child.* 46:623–32
17. Dunnill, M. S. 1962. Postnatal growth of the lung. *Thorax.* 17:329–333
18. Gamsu, G., Thurlbeck, W. M., Macklem, P. T., Fraser, R. G. 1971. Peripheral bronchographic morphology in the normal human lung. *Invest. Radiol.* 6:161–70
19. Hayek, H. 1960. *The Human Lung,* transl. V. E. Krahl. New York: Hafner
20. Hildebrandt, J. 1972. Models of pressure-volume hysteresis. *Bull. Physio-path. Resp.* 8:337–50
21. Hills, B. A. 1971. Geometric irreversibility and compliance hysteresis in the lung. *Resp. Physiol.* 13:50–61
22. Hogg, J. C. et al 1972. Distribution of airway resistance with developing pulmonary edema in dogs. *J. Appl. Physiol.* 32:20–24
23. Horie, T., Hildebrandt, J. 1971. Dynamic compliance, limit cycles, and static equilibria of excised cat lung. *J. Appl. Physiol.* 31:423–30
24. Horsfield, K., Cumming, G. 1968. Morphology of the bronchial tree in man. *J. Appl. Physiol.* 24:373–83
25. Horsfield, K., Dart, G., Filley, G. F., Olson, D. E., Cumming, G.

1971. Models of the human bronchial tree. *J. Appl. Physiol.* 31:207–17

26. Hughes, J. M. B., Hoppin, F. G., Jr., Mead, J. 1972. Effect of lung inflation on bronchial length and diameter in excised lungs. *J. Appl. Physiol.* 32:25–35

27. Hyatt, R. E., Flath, R. 1966. Influence of lung parenchyma on pressure-diameter behavior of dog bronchi. *J. Appl. Physiol.* 21:1448–52

28. Hyatt, R. E., Sittipong, R., Olafson, S., Potter, W. A., 1970. Some factors determining pulmonary pressure-flow behavior at high rates of flow. *Airway Dynamics,* ed. A. Bouhuys, 43–60. Springfield, Illinois: Thomas

29. Johanson, W. G., Jr., Pierce, A. K. 1972. Effects of elastase, collagenase, and papain on structure and function of rat lungs in vitro. *J. Clin. Invest.* 51:288–93

30. Johnson, R. M., Lindskog, G. E. 1971. Further studies on factors influencing collateral ventilation. *J. Thorac. Cardiov. Surg.* 63:321–29

31. Kahana, L. M., Thurlbeck, W. M. 1972. Surface tension and static volume pressure hysteresis in pulmonary emphysema and other conditons. *Am. Rev. Resp. Dis.* 105:217–28

32. Lacourt, G., Polgar, G. 1971. Interaction between nasal and pulmonary resistance in newborn infants. *J. Appl. Physiol.* 30:870–73

33. Laurell, C. B., Eriksson, S. 1963. The electrophoretic alpha$_1$-globulin pattern of serum in alpha$_1$-antitrypsin deficiency. *Scand. J. Clin. Lab. Invest.* 15:132–40

34. Lempert, J., Macklem, P. T. 1971. Effect of temperature on rabbit lung surfactant and pressure-volume hysteresis. *J. Appl. Physiol.* 31:380–85

35. Matsubu, K., Thurlbeck, W. M. 1971. The number and dimensions of small airways in nonemphysematous lungs. *Am. Rev. Resp. Dis.* 104:516–24

36. Mead, J., Takishima, T., Leith, D. 1970. Stress distribution in lungs: a model of pulmonary elasticity. *J. Appl. Physiol.* 28:596–608

37. Menkes, H., Gardiner, A., Gamsu, G., Lempert, J., Macklem, P. T.,

1971. Influence of surface forces on collateral ventilation. *J. Appl. Physiol.* 31:544–49

38. Menkes, H., Lindsay, D., Wood, L., Muir, A., Macklem, P. T. 1972. Interdependence of lung units in intact dog lungs. *J. Appl. Physiol.* 32:681–86

39. Menkes, H., Gamsu, G., Schroter, R., Macklem, P. T. 1972. Interdependence of lung units in isolated dog lungs. *J. Appl. Physiol.* 32:675–80

40. Mittman, C., Lieberman, J., Marasso, F., Miranda, A. 1971. Smoking and chronic obstructive lung disease in alpha$_1$-antitrypsin deficiency. *Chest* 60:214–21

41. Murtagh, P. S., Proctor, D. F., Permutt, S., Kelly, B. L., Evering, S. 1971. Bronchial mechanics in excised dog lobes. *J. Appl. Physiol.* 31:403–8

42. Murtagh, P. S., Proctor, D. F., Permutt, S., Kelly, B., Evering, S., 1971. Bronchial closure with mecholyl in excised dog lobes. *J. Appl. Physiol.* 31:409–15

43. Nadel, J. A., Wolfe, W. G., Graf, P. D., 1968. Powdered tantalum as a medium for bronchography in canine and human lungs. *Invest. Radiol.* 3:229–38

44. Olsen, C. R., Stevens, A. E., McIlroy, M. B. 1967. Rigidity of trachea and bronchi during muscular constriction. *J. Appl. Physiol.* 23:27–34

45. Otis, A. B. 1972. Man's urge to model. *Bull. Physio-Path. Resp.* 8:181–98

46. Parker, H., Horsfield, K., Cumming, G. 1971. Morphology of distal airways in the human lung. *J. Appl. Physiol.* 31:386–91

47. Peslin, R., Hixon, T., Mead, J. 1971. Variations des resistances thoraco-pulmonaires au cours du cycle ventilatoire etudiees par methode d'oscillation. *Bull. Physio-Pathol. Resp.* 7:173–86

48. Rattenborg, C. 1961. Laryngeal regulation of respiration. *Acta Anaesthesiol. Scand.* 5:129–40

49. Schroter, R. C., Pedley, T. J., Dudlow, M. F. 1972. The design of a model in physics and physiology. *Bull. Physio-path. Resp.* 8:209–23

50. Setnikar, I. 1955. "Meccanica respiratoria." *Aggiornamenti di Fi-*

siologica, Vol. 3, ed. L. Macri, Florence, Italy

51. Setnikar, I. 1955. Origine e significate delle propriate meccacische del pulmone. *Arch. Fisiol.* 55:349

52. Spann, R. W., Hyatt, R. E. 1971. Factors affecting upper airway resistance in conscious man. *J. Appl. Physiol.* 31:708–12

53. Stănescu, D. C., Pattijn, J., Clement, J., van de Woestijne, K. P. 1972. Glottis opening and airway resistance. *J. Appl. Physiol.* 32:460–66

54. Sterling, G. M., Holst, P. E., Nadel, J. A. 1972. Effect of CO_2 and pH on bronchoconstriction caused by serotonin vs. acetylcholine. *J. Appl. Physiol.* 32:39–43

55. Stubbs, S. E., Hyatt, R. E. 1972. Effect of increased lung recoil pressure on maximal expiratory flow in normal subjects. *J. Appl. Physiol.* 32:325–31

56. van Allen, C. M., Lindskog, G. E., Richter, H. G. 1930. Gaseous interchange between adjacent lung lobules. *Yale J. Biol. Med.* 2: 297–300

57. Vincent, N. J., Knudson, R., Leith, D. E., Macklem, P. T., Mead, J. 1970. Factors influencing pulmonary resistance *J. Appl. Physiol.* 29:236–43

58. Weibel, E. R. 1963. *Morphometry of the Human Lung.* Berlin: Springer.

Ann. Rev. Physiol. 1973. 35:193–220

THE PHYSIOLOGY OF EXERCISE 1094
UNDER HEAT STRESS

Cyril H. Wyndham

*Human Sciences Laboratory, Chamber of Mines of South Africa and
University of Witwatersrand, Johannesburg, South Africa*

Introduction

The four-year period of the review—mid 1968 to mid 1972—was one of considerable activity in the field of heat and exercise physiology. Major conferences have been held annually, resulting in the following notable publications: *Physiological and Behavioral Temperature Regulation* (22); *Proceedings of the Fifth International Biometeriological Congress* (91); *Proceedings of the International Symposium on Behavioral Temperature Regulation* (10); *Essays on Temperature Regulation* (7); and *Proceedings of the Dublin Symposium on Temperature Regulation* (92). The amount of research is too great to review effectively in the space allotted; consequently no effort was made to consider all papers in the period assigned.

I have, therefore, confined myself to three aspects of acclimatization to heat—the mechanisms, the role of physical conditioning, and certain practical aspects; three aspects of physiological responses to exercise in heat—the central circulatory and body fluid shifts, capacitance vessels, and core temperature; and three aspects of temperature regulation—the statistical evaluation of the effects on sweating and heat conductance of the input signals from T_{core}, $\overline{T}_s$, and other thermal sources, the use of Bullard's resistance hygrometer in holding local skin temperature, T_{sl}, constant while varying other inputs and vice-versa, and the influence of modeling upon our concepts of temperature regulation.

Abbreviations

Abbreviations used in this article are: Es—evaporative sweat; T_{core}—core temperature; T_{es}—esophageal temperature; T_{fem}—femoral vein temperature; T_m—muscle temperature; T_r—rectal temperature; T_{saph}—saphenous vein temperature; $\overline{T}_s$—skin temperature; T_{sd}—skin temperature, deep; T_{sl}—skin temperature, local; T_{ty}—tympanic temperature; SGOT—serum glutamic oxaloacetic acid; SGPT—serum glutamic pyruvic transaminase; LDH—lactic dehydrogenase; ATP—adenosine triphosphate; 5-HT—5-hydroxytryptamine; Q_{10}—increase in metabolism per 10°C rise in tissue temperature.

ACCLIMATIZATION

Mechanisms.—Rowell et al (59) and Wyndham and his associates (115) studied the central circulation during heat acclimatization and, although different techniques were used for measuring cardiac output, the results of these studies were similar. Cardiac output and arteriovenous oxygen difference did not change significantly over the period of acclimatization; oxygen consumption increased significantly in the first day or two of exposure but thereafter returned to control levels. Significant increases in heart rate and decreases in stroke volume occurred in the first few days of acclimatization, but by about the tenth day of the procedure both had returned towards, but had not reached, control levels.

Three possible explanations have been put forward for the heart-rate/stroke-volume adjustments. One is that there is a rapid expansion in plasma volume. A 16% increase on day 5 was shown by Bass et al (3) some years ago using T-1824 and a 10% increase by Wyndham et al (115) on day 3 using ^{131}I. Both noted some subsequent decrease in the expansion of plasma volume but not a return to control values.

Another possible explanation is that venous tone increases. Wood & Bass (106) put forward evidence for this mechanism but in my view their method, the measurement of pressure/volume curves of an extremity, is unacceptable. The expansion in volume of a limb when the venous pressure is raised is not solely due to venous distension. More acceptable methods (Rowell et al 64, Zitnick et al 122) are now available for measuring venous tone and have shown clearly that venous tone is lost when there is an increase either in skin temperature or in core temperature.

The third possible explanation was put forward by Rowell et al (59), namely, that the change in heart rate is the primary event, due to decrease in core temperature T_{core} and skin temperature $\overline{T}_s$, as a result of acclimatization, and that the increase in stroke volume is secondary to the decrease in heart rate. This explanation is unlikely because the major fall in heart rate usually occurs in the first two to three days and precedes the decrease in T_{core} and $\overline{T}_s$.

The reason for the rapid expansion in plasma volume is not yet clear. Both Bass et al and Wyndham et al reported an expansion of the extracellular volume and postulated that this expansion could be explained by the retention of Na^+ as a result of an increase in the secretion of aldosterone. Wyndham et al (115) postulated further that it is the central circulatory instability on day 1 of acclimatization that "triggers" the volume receptors. This, in turn, is the stimulus to the renin-angiotensin mechanism which leads to the increased secretion of aldosterone. In the absence of an increase in the secretion of anti-diuretic hormone, an increase in the secretion of aldosterone should lead to an isotonic expansion of the extracellular space. Bass et al and Wyndham et al both found that the percentage increase in extravascular space is less than that of plasma volume, which should have indicated to them that the aldosterone mechanism was not the main factor. Furthermore, according to Collins & Weiner (11) and Smiles & Robinson (80) there is no certainty that the secretion of either aldosterone or anti-diuretic hormone is increased during acclimatization to heat in men in Na^+ and water balance.

Senay (76) has recently made a notable contribution to our understanding of the changes in fluid spaces during acclimatization. He measured total protein and hematocrit in men during mild exercise at 40°C before and after they were heat-acclimatized. He showed that in the unacclimatized state there was hemoconcentration and a loss of protein from the vascular space by the end of 45 min. After acclimatization the picture was completely different. There was hemodilution, and protein entered the intravascular space. Protein concentrations and hematocrit values, therefore, changed in opposite directions. These findings are a clear indication that the use of substances such as T-1824 or ^{131}I which are tagged to protein can give misleading results on the fluid shifts during acclimatization. Senay's results throw into doubt the percentage increases in plasma volume reported by both Bass et al and Wyndham et al.

Senay's explanation for the hemodilution and increase in concentration of protein in plasma with acclimatization is that there is either some modification in the content of the cutaneous interstitial space, perhaps a change in the sol:gel ratio. Or there might be an increased tendency for the translocated protein to remain within the vascular volume due to reduced permeability of the cutaneous capillaries to large molecules. A third possibility is that on first exposure to heat there is often circulatory instability with conflicting baroreceptor and thermoregulatory responses. Rowell et al (57) have noted on day 1 that "pronounced oscillations in skin color were sometimes observed as if a 'hunting' reaction for optimum distribution of cardiac output were occurring." It seems that it takes two to three days for the proper redistribution of blood flow between splanchnic, muscle, and cutaneous areas to occur and for the optimum blood flow in cutaneous regions to be established. This would fit in with Senay's observation that it takes a few days for the hemodilution of blood and the increase in protein concentration in plasma to take place during heat acclimatization.

Robinson and his associates (80) looked into the plasma volume changes during acclimatization from the point of view of Na^+ and water balances. One group of subjects had a total NaCl intake of 140 meq Na^+ per day and 1 liter of low Na^+ tap water—the low salt intake group. The other group had this basic Na^+ and water intake, plus replacement of all sweat Na^+ and water lost during heat exposure. The results showed that when the men were on full salt and water replacement they were in positive Na^+ balance but when they were on low salt and water intakes they developed Na^+ deficits of 140–320 meq. The weights of the subjects correlated well with the state of Na^+ balance, indicating that the weight changes were mainly due to changes in extracellular volume. On low salt and water intakes, the urinary output of Na^+ fell sharply during the first day of heat exposure but the sweat output of Na^+ decreased more slowly. The men on the low intakes also had a marked increase in tetrahydroaldosterone excretion; the hematocrits increased, indicating a decrease in plasma volume; and the sweat rate decreased and rectal temperatures rose to higher levels than when the men were on full salt and water replacements. The men on full water and salt replacement had no decrease in urinary or sweat Na^+: there was no increase in mineralo-corticoid secretion and the hematocrits decreased, indicating an increase in plasma volume; and, the sweat rates were higher and rectal temperatures were lower than in the men on low salt intakes. It seems clear from this study that hemodilution and the increase in plasma volume occur only when men are in salt and water balance. There was also no evidence that an increase in the secretion of aldosterone occurs or that urinary Na^+ decreases in men on full water and salt replacement. There is, therefore, no support in Robinson's study for the suggestion that Na^+ retention by the kidney occurs during acclimatization and results in isotonic expansion of the plasma volume unless there is concomitant low salt intake. Senay's hypothesis that the increase in concentration of plasma proteins causes the expansion of the intravascular volume during acclimatization is a more acceptable explanation.

The role of physical conditioning.—A dispute which began in 1965 continued into the period under review. Piwonka et al (51) claimed that university track-men were heat-acclimatized, whereas untrained subjects were not, as demonstrated when both groups walked on a treadmill in heat. Strydom et al (85) exposed a group of men to a standard heat test before and after a mild physical conditioning program and could show no evidence of heat-acclimatization, as manifested by sweat rate, rectal temperature, and heart rate changes. They criticized Robinson et al's comparison between university trackmen and untrained subjects as invalid, firstly because the trackmen weighed much less than the others and therefore had lower metabolic rates: rectal temperatures are directly proportional to metabolic rate. Secondly, the maximum oxygen intakes of the trackmen were much higher than those of the untrained subjects and the rectal temperatures during exercise in heat have been shown to be proportional to the percentage of maximum oxygen intake. Robinson et al's next paper (52) bore out Strydom et al's criticism because the university trackmen showed rapid improvement in rectal temperature and sweat rate over four days of daily exposure to exercise in heat, indicating that initially they were not heat-acclimatized.

Strydom et al (87) then studied the responses to heat stress of a group of men, before and after 12 days of more severe physical conditioning than in their first experiment. This comprised four hours per day of exercise at 1.6 liters/min oxygen consumption. Their study demonstrated that the strenuous physical conditioning program reduced rectal temperature and heart rate for the first two hours in standard heat tests, but thereafter rectal temperature and heart rate rose to the preacclimatization levels; sweat rate was not significantly changed. In Robinson et al's latest paper (16) a group of unfit men were physically conditioned; their physiological responses were improved when they exercised under hot conditions but were not as good as those of the university trackmen. Once again the comparison between the university trackmen and the others is invalid because of the differences between the two groups in body weights and in maximum oxygen intakes. A further criticism of Robinson et al's conclusion is that it is based upon only 90 min of heat exposure, whereas Strydom et al showed clearly that after two hours the physiological responses of the physically conditioned men were the same as those of the untrained men. A general conclusion that can be drawn from these studies is that physical conditioning improves the initial circulatory responses to exercise in heat but it does not alter sweat rate. Furthermore, in our view, acclimatization by means of controlled elevation of body temperature as proposed by Fox et al (15a) is also inadequate for conditioning at elevated temperatures because adaptation of both the circulatory system and the sweat glands is required, and for these adaptations *exercise* in heat is essential.

Practical considerations.—In the armed forces and in hot industries with a rapid turnover in the labor force, the problem of the most rapid and efficient method of acclimatizing large numbers of men is of practical importance. Wyndham & Strydom (116) have recently published their experience of acclimatizing some 280,000 new recruits per annum for physical work in hot and humid air conditions. These men are acclimatized in some 32 climatic chambers spread out over the gold mines in South Africa. The temperature of the air in these chambers is controlled at 31.7°C (in air saturated with water vapor) with an air movement of 0.4 m/sec.

The procedures employed for acclimatization to heat in the climatic rooms are based upon the following research: (a) Studies (89) to establish the minimum number of hours each day and the minimum number of days required for acclimatization showed that men cannot be acclimatized *adequately* for a normal work shift of 6 to 8 hours, in less than 4 hours per day and in less than 8 to 9 days. The often-quoted period of 90 min per day as adequate for acclimatization, according to Lind & Bass (33), was never validated in men working a full shift. (b) Studies (119) have been made to establish the combinations of wet bulb temperatures (in air saturated with water vapor and an air movement of 0.4 m/sec) and rates of oxygen consumption for "optimum" acclimatization. Optimum acclimatization is defined as the combination of heat stress conditions in which few men develop hyper-pyrexia (40°C) during the procedure and all are well adapted to work at an oxygen consumption of 1.0 liter/min at 32.2°C wet bulb temperature. The following conditions gave optimum acclimatization:

Oxygen consumption (liter/min)	Wet-bulb temperature (°C)
0.65 (light work)	34
0.95 (moderate work)	32
1.45 (hard work)	30.5

As a result of these studies the procedure used for acclimatization is a gradual increase in work rate and hence in the rate of oxygen consumption: from 1.0 to 1.4 liters/min over an 8–9 day period (obtained by having the men step on and off benches at 24 steps per min at heights which are adjusted to give the required work rates). The oxygen consumption of 1.4 liters/min was chosen because it is equivalent to the hardest physical task in the mine, shoveling rock (Morrison et al 40). Oral temperatures are measured every hour on each subject on each day of acclimatization, in order to detect and treat any man developing hyperpyrexia (oral temperature higher than 38°C). It is found that between 2 and 4% of the recruits are heat intolerant in that they develop hyperpyrexia every day of the procedure but are not found on medical examination to be suffering from any overt disease process. Heat intolerance will be dealt with in a later section.

PHYSIOLOGICAL REACTIONS TO EXERCISE IN HEAT

Central circulatory responses and body fluid shifts.—Wyndham and his colleagues (111) had shown earlier that in heat-acclimatized men, at different work rates up to their maximum oxygen intake, there is no significant difference in cardiac output at the same levels of oxygen consumption in hot compared with cool air conditions. Rowell et al (58) confirmed these findings and suggested that "metabolic requirements may be prepotent in the regulation of cardiac output during exercise in heat." They found that cardiac output was minimally affected by heat, when compared with cool conditions, up to 60% of maximum oxygen intake and that the main adjustment in the central circulation was a reduction in central blood volume and stroke volume which was compensated by a faster heart rate. Damato et al (12), using the direct Fick method, agreed with these findings in mild heat but in more severe heat they reported an increase in cardiac output both at rest and at mild exercise.

Rowell et al (58) demonstrated that the ability to maintain cardiac output in the face of a fall in stroke volume was lost when the combined stress of exercise and heat caused heart rate to rise to 180–190 beats/min. This occurred at about 60% of maximum oxygen intake in Rowell et al's subjects at 43°C. Under these circumstances the metabolic requirements of working muscle was supplied by a widening of the arteriovenous oxygen difference. However, as pointed out earlier by Wyndham et al (111), such a circulatory state is very unstable because if more blood is pooled in the veins of the lower extremities when, for example, the individual stands still after exercise or stands up after sitting at rest, then the venous return to the right heart decreases, right auricular pressure falls, and stroke volume is reduced. Heart rate being at its maximum cannot increase further; therefore cardiac output decreases, blood pressure falls precipitately, and syncope results.

In one case of severe heat syncope, Wyndham (108) observed a sharp fall in heart rate and a massive increase in forearm blood flow in association with the fall in blood pressure. He concluded that heat syncope is similar to the vasovagal faint seen in hemorrhage. Lind et al (34), in a recent study of syncope on tilting men in heat, were unable to substantiate this finding. One of their cases showed a sharp fall in heart rate but, with the fall in blood pressure, forearm blood flow decreased markedly, unlike that in the vasovagal faint. Lind postulated that, because blood flow in skin and muscle was reduced, there must be pooling of blood in the splanchnic region. This would be surprising in the light of Rowell et al's findings on hepatic blood flow which will be discussed below. Also contrary to Lind's hypothesis are the results of Shvartz's study (78) in which the syncope of tilting in heat was prevented by inflating a pneumatic cuff around either the lower abdomen or the legs. The mechanism of heat syncope is therefore still open.

The fact that cardiac output during exercise in heat does not increase above the level in cool conditions raises the question of how the increase in blood flow through the skin due to vasodilation of subcutaneous blood vessels is met. There could be a shunt of blood flow away from exercising muscles or a shunt of blood flow away from the splanchnic region. Wyndham et al (111) produced indirect evidence for the former mechanism in that blood lactate rose under hot conditions at oxygen intakes below 50% of maximum. This question, however, has been put upon a sound footing by the excellent research of Rowell and his group (57). They measured the hepatic clearances of indocyanine green and calculated hepatic blood flows on unacclimatized men during short exposures to exercise, at different percentages of maximum oxygen intake, at 25.6°C and at 43°C. They showed that hepatic blood flow decreased in inverse proportion to the percentage of maximum oxygen intake in both cool $(R = -0.78)$ and hot $(R = -0.81)$ conditions and, further, that in cool conditions hepatic blood flow only began to decrease when the subjects worked at 26% of maximum oxygen intake whereas in hot conditions hepatic blood flow at rest had already decreased below control values. At maximum oxygen intake at 25.6°C hepatic blood flow decreased by 72% and at 43°C the same percentage decrease in hepatic blood flow occurred at 80% of maximum oxygen intake. Rowell et al (60) also studied hepatic-splanchnic blood flow and metabolism during exercise in heat over a period of one hour in experiments which were designed to induce maximum reduction in hepatic-splanchnic blood flow. Subjects were exercised to exhaustion in an ambient air temperature of 48.9°C at workloads which required oxygen consumptions, ranging from 42 to 56% of maximum oxygen intake. These heat stress conditions reduced hepatic blood flow to a mean of 667 ml/min from the normal resting value of 1600 ml/min at a mean oxygen consumption of 2.02 liters/min, and hepatic blood flow was stable over the period of exposure. Hepatic oxygen consumption rose 1.4 times and hepatic venous oxygen fell to 0.6 ml/100 ml, probably as a result of the Q_{10} effect of the rise in hepatic vein temperature to 41.7°C (mean rectal temperature was 40.2°C). Evidence of abnormal hepatic metabolism was seen in the outpouring of hepatic glucose from 351 mg/min at 10 min to 749 mg/min at exhaustion and in the subnormal extraction of lactate by the liver of only 26%, which was associated with an abnormally high arterial blood lactate level. These results suggest hepatic ischaemia or anoxia; however, the unaltered K^+ levels in hepatic venous blood do not support this hypothesis.

The maintenance of the central circulation of blood during exercise in heat can be compromised, as suggested above, if the stroke volume falls excessively. This can occur if the plasma volume decreases, particularly during dehydration. Senay (73, 74) has pioneered a novel approach to the study of plasma volume during heat exposure. He measured the changes in hematocrit, plasma proteins, and crystalloids in men at rest or work when exposed to heat in the hydrated or dehydrated states. From these measurements he has been able to infer what the movements of fluid are between the vascular and extravascular spaces. During heat exposure, in various states of hydration, there were disproportionate changes in osmolarity, proteins, and hematocrit in plasma (73, 74, 75). For example, in his dehydration studies the percentage changes in protein concentrations in plasma were greater than the percentage changes in hematocrit. The dye T-1824 is bound to certain of the protein fractions; Senay's findings indicate that the two- to fivefold greater loss of water from the vascular space than from the total body reported by Saltin (67) and by Kozlowski & Saltin (30) using T-1824 is in error. Their calculations of the water losses, based on hematocrit values, correlated closely with those from the whole body. Senay's findings in this regard throw considerable doubt on all the previous studies of plasma volume changes during exposure to heat by markers which bind with proteins.

Senay suggests that protein enters the vascular space during exposure to heat at a greater rate than it escapes from the space. His hypothesis is that cutaneous vessels dilate when the body is exposed to heat; this increases the capillary filtration coefficient and increases the amount of fluid flowing through the interstitial spaces in the cutaneous bed. Cutaneous lymph contains considerable amounts of protein which would be washed into the vascular space through the main lymph ducts. Because of the molecular size of the proteins they would escape slowly from the intravascular space. The increased oncotic pressure of the protein in this space results in hemodilution. In Senay's studies, hemodilution was shown at rest in the hydrated state throughout the period of exposure to heat and for 2 to 3 hours in the dehydrated state also. When men exercise in heat there are opposing tendencies with regard to the movement of water between the intra- and extravascular spaces. Mild exercise in cool conditions causes hemodilution but more severe exercise results in hemoconcentration. When men exercise in heat, hemodilution may be prevented and the net movement of water between these spaces may result in hemoconcentration, as shown in Senay's dehydration study (75).

Capacitance vessels.—Shepherd and his associates have advanced our knowledge of the effects of local and central heating and cooling on capacitance vessels in the cutaneous and splanchnic regions. Rowell and his associates examined the effects on the central circulation of dilation of capacitance vessels, resulting from controlled changes in T_s.

Bevegard & Shepherd (5, 6) studied capacitance vessels of the forearm and hand in man during supine exercise with the legs. They measured the change in volume of the forearm and hand with plethysmographs, with a pneumatic cuff placed proximal to the plethysmograph and inflated to the single pressure of 30–40 mm Hg. They demonstrated that over the work rate range 220–810 kgm/min, transient venoconstriction occurred in the capacitance vessels of the forearm and hand, via the sympathetic nerves, and that the degree of venoconstriction was proportional to the workload. However, if the forearm and hand were heated to 44°C the venomotor reflex was abolished.

Zitnick, Ambrosioni & Shepherd (122) examined the effects of changes in local skin temperatures T_{sl} and core temperature T_{core} on venomotor tone during exercise in man by measuring the pressure in the dorsal vein of the hand during temporary occlusion of the circulation of the hand. Local heating of the hand from 34° to 42°C abolished venoconstriction, as did an increase in T_{core} from 36.6° to 38.4°C. The effect of change in T_{core} was more marked than change in T_{sl}. They also showed that the initial venoconstriction, at the onset of exercise, disappeared when T_{core} increased as a result of the exercise.

Rowell et al (65) used a similar technique for measuring the venous tone in the wrist vein of man in a study in which local arm temperature T_{sl} and whole body temperature $\bar{T}_s$ were changed separately and independently. The latter was done by varying the temperature of water flowing through a "space" suit worn by the subjects. The men exercised at 300 kpm/min during each of the four phases of the experiments. Change of arm T_{sl} at a constant $\bar{T}_s$ of 34°C altered venous tone, but with a larger latency and more gradually than when $\bar{T}_s$ was changed at constant T_{sl}. Change in $\bar{T}_s$ over 3–4°C changed venous tone in a cool arm ($T_{sl}=31$°C) rapidly and markedly. Central body temperature (measured in the right atrium) was unchanged during these procedures so that the changes in venous tone are entirely attributable to changes in $\bar{T}_s$ and T_{sl}. The venomotor responses to exercise at $\bar{T}_s$ of 34°C, before and after the series of experiments, were normal and this shows that the veins in the forearm retained their normal venomotor tone throughout the period of the experiment.

Rowell et al concluded that these responses are consistent with, firstly, changes in the adrenergic neural stimulation to cutaneous vein from altered $\bar{T}_s$; raising $\bar{T}_s$ reduces the rate of neural impulses so that even when veins are under local conditions for maximum constriction, no constriction occurs. Secondly, altering T_{sl} "modulates" the reactivity of cutaneous veins to a given level of sympathetic impulse traffic. Rowell et al were, therefore, the first to show in man that local changes in temperature modulates peripheral venomotor tone. Webb-Peploe & Shepherd had shown this earlier in the lateral saphenous vein of the dog.

Webb-Peploe & Shepherd carried out an elegant series of experiments in which perfusion pressures, measured in the lateral saphenous vein of the dog at constant flow rate, were used as an index of venomotor tone (101–103). They demonstrated that in the range of perfusate temperature from 47° to 17°C, cooling the perfusate caused venoconstriction and heating venodilation. Sensitivity to cooling was maximal between 42° and 27°C. The combined effects of central and local heating and cooling were studied in a crossperfusion experiment. Central heating reduced the response of cooling the perfusate from 42° to 22°C and central cooling enhanced it. This effect is not merely additive. A reduction in central temperature from 38° to 34°C increased the response to local cooling from 42° to 22°C by a factor of ten. Next, they examined the effects on venomotor tone of stimulating the distal end of the cut sympathetic chain at 2 and 6 cps at perfusate temperatures between 27° and 47°C and norepinephrine in the perfusate. They found a marked change in thermosensitivity to both forms of stimulation of smooth muscle in the vein when local temperature was changed. For example, an increase of 5°C in perfusate temperature reduced venomotor tone by 60% and a decrease of 10°C in perfusate temperature increased the response by a similar percentage. This profound effect of local temperature change on the response of smooth muscle in the vein to arriving sympathetic nerve impulses suggests that local temperature, in control theory parlance, "modulates" the effect of central heating or cooling.

Webb-Peploe & Shepherd studied the efferent pathways of the peripheral venomotor response to temperature and demonstrated that maximum veno-constrictor responses to cooling were reduced by 60% by lumbar sympathectomy and were largely abolished by alpha receptor (phenoxybenzamine) and ganglionic (pentolinium) blockade. Warming the perfusate to 47°C did not result in veno-dilation in excess of that due to these two blocking agents, which indicates that there are no venodilator fibers in the sympathetic supply to the saphenous veins. They also studied the efferent pathways by removing the skin and dissecting the vein free from surrounding connective tissue. Neither this operation nor cutting the dorsal nerve roots from L_1 downwards changed the thermosensitive response of the vein. They therefore concluded that the thermosensitivity resides in the vein walls and that the afferent impulses do not run in the sensory nerves. The nature of the afferent pathway of the venomotor response in the intact animal is still obscure.

Webb-Peploe (104) also investigated the site and mechanism of the tempera-ture effect on smooth muscle of veins. He showed that the typical thermosensitive response occurs: (a) with adrenergic drugs such as norepinephrine, 5-HT, etc., (b) with molar solutions of KCl, (c) in acutely and chronically denervated veins, and (d) in cocaine-treated veins where the re-entry of released norepinephrine is blocked. These findings indicate that neither the adrenergic receptors nor the chain of reactions leading from receptor activation to muscle contraction is re-sponsible for the thermosensitive response of the veins. The thermosensitive re-sponse to a molar solution of KCl suggests, further, that the thermal effect is not at the cell membrane but either involves excitation-contraction coupling or the process of contraction.

Vanhoutte & Shepherd (96, 97, 99) also examined this question in their studies on isolated, excised segments of dogs' saphenous veins perfused at con-stant flow with either autologous blood or Kreb's-Ringer solution. Change in perfusion pressure was the measure of change in venomotor tone. This prepara-tion reacted vigorously to electric stimulation and to norepinephrine infusion. The constriction caused by electric stimulation was abolished by bretylium tosylate, reserpine pretreatment, and alpha-adrenergic blockage—from which it could be concluded that electric stimulation causes venoconstriction by the release of norepinephrine from nerve terminals in the vein wall.

The venoconstriction caused by electric stimulation and by norepinephrine was augmented by cooling perfusate from 37° to 25°C and reduced by warming it to 42°C. Since the thermosensitivity of the isolated segments was still present when Kreb's-Ringer solution was used instead of autologous blood to perfuse the veins, the response is not due to temperature-dependent properties of the blood. These thermosensitivity responses are not specific for adrenergic drugs. They were also seen with substances such as 5-HT, ATP, and acetylcholine which, in vitro, constrict cutaneous veins. Thus neither the sympathetic nerves nor functional adrenergic effectors are essential for the potentiation of constriction with cooling. These findings led Vanhoutte & Shepherd to postulate, like Webb-Peploe, that local temperature acts in a nonspecific way on smooth muscle without interference with adrenergic receptor mechanisms. However they had to reconcile this interpretation of their results with their own observations in a later paper (98) that the spontaneous activity of the unstimulated preparation decreased with cooling and increased with warming. It is a fundamental biological property of all muscle that contraction is enhanced by warming. Their views also had to be reconciled with their observation that when the perfusate contained depolarizing doses of KCl, the stimulated vein showed marked enhancement of the fundamental biological property of smooth muscle, i.e. increased tone in warming and the reverse on cooling. Barium chloride in the perfusate led to a similar result; barium chloride is believed to release bound intracellular calcium and it is this calcium which leads to the shortening of the contractile protein. Their later interpretation of these various findings was that temperature affects the excitation mechanisms of smooth muscle in a manner opposite to its action on the contractile process itself. The final response of the venous smooth muscle cell will be determined by the summation of these opposing effects of temperature. With physiological stimuli, the facilitating and inhibiting action of temperature on the excitation mechanisms dominates. Further elucidation of the site and mechanism of thermosensitivity in peripheral veins is thus still an open challenge.

The specificity of the thermosensitive response of different veins was examined by Webb-Peploe (105). He used the technique described above for measuring venomotor tone in the lateral saphenous vein of the dog and changes in venous pressure in the isovolumetric spleen, in which blood flow had been arrested, to determine the behavior of capacitance vessels in the spleen. Decrease in central temperature from 38° to 34°C caused venoconstriction in the saphenous vein which was abolished by sympathectomy but there was no effect of central cooling upon the smooth muscle of veins of the spleen. Vanhoutte & Shepherd's results (98) are confusing. They showed that isolated segments of saphenous, mesenteric, and femoral veins, in the unstimulated state, had normal biological responses to cooling and warming, i.e. a decrease and an increase in tone, respectively. However, the electrically stimulated preparations gave different results. Saphenous and mesenteric vein segments showed increases in tension with cooling to 29°C and decreases in tension with heating to 42°C, compared with the response at 37°C. This result in mesenteric veins is in direct conflict with Webb-Peploe's findings on the intact splenic veins. Even more confusing is the fact that the femoral vein gave a reversal of the thermosensitivity response shown by the other two veins. The tone of the femoral vein decreased on cooling and increased on heating. These responses of the femoral vein were inhibited by bretylium tosylate. It cannot be argued therefore that the femoral vein lacks adrenergic nerve terminals. Vanhoutte & Shepherd's explanation that in the femoral vein there must be a preponderance of the direct effect of temperature on the contractile process over the temperature effect on the excitation mechanisms lacks supporting evidence.

In discussing the role of the peripheral venous system in heat physiology in man, Shepherd and his associates (99) refer only to countercurrent heat exchange between artery and veins. However, Mitchell et al (39) have effectively shown in a neat quantitative analysis of heat exchange by countercurrent flow that it plays a negligible role in temperature regulation. It is Rowell and his associates who, in my view, have grasped the real significance of the capacitance vessels in heat physiology. Rowell and his associates (61, 62) studied the central circulation, the splanchnic circulation and venomotor responses of men in "space" suits through which water could be circulated at different temperatures and so control skin temperature at any preselected temperature. They followed the changes in central circulation when, after 30 min at a skin temperature of 33°C, skin temperature was raised abruptly to 38–39°C for a further 30 min and then decreased rapidly to 33°C again. The abrupt rise in skin temperature during mild exercise (0.9–1.5 liters/min oxygen consumption) caused cardiac output to increase by approximately 3.0 liters/min and heart rate to increase to 150 beats/min. Central blood volume, stroke volume, right atrial pressure, aortic mean pressure, and total peripheral resistance all fell. Sudden cooling of skin temperature reversed these changes. At higher rates of exercise (oxygen consumptions of 2.0–2.5 liters/min) similar central circulatory changes were observed with certain exceptions. Stroke volume fell more and heart rate rose higher than during heating at the lower rate of exercise; further, on sudden cooling, aortic mean pressure fell markedly and transiently in most of the subjects, but in one man it remained low and the subject was giddy and complained of blurred vision. Rowell et al based their explanation of these various findings on the observation that abrupt skin heating abolishes peripheral venomotor tone. Blood pools in peripheral veins resulting in a reduction in both central blood volume and stroke volume. Peripheral resistance vessels also dilate and this results in increased cardiac output, which is achieved by the increase in heart rate.

When skin temperature was raised even higher in resting men to the unphysiological levels of 40–41°C for 40–53 minutes, the increase in cardiac output was even greater, being 7–10 liters/min in three of four subjects. Central blood volume and stroke volume were not decreased in these subjects but heart rate increase was, again, the main mechanism responsible for the increase in cardiac output. Right auricular pressure, aortic mean pressure, and total peripheral resistance all fell. Rowell et al (62) were surprised at the large increase in cardiac output (about twice that reported by other workers) and considered that hyperventilation might, in part, be responsible or that venoconstriction might not have occurred in the splanchnic region (arterial temperature was 39°C).

In subsequent papers (63, 66), however, they demonstrated intense venoconstriction in the splanchnic region by measuring hepatic and renal blood flow. In my view the larger than usually observed increase in cardiac output in man exposed to heat is due to the very high skin temperature of Rowell et al's subjects. A paradoxical finding was the lack of change in central blood volume and stroke volume in spite of a fall in right auricular pressure and peripheral venodilation. Rowell et al concluded that this paradox is due to the fact that peripheral veins in men at rest are not constricted as they are during exercise and therefore the degree of venodilation on skin heating is not as great as during exercise. The shift in blood in peripheral veins would therefore not be as great during rest as it would be in exercise. Another possible explanation is that as these subjects were studied in the supine position there was no orthostatic pooling of blood in dilated peripheral veins such as would occur in the men exercising in the vertical position.

Direct evidence of the role of peripheral venomotor tone on these central circulatory adjustments with sudden changes in skin temperature in "space" suits was obtained by Rowell (64) by recording pressure in a superficial wrist vein in a temporarily occluded limb. Men exercised at 300 and 600 kpm/min when their skin temperature was "clamped" at 33–34°C and showed the typical venoconstrictor responses to exercise noted earlier by Bevegard & Shepherd (5,6). When skin temperature was suddenly raised to 38°C, venomotor responses to exercise were either abolished or were markedly attenuated. When skin temperature was cycled between 33 and 38°C during exercise at 300 kpm/min, the venomotor responses disappeared during skin heating and reappeared during skin cooling. Not all of the subjects showed the full range of these responses. These findings confirmed Rowell et al's (62) earlier hypothesis that the decrease in central blood volume and stroke volume, when $\overline{T}_s$ is suddenly raised during exercise, is due to the relaxation of venomotor tone in cutaneous regions and to a shift of blood into the cutaneous veins.

Core temperature.—In his classic 1938 paper M. Nielsen (49) demonstrated that over a 60-min period of exercise T_r rose to a new steady level, that this level was directly related to metabolic rate, and that the level was unaffected by air temperature over a wide range (from 5° to 30°C). Nielsen & Nielsen (42) and Kitzing et al (28) have since produced evidence that T_{es} reaches a new steady level in the much shorter time of from 15–20 minutes than does T_r. Wyndham et al (109) and Lind et al (32) showed that the relationship between T_r and metabolic rate holds true only up to certain critical air temperatures which are different for different metabolic rates. The higher the metabolic rate, the lower is the critical air temperature. Above the critical air temperature T_r rises to a new, higher, steady level, or in even higher air temperatures T_r may continue to rise to dangerous levels. In the steady state of exercise in heat, T_r is as good a measure of T_{core} as is T_{es} or T_{ty} according to Saltin et al (68) and Nielsen & Nielsen (42).

That the increase in T_r during exercise is not solely dependent upon metabolic rate was first shown by Astrand in 1960 (2). Her subjects, working at 50% of Vo_{2max} all had rectal temperatures of about 38.0°C but their oxygen consumptions varied from 1.1 to 2.7 liters/min. Her findings were confirmed by Saltin & Hermansen (68). These findings led Greenleaf et al (18) and B. Neilsen (48) to study the effects upon T_r during exercise of acutely reducing Vo_{2max}, in the former case by simulating an altitude of 4000 m above sea level and in the latter case by inhalation of carbon monoxide. The results are conflicting. No change in T_r occurred at high altitude in spite of a marked decrease in Vo_{2max} but T_r rose by 0.5° to 0.7°C with 25–33% of the oxygen carrying capacity of blood blocked by CO.

Wyndham et al (118) studied the effects of heat on the T_r/Vo_{2max} relationship in both the unacclimatized and the acclimatized states. They found that T_r of men working at 1.0 liter/min oxygen consumption in 32°C wet bulb temperature was significantly correlated with Vo_{2max}. With acclimatization the slope and intercept of the regression line of T_r on Vo_{2max} decreased. Wyndham et al (118) differ from Davies et al (14) in their finding that this relationship is significant in both the unacclimatized and acclimatized states. Wyndham et al (118) raise the question of whether the T_r/Vo_{2max} relationship is not dependent upon the high correlation between Vo_{2max} and the two body size parameters, body weight and surface area. The residual variance of the $T_r/$surface area relationship is smaller than that for the T_r/Vo_{2max} relationship which suggests that in hot, humid conditions, surface area is the main determinant of T_r at a single metabolic rate.

The T_r/Vo_{2max} relationship during exercise in heat is of some practical importance in selecting men for work in hot mines who will have less risk of developing heat stroke than does the average man. Lavenne and his colleagues (31) studied the heat responses and Vo_{2max} of 50 Belgian mine workers and concluded that at "a value of 40 ml/kg/min, Vo_{2max} may be considered the dividing line between those who are able to tolerate high temperatures and those who are adversely affected." Wyndham et al (113) in a study of 59 mine rescue workers found that 55% of the men with Vo_{2max} values of less than 3.2 liters/min (the median value for the sample) had T_r of 39.0°C and above, after two hours of work at 1.0 liter/min at 32°C wet bulb temperature, compared with only 17% of the men with Vo_{2max} values of 3.2 liters/min and above. In a recent study by Wyndham et al (120) of the T_r/Vo_{2max} relationship of 40 men before and after acclimatization, in the same heat stress conditions, significant negative correlation coefficients of -0.50 and -0.51 were found for the men in the unacclimatized and acclimatized states, respectively. Using a log-normal mathematical model to fit the skew distributions of T_r in these two states, the probability of men in the samples reaching heat stroke levels of body temperature were calculated in 0.5 liter/min Vo_{2max} class intervals with the following results:

Unacclimatized state

n	Vo_{2max}	Probability of exceeding 40°C
9	less than 2.0 liters/min	0.17
19	2.0 to 2.5 "	0.045
7	2.5 to 3.0 "	0.018
6	more than 3.0 "	0.009

Acclimatized state

n	Vo_{2max}	Probability of exceeding 40°C
4	less than 2.0 liters/min	no estimate possible
13	2.0 to 2.5 "	0.03
12	2.5 to 3.0 "	0.0003
12	more than 3.0 "	less than 0.0001

Kok et al (29) studied samples of heat tolerant men and heat intolerant men (i.e., men who in the acclimatization procedure had had ten successive days of oral temperature above 38°C and in whom no overt medical disease had been found) and found that the Vo_{2max} of the heat tolerant group was 3.2 liters/min and the Vo_{2max} of the heat intolerant group was 2.4 liters/min. However, when the two groups worked at 30 and 50% of Vo_{2max} at 32°C wet bulb temperature both the heat tolerant and the heat intolerant groups had similar rectal temperatures. These were higher at 50% Vo_{2max} than at 30% Vo_{max}, confirming once again that T_r is determined by the percentage of Vo_{2max} and not by the absolute level of metabolic rate.

There are other factors, of course, which affect the level of T_r during exercise in heat. Strydom (88) showed that 50% of the heat stroke deaths in the gold mining industry in South Africa were in men of 40 years and older. Strydom et al (90) have also shown that men of less than 50 kg in weight develop higher levels of T_r than do heavier men when they work at either 1.0 or 1.5 liters/min oxygen consumption at 32°C wet bulb temperature (the lighter men also have lower Vo_{2max} and smaller surface areas). Finally, the state of hydration plays an important role: T_r is higher in the dehydrated state and lower in the fully hydrated state, than when men drink water ad libitum and generally end the experiment in a water deficit of about 1 liter (15, 86, 121).

Another important practical aspect of the T_{core}/metabolic rate relationship is the fact that men can develop very high body temperatures during prolonged exercise of high intensity, such as marathon running or cycling, in warm weather. Robinson (54) many years ago reported T_r of 41.1°C in two world class runners after races lasting 14 and 30 min in warm, humid weather. Recently, Pugh et al (53) and Wyndham et al (117) noted T_r of 41.1 and 40.9°C in the winners of marathon races in relatively cool air temperatures. These men had water deficits of 6.7 and 4.3%, respectively. Wyndham et al (117) reported a correlation between elevation in T_r and percentage water deficit, above water deficits of 3%.

That heat injury occurs in heat-susceptible body organs in such circumstances was well documented in this period. A heat stroke death occurred with a T_r of 43°C in a marathon cyclist during a "Tour de France" (4) and an increasing number of heat stroke cases are being reported in sports events, lasting an hour or more, in warm and humid weather. Two cases of nephropathy were reported in marathon runners by Dancaster et al (13). One collapsed during the race and was anuric for 48 hr and had a blood pressure of 200/130 and a blood urea of 186 mg/100 ml. The other passed only 400 ml of urine in the first 4 days after the race, his blood urea was 176 mg/100 ml, his SGOT level was 135, SGPT was 180, and LDH 1500 units. Both men recovered completely. McKechnie et al (36) studied ECG and serum enzyme levels in 20 50-mile marathon runners. None showed any pathological changes in ECG. Serum aldose levels were raised in all the runners, and SGOT, SGPT, and LDH levels were raised in about half of them. Rose et al (56) measured LDH fractions in marathon runners and found that LDH 3, 4, and 5 fractions were elevated, but not LDH 1 and 2, the myocardial and renal enzymes. The enzyme studies suggest that the heat injury is in muscle itself.

There has also been increasing evidence that in healthy young men physical exercise is an essential factor in the development of heat stroke which occurs in hot industries and in the armed forces (Wyndham et al 112, Shibolet et al 77, and Schrier et al 72). In this period the pathophysiology of organ damage due to heat stroke was advanced considerably. Renal function and damage was studied by Kew et al (24), Schrier et al (71), Shibolet et al (77), and Vertel et al (100). Serum enzyme levels in heat stroke were reported by Kew et al (27), and are amongst the highest recorded in the medical literature. The damage to heart and liver were studied by Kew et al (25, 26) and the change in clotting mechanism by Schrier et al (72) and by Shibolet et al (77). It is still not clear what are the relative roles of high temperature per se, of metabolic acidosis, and of cellular anoxia, due to decreased local blood flow, in the cell damage which occurs in heat stroke. Information on these points is essential in guiding the treatment of heat stroke cases.

TEMPERATURE REGULATION DURING EXERCISE IN HEAT

During the period under review the major advances, in my view, came from the following lines of research: Firstly, there was the application of statistical techniques to determine the relative contributions of changes in $\overline{T}_s$ and T_{core}, and of other thermal and nonthermal factors, to changes in sweat rate and heat conductance. Secondly, Bullard's (9) resistance hygrometer with its built-in heating system was employed to study sweat gland physiology with local skin temperature T_{st} "clamped" at specific temperatures. Thirdly, new ideas were generated from the development and the testing of mathematical-physical models of temperature regulation in man.

Much of the research in this area flows from the earlier studies by Robinson and his colleagues (55) and by Nielsen & Nielsen (43) in which, on the one hand, they varied the metabolic rate, by having the men exercise at different rates, in one hot air temperature and showed that T_{core}, sweat rate, and heat conductance all increased with increase in metabolic rate, but $\overline{T}_s$ either remained constant or decreased. On the other hand, they varied air temperature at one metabolic rate and showed that $\overline{T}_s$, sweat rate, and heat conductance all increased with air temperature but T_r remained constant. Thus they demonstrated that both T_r and $\overline{T}_s$, independently, are important inputs to the temperature regulator. They also showed that for comparable values of $\overline{T}_s$ and T_r, sweat rate and heat conductance are higher during exercise than during rest. This latter observation suggested that some factor associated with exercise, other than changes in $\overline{T}_s$ and T_r, is responsible for the higher sweat rates and heat conductances during exercise in heat.

Robinson and colleagues (17) searched for factors, other than T_{core} and $\overline{T}_s$, which regulate sweat rate during intermittent rest and exercise in cool and hot conditions. They monitored sweat rate with a resistance hygrometer and, in addition to $\overline{T}_s$ and T_r, measured the temperature of working muscle, T_m, the femoral vein, T_{fem}, and the saphenous vein, T_{saph}. They confirmed Bullard and van Beaumont's earlier observations (93, 94) that in men with either warm skin ($\overline{T}_s > 33°C$) or warm core ($T_{core} > 38°C$), sweating starts within 1–2 sec of the commencement of exercise and decreased as rapidly on its cessation. They found that although T_{fem} followed the rapid changes in sweat rate in certain experiments it did not do so under other circumstances. None of the other temperatures measured were associated with the abrupt changes in sweat rate. They, therefore, concluded that the predominant factor in the abrupt changes in sweat rate at the start and end of exercise must be the activation and cessation of neuromuscular reflexes, whereas the more gradual rise as the work continued was dependent on the gradually rising central temperatures, including T_m and T_{fem}.

Nielsen & Nielsen showed (44) that, in the steady state, the sweat rate/$\overline{T}_s$ and heat conductance/$\overline{T}_s$ relationships were closely similar in experiments conducted over a wide range of air temperatures in which T_{es} and T_r were elevated to similar levels either by passive (diathermy) or active (exercise) heating. B. Nielsen (46) then measured sweat rate and heat conductance at similar metabolic rates when men exercised with either their arms or legs and either continuously or intermittently, and showed that the sweat rate/total heat production and heat conductance/total heat production relationships were identical in the different experimental situations, even though the mechanical tensions and afferent impulse traffic from exercising muscle were different. She concluded from these two experiments that "in the steady state of exercise the thermoregulatory responses are only to a minor degree influenced by special work factors."

B. Nielsen looked for thermal factors other than $\overline{T}_s$ and T_{core} which are involved in temperature regulation during exercise in heat. In the first paper of a series (47) she tested Kerslake's hypothesis that the important input temperature signal is a "calculated" deep skin temperature. She measured sweat rate and heat conductance (and estimated skin blood flow by means of a new equation) and measured, in addition to $\overline{T}_s$, T_r, and T_{es}, a temperature at a depth in the subcutaneous tissue corresponding to half skinfold thickness T_{sd}. These measurements were made towards the end of 60 min of exposure at three different metabolic rates in three air temperatures which were different for each of the metabolic rates. She demonstrated, in confirmation of her earlier paper (46), that the sweat rate/$\overline{T}_s$ relationship is different for the different metabolic rates, the sweat rate and T_r being higher, for the same $\overline{T}_s$, at the higher metabolic rates. The sweat rate/T_{sd} relationship had the same characteristics but the curves were displaced to the right. Thus she was unable to confirm Kerslake's hypothesis.

In her next experiment in the series (47) Nielsen studied positive and negative exercise in an endeavor to separate the input/output relationships in experiments where the metabolic rates and total heat productions were markedly different. In agreement with an earlier paper on this subject (45) she found that T_{es} was directly related to metabolic rate whereas sweat rate and heat conductance were more closely correlated with total heat production. Sweat rate and heat conductance have separate curves for positive and negative work when plotted against T_{es}, T_r, and T_{sd}. Only $T_{sd}-T_s$, which is a function of heat flow, showed a close correlation with data from positive and negative work together, as one would anticipate from the correlation with total heat productions, but this is at odds with the results in her previous paper.

By regression analysis Nielsen demonstrated that $\overline{T}_s$ and T_{es}, either singly or in combination, could not predict adequately variations in sweat rate. However, when she included T_{sd} and T_m in the regression equation she could account for 76% of the variation in sweat rate. These results led Nielsen to postulate that core temperature provides an input to the thermoregulator proportional to metabolic rate and that other temperature receptors in the region of exercising muscle provide an input proportional to total heat production, and led her to hypothesize that sweat rate during exercise is determined by the summed inputs from thermoreceptors in all parts of the body.

This hypothesis is similar to the conclusion reached by Snellen (81) that mean body temperature is the main input signal in temperature regulation. Neilsen's hypothesis is also supported by Mitchell's recent study (38) on men at rest over a wide range of heat stress conditions in which he showed that for a fixed skin temperature, sweat rate (in g/min) is more closely correlated with mean body temperature, determined calorimetrically (R=0.68 and 0.98) in two different subjects than with T_r (R=0.57 and 0.71). When either T_r or mean body temperature was held constant by calculating partial correlation coefficients it was clear that the main determinant of sweat rate was mean body temperature. Similar results were found for heat conductance. Mitchell also showed, in agreement with Snellen, but with more reliable calorimetric determinations of mean body temperature, that mean body temperature during exercise in heat cannot be determined from any fixed ratio of $\overline{T}_s$ and T_r.

Robinson and his colleagues (79) also used positive and negative work, but in a cool environment, in their search for other factors which influence sweat rate. They confirmed Nielsen's (47) finding that there was a high correlation between sweat rate and total heat production (R=0.94). Smiles & Robinson (79) do not seem to appreciate that the First Law of Thermodynamics must hold true in both positive and negative work, and hence this high correlation coefficient is implicit. They differ from Nielsen in that T_r was significantly correlated with both metabolic rate and total heat production (R>0.71) but with significantly different regression lines for positive and negative work, in both instances. They also differ from Nielsen in their finding that sweat rate was significantly correlated with T_r for positive and negative work taken together (R=0.54). Their multiple correlation coefficient is 0.56 between sweat rate and $\overline{T}_s$ and T_r, in combination, and the regression equation is:

$$Es(g/min) = 207T_r - 30.5\overline{T}_s - 6550$$

The negative sign for $\overline{T}_s$ is surely a misprint. From this it is clear that these two body temperatures only account for a small proportion of the variance in sweat rate during exercise in cool conditions. In their search for nonthermal factors Robinson et al showed that sweat rate could also be predicted from speed of walking and metabolic rate (R=0.95) as from metabolic rate and external work (R=0.96). The partial correlation coefficient between sweat rate and speed, with metabolic rate held constant, was 0.91. Thus they concluded that sweat rate is the result of a stimulus proportional to metabolic rate, probably T_r, and of a neuromuscular stimulus proportional to the speed of walking.

In striking contrast to findings that factors, additional to T_r and T_{core}, play a significant role in the control of sweating and heat conductance are the results published by Saltin and his associates at the Pierce Laboratory (69, 84). They studied men exercising at 25, 50 and 75% of maximum oxygen intake in air temperatures of 10°, 20° and 30°C, both in the steady state (after 30–45 min) and in the thermal transient state (using a sensitive, fast-responding balance). The multiple correlation coefficient, in the steady state, between evaporative heat loss and T_r and $\overline{T}_s$, combined, was 0.92 and the linear regression equation:

$$Es(W/m^2) = 132(T_r - 36.6) + 19(\overline{T}_s - 33.3)$$

In their studies on thermal transient state, the same metabolic rate/air temperature combinations were used but the men rested for 30 min before exercising and also rested for 30 min between bouts of exercise, all rest being in the air temperature of the test. Sweat rate and T_r, T_{es} and T_m were measured continuously. Unlike Robinson et al (17) and Bullard et al (9), Saltin et al (69) found that even in the warm environment, sweating was delayed for 2 to 5 minutes after the start of exercise probably because the subjects were unacclimatized, and then a rapid increase occurred which was associated with the rise in T_{es}. Statistical analysis of the data showed that during exercise at 30°C sweat rate was most highly correlated with T_r (R=0.85); at 20°C, T_{es} was predominant (R=0.89); and at 10°C, T_m was predominant (R=0.76). Multiple correlation coefficients were calculated between sweat rate and T_{es} and $\overline{T}_s$, for T_{es} and $\overline{T}_s$ in different ratios. That for exercise and recovery was 0.81 (with a $\overline{T}_s:T_r$ ratio of 1:8) and the highest multiple correlation for exercise alone was 0.93 (with a $\overline{T}_s:T_r$ ratio of 1:7.5). The two regression equations are

$$Es(W/m^2) = 93.0(T_{es} - 37) + 11.8(\overline{T}_s - 27.7)$$
$$= 109.9(T_{es} - 37) + 14.3(\overline{T}_s - 29.7)$$

(Threshold temperatures were arbitrarily selected from factoring intercept from regression equation.) Saltin et al later (70) studied these relationships at maximum oxygen intake and gave multiple correlation coefficients of 0.90 for exercise and recovery; of 0.82 for the 3 to 15 min of exercise; and 0.88 for recovery. The exercise regression equation is:

$$Es(g/min) = 3.12(T_r - 37.0) + 0.70(\overline{T}_s - 26.6)$$

Thus in the steady state and in the thermal transients, at submaximal levels of exercise, in cool and warm environments, Saltin et al were able to predict at least 80% of the variation in sweat rate from the two body temperatures, $\overline{T}_s$ and T_{es}. Saltin et al's much higher correlation coefficients than those of other workers are difficult to explain but may be due to the fact they choose their air temperatures and work rates in ranges where there is a high correlation between air temperature and $\overline{T}_s$, on the one hand, and metabolic rate and T_{es}, on the other hand.

It is also surprising that Saltin et al and others examined only the predictive capacity of linear regression equations. Because of the local modulation $Es = F(\overline{T}_s)$ will always be nonlinear. Hardy & Stolwijk (21) earlier had shown, in the thermal transient state of men at rest, that a multiplicative model is a better representation of the relationships. Wyndham & Atkins (114) also demonstrated that the relationships between sweat rate and heat conductance, on the one hand, and T_r and $\overline{T}_s$, on the other hand, are nonlinear. They studied men at four metabolic rates from 44 to 324 kcal/m² hr and at four different air temperatures of 10°, 25°,

38°, and 49°C with a low humidity. They gave the following nonlinear regression equation:

$$Es(g/min) = 9.1(T_r - 36.5) - 7.6[(T_r - 36.5)(1 - \exp 2.7(T_s - 33))]$$

or approximately,

$$Es = (T_r - 36.5)[1.7 + 7.6 \exp 2.7(\overline{T}_s - 33)]$$

These equations have not been tested to determine how much of the variation in sweat rate in different combinations of exercise and environmental heat stress could be accounted for by $\overline{T}_s$ and T_r.

Next we should consider Bullard and his colleagues' contributions to our understanding of temperature regulation during exercise in heat. Bullard and van Beaumont demonstrated some years back (93–95), firstly, that there was an abrupt increase in sweating with the onset of exercise in men who were already sweating; secondly, that the local temperature markedly affected the extent of increase in sweat rate; and, thirdly, that this response was reflex in origin—it was demonstrated in a limb in which the circulation had been occluded by a blood pressure cuff.

In 1967 Bullard et al (9) published an important paper in which they reported the effects on local sweat rates of changes in local temperatures (T_{sl}) from 20° to 40°C in subjects after they had been sitting at rest for 60 min at air temperatures from 31° to 39°C. The sweat rates were measured during the last 5 min of 20 min at a particular local temperature. The sweat rate/T_{sl} relationships were nonlinear, being displaced upwards and to the left with increase in air temperature. The Q_{10} of the sweat rate response was approximately 5–6. When $\overline{T}_s$ was warm there was a rapid augmentation of sweating when T_{sl} exceeded 32–34°C. But when $\overline{T}_s$ was low, as in the air temperature of 31°C, local sweating only occurred when T_{sl} exceeded 42°C. Bullard et al's interpretation of these findings was that when neural impulses are arriving at the sweat glands under the capsule, as a result of an increase in T_s, local cooling or heating modulates the effect of the arriving neural impulses. In a control system model this effect would be represented as a multiplier. The hypothetical mechanism they proposed is that the number of molecules of acetylcholine released per neural impulse arriving at the neuroglandular junction is altered by local cooling or heating.

MacIntyre et al (35) looked for evidence to support Bullard et al's hypothesis by studying the effect upon local sweat rate of warming T_{sl} from 36° to 40°C in a warm room when parasympathetic drugs were iontophoresed locally and when arterial flow to the limb was occluded. They showed that local heating augmented sweating in a warm room but not in a cool room. Rather surprisingly, pilocarpine iontophoresis did not augment the sweating due to local heating in the warm room nor did it elicit sweating in the cool room. By contrast physostigmine, an anticholinesterase, which allows acetylcholine to accumulate at the site of neuroglandular transmission, enhanced sweating on local heating. Only the effect of physostigmine can be said to support Bullard et al's hypothesis for the mechanism. They also showed that the local increase in sweating with increase in T_{sl} was blocked by iontophoresis with atropine and hemicholonium and by arterial occlusion. Pilocarpine elicited sweating in these preparations which merely indicates that the sweat glands were susceptible to postsynaptic stimulation, but this has no bearing on the Bullard et al hypothesis.

Ogawa's experiments (50) also do not support Bullard et al's hypothesis. He showed that local heating reduced the threshold dose at which sweating occurred with local injection of acetylcholine and pilocarpine and that this response was unaltered when efferent sympathetic impulses to the sweat glands were blocked by injecting a local anaesthetic into the sensory nerve supplying the area. His result suggests that high skin temperature exerts a local facilitating effect by acting on specific receptor mechanisms of the sweat glands and by increasing their sensitivities to local thermal stimuli; i.e. the effect is postsynaptic. However, the mechanism still results in a modulation by local skin temperature of the central control of sweat rate.

Nadel, Bullard & Stolwijk (41), used the Bullard resistance hygrometer in studies of the effect of independent variations in T_{sl}, $\overline{T}_s$ and T_{core} upon local and general sweating. They used longwave infrared heating to change $\overline{T}_s$ cyclically, exercise to raise T_{es}, and the resistance hygrometer with an inbuilt heating device to vary T_{sl}. Their result throws light on the regulation of body temperature in exercise when $\overline{T}_s$ is raised. They showed, firstly, that in the presence of an elevated T_{es}, due to exercise, local sweating was linearly related to $\overline{T}_s$ but the slope of the sweat rate/$\overline{T}_s$ relationship was reduced. Secondly, that at constant T_{sl}, sweat rate is linearly related to T_{es}, with increase in $\overline{T}_s$ shifting the regression line upwards and to the left. Thirdly, that when T_{sl} is clamped at different levels, during changes in $\overline{T}_s$, the slope of the sweat rate/$\overline{T}_s$ relationship is altered but not the threshold of T_{sl} at which sweating occurs. Fourthly, that there is a nonlinear relationship between sweat rate and T_{sl}, for given levels of $\overline{T}_s$. They also demonstrated an effect of rate of change in $\overline{T}_s$ on sweat rate when $\overline{T}_s$ is cooling but not when it is rising, which is in accord with Wurster & McCook's findings in this regard (107). From these results they concluded that there are both additive and multiplicative aspects of the integration of central and peripheral input signals in the determination of the sweat response. The relationship between local sweat rate and change in T_{es} and $\overline{T}_s$ is considered to be additive while the T_{sl} effect is that of a multiplier. Rate of change of $\overline{T}_s$ has an effect upon the integrator only during skin cooling. Nadel et al concluded that other thermal and nonthermal effects probably only operate during exceptional circumstances. They gave the following nonlinear regression equation for total body sweating:

$$E_s(\text{W/m}^2) = [197(T_{es} - 36.7) + (\overline{T}_s - 34)] \exp (\text{weighted } T_{sl}/10)$$

Nadel et al's equation consists of a term representing the nervous drive to sweating, multiplied by a modulation term. In order to show that $\overline{T}_s$ contributed a linear additive component to the nervous term they used a special technique in which they measured the sweat rate from the local area under the resistance hygrometer, with a fixed T_{sl}, while changing $\overline{T}_s$. Nadel et al must receive full credit for being the first to demonstrate conclusively that the relationship between $\overline{T}_s$ and local sweat rate is linear. However, it must be appreciated that if the relationship between T_{sl} and local sweating is nonlinear then the relationship between

$\overline{T}_s$ and whole body sweating must of necessity also be nonlinear. In other words Stolwijk & Hardy in 1966 (83), and Stolwijk et al in 1968 (84) were incorrect in fitting a regression equation, linear in $\overline{T}_s$, between sweat rate and $\overline{T}_s$ and T_{core}. One must, however, sound a word of caution about the use of Nadel et al's equation for predicting whole body sweating during exercise in heat. While it is theoretically correct to distinguish between the linear and nonlinear components of the $\overline{T}_s$ effects upon sweat rate, it would be very difficult to develop a general equation, including a term which was based upon "weighted T_{st}". Therefore the approach adopted by Wyndham & Atkins (114) of using a nonlinear term for the effect of $\overline{T}_s$ upon sweat rate is of more practical use for predicting sweat rates.

Finally let us consider the influence of models of temperature regulation on our understanding of the mechanisms involved. During the last decade physiologists have accepted that negative feedback control provides a useful model of human temperature regulation. However, most descriptions of temperature as a control system have been confined to resting men: Stolwijk & Hardy's 1966 model (82) is an example. An analog computer capable of simulating the thermal responses of resting men was reported as long ago as 1960 by Wyndham & Atkins (110), but the first successful analog simulation of the responses of exercising men was reported at the Dublin symposium by Atkins & Mitchell (1).

There can be little doubt that the same general type of control operates both in rest and exercise. The thermal disturbances resulting from the release of metabolic heat causes body temperatures to rise. Neurones sensitive to rising temperature transmit nervous information to the brain. Efferent nervous signals emerge which stimulate the control actions of circulatory adjustment and sweating, which results in dissipation of heat to the environment.

Whether the temperature regulatory system operates in exactly the same way during rest and exercise is the subject of current controversy. One often encounters the statement, originating from Hammel in 1963 (20) that the "set-point" on the control system is elevated during exercise. This statement results from a misinterpretation of M. Nielsen's classic 1938 observation that, during exercise, body core temperature reaches a regulated but elevated level (49). As Bradbury et al (8), Kitzing et al (28), and Wyndham & Atkins (114) have pointed out, the stable but elevated body core temperature is a necessary consequence of the proportional nature of the control system. During steady state exercise the outputs from the system (such as sweat rate) reach steady levels elevated above resting levels. To achieve the increase in output, the inputs to the system (one of which is a temperature related to core temperature) must do likewise.

There is also controversy, as discussed earlier, on the role of nonthermal inputs to the control system during exercise. In the transient phase of the change from rest to exercise, evidence for a nonthermal input is strong. Gisolfi & Robinson (17) have demonstrated that the abrupt increase in sweating in a warm man at the onset of exercise does not seem to depend upon a thermal stimulus. The stimulus seems to be neural or mechanical according to Jequier (23).

In steady-state exercise the situation is less clear-cut. Statistical analyses of the relationships between body temperatures and control actions fail to reveal any difference between rest and exercise (38, 81). More critical experiments do, however, reveal differences between steady-state rest and steady-state exercise. Mitchell (37, 38) conducted experiments in which nude subjects went from a steady-state of rest to a steady-state of exercise and returned to a steady-state of rest in the same hot environment. He observed that: (a) The increase in body temperature associated with a constant or rising output from the control system decreased with increasing environmental temperature. (b) An increase in sweat rate or conductance could occur with no change, or indeed a fall, in body temperature. (c) The change in body temperature associated with a drop in output at the cessation of exercise was significantly smaller than the change associated with a rise in output by the same amount at the onset of exercise. (d) The deviation in body temperature which persisted after exercise was significantly correlated with the deviation during exercise.

Mitchell interpreted his observations as support for Robinson's concept (55) that the gain, or sensitivity, of the control system increases during exercise. The elevation of body temperature after exercise in man has also been observed by Haight & Keatinge (19) who report a persistance in the temperature rise for at least five hours.

Although much progress has been made since 1968 in our understanding of the temperature regulatory system when men exercise in heat, more research is required before the control system is fully understood. It seems probable that it would be profitable to combine a number of different lines of approach: to measure mean body temperature calorimetrically to determine its importance as an input signal; to use positive and negative exercise to sort out the influence of metabolic heat and total heat production on the input/output relationships; to design experiments in such a way that multiple regression analysis could be used to determine the proportion of the total variances in sweat rate and heat conductance that could be accounted for by the measured parameters and the proportion which remains in the residual variance and is therefore unaccounted for by the measured parameters; and to use a nonlinear mathematical term in the regression equation for the effect of $\bar{T}_s$ on sweat rate and heat conductance.

ACKNOWLEDGMENTS

I wish to thank Dr. Duncan Mitchell for much helpful and constructive criticism and Mr. D. Rabe for his careful editing of the text.

LITERATURE CITED

1. Atkins, A. R., Mitchell, D. 1971. Simulating the thermal responses of a working man with a computer. *Int. J. Biometeorol.* 15(2-4):183-88
2. Astrand, I. 1960. Aerobic work capacity in men and women with special reference to age. *Acta Physiol. Scand. #49*: Suppl. 169
3. Bass, D. E., Kleeman, C. R., Quinn, M., Henschel, A., Hegnauer, A. H. 1955. Mechanisms of acclimatization to heat. *Medicine* 34:323-80
4. Bernheim, J., Cox, J. N. 1960. Coup de chaleur et intoxication amphetamine chez un sportif. *Schweiz. Med. Wochenschr.* 90:322-31
5. Bevegard, B. S., Shepherd, J. T. 1965. Changes in tone of limb veins during supine exercise. *J. Appl. Physiol.* 20(1):1-8
6. Bevegard, B. S., Shepherd, J. T. 1966. Reaction in man of resistance and capacity vessels in forearm and hand to leg exercise. *J. Appl. Physiol.* 21(1):123-32
7. Bligh, J., Moore, R., Eds. 1972. *Essays on Temperature Regulation.* Amsterdam:North Holland
8. Bradbury, P. A., Fox, R. H., Goldsmith, R., Hampton, I. F. G. 1964. The effect of exercise on temperature regulation. *J. Physiol. London.* 171:384-96
9. Bullard, R. W., Banerjee, M. R., MacIntyre, B. A. 1967. The role of the skin in negative feedback regulation of eccrine sweating. *Int. J. Biometeorol.* 11(1):93-104
10. Cabanac, M., Ed. 1971. *Proc. Int. Symp. Behav. Temp. Regul., J. Physiol. Paris* 63:189-472
11. Collins, K. J., Weiner, J. S. 1968. Endocrinological aspects of exposure to high environmental temperatures. *Physiol. Rev.* 48(4):785-839
12. Damato, A. N. et al 1968. Cardiovascular response to acute thermal stress (hot environment) in unacclimatised normal subjects. *Am. Heart J.* 76(6):769-74
13. Dancaster, C. P., Duckworth, W. C., Roper, C. J. 1969. Nephropathy in marathon runners. *S. Afr. Med. J.* 43:758-60
14. Davies, C. M. T., Barnes, C., Sargent, A. J. 1971. Body temperature in exercise. *Int. Z. angew. Physiol.* 30:10-19

15. Ekblom, B., Greenleaf, C. J., Greenleaf, J. E., Hermansen, L. 1970. Temperature regulation during exercise dehydration in man. *Acta Physiol. Scand.* 79:475-83
15a. Fox, R. H., Goldsmith, R., Kidd, D. J., Lewis, H. E. 1963. Acclimatization to heat by controlled elevation of body temperature. *J. Physiol. London* 166:530-47
16. Gisolfi, C., Robinson, S. 1969. Relations between physical training, acclimatisation and heat tolerance. *J. Appl. Physiol.* 26(5):530-34
17. Gisolfi, C., Robinson, S. 1970. Central and peripheral stimuli regulating sweating during intermittent work in man. *J. Appl. Physiol.* 29(6):761-68
18. Greenleaf, J. E., Greenleaf, C. J., Card, D. H., Saltin, B. 1969. Exercise-temperature regulation in man during acute exposure to simulated altitude. *J. Appl. Physiol.* 26(3):290-96
19. Haight, J. S. J., Keatinge, W. R. 1969. Human temperature regulation after prolonged intermittent exercise. *J. Physiol. London* 206:20P-21P
20. Hammel, H. T., Jackson, D. C., Stolwijk, J. A. J., Hardy, J. D., Stromme, S. B. 1963. Temperature regulation by hypothalamic proportional control with an adjustable set point. *J. Appl. Physiol.* 18(6):1146-54
21. Hardy, J. D., Stolwijk, J. A. J. 1966. Partitional calorimetric studies of man during exposures to thermal transients. *J. Appl. Physiol.* 21(6): 1799-1806
22. Hardy, J. D., Gagge, A. P., Stolwijk, J. A. J., Eds. 1970. *Physiological and Behavioral Temperature Regulation.* Springfield, Illinois:Thomas
23. Jequier, E. 1970. Reduced hypothalamic set-point temperature during exercise in man. *Experientia* 26:681
24. Kew, M. C. et al 1967. The effects of heat stroke on the function and structure of the kidney. *Quart. J. Med.* 36:277-300
25. Kew, M. C., Tucker, R. B. K., Bersohn, I., Seftel, H. C. 1969. The heart in heat stroke. *Am. Heart J.* 77:324-35
26. Kew, M. C., Bersohn, I., Seftel, H. C., Kent, G. 1970. Liver dam-

age in heat stroke. *Am. J. Med.* 49:192-202
27. Kew, M. C., Bersohn, I., Seftel, H. C. 1971. The diagnostic and prognostic significance of serum enzyme changes in heat stroke. *Roy. Soc. Trop. Med. Hyg.* 65(3): 325-30
28. Kitzing, J., Kutta, D., Bleichert, A. 1968. Thermoregulation during prolonged, strenuous exercise. *Pfluegers Arch.* 301:241-53
29. Kok, R., Wyndham, C. H., Strydom, N. B., Rogers, G. G. 1972. A comparison of certain physiological and anthropometrical characteristics of heat intolerant and heat tolerant Bantu from climatic room acclimatization. *COM Res. Rept. No. 14/72, Johannesburg*
30. Kozlowski, S., Saltin, B. 1964. Effect of sweat loss on body fluids. *J. Appl. Physiol.* 19(6):1119-24
31. Lavenne, F., Belayew, D. 1966. Exercise tolerance test at room temperature for the purpose of selecting rescue teams for training in a hot climate. *Rev. Inst. Hyg. Mines* 21(1):48-58
32. Lind, A. R. 1963. A physiological criterion for setting thermal environmental limits for everyday work. *J. Appl. Physiol.* 18(1):51-56
33. Lind, A. R., Bass, D. E. 1963. Optimum exposure time for the development of acclimatisation to heat. *Fed. Proc.* 22:704-8
34. Lind, A. R., Leithead, C. S., McNicol, G. W. 1968. Cardiovascular changes during syncope induced by tilting men in heat. *J. Appl. Physiol.* 25(3):268-76
35. MacIntyre, B. A., Bullard, R. W., Banerjee, M., Elizondo, R. 1968. Mechanism of enhancement of eccrine sweating by localized heating. *J. Appl. Physiol.* 25(3):255-60
36. McKechnie, J. K., Leary, W. P., Joubert, S. M. 1967. Some electrocardiographic and biochemical changes recorded in marathon runners. *S. Afr. Med. J.* 41:722-25
37. Mitchell, D., Atkins, A. R., Wyndham, C. H. 1972. Mathematical and physical models of temperature regulation. *Essays on Temperature Regulation*, ed. J. Bligh, R. Moore, 37-54. Amsterdam:North Holland
38. Mitchell, D. 1972. *Human surface temperature: its measurement and its significance in thermoregulation.*

PhD thesis. Univ. Witwatersrand, Johannesburg
39. Mitchell, J. W., Myers, G. 1968. An analytical model of the countercurrent heat exchange phenomena. *Biophys. J.* 8:897-911
40. Morrison, J. F., Wyndham, C. H., Mienie, B., Strydom, N. B. 1968. Energy expenditure of mining tasks and the need for the selection of labourers. *J. S. Af. Inst. Mining Met.* 69:185-91
41. Nadel, E. R., Bullard, R. W., Stolwijk, J. A. J. 1971. Importance of skin temperature in the regulation of sweating. *J. Appl. Physiol.* 31(1):80-87
42. Nielsen, B., Nielsen, M. 1962. Body temperature during work at different environmental temperatures. *Acta. Physiol. Scand.* 56:120-29
43. Nielsen, B., Nielsen, M. 1965. On the regulation of sweat secretion in exercise. *Acta. Physiol. Scand.* 64: 314-22
44. Nielsen, B., Nielsen, M. 1965. Influence of passive and active heating on temperature regulation of man. *Acta Physiol. Scand.* 64:323-31
45. Nielsen, B. 1966. Regulation of body temperature and heat dissipation at different levels of energy- and heat production in man. *Acta. Physiol. Scand.* 68:215-27
46. Nielsen, B. 1968. Thermoregulatory responses to arm work, leg work and intermittent leg work. *Acta. Physiol. Scand.* 72:25-32
47. Nielsen, B. 1969. Thermoregulation in rest and exercise. *Acta. Physiol. Scand.* 76: Suppl. 323, 1
48. Nielsen, B. 1971. Thermoregulation during work in carbon-monoxide poisoning. *Acta. Physiol. Scand.* 82:98-106
49. Nielsen, M. 1938. Die Regulation der Körpertemperatur bei Muskelarbeit. *Skand. Arch. Physiol.* 79:193-230
50. Ogawa, T. 1970. Local effect of skin temperature on threshold concentration of sudorific agents. *J. Appl. Physiol.* 28(1):18-22
51. Piwonka, R. W., Robinson, S., Gay, V. L., Manalis, R. S. 1965. Preacclimatization of men to heat by training. *J. Appl. Physiol.* 20(3): 379-84
52. Piwonka, R. W., Robinson, S. 1967. Acclimatization of highly trained men to work in severe heat. *J. Appl. Physiol.* 22(1):9-12

53. Pugh, L. G. C. E., Corbett, J. L., Johnson, R. H. 1967. Rectal temperatures, weight losses and sweat rates in marathon running. *J. Appl. Physiol.* 23(3):347–52

54. Robinson, S. 1949. *Physiological Adjustments to Heat*, ed. L. H. Newburgh, 193–231. Philadelphia: Saunders

55. Robinson, S. 1963. Temperature regulation in exercise. *Pediatrics* 32(4):691–702

56. Rose, L. I., Bousser, J. E., Cooper, K. H. 1970. Serum enzymes after marathon running. *J. Appl. Physiol.* 29(3):355–57

57. Rowell, L. B., Blackmon, J. R., Martin, R. H., Mazzarella, J. A., Bruce, R. A. 1965. Hepatic clearance of indocyanine green in man under thermal and exercise stresses *J. Appl. Physiol.* 20(3):384–94

58. Rowell, L. B., Marx, H. J., Bruce, R. A., Conn, R. D., Kusumi, F. 1966. Reductions in cardiac output, central blood volume, and stroke volume with thermal stress in normal men during exercise. *J. Clin. Invest.* 45(11):1801–16

59. Rowell, L. B., Kraning, K. K., Kennedy, J. W., Evans, T. O. 1967. Central circulatory responses to work in dry heat before and after acclimatisation. *J. Appl. Physiol.* 22(3):509–18

60. Rowell, L. B., Brengelmann, G. L., Blackmon, J. R., Twiss, R. D., Kusumi, F. 1968. Splanchnic blood flow and metabolism in heat stressed man. *J. Appl. Physiol.* 24(4):475–84

61. Rowell, L. B, Murray, J. A., Brengelmann, G. L., Kraning, K. K. 1969. Human cardiovascular adjustments to rapid changes in skin temperature during exercise. *Circ. Res.* 24:711–24

62. Rowell, L. B., Brengelmann, G. L. Murray, J. A. 1969. Cardiovascular responses to sustained high skin temperature in resting man. *J. Appl. Physiol.* 27(5):673–80

63. Rowell, L. B., Brengelmann, G. L. Blackmon, J. R., Murray, J. A. 1970. Redistribution of blood-flow during sustained high skin temperature in resting man. *J. Appl. Physiol.* 28(4):415–20

64. Rowell, L. B., Brengelmann, G. L., Detry, J. M. R., Wyss, C. 1971. Venomotor responses to rapid changes in skin temperature in

65. Rowell, L. B., Brengelmann, G. L., Detry, J. M. R., Wyss, C. 1971. Venomotor responses to local and remote thermal stimuli to skin in exercising man. *J. Appl. Physiol.* 30(1)72–77

66. Rowell, L. B., Detry, J. M. R., Profant, G. R., Wyss, C. 1971. Splanchnic vasoconstriction in hyperthermic man—role of falling blood pressure *J. Appl. Physiol.* 31(6):864–69.

67. Saltin, B. 1964. Circulatory response to submaximal and maximal exercise after thermal dehydration. *J. Appl. Physiol.* 19(6):1125–32

68. Saltin, B., Hermansen, L. 1966. Esophageal, rectal and muscle temperature during exercise. *J. Appl. Physiol.* 21(6):1757–62

69. Saltin, B., Gagge, A. P., Stolwijk, J. A. J. 1970. Body temperature and sweating during thermal transients caused by exercise. *J. Appl. Physiol.* 28(3):318–27

70. Saltin, B , Gagge, A. P. 1971. Sweating and body temperatures during exercise. *Abstr., Int. Symp. Environ. Physiol. Dublin*, 84

71. Schrier, R. W., Henderson, H. S., Tisher, C. C., Tannen, R. L. 1967. Nephropathy associated with heat stress and exercise. *Ann. Intern. Med.* 67:356–76

72. Schrier, R. W. et al 1970. Renal, metabolic and circulatory responses to heat and exercise. *Ann. Intern. Med.* 73(2):213–23

73. Senay, L. C., Christensen, M. L. 1965. Changes in blood plasma during progressive dehydration. *J. Appl. Physiol.* 20(6):1136–40

74. Senay, L. C., Christensen, M. L. 1968. Variations of certain blood constituents during acute heat exposure. *J. Appl. Physiol.* 24(3): 302–9

75. Senay, L. C. 1970. Movement of water, protein and crystalloids between vascular and extra-vascular compartments in heat exposed men during dehydration and following limited relief of dehydration. *J. Physiol. London* 210:617–35

76. Senay, L. C. 1972. Changes in plasma volume and protein content during exposures of working men to various temperatures before and after acclimatisation to heat: separation of the roles of cutaneous and

skeletal muscle circulation. *J. Physiol. London* 224:61–81

77. Shibolet, S., Coll, R., Gilat, T., Soher, E. 1967. Heat stroke: its clinical picture and mechanism in thirty-six cases. *Quart. J. Med.* 36: 525–48

78. Shvartz, E. 1970. Prevention of heat syncope by the inflation of cuffs around the legs or around lower abdomen. *Aerosp. Med.* 41(10): 1143–44

79. Smiles, K. A., Robinson, S. 1971. Regulation of sweat secretion during positive and negative work. *J. Appl. Physiol.* 30(3):409–12

80. Smiles, K. A., Robinson, S. 1971. Sodium ion conservation during acclimatisation of men to work in the heat. *J. Appl. Physiol.* 31(1): 63–69

81. Snellen, J. W. 1966. Mean body temperature and the control of thermal sweating. *Acta Physiol. Pharmacol. Neerl.* 14:99–174

82. Stolwijk, J. A. J., Hardy, J. D. 1966. Temperature regulation in man— a theoretical study. *Pfluegers Arch.* 291:129–62

83. Stolwijk, J. A. J., Hardy, J. D. 1966. Partitional calorimetric studies of responses of man to thermal transients. *J. Appl. Physiol.* 21(3):967–77

84. Stolwijk, J. A. J., Saltin, B., Gagge, A. P. 1968. Physiological factors associated with sweating during exercise, *Aerosp. Med.* 39:1101–05

85. Strydom, N. B. et al 1966. Acclimatisation to humid heat and the role of physical conditioning. *J. Appl. Physiol.* 21(2):636–42

86. Strydom, N. B., Holdsworth, L. D. 1968. The effects of different levels of water deficit on physiological responses during heat stress. *Int. Z. angew. Physiol.* 26:95–102

87. Strydom, N. B., Williams, C. G. 1969. Effect of physical conditioning on state of heat acclimatisation of Bantu labourers. *J. Appl. Physiol.* 27(2):262–65

88. Strydom, N. B. 1971. Age as a causal factor in heat stroke. *J. S. Afr. Inst. Mining Met.* 72(4):112–14

89. Strydom, N. B., Benade, A. J. S., Swanepoel, H. J., Heyns, A. J. A. 1971. A comparison of the effectiveness of 5, 7, 8 and 9-day acclimatization procedures. *J. S. Afr. Inst. Mining Met.* 72(4):105–07

90. Strydom, N. B., Wyndham, C. H., Benade, A. J. S. 1971. The responses of men weighing less than 50 kg to standard climatic room acclimatization procedures. *J. S. Afr. Inst. Mining Met.* 72(4)101–04

91. Tromp, S. E., Weihe, W. H., Eds. 1970. *Proc. 5th Int. Biometeorol. Congr., Int. J. Biometeorol.* 14(1,2)

92. Tromp, S. W., Weihe, W. H., Eds. 1971. *Proc. Symp. Temp. Regul., Dublin, Int. J. Biometeorol.* 15(2, 3,4)

93. van Beaumont, W., Bullard, R. W. 1963. Sweating: its rapid response to muscular work. *Science* 141: 643–46

94. van Beaumont, W., Bullard, R. W. 1965. Sweating: direct influence of skin temperature. *Science* 147: 1465–67

95. van Beaumont, W., Bullard, R. W. 1966. Sweating: exercise stimulation during circulatory arrest. *Science* 152:1521–23

96. Vanhoutte, P. M., Leusen, I. 1969. The reactivity of isolated venous preparations to electrical stimulation. *Pfleugers Arch.* 306:341–53

97. Vanhoutte, P. M., Shepherd, J. T. 1970. Effect of temperature on reactivity of isolated cutaneous veins of the dog. *Am. J. Physiol.* 218(1):90

98. Vanhoutte, P. M., Lorenz, R. R. 1970. Effect of temperature on reactivity of saphenous, mesenteric and femoral veins of the dog. *Am. J. Physiol.* 218(6):1746–50

99. Vanhoutte, P. M., Shepherd, J. T. 1970. Thermosensitivity and veins. *J. Physiol. Paris* 63:449–51

100. Vertel, R. M., Knochel, J. P. 1967. Acute renal failure due to heat injury. *Am. J. Med.* 43:435–51

101. Webb-Peploe, M. M., Shepherd, J. T. 1968. Response of superficial limb veins of the dog to changes in temperature. *Circ. Res.* 22:737–46

102. Webb-Peploe, M. M., Shepherd, J. T. 1968. Response of dogs' cutaneous veins to local and central temperature changes. *Circ. Res.* 23:693–99

103. Webb-Peploe, M. M., Shepherd, J. T. 1968. Peripheral mechanism involved in response of dogs' cutaneous veins to local temperature change. *Circ. Res.* 23:701–08

104. Webb-Peploe, M. M. 1969. Cutaneous venoconstrictor response to local cooling in the dog. *Circ. Res.*

24:607–15

105. Webb-Peploe, M. M. 1969. Effect of changes in central body temperature on capacity elements of limb and spleen. *Am. J. Physiol.* 216(3): 643–46

106. Wood, J. E., Bass, D. E. 1960. Responses of the veins and the arterioles of the forearm to walking during acclimatization to heat in man. *J. Clin. Invest.* 39:825–33

107. Wurster, R. D., McCook, R. D. 1969. Influence of rate of change in skin temperature on sweating. *J. Appl. Physiol.* 27(2):237–40

108. Wyndham, C. H. 1951. Effect of acclimatization on circulatory responses to high environmental temperatures. *J. Appl. Physiol.* 4: 383–95

109. Wyndham, C. H., Bouwer, W. van der M., Paterson, H. F., Devine, M. G. 1953. Practical aspects of recent physiological studies in Witwatersrand Gold Mines. *J. Chem., Met. Mining Soc. S. Afr.* 53:287–313

110. Wyndham, C. H., Atkins, A. R. 1960. An approach to the solution of the human biothermal problem with the aid of an analogue computer. *Trans. 3rd Int. Conf. Med. Electron., London*, 32–38

111. Wyndham, C. H. et al 1962. Circulatory and metabolic reactions to work in heat. *J. Appl. Physiol.* 17(4):625–38

112. Wyndham, C. H. 1965. A survey of the causal factors in heat stroke and of their prevention in the gold mining industry. *J. S. Afr. Inst. Mining Met.* 66(4):125–55

113. Wyndham, C. H., Strydom, N. B., Williams, C. G., Heyns, A. 1967. An examination of certain individual factors affecting the heat tolerance of mine workers. *J. S. Afr. Inst. Mining Met.* 68:79–91

114. Wyndham, C. H., Atkins, A. R.

1968. A physiological scheme and mathematical model of temperature regulation in man. *Pfluegers Arch.* 303:14–30

115. Wyndham, C. H. et al 1968. Changes in central circulation and body fluid spaces during acclimatization to heat. *J. Appl. Physiol.* 25(5):586–93

116. Wyndham, C. H., Strydom, N. B. 1969. Acclimatizing men to heat in climatic rooms in mines. *J. S. Afr. Inst. Mining Met.* 70:60–64

117. Wyndham, C. H., Strydom, N. B. 1969. The danger of an inadequate water intake during marathon running. *S. Afr. Med. J.* 43:893–96

118. Wyndham, C. H., Strydom, N. B., van Rensburg, A. J., Benade, A. J. S., Heyns, A. J. 1970. Relation between $V_{O_{2max}}$ and body temperature in hot, humid conditions. *J. Appl. Physiol.* 29(1)45–50

119. Wyndham, C. H., Strydom, N. B., Benade, A. J. S., van Rensburg, A. J. 1971. Limiting rates of work for acclimatization at high wet bulb temperatures. *COM Res. Rep. No. 11/71, Johannesburg*

120. Wyndham, C. H., Strydom, N. B., Benade, A. J. S., van Rensburg, A. J., Rogers, G. G. 1972. Heat stroke risks in unacclimatized and acclimatized men of different $V_{O_{2max}}$ working under hot and humid conditions. *COM Res. Rep. No. 12/72, Johannesburg*

121. Wyndham, C. H., Strydom, N. B., Benade, A. J. S., van Rensburg, A. J. 1972. The influence of the state of hydration on physical responses of men during work in heat. *COM. Res. Rep. No. 13/72, Johannesburg*

122. Zitnik, R. S., Ambrosioni E., Shepherd J. T. 1971. Effect of temperature on cutaneous venomotor reflexes in man. *J. Appl. Physiol.* 31(4):507–12

Ann. Rev. Physiol. 1973. 35:221–242

COMMUNICATION AMONG PRIMATES 1095

MICHAEL PETERS AND DETLEV PLOOG

Max Planck Institute for Psychiatry
Munich, Germany

INTRODUCTION

The term "communication" enjoys a wide variety of meanings. Here, it shall be used as defined by Scheflen (139): "Communication includes all behaviors by which a group forms, sustains, mediates, corrects and integrates its relationships." Only nonverbal communication shall be considered. A number of articles provide general reviews of primate communication (4, 95) or treat selected aspects of the topic (5, 6, 31, 60, 62, 112, 122). In the past, research on primate social interactions has concentrated on the genus *Macaca*. Relevant papers published in the period covered by this review, September 1967 to May 1972, show a continued emphasis on *Macaca*. Of the 400 papers surveyed, over half deal with but a few species of *Macaca*. Adding to this *Pan, Papio, Presbytis,* and *Saimiri,* one has exhausted the primate genera which have been studied in detail. Intensive investigation of many more genera has begun during the last decade and a more representative view of primate behavior will hopefully result. A noteworthy development is the increase in excellent field studies.

While the review will not deliberately attempt to point out areas of mutual concern to physiologists and behavioral primatologists, such areas exist. As an example, work on the physiology of reproduction inevitably involves questions about behaviors indicative of receptive status and social stimuli involved in the synchronization of breeding cycles.

The review consists of three parts. First, the methods of studying primate social interactions are discussed. The second part describes the means of communication available to primates. The third part focuses on social interactions in the specific context of sexual behavior, which were chosen because collaboration between physiologists and behavioral primatologists in this area has been fruitful. Social interactions not referred to in this paper are discussed in the general sources cited above.

METHODS

Primate social interactions are studied in a variety of contexts. A basic requirement of all approaches is the establishment of a behavioral repertoire

of the species under observation. Usually, the repertoire is established by observing groups of primates in the field, the semi-free environment, and the
laboratory, without attempting to interfere actively with the group. The repertoire is then recorded in the form of a catalogue of behaviors. The catalogue contains a number of distinct motor behaviors (i.e. screaming, lip-
smacking, grooming) which are stereotyped to the extent that they occur repeatedly in similar form and can be described in similar terms by independent observers. Catalogue items are commonly referred to as "behavioral
units."

For some purposes, the communicative meaning of repertoire items is not
of primary interest; rather it is sufficient to characterize the overall frequencies of interactions between and within different age-sex classes (2). Often
the communicative meaning of a given behavior is simply estimated on the
basis of its real or imagined occurrence in certain contexts, and interactions
are described in terms of frequencies with which given behaviors occur between specified animals (who does what to whom how often). Establishing
the exact communicative significance of a given item, however, poses severe
problems. Normally, the "what" in "who does what to whom" is a catalogue
item such as "lip-smacking." It is inferred that the lip-smacking has a certain
communicative function, although in reality "lip-smacking'" may occur with a
certain body orientation and a specific vocalization. By recording only frequencies of "lip-smacking," the reaction of the receiving animal to the signal
would appear to be unpredictable in the statistical analysis of the occurrence
of signal and response. The problem of defining this "what" is generally recognized. Marler (95) comments that primates rarely use just one signal, but
rather combinations of visual and vocal signals in interaction. Therefore, in
behavioral recording, combinations of signals rather than single unitary signals should ideally be registered. In practice, this is very difficult; use of catalogue items which combine under one code number a constellation of signals
(3) is rare.

In addition to the problem of observing and recording several simultaneously emitted signals, the question of what constitutes a meaningful behavioral sequence in terms of signals emitted in a temporal order (when is a
message begun and when is it terminated) must be considered. This question
is known to investigators as the "where to split and where to lump" problem
(7). The above difficulties arise through the desire of primatologists to quantify behavioral interactions. Quantification is essential for the establishing and
testing of models of communication and the accurate measuring of change in
communication after experimental manipulation. The objective of quantify-
ing social interactions has been met so far only in very few cases in very
simple behavioral contexts. In the following discussion of methods by means
of which social interactions are studied, therefore, it should be kept in mind
that changes in social interactions are judged in most cases on an intuitive
basis and that catalogues, where such were used, contain behavioral units the
communicative meaning of which has not been rigorously documented.

Observation of undisturbed groups of primates.—This is one of the simplest methods of studying social interactions. While earlier studies have relied heavily on shorthand or telegraph style recording, widespread use of checklists, tape recording and filming is common in contemporary work. The advantage of field observation is studying animals under "natural" conditions. However, many free-living primates exist in environments changed drastically by man; the social structure and social interactions may have evolved to meet the demands of environments which are no longer present. One of the main disadvantages of field observation is the low frequency of spontaneous social interactions. In the laboratory, crowding and provisioning result in an increase in social interactions. A further increase or change in the quality of social interactions can be achieved by actively interfering with group composition, with the environment, or with the behaviors of individual group members, as will be discussed below.

Brain stimulation.—Stimulation of certain portions of the brain of animals freely moving within a social group elicits social interactions through the behavioral changes of the stimulated animal (29, 97, 131). Behavioral interactions can be produced repeatedly and are amenable to quantification. Careful analysis of social interactions following brain stimulation led Maurus & Pruscha (98) to the conclusion that many of the catalogue items thought to have a communicative function actually occurred randomly in social interactions, thus suggesting that catalogue items should be reformulated. The potential of this method as a tool for testing the communicative significance of catalogue items is considerable. The method is less suited for the correlation of specific elicited social behaviors with the location of effective stimulation sites, as stimulation of a given site with constant parameters gives rise to different behaviors in differing social contexts. The work (97, 98) indicates that some *Saimiri sciureus* communicative signals are imperceptible to human observers, producing further difficulties in the study of nonhuman primate communication. Brain stimulation has also been used to affect dominance ranking in *Macaca mulatta* by Robinson et al (131).

Brain lesions.—Lesion studies have been carried out in the laboratory and free environments. Lesions of the amygdala and anterior temporal lobe in *Macaca mulatta* and *Cercopithecus aethiops* severely reduce survival chances in the free environment (33, 78, 116) although survival changes in the laboratory are adequate (77). With temporal lobe lesions the small survival chance was possibly related to aggression of normal animals towards lesioned animals; it seems to have been the case with animals lesioned in the amygdala. Generally, studies in the free environment have contributed relatively little information as histological documentation was not available and opportunity to observe behavioral interactions limited.

Laboratory lesion studies have commonly focused on changes in restricted aspects such as fear, aversion, and aggression. Supporting earlier reports, Plotnik (123) and Bucher, Myers & Southwick (19) found that lesions of the anterior temporal lobe in *Saimiri sciureus* and *Macaca mulatta* reduced the incidence of aggressive behavior. Bucher et al (19) stated that lesioned animals appeared to have lost awareness of their social status. Amygdalectomy in infant *Macaca mulatta* (150) led to greater fear responses towards conspecifics, but this was not seen in *Cercopithecus aethiops* (77). In *Cercopithecus aethiops,* fear responses towards man were presumably reduced after amygdalectomy. In *Macaca mulatta,* amygdalectomy can result in "hypersexuality" (75), although this is not so in *Cercopithecus aethiops.* The species differences have been attributed to baseline differences in the frequency of mounting and presenting in the two species, the frequency being much higher in *Macaca mulatta.* Changes in mounting behavior were also seen in *Macaca fuscata* after lesions of the superior temporal lobe. The lesioned animals attempted to mount dominant animals and showed an increase in play behavior (72). Lesions of the frontal agranular cortex in *Macaca mulatta* lead to behavioral changes which can be recognized by conspecifics and human observers (28, 148). In one of the few studies in which behavioral changes were assessed with the help of a behavioral catalogue (28), lesioned animals showed inappropriate aggressive behavior towards normal animals. Unfortunately, in the studies of Suomi et al (148), and Deets et al (28), most of the frontal granular cortex was removed, although it is highly probable that lesions of the orbitofrontal and dorsolateral frontal cortex yield different effects on social behavior (20, 21).

Some caution is warranted in evaluating even simple unidimensional behavior changes after brain lesions. Butter et al (21) stated that *Macaca mulatta* with orbitofrontal lesions do not show noticeable changes in aversion reactions towards man; but in a different paper (20) Butter et al stated that they do. The discrepancy is apparently due to differing familiarity of animals with the human observers (21).

While the papers cited above provide evidence that lesions may produce abnormal social behavior with consequent changes in social interactions between lesioned and unlesioned animals, some questions remain. First, few of the papers give adequate documentation of the lesions; many provide none at all. Second, the structures lesioned were treated as if having unitary function. Third, very few experiments used adequate controls for general effects of surgery. Fourth, the reintroduction of operated animals is problematic. Postoperative weakness, group reaction to long absence of the operated animal (76, 156), and time course of lesion effects are factors to be considered. Finally, as the work of Kling & Cornell (76) on amygdala lesions in *Macaca speciosa* emphasizes, interpretation of lesion effects must take into account the normal behavior of the subject species.

Drug application.—Abnormal behavior has also been induced by drug application. As with lesion studies, behavioral analysis in this area has been limited. Nevertheless, the method has some potential for manipulation of social interactions. Doses of L-dopa, for example, result in higher incidence of aggressive and threat behaviors in *Macaca mulatta*. L-Dopa treated animals also show pronounced orienting behavior (138). A reversed effect was reported by Redmond et al (129), who treated *M. speciosa* with an inhibitor of dopamine and norepinephrine synthesis. The treated animals initiated fewer social interactions, and showed retarded motor activity and withdrawal postures. The animals gave the impression of lacking interest in the environment. Young *M. mulatta* exhibited increased hostility and greater withdrawal after they were fed a high phenylalanine diet (27). As with other experimental treatments, animals show great variability in response to drugs (92). A number of drawbacks are associated with drug studies in this area. If the drugs are added to the diet, accurate dosing is not possible. If they are injected, the ensuing excitement may interact with the drug effects or produce changes in social interaction by itself. When the animal is used as its own control by injecting the effective drug or neutral solutions at different times, there is considerable danger that the drug effect will be conditioned to the control injection (92).

Deprivation rearing and separation studies.—Animals raised in social isolation become deficient in social interactive skills. Social interactions between deprivation-raised animals and normal animals can be studied to detect abnormal behavior through reactions of normal towards deprivation-reared animals. Interesting recent work has been directed at determining the presence of disturbed social behavior after isolation-rearing and how such disturbances can be combated (56).

In assessing social behavior of isolates it is important to remember that isolates have no opportunity to learn under what conditions species-specific motor patterns involved in communication are performed; they also lack opportunity to learn how to synchronize their motor behavior with that of social partners. "Motor deprivation" could well be one of the determining factors in the disturbed social interactions of isolation-reared animals. Behavioral disturbances can also be produced by separating monkey infants from their mothers. Such separations result in changes resembling depressive states in humans; this type of work can serve as a model for the study of human psychopathology (100). Psychopathology is characterized by disturbances in social interactions, frequently expressed nonverbally. In the future, increasing use will be made of nonhuman primates to develop methods of identifying and rating abnormal social interactions.

Manipulation of group structure and space.—Social interactions are, to some extent, a function of the size and composition of the group. By introducing animals into a group, removing animals from a group (12, 83, 147, 156), or arranging group encounters (24, 96), the frequency and quality of social interactions can be manipulated. Field work shows considerable variability in group size and composition within species, and attempts have been made to correlate these factors with social interactions (10, 158, 167). Labo-

ratory groups which are randomly assembled may show different interactions
than groups which are formed in a more natural way (70, 133). Social interactions can also be manipulated by reducing spatial distance between animals. This can be achieved by acute crowding (1, 143) or by provisioning
free-living animals. Central feeding stations in the wild (83) lead to reduction of interindividual distance of animals which would normally be spaced
out. The effects of reducing spatial distance on social interaction are drastic
(82). Provisioning also provides more time and energy for social interactions;
free-living animals often devote so much time to foraging that little is left for
social interactions.

MEANS OF COMMUNICATION

Auditory signals.—Primates make use of vocal and nonvocal auditory
signals. The nonvocal are produced with hands and feet (chest drumming,
branch shaking and breaking, slapping or stamping on the ground, drumming
on tree roots) or with lips, tongue and teeth (tongue clicking, tongue smacking, lip smacking, teeth chattering, teeth grinding). The literature describing
the occurrence of these signals is concentrated on cartarrhines (16, 25, 42,
125, 146, 153, 155), but platyrrhines and lemuriformes also use nonvocal
auditory signals (8, 65, 162).

A tendency to elaborate the ventriculi laryngis is characteristic of many
primates although the vocal apparatus exhibits great diversity among species.
While the general anatomy of the vocal apparatus has been investigated in
various species (42, 141, 142, 144), little is known about the physiological
mechanisms of sound production in nonhuman primates. The vocal apparatus
of man is distinguished by the great thickness and mobility of the root of the
tongue and a lowering of the larynx in relation to the root of the tongue.
Computer simulated sound production, using a cast of the buccopharyngeal
region of a *Macaca mulatta* (88), has shown that this primate, as it lacks ability to modulate sounds by varying the cross-sectional area of the pharynx
above the larynx, cannot produce the entire range of human speech sounds.
This finding probably applies to other primates as well (87).

In studying the communicative function of vocalizations, the calls must
be related to the behavioral context. The success of this approach depends
not only on accurate description of behavior but also on the ability of human observers to discriminate between different vocalizations. Many of the
vocal sounds of catarrhines lie well within the human range of auditory sensitivity and, to some extent, can be transcribed into spoken combinations of
consonants and vowels (149). Descriptions of vocalizations in terms of familiar sounds, such as barking, screaming, and roaring, are also common.
More useful than the mere description of sounds is the characterization of
vocal sounds with the aid of sound spectrographs which enable researchers to
agree on a common terminology of vocalizations. Such spectrographs allow
discrimination of call features which elude the human ear and provide a
means to assess variability of given call types. Spectrographs are available for

a variety of species (15, 25, 44, 52, 54, 84, 94, 114, 134, 163, 164), but extensive recordings exist only for *Saimiri sciureus, Macaca mulatta, Macaca nemestrina,* and a few species of *Cercopithecus* and *Colobus.*

When the vocalizations of ground dwelling and arboreal primates are compared, the former appear to use graded vocalizations to a greater extent than the latter. Explanations of this difference have stressed environmental factors. Visual contact is often lacking with arboreal primates; spatial distance and background noise favor discreteness of vocal signals. Moynihan (113) has suggested that smaller arboreal primates risk detection and localization by predators when vocalizing; brief calls, again favoring discreteness, presumably reduce that risk. Field recording is biased in favor of discrete vocalizations since the recording distance is usually appreciable. Arboreal primates in close contact may well use graded vocalizations of lower intensity (166, p. 56). Such vocalizations do not register on recording devices in the field. Use of the term "discrete" should not imply that transitional forms do not occur between discrete call types. Winter, Ploog & Latta (164) described 26 discrete calls in *Saimiri sciureus,* but analysis of over 6000 *Saimiri* sound spectrographs in the same laboratory (142) has shown transitional forms between all call types.

Spectrographic analysis forces the question of "where to split and where to lump" calls. To answer that question one would have to know what portions of vocal transmissions carry communicative meaning. Marler (166, p. 56) has speculated that even small portions of vocal transmissions may carry information, but no published data are available so far. Grimm (54) has stated that *Macaca nemestrina* readily combines different fragments of vocal signals and has suggested that information is contained not only in the shape of the fragments but also in their various combinations. Here, too, data are not available. The recent development of miniature sound transmitting devices (99) which can transmit even low intensity vocalizations of freely moving animals will do much to further work in this area. The transmitters will enable investigators to accurately identify vocalizing animals and will allow synchronized recording of visual and vocal behavior.

With restrained animals, vocalizations can be elicited by stimulation in the brain of regions from which other species-specific behaviors can be elicited as well (68, 69, 130). In *Saimiri sciureus,* it has been possible to elicit many of the calls contained in the normal vocal repertoire (69). In the same species, some cells of the auditory cortex respond selectively to certain *Saimiri* calls (165).

Nonhuman primates, unlike man, have marked difficulties in an operant conditioning situation in bringing vocalizations under control (115) or in using acoustic stimuli as discriminative cues (32). Failure to demonstrate voluntary control of vocalization may be due in part to inappropriate experimental design which employs reinforcers having no biological relevance to the response which is to be reinforced. Attempts to elicit voluntary vocalization in nonhuman primates have mostly made use of food reinforcers. Vocalization in nonhuman primates, however, is commonly considered to be emotional signaling. Emotional signaling is social signaling whose effective control requires social reinforcers. Randolph & Brooks (128) reinforced a certain vocalization in *Pan* with a 15 sec period of play, and showed that under these conditions voluntary emission of vocalizations could be demonstrated. Speaking, apart from the message transmitted, is in itself a social (emotional) signal: the initiation or sustaining of vocalization in man is probably governed by much the same mechanisms which effect vocalization in nonhuman primates. Strong emotional arousal interferes with the voluntary control of vocalization. Examples are rising pitch, faltering of speech during intense excitement, exclamations during startle, and, sometimes, laughter.

Visual signals.—Primates, like other mammals, signal species identity with body features. Where these features do not allow clear species differentiation, other cues, such as vocalization, operate (145). Sex differences, apart from the primary sexual organs, are signaled by dimorphism in body shape, pelage, and dentition. Supposed lack of dimorphism may be a function of subtleness of signals rather than of their absence, as the example of *Cebus capuchinus* shows (118). In field observation, when subtle visual signals evade detection, sex recognition is aided by vocalizations (84, 145) or patterns of body movements and postures (36). Body shape and pelage also signal age of an individual. In *Papio hamadryas*, for example, the age of males can be gauged quite accurately by visual cues.

While the above visual signals are used by mammals in general, primates make more use of visual communicative signals involving facial features and expressions than do other mammalian orders. This statement applies to higher primates only; advanced carnivores make greater use of facial expressions than lower primates (117). The facial musculature of higher primates has undergone a remarkable differentiation, permitting a variety of movements elaborated from those made during feeding, attack, defense, and respiration (8). The movements of the facial musculature are often accentuated by conspicuous features of the overlying skin. These features and other aspects of facial morphology may in some cases have a signal function independent of movement. Many facial expressions of higher primates can be described in similar terms by independent observers and appear to have species-specific character. Descriptions of such facial expressions are available for various species and form part of the behavioral catalogue of these species (15, 16, 71, 126, 153, 155). Some facial expressions appear in similar form in more than one genus and have tempted speculations about their phylogenetic history (8, 154).

When communicating, primates are not bound to specific signals and similar signals assume different meaning in different contexts. This flexibility is also characteristic of facial expressions. An indirect example of flexibility in communication is Bernstein's (14) observation that hybrids between *Ma-*

caca irus and *M. nemestrina* function well within a *M. irus* group. Because of this flexibility, the communicative meaning of a given visual signal (and this applies to other channels as well) can be given in probabilisitic terms only. Meaningful probabilistic statements are warranted only after very time consuming observation, as shown, for example, by Jensen & Gordon's study (64) in *M. nemestrina* of the facial "LEN" expression, characterized by rhythmic smacking of the protruded lips. Jensen & Gordon documented this expression as a maternal beckoning gesture.

Experimental approaches to primate visual communication have also been employed. Miller (109) demonstrated that *Macaca mulatta* can use, as the cue for initiation of an instrumental shock avoidance response, the facial expression of conspecifics which are anticipating shock. The approach is useful for a narrow range of facial expressions only; a similar paradigm, using food instead of shock as reinforcer, proved far less effective. Miller, Carl & Mirsky (110) showed that *M. mulatta* reared in social isolation for one year after birth proved bad senders and receivers of communicative signals in the shock avoidance paradigm. Their failure to function as senders was not caused by an inability to produce appropriate facial expressions. Rather, they made frequent fear expressions which led normal receivers to initiate unnecessary responses. As receivers, isolation-reared animals may have failed because of a tendency to avoid looking at the stimulus animal. Sackett (137) investigated the response of isolation-reared macaques to pictures of conspecifics of different age-sex classes with differing facial expressions. His findings suggest that a threat expression, for example, can function as a releasing stimulus which is recognized by a socially naive animal. The isolation-reared animal reacts to the picture of a threatening animal with fear, suggesting operation of an innate releasing mechanism.

For both *Homo* and other primates the accurate description of facial expressions presents difficulties; not all muscle movements involved in facial expressions are visible and subtle facial movements elude description. Facial expressions may involve rapid movements, such as ear movements in *Saimiri sciureus,* which have communicative significance (50) but are difficult to detect. Efficient perception of a given facial expression may involve the ability of the receiver to produce that expression.

While facial expressions are known to be involved in the communication of affect in *Homo,* systematic investigation has only recently begun (9, 40, 157). Principal problems have been the description of facial expressions and their measurement (57), the dependence of interpretation on context, and the possibility of differing affective states giving rise to similar facial expressions. Consequently, investigation has centered on a few, relatively uncomplicated affective states (happiness, anger, fear, disgust, sadness) and their corresponding facial expressions. According to suggestive evidence, facial expressions associated with these affective dimensions have species-specific character (40, 41). Future research in this area might well concentrate on the ontogeny of facial expression in children since cultural demands on hiding certain affects and amplifying others (37) are not yet internalized at early age.

Together with facial expression, body posture and movement also function in nonverbal communication. Depressive states and joyous exhilaration are both accompanied by characteristic changes in postural tonus, and normal social interaction involves delicate adjustment of interindividual distance and postures (35, 101, 155). Man also uses facial expressions and body movements to modify the content of verbal messages or to synchronize verbal interactions (73, 89). Efficient use of visual communicative signals requires some interactive skill which is not necessarily equally commanded by all individuals. Individual variability in social skills is not unique to man. Miller, Caul & Mirsky (110) found, in the experiment mentioned above, large individual differences in the extent to which normal control animals could act as senders and receivers of visual signals.

Little is known about the neural substrate underlying visual communication. Observation of anencephalic babies (67), blind and deaf human children (39), and isolation-reared *Macaca mulatta* (18) confirms that facial expressions are species-specific and occur in basic form without learning. Facial expressions, or fragments thereof, which may or may not be accompanied by corresponding affective states can be elicited by brain stimulation (30). Over the years, clinical evidence has provided numerous examples of patients with brain damage in which voluntary facial movements are abolished but affective expression is intact, and vice versa (115, 124). This suggests that the motor systems subserving affective facial expression are different from those subserving voluntary facial movement (152).

While both man and other primates react sensitively to communicative signals, attempts to define, isolate, and quantify their essential characteristics have met with little success. Much work must be carried out in this area, because visual communicative signals are assuming increasing importance in the assessment of behavioral changes and the identification of abnormal social behavior (53, 61, 92).

Tactile signals.—Higher primates make extensive use of body contact and touching behavior during interactions involving expression of dominance, reassurance, or affinity (95). Much of the body contact behavior is used in maintaining affinitive ties (133) and consists of various forms of huddling or embracing. In catarrhines, grooming is a commonly observed behavior. While grooming may have evolved for reasons of hygiene and probably still functions in this context at times there is little doubt that it is instrumental in establishing and maintaining peaceful social relations (17, 135) in many species. Subtle dominance interactions may involve the use of light touches of the hand, together with appropriate body orientation and movement (63, 121).

Of the nonhuman primates, *Pan* deserves special mention because a great variety of tactile cues in social interaction (155) have been observed.

Extensive use of touching with the hand of selective body parts of social partners is common. A striking morphological and behavioral specialization involving tactile communication can be seen in *Perodicticus potto* (160). In
this species, a specialized area overlying several anterior vertebrae is sensitive
to touch; contact with this area is important in the establishment of peaceful
relations between interacting animals. The importance of contact behavior
in the ontogeny of nonhuman primates is vividly illustrated by studies of isolation-reared *Macaca mulatta* (55) which were raised with surrogate cloth
mothers. Contact behavior is of extreme importance for normal development
in human infants as well. With adult man, touching behavior and body contact, though culture dependent in frequency and form, is observed univer-
sally. Jourard (66) studied preferential touching of body parts by various
combinations of interacting social partners and found that considerable sex
differences in body contact patterns exist.

Man also makes extensive use of self-touching behavior, much of which
is meaningful to interactants or observers. In some cultures the upper part of
the face and eyes are covered with the hand during expression of grief and
covering of the mouth during laughter is also observed. Hand touches to the
face occur considerably more often than touches of other parts of the body
(49). Face touches seem to fulfill a variety of functions. They may hide affect expressed on the face (38), or self-reassure and comfort. Self-touching
as a reassurance mechanism is also observed in the behavioral repertoire of
isolation-raised *Macaca mulatta*.

Autonomic signals.—The principal overt autonomic correlates of social
interaction are pupillary dilation, piloerection, penile erection, changes in
blood supply to facial regions, defecation, and urination. Pupillary dilation, a
well known corollary of sympathetic discharge, may have a signal function
(actors at times use artifical means to dilate the pupils, presumably to increase intensity of projected emotion).

Piloerection, while not of importance in man, is often alluded to: "his
hair stood on end." It is readily observed in many nonhuman primates during
stressful social interactions (155) and may function to increase the apparent
size of an animal. In *Tupaia glis,* piloerection serves as a fine gauge of
autonomic responses to social stress (159), allowing judgments of severity
of stress experienced by animals exposed to each other and permitting predictions of effects on fertility and survival. Penile erection, the result of local
parasympathetic discharge, is observed in displays of many primate species
(86, 120, 161). It can be elicited through brain stimulation from a variety of
limbic and diencephalic sites (93). Changes in blood supply to facial regions
are very conspicuous in lightly pigmented varieties of *Homo* where such
changes, according to context, are interpreted as signs of rage or embarrass-
ment.

Primates, like other mammals, may defecate or urinate in response to
stress. During such defecation, feces from upper intestinal regions are also

expelled. As these feces have not been fully processed they differ in smell and consistency from normal feces (65).

While the autonomic responses considered above are correlated with social interactions, their communicative function remains to be established. In addition to overt autonomic responses, covert autonomic correlates of social interactions have also been investigated. These include heart rate changes during social encounters in *Saimiri sciureus* (22) and change in adrenal corticosteroid levels in *Macaca mulatta* (132). Measurement of adrenal corticosteroid levels, limited mostly to urinary 17-hydroxycorticosteroid, has provided little information to date. Problems in this area lie in the marked individual differences in adrenal responses which tend to mask experimental manipulation, sampling procedures, and creation of appropriate stress conditions. Certain primate species, such as *Saimiri sciureus,* appear particularly suited for this type of study as their adrenocortical system is highly reactive (119).

Olfactory signals.—Primates use olfactory signals for communicative purposes, as do other mammals (127). Prosimians (111) and platyrrhine monkeys (45, 114) have well developed scent glands, but these are also found in catarrhines. Primate scent glands are found mainly in the epigastric-sternal region, axillary region, and the genital region. Olfactory substances originate from specialized scent glands but may be present also in saliva, sweat, and urine. Observation of primates suggests that olfactory cues may function in the demarcation of territory and communication of sex, state of sexual receptivity, individual identity, and dominance status (45, 47, 51, 80, 103, 114, 140). Epple & Lorenz (45) have stated that in *Hapalidae,* low ranking animals show poor or no development of the sternal glands. The social importance of scent marking is further emphasized by the increased marking behavior of high ranking females in the presence of other females; the same applies to males (43). Poor development of some scent glands under certain social conditions may explain failure to detect scent glands in individuals of species known to possess such glands. Urine washing, a behavior which occurs in different situations in various species (23, 34) could be related to olfactory communication. By spreading the urine over the surfaces of the feet, the area from which olfactory cues act is increased. The olfactory stimuli may be contained in the urine or brought into the urine from scent glands located in the genital area.

Sniffing of the genital region is a common behavior in primates, and a series of experiments has shown olfactory stimuli to signal sexual attractiveness in *Macaca mulatta* females (102, 103). It was shown that male *M. mulatta,* rendered anosmic, did not respond with sexual interest towards ovariectomized females treated with estrogen. Upon restoration of olfaction, the males showed renewed sexual interest in such females. The search for olfactory substances which signal sexual attractiveness, and, under normal conditions, sexual receptivity, led to the isolation of a mixture of short chained

aliphatic acids which was extracted from vaginal washings of normal receptive females (103). A similar, synthetically produced mixture, applied to the
sexual skin of non-receptive females, caused strong sexual excitement and
activity of the males. The conditions for studying the neurophysiology of this
particular "releasing stimulus" are favorable.

Although an enormous deodorant and perfume industry attests to the importance of olfactory stimuli to man, little is known about the communicative
function of these stimuli. An often cited study by Le Magnen (11, p. 44)
showed that adult women can detect a particular macrocyclic musk odor far
more readily than adult men or young boys or girls, suggesting an interaction
between olfactory sensitivity and hormone activity.

Although olfactory signals are considered a somewhat primitive means of
communication, further work may show that they involve very complicated
mechanisms, including the recognition, by olfaction, of individuals (79). In
discussing the use of olfactory signals in *Lemur catta,* Evans & Goy (47)
speculated that "Ringtails may prove to possess an olfactory repertoire whose
complexity rivals the more sophisticated visual and acoustic systems of larger
brained primates" (p. 195).

COMMUNICATION IN SEXUAL BEHAVIOR

In discussing sexual behavior, a distinction must be made between behavior which is directly related to reproduction and that which is not. In numerous primate species the genital organs of conspecifics are presented, touched,
and visually inspected not only in reproductive behavior but also in the initiation of contact ("greeting"), expression of submission, or expression of dominance status (26, 120, 155).

This section will be concerned only with communicative processes involved in sexual reproductive behavior. Communication in this context is studied for two principal reasons. First, in females of many species outward physiological signs of receptive status, such as the genital swelling observed in *Macaca* and *Papio,* are subtle or not present. Therefore, knowledge of the postures or movements, as well as olfactory cues, by means of which females
communicate receptive status, is important. Secondly, behaviors related to
reproduction are important variables in the study of hormone activity-mating
behavior. Systematic studies of mating behavior have been carried out on a
very limited number of primate species, not only because the natural habitat
often precludes detailed observation of mating behavior (8) but also because
mating behavior occurs very infrequently (74, 81, 85, 125) in most species or
only during very restricted periods (47).

In primates which do not show the familiar presenting behavior of *Macaca, Papio, Cercocebus,* and *Pan,* the identification of behavioral indices of
female receptive status has been quite difficult. Examples of such indices are
the lateral shaking of the head seen in *Presbytis* (13, 63) and the upward
tail-coiling movement in *Saguinus geoffroyi* (114). Far more characteristic of
present incomplete knowledge about receptive signaling in anthropoidea than

the above examples, is the unclear situation with regard to receptive behavior seen, for example, in *Ateles geoffroyi* and *Ateles belzebuth* (74). Less yet is known about female signaling of receptive status in prosimians; in *Lemur catta* (47) and *Galago senegalensis* (34) olfactory cues seem of predominant importance.

Even the presenting behavior of catarrhines is not without ambiguity (26). With the possible exception of captive *Cercocebus* (26), occurrence in contexts not associated with reproduction is very frequent. In *Macaca mulatta*, behaviors which are more specifically related to mating than is presentation have been identified. Michael & Zumpe (107) reported that the correlation of head-bob, head-duck, and hand-reaching with mating behavior is higher than is the correlation of presentation with these activities or with mating behavior. Support for the mating-specific character of these behaviors is offered by the observations of Zumpe & Michael (168), who increased the frequency of occurrence of head-ducks, head-bobs, and hand-reaching by treating ovariectomized females with estradiol, and reduced their frequency by administering progesterone. Progesterone was shown by Michael, Saayman & Zumpe (106) to decrease female presenting and to increase male refusal of female presentations; it appeared to reduce the attractiveness of females for males.

The relative unreliability of female presenting behavior as an indicator of receptive status in *M. mulatta* may account for the discrepancy between the reports by Zumpe & Michael (168) and Herbert & Trimble (59). The former stated that subcutaneous injection of estradiol increased the female presenting behavior, together with head-ducks, head-bobs, and hand-reaching. Herbert & Trimble reported, on the other hand, that subcutaneous injections of estrogen, while not increasing the frequency of presentation, did apparently increase the attractiveness of females to the males. Apart from the differences reported for presenting behavior, the studies agree that estradiol injections increase the attractiveness of the female to the male. If estradiol is applied to the sexual skin of females, their attractiveness to males (104) is increased but not their willingness to mate; this leads to increased frequency of aggressive interactions. Herbert & Trimble (59) reported a reversed effect when females were treated with testosterone. With testosterone, the females presented more frequently although their attractiveness to males did not seem increased. These reports lead to the conclusion that the sex pheromones are more important in signaling female attractiveness than is female presenting behavior. It would be interesting to see if this also holds for the head-duck, head-bob, and hand-reaching behavior (168).

In view of the established role of sex pheromones in signaling female attractiveness (103) the question of the relationship between the preference shown by males for certain females (58, 90), and the action of pheromones, arises. Everitt & Herbert (48) showed that while pheromones play a role in preference behavior, other factors must also be involved. Hormone levels of ovariectomized females were manipulated and the preference behavior of males towards a pair of such feamles was observed. When the estrogen dose for the preferred female was reduced, the male's preference for the preferred female was reducd, but there was no increased preference for the non-preferred female which received the normal dose of estrogen. Application of progesterone had the same effect on the preferred female as reduction of the estrogen dose. When the preferred female's estrogen dose was reduced, the nonpreferred female showed an increased occurrence of presentations. One unanswered question is the influence of female-female behavioral interactions on the initial preference behavior of the male. With wolves, for example, high ranking females achieve a "preferred" status by driving lower ranking females away from the male mate. Herbert (58), however, stated that only after a female was chosen did she show a marked increase in aggression towards the nonpreferred female. Thus, the cues which determine the preferences of males for some females remain to be defined.

When primate mating activity is observed, conclusions about estrous condition are inferred from instances of copulatory behavior. Nevertheless, the occurrence of neither full copulatory behavior nor female presentation (46, 91, 107, 136) justifies the unqualified deduction of female estrous status; copulation occurs during perimenstrual days as well as during the follicular phase. However, it is possible to draw conclusions about the estrous states of females with use of more differentiated observation methods. Michael & Zumpe (108) stated that no rhythmicity of copulatory behavior could be detected during the estrous cycle when full copulatory behavior was considered the dependent variable, but that rhythmicity emerged when the mean number of ejaculations per test was considered. It appears that the female reacts somewhat differently to copulation during the follicular phase and the male is responsive to this. Apart from maximal production of sex pheromones during the follicular phase, the vaginal response of the female at this time may be more conductive to male ejaculation (46, 105, 169). In man (151), rhythmic variation of receptivity is also observed during estrous cycles but it is probable that initiation of mating is based not so much on olfactory stimuli which render the female attractive to the male, but on soliciting behavior.

LITERATURE CITED

1. Alexander, B. K., Roth, E. M. 1971. The effects of acute crowding on aggressive behavior in Japanese monkeys. *Behaviour* 39:73–90
2. Altmann, S. A. 1968. Sociobiology of rhesus monkeys. III. The basic communication network. *Behaviour* 32:17–32
3. Altmann, S. A. 1968. Sociobiology of rhesus monkeys. IV. Testing Mason's hypothesis of sex differences in affective behavior. *Behaviour* 32:49–69
4. Altmann, S. A. 1968. Primates. In *Animal Communication,* ed. T. A. Seboek, 466–522. London, Indiana: Indiana Univ. Press. 686 pp.
5. Altmann, S. A. 1967. *Social Communication Among Primates.* Chicago: Univ. Chicago Press. 392 pp.
6. Altmann, S. A. 1967. The structure of primate communication. See ref. 5, 325–62
7. Altmann, S. A. 1965. Sociobiology of rhesus monkeys. II. Stochastics of social communication. *J. Theor. Biol.* 8:490–522

8. Andrew, R. J. 1963. Evolution of facial expression. *Science* 142: 1034–41

9. Argyle, M. 1969. *Social Interaction*. London: Methuen. 504 pp.

10. Baldwin, J. D., Baldwin, J. I. 1971. Squirrel monkeys (Saimiri) in natural habitats in Panama, Colombia, Brazil and Peru. *Primates* 12:45–61

11. Beets, M. G. J. 1964. A molecular approach to olfaction. *Mol. Pharmacol.* 2:3–51

12. Bernstein, I. S. 1969. Introductory techniques in the formation of pigtail monkey troops. *Folia Primatol.* 10:1–19

13. Bernstein, I. S. 1968. The Lutong of Kuala Selangor. *Behaviour* 14:136–63

14. Bernstein, I. S. 1968. Social status of two hybrids in a wild troop of Macaca irus. *Folia Primatol.* 8:121–31

15. Bertrand, M. 1969. The behavioral repertoire of the stumptail macaque. *Bibl. Primatol.* 11:1–123. Basel, Switzerland: Karger

16. Blurton-Jones, N. G., Trollope, J. 1968. Social behaviour of stumptailed macaques in captivity. *Primates* 9:365–94

17. Bramblett, C. A. 1970. Coalitions among Gelada Baboons. *Primates* 11:327–33

18. Brandt, E. M., Stevens, C. W., Mitchell, G. 1971. Visual social communication in adult male isolate-reared monkeys (Macaca mulatta). *Primates* 12:105–12

19. Bucher, K., Myers, R. E., Southwick, C. 1970. Anterior temporal cortex and maternal behavior in monkey. *Neurology* 20:415

20. Butter, C. M., Mishkin, M., Mirsky, A. F. 1968. Emotional responses toward humans in monkeys with selective frontal lesions. *Physiol. Behav.* 3:213–15

21. Butter, C. M., Snyder, D. R., McDonald, J. A. 1970. Effects of orbital frontal lesions on aversive and aggressive behavior in rhesus monkeys. *J. Comp. Physiol. Psychol.* 72:132–44

22. Candland, D. K., Bryan, D. C., Nazar, B. L., Kopf, K. J., Sendor, M. 1970. Squirrel monkey heart rate during formation of status orders. *J. Comp. Physiol.*

Psychol. 70:417–23

23. Castell, R., Maurus, M. 1967. Das sogenannte Urinmarkieren von Totenkopfaffen (Saimiri sciureus) in Abhängigkeit von umweltbedingten und emotionalen Faktoren. *Folia Primatol.* 6:170–76

24. Castell, R., Ploog, D. 1967. Zum Sozialverhalten der Totenkopf-Affen (Saimiri sciureus): Auseinandersetzung zwischen zwei Kolonien. *Z. Tierpsychol.* 24: 625–41

25. Chalmers, N. R. 1968. The visual and vocal communication of free living mangabeys in Uganda. *Folia Primatol.* 9: 258–80

26. Chalmers, N. R., Rowell, T. E. 1971. Behavior and female reproductive cycles in a captive group of mangabeys. *Folia Primatol.* 14:1–14

27. Chamove, A. S., Waisman, H. A., Harlow, H. F. 1970. Abnormal social behavior in phenylketonuric monkeys. *J. Abnorm. Soc. Psychol.* 76:62–8

28. Deets, A. C., Harlow, H. F., Singh, S. D., Bloomquist, A. J. 1970. Effects of bilateral lesions of the frontal granular cortex on the social behavior of rhesus monkeys. *J. Comp. Physiol. Psychol.* 72:452–61

29. Delgado, J. M. R. 1967. Social rank and radio-stimulated aggressiveness in monkeys. *J. Nerv. Ment. Dis.* 144:383–90

30. Delgado, J. M. R., Mir, D. 1969. Fragmental organization of emotional behavior in the monkey brain. *Ann. NY. Acad. Sci.* 158:731–51

31. DeVore, I., Ed. 1965. *Primate Behavior*. New York: Holt, Rinehart Winston. 654 pp.

32. Dewson, J. H., Cowey, A. 1969. Discrimination of auditory sequences by monkeys. *Nature* 222:695–97

33. Dicks, D., Myers, R. E., Kling, A. 1969. Uncus and amygdala lesions: Effects on social behavior in the free-ranging rhesus monkey. *Science* 165:69–71

34. Doyle, G. A., Pelletier, A., Bekker, T. 1967. Courtship, mating and parturition in the lesser bushbaby (Galago senegalensis moholis) under seminatural

conditions. *Folia Primatol.* 7: 169–97

35. Duncan, S. 1969. Nonverbal communication. *Psychol. Bull.* 72: 118–37

36. Durham, N. M. 1969. Sex differences in visual threat displays of West African vervets. *Primates* 10:91–5

37. Eibl-Eibesfeldt, I. 1972. *Die !Ko Buschmann Gesellschaft.* Munich: Piper. 223 pp.

38. Eibl-Eibesfeldt, I. 1972. Similarities and differences between cultures in expressive movements. See ref. 60, 297–312

39. Eibl-Eibesfeldt, I. 1973. The expressive behaviour of the deaf and blind born. In *Non-Verbal Behaviour and Expressive Movements,* ed. M. von Cranach, I. Vine. London: Academic. In press

40. Ekman, P. 1970. Universal facial expressions of emotion. *Calif. Ment. Health Res. Dig.* 8(4): 151–58

41. Ekman, P., Friesen, W. V., Tomkins, S. S. 1971. Facial affect scoring technique: A first validity study. *Semiotica* 1:37–58

42. Ellefson, J. O. 1968. Territorial behavior in the common white-handed Gibbon, Hylobates lar Linn. See ref. 62, 180–99

43. Epple, G. 1970. Quantitative studies on scent marking in the Marmoset (Callithrix jacchus) *Folia Primatol.* 13:48–62

44. Epple, G. 1968. Comparative studies on vocalization in Marmoset monkeys (Hapalidae). *Folia Primatol.* 8:1–40

45. Epple, G., Lorenz, R. 1967. Vorkommen, Morphologie und Funktion der Sternaldrüse bei den Platyrrhini. *Folia Primatol.* 7:98–126

46. Erikson, L. B. 1967. Relationship of sexual receptivity to menstrual cycles in adult rhesus monkeys. *Nature* 216:299–301

47. Evans, C. S., Goy, R. W. 1968. Social behavior and reproductive cycles in captive ring-tailed lemurs (Lemur catta). *J. Zool.* 156:181–97

48. Everitt, B. J., Herbert, J. 1969. The role of ovarian hormones in the sexual preference of rhesus monkeys. *Anim. Behav.* 17: 738–46

49. Fischer, S., Cleveland, S. F. 1968. *Body Image and Personality.* New York: Dover. 182 pp.

50. Francois, G. R., Barratt, E. S., Harris, C. S. 1970. Assessing the spontaneous cage behavior of the squirrel monkey (Saimiri sciureus). *Primates* 11:89–92

51. Gartlan, J. S., Brain, C. K. 1968. Ecology and social variability in Cercopithecus aethiops and Cercopithecus mitis. See ref. 62, 253–92

52. Gautier, J. P. 1971. Etude morphologique et fonctionelle des annexes extra-laryngees des Cercopithecinae; Liaison avec les cris d'espacement. *Biol. Gabonica* 7(2):229–68

53. Grant, E. C. 1972. Non-verbal communication in the mentally ill. See ref. 60, 349–58

54. Grimm, R. J. 1967. Catalog of sounds of the pigtailed macaque (Macaca namestrina). *J. Zool.* 152:361–73

55. Harlow, H. F., Zimmermann, R. R. 1959. Affectional responses in the infant monkey. *Science* 130:431–32

56. Harlow, H. F., Suomi, S. J. 1971. Social recovery by isolation-reared monkeys. *Proc. Nat. Acad. Sci. USA* 68:1534–38

57. Heimann, H., Lukacs, G. 1966. Eine Methode zur quantitativen Analyse der mimischen Bewegungen. *Arch. Ges. Psychol.* 118:1–17

58. Herbert, J. 1968. Sexual preference in the rhesus monkey Macaca mulatta in the laboratory. *Anim. Behav.* 16:120–28

59. Herbert, J., Trimble, M. R. 1967. Effect of oestradiol and testosterone on the sexual receptivity and attractiveness of the female rhesus monkey. *Nature* 216: 165–66

60. Hinde, R. A., Ed. 1972. *Non-Verbal Communication.* Cambridge: Cambridge Univ. Press. 443 pp.

61. Hinde, R. A., Spencer-Booth, Y. 1970. Individual differences in responses of rhesus monkeys to a period of separation from their mothers. *J. Child Psychol.* 11:159–76

62. Jay, P. C., Ed. 1968. *Primates.* New York: Holt, Rinehart and Winston. 529 pp.

63. Jay, P. C. 1965. The common Langur of North India. See ref. 31, 197–249

64. Jensen, G. D., Gordon, B. N. 1970. Sequences of mother-infant behavior following a facial communicative gesture of pigtail monkeys. *Recent Adv. Biol. Psychiat.* 2:267–72

65. Jolly, A. 1966. *Lemur Behavior.* Chicago: Univ. Chicago Press. 187 pp.

66. Jourard, S. M. 1966. An exploratory study of body accessibility. *Brit. J. Soc. Clin. Psychol.* 5:221–31

67. Jung, R., Hassler, R. 1960. The extrapyramidal motor system. In *Neurophysiology,* ed. H. W. Magoun, 2:863–927. Washington, DC: Am. Physiol. Soc.

68. Jürgens, U., Maurus, M., Ploog, D., Winter, P. 1967. Vocalization in the squirrel monkey (Saimiri sciureus) elicited by brain stimulation. *Exp. Brain. Res.* 4:114–7

69. Jürgens, U., Ploog, D. 1970. Cerebral representation of vocalization in the squirrel monkey. *Exp. Brain. Res.* 10:532–54

70. Kaufman, I. C., Rosenblum, L. A. 1969. Effects of separation from mother on the emotional behavior of infant monkeys. *Ann. NY Acad. Sci.* 159:681–95

71. Kaufman, I. C., Rosenblum, L. A. 1966. A behavioral taxonomy for Macaca nemestrina and Macaca radiata: Based on longitudinal observation of family groups in the laboratory. *Primates* 7:205–58

72. Kawai, J. 1966. Changes in social behavior following bilateral removal of the posterior parts of the superior temporal gyri in Japanese monkeys. *Primates* 7: 1–20

73. Kendon, A. 1967. Some functions of gaze direction in social interaction. *Acta Psychol.* 26:22–63

74. Klein, L. L. 1971. Observations on copulation and seasonal reproduction of two species of spider monkey, Ateles belzebuth and Ateles geoffroyi. *Folia Primatol.* 15:233–48

75. Kling, A. 1968. Effects of amygdalectomy and testosterone on sexual behaviour of male juvenile macaques. *J. Comp. Physiol. Psychol.* 65:466–71

76. Kling, A., Cornell, R. 1971. Amygdalectomy and social behavior in the caged stump-tailed macaque (Macaca speciosa). *Folia Primatol.* 14:190–208

77. Kling, A., Dicks, D., Gurowitz, E. M. 1969. Amygdalectomy and social behavior in a caged group of vervets (C. aethiops). *Proc. 2nd Int. Congr. Primatol., Atlanta, 1968* 232–41. Basel, Switzerland: Karger

78. Kling, A., Lancaster, J., Benitone, J. 1970. Amygdalectomy in freeranging vervet (C. aethiops). *J. Psychiat. Res.* 7(3): 191

79. Klopfer, P. H. 1970. Discrimination of young in galagos. *Folia Primatol.* 13:137–43

80. Klopfer, P. H., Jolly, A. 1970. The stability of territorial boundaries in a lemur troop. *Folia Primatol.* 12:199–208

81. Koyama, N. 1971. Observations on mating behavior of wild Siamang Gibbons at Fraser's Hill, Malaysia. *Primates* 12: 183–90

82. Kummer, H. 1970. Spacing mechanisms in social behavior. *Soc. Sci. Inform.* 9(6):109–22

83. Kummer, H. 1968. Social organization of hamadryas baboons. *Bibl. Primatol.* 6:1–189

84. Lamprecht, J. 1970. Duettgesang beim Siamang, Symphalangus syndactylus. *Z. Tierpsychol.* 27: 186–204

85. Lancaster, J. B. 1971. Play-mothering: The relations between juvenile females and young infants among free-ranging vervet monkey (Cercopithecus aethiops). *Folia Primatol.* 15: 161–82

86. Latta, J., Hopf, S., Ploog, D. 1967. Observation on mating behavior and sexual play in the squirrel monkey (Saimiri sciureus). *Primates* 8:229–46

87. Lieberman, P., 1969. On the acoustic analysis of primate vocalizations. *Behav. Res. Method. & Instrum.* 1:169–74

88. Lieberman, P. H., Klatt, D. H., Wilson, W. H. 1969. Vocal tract limitations on the vowel repertoires of rhesus monkey and other nonhuman primates. *Science* 164:1185–87

89. Lindenfold, J. 1971. Verbal and

non-verbal elements in discourse. *Semiotica,* 3:223–33

90. Loy, J. 1971, Estrous behavior of free-ranging primates (Macaca mulatta). *Primates* 12:1–31

91. Loy, J. 1970. Peri-menstrual sexual behavior among rhesus monkeys. *Folia Primatol.* 13: 286–97

92. Machiyama, Y., Utena, H., Kikuchi, M. 1970. Behavioral disorders in Japanese monkeys produced by the long-term administration of metaamphetamine. *Proc. Jap. Acad.* 46:738–43

93. MacLean, P. D., Ploog, D. W. 1962. Cerebral representation of penile erection. *J. Neurophysiol.* 25:29–55

94. Marler, P. 1970. Vocalizations of East African monkeys. I. Red Colobus. *Folia Primatol.* 13: 81–91

95. Marler, P. 1965. Communication in monkeys and apes. See ref. 31, 544–84

96. Marsden, H. M. 1968. Behavior between two social groups of rhesus monkeys within two tunnel-connected enclosures. *Folia Primatol.* 8:240–46

97. Maurus, M., Ploog, D. 1971. Social signals in squirrel monkeys: analysis by cerebral radio stimulation. *Exp. Brain. Res.* 12: 171–83

98. Maurus, M., Pruscha, H. 1972. Quantitative analysis of behavioral sequence elicited by automated telestimulation in squirrel monkeys. *Exp. Brain. Res.* 14:372–94

99. Maurus, M., Szabolcs, J. 1971. Kleinstsender für die Übertragung von Affenlauten. *Naturwissenschaften* 58:273–74

100. McKinney, W. T., Harlow, H. F., Suomi, S. J. 1971. Primate models for human depression. *World Congr. Psychiat., Mexico City*

101. Mehrabian, A. 1969. Significance of posture and position in the communication of attitude and status relationships. *Psychol. Bull.* 71:359–72

102. Michael, R. P., Keverne, E. B. 1968. Pheromones in the communication of sexual status in primates. *Nature* 218:746–49

103. Michael, R. P., Keverne, E. B., Bosnell, R. W. 1971. Pheromones: Isolation of male sex at-

tractants from primate females. *Science* 172:964–66

104. Michael, R. P., Saayman, G. S. 1968. Differential effects on behavior of the subcutaneous and intravaginal administration of oestrogen in the rhesus monkey (Macaca mulatta). *J. Endocrinol.* 41:231–46

105. Michael, R. P., Saayman, G. S. 1967. Individual differences in the sexual behavior of male rhesus monkeys (Macaca mulatta) under laboratory conditions. *Anim. Behav.* 15:460–66

106. Michael, R. P., Saayman, G. S., Zumpe, D. 1967. Inhibition of sexual receptivity by progesterone in rhesus monkeys. *J. Endocrinol.* 39:309–10

107. Michael, R. P., Zumpe, D. 1970. Sexual initiating behavior by female rhesus monkeys (Macaca mulatta) under laboratory conditions. *Behaviour* 36:168–86

108. Michael, R. P., Zumpe, D. 1970. Rhythmic changes in copulatory frequency of rhesus monkeys (Macaca mulatta) in relation to menstrual cycle and a comparison with human cycle. *J. Reprod. Fert.* 21:199–201

109. Miller, R. E. 1967. Experimental approaches to the physiological and behavioral concomitants of affective communication in rhesus monkeys. See ref. 5, 125–34

110. Miller, R. E., Caul, W. F., Mirsky, J. A. 1967. Communication of affects between feral and socially isolated monkeys. *J. Pers. Soc. Psychol.* 7:231–39

111. Montagna, W. 1962. The skin of lemurs. *Ann. NY. Acad. Sci.* 102:190–209

112. Morris, D., Ed. 1969. *Primate Ethology.* Garden City, NY: Doubleday. 471 pp.

113. Moynihan, M. 1967. Comparative aspects of communication in New World Primates. See ref. 112, 306–42

114. Moynihan, M. 1970. Some behavior patterns of platyrrhine monkeys II. Saguinus geoffroyi and some other tamarins. *Smithson. Contrib. Zool.* 28:1–77

115. Myers, R. E. 1969. Neurology of social communication in primates. *Proc. 2nd Int. Congr.*

Primatol., Atlanta, 1968, 3:1–9. Basel, Switzerland: Karger

116. Myers, R. E., Swett, C. 1970. Social behavior deficits of free-ranging monkeys after anterior temporal cortex removal: a preliminary report. *Brain Res.* 18: 551–6

117. Newell, T. G. 1971. Social encounters in two prosimian species: Galago crassicaudatus and Nycticebus coucang. *Psychon. Sci.* 24:128–30

118. Oppenheimer, J. R. 1969. Changes in forehead patterns and group composition of the white-faced monkey (Cebus capuchinus). *Proc. 2nd Int. Congr. Primatol., Atlanta, 1968,* 1:36–42. Basel, Switzerland: Karger

119. Penney, D. P., Brown, G. M. 1971. The fine structural morphology of adrenal cortices of normal and stressed squirrel monkeys. *J. Morphol.* 134: 447–65

120. Ploog, D. W., Blitz, J., Ploog, F. 1963. Studies on social and sexual behavior of the squirrel monkey (Saimiri sciureus). *Folia Primatol.* 1:29–66

121. Ploog, D., Hopf, S., Winter, P. 1967. Ontogenese des Verhaltens von Totenkopf-Affen (Saimiri sciureus). *Psychol. Forsch.* 31:1–41

122. Ploog, D., Melnechuk, T. 1969. Primate communication. *Neurosci. Program Res. Bull.* 7(5): 419–510

123. Plotnik, R. 1968. Changes in social behavior of squirrel monkeys after anterior temporal lobectomy. *J. Comp. Physiol. Psychol.* 66:369–77

124. Poeck, K. 1969. Pathophysiology of emotional disorders associated with brain damage. In *Handbook of Clinical Neurology,* ed. P. J. Vinken, G. W. Bruyn, 3:343–67. Amsterdam: North-Holland

125. Poirier, F. E. 1970. The Nilgiri Langur (Presbytis johnii) of South India. In *Primate Behavior,* ed. L. A. Rosenblum, 254–383. New York: Academic

126. Rahaman, H., Parthasarathy, M. D. 1968. The expressive movements of the Bonnet macaque. *Primates* 9:259–72

127. Ralls, K. 1971. Mammalian scent marking. *Science* 171:443–9

128. Randolph, M. C., Brooks, B. A. 1967. Conditioning of a vocal response in a chimpanzee through social reinforcement. *Folia Primatol.* 5:70–9

129. Redmond, D. E., Maas, J. W., Kling, A., Dekirmenjian, H. 1971. Changes in primate social behavior after treatment with alpha-methyl-paratyrosine. *Psychosom. Med.* 33:97–113

130. Robinson, B. W. 1967. Neurological aspects of evoked vocalizations. See ref. 5, 135–47

131. Robinson, B. W., Alexander, M., Browne, G. 1969. Dominance reversal resulting from aggressive responses evoked by brain telestimulation. *Physiol. Behav.* 4:749–52

132. Rose, R. M., Mason, J. W. Brady, J. V. 1969. Adrenal responses to maternal separation and chair adaption in experimentally-raised rhesus monkey (Macaca mulatta). *Proc. 2nd Int. Congr. Primatol., Atlanta, 1968,* 1:211–18. Basel, Switzerland: Karger

133. Rosenblum, L. A. 1971. Kinship interaction patterns in pigtail and bonnet macaques, *Proc. 3rd Int. Congr. Primat., Zürich, 1970,* 3:79–84. Basel, Switzerland: Karger

134. Rowell, T. E., Hinde, R. A. 1962. Vocal communication by the rhesus monkey (Macaca mulatta). *Proc. Zool. Soc. Lond.* 138:279–94

135. Saayman, G. S. 1971. Grooming behavior in a troop of free-ranging Chacma baboons (Papio ursinus). *Folia Primatol.* 16:161–71

136. Saayman, G. S. 1970. The menstrual cycle and sexual behavior in a troop of free ranging chacma baboons (Papio ursinus). *Folia Primatol.* 12:81–110

137. Sackett, G. P. 1966. Monkeys reared in isolation with pictures as visual input. *Science* 154:1468–72

138. Sassini, J., Taub, S., Weitzman, E. 1971. Abnormal behavior patterns produced in normal monkeys by L-Dopa. *Neurology* 21:403

139. Scheflen, A. E. 1964. The signifi-

cance of posture in communication systems. *J. Psychiat. Res.* 27:316–31

140. Schifter, H. 1968. Sicht und Markierungsverhalten von Wollaffen im Zoologischen Garten Zürich. *Zool. Gart. (Leipzig)* 36:107–36

141. Schön, M. A. 1971. The anatomy of the resonating mechanism in howling monkeys. *Folia Primatol.* 15:117–32

142. Schott, D. 1972. Quantitative Untersuchungen der Vokalisationen von Totenkopfaffen (Saimiri sciureus). PhD Thesis. Faculty of Sciences, Univ. Munich

143. Southwick, C. H. 1967. An experimental study of intragroup agonistic behavior in rhesus monkey (Macaca mulatta). *Behaviour* 28:182–209

144. Starck, D., Schneider, R. 1960. Respirationsorgane. A Larynx. In *Primatologia*, ed. H. Hofer, A. H. Schultz, D. Starck, 3: 423–587. Basel, Switzerland: Karger

145. Struhsaker, T. T. 1970. Phylogenetic implications of some vocalizations of Cercopithecus monkeys. In *Old World Monkeys*, ed. J. R. Napier, P. H. Napier, 365–444. New York: Academic. 660 pp.

146. Sugiyama, Y. 1969. Social behavior of chimpanzees in the Budongo Forest, Uganda. *Primates* 10:197–225

147. Sugiyama, Y. 1966. An artificial social change on a Hanuman Langur troop (Presbytis entellus). *Primates* 7:41–72

148. Suomi, S. J., Harlow, H. F., Lewis, J. K. 1970. Effect of bilateral frontal lobectomy on social preferences of rhesus monkeys. *J. Comp. Physiol. Psychol.* 70: 448–53

149. Takeda, R. 1965. Development of vocal communication in Man-raised Japanese monkeys. I. From birth until the sixth week. *Primates* 6:337–80

150. Thompson, C. I., Schwartzbaum, J. S., Harlow, H. F. 1969. Development of social fear after amygdalectomy in infant rhesus monkeys. *Physiol. Behav.* 4: 249–54

151. Udry, J. R., Morris, N. M. 1968. Distribution of coitus in the menstrual cycle. *Nature,* 220: 593–96

152. Vanderwolf, C. H. 1971. Limbic-diencephalic mechanisms of voluntary movement. *Psychol. Rev.* 78:83–113

153. Van Hooff, J. A. R. A. M. 1967. The facial displays of catarrhine monkeys and apes. See ref. 112, 9–88

154. Van Hooff, J. A. R. A. M. 1972. A comparative approach to the phylogeny of laughter and smiling. See ref. 60, 209–38

155. VanLawick-Goodall, J. 1968. A preliminary report on expressive movements and communication in the Gombe Stream Chimpanzees. See ref. 62, 313–74

156. Vessey, S. H. 1971. Free-ranging rhesus monkeys: behavioral effects of removal, separation and reintroduction of group members. *Behaviour* 40:216–27

157. Vine, I. 1970. Communication by facial-visual signals. In *Social Behaviour in Birds and Mammals*, ed. J. H. Crook, 279–354. London: Academic. 492 pp.

158. Vogel, C. 1971. Behavioral differences of Presbytis entellus in two different habitats. *Proc. 3rd Int. Congr. Primat., Zürich, 1970,* 3:41–47. Basel, Switzerland: Karger

159. Von Holst, D. 1969. Sozialer Stress bei Tupajas (Tupaia belangeri). Die Aktivierung des sympathischen Nervensystemes und ihre Beziehung zu hormonal ausgelösten ethologischen und physiologischen Veränderungen. *Z. Vergl. Physiol.* 63: 1–58

160. Walker, A. 1970. Nuchal adaptions in Perodicticus potto. *Primates* 11:135–44

161. Wickler, W. 1967. Socio-sexual signals and their intra-specific initiation among primates. See ref. 112, 89–189

162. Williams, L. 1968. Der Affe wie ihn keiner kennt. Vienna: Molden. 238 pp.

163. Winter, P. 1969. The variability of peep and twit calls in captive squirrel monkeys (Saimiri sciureus). *Folia Primatol.* 10: 204–15

164. Winter, P., Ploog, D., Latta, J.

1966. Vocal repertoire of the squirrel monkey (Saimiri sciureus). *Exp. Brain. Res.* 1:359–84

165. Wollberg, Z., Newman, J. D. 1972. Audtiory cortex of squirrel monkey: response patters of single cells to species-specific vocalizations. *Science* 175:212–14

166. Worden, F. G., Galambos, R., 1972. Auditory processing of biologically significant sounds. *Neurosci. Res. Program Bull.* 10:2–119

167. Yoshiba, K. 1968. Local and intertroop variability in ecology and social behavior of common Indian Langurs. See ref. 62, 217–42

168. Zumpe, D., Michael, R. P. 1970. Ovarian hormones and female sexual invitations in captive rhesus monkey (Macaca mulatta). *Anim. Behav.* 18:293–301

169. Zumpe, D., Michael, R. P. 1968. The clutching reaction and orgasm in the female rhesus monkey (Macaca mulatta). *J. Endocrinol.* 40:117–23

Ann. Rev. Physiol. 1973. 35:243–272

CNS: AFFERENT MECHANISMS WITH EMPHASIS ON 1096 PHYSIOLOGICAL AND BEHAVIORAL CORRELATIONS

JUHANI HYVÄRINEN[1]

Institute of Physiology, University of Helsinki, Finland

Although it has always been clear that the function of the brain is connected with behavior, it has not been possible to make direct observations on this connection until recently. Clinical and experimental knowledge based on lack of function in some parts of the nervous system has supplied neuroscientists with basic knowledge of the role that various structures play in behavior. However, the very question of the mechanisms by which external stimuli interact with nervous tissue to produce behavioral output or, vice versa, how behavior influences the action of the nervous tissue, has remained an enigma. The correlation between the function of afferent mechanisms of the CNS and behavior has in recent years been studied in separate physiological experiments on animals for comparison with psychophysical data from similar experiments on humans. In this way important evidence has been gained of the role of various receptors and sensory systems in sensation (e.g. 82, 83, 121).

In the past, it was possible to study the function of the CNS of behaving subjects with electroencephalographic techniques, but in recent years, with the application both of improved microphysiological techniques and of the behavioral training techniques of experimental psychology to neurophysiological experiments, new hopes have risen over clarification of the neural mechanisms involved in the control of behavior. Such studies have now been started on sensory mechanisms of the CNS—a field in which combined experiments with neurophysiological and behavioral observations previously were limited to observations of gross electrical phenomena.

The Editorial Committee has asked for a review on the afferent mechanisms with particular emphasis on simultaneous behavioral and neurophysiological observations of sensory phenomena. Through methodological advances it has become possible to study afferent mechanisms on the cellular level in unanesthetized behaving animals and humans (5, 26, 27, 31, 40, 41, 43, 46, 49, 57, 63, 67, 71, 72, 100, 102, 114). In contrast to experiments made

[1] Research Fellow of the Finnish National Research Council for Medical Sciences. This review was supported in part by a grant from the Foundations' Fund for Research in Psychiatry.

on anesthetized preparations, observations on unanesthetized animals have emphasized the importance of higher nervous mechanisms in sensory function. It is the aim of this review to introduce the reader to recent results of study of afferent mechanisms in behaving animals and to point out the potential significance of such studies for the understanding of brain function. Progress in this field is likely to be rapid in the future, but since most work in this area is now in an early phase this review is an introduction rather than a critical appraisal. Obviously, a specialist in a particular modality could present a more concise picture of one modality, but for the behavioral emphasis I shall briefly refer to all six modalities. A student of afferent mechanisms in one modality is likely to benefit from work in other modalities since the behavioral influences are then viewed in another framework facilitating extraction of common principles.

VISION

New important fields of vision research were reviewed by Rodieck (103) and McIlwain (78). An enjoyable lecture on color vision was recently published by Rushton (107).

Recent electrophysiological evidence from the laboratories in Canberra has clarified the connections of cells in visual pathways and has led to the following conclusions. Each relay cell in the lateral geniculate nucleus (*LGN*) receives its major excitatory retinal input via optic tract axons of one particular conduction velocity, and from each an axon of similar conduction velocity projects to the visual cortex (118). Moreover, the connections are specific with respect to adaptational properties of the cells (16) as well as to on- or off-center properties. Cat retinal ganglion cells may be subdivided into sustained and transient response types; this classification also applies to LGN cells. Sustained response type ganglion cells which have slower conduction velocities project to similar LGN cells; transient response type ganglion cells project to transient type LGN cells. On-center cells project to on-center cells and off-center cells to off-center cells. Thus the pathways carrying sustained and transient information remain essentially separate from the retina through the LGN to the striate cortex.

Moreover, studies on the conduction velocity of afferents to the visual cortex indicate that a large proportion of complex cells are activated monosynaptically from the optic radiation (47). Stimulation of slow afferents appeared to activate some of the simple and hypercomplex cells in the cat. This finding suggests that at least some of the simple, complex, and hypercomplex cells process visual information simultaneously in parallel and not sequentially in series as proposed originally by Hubel & Wiesel (50, 51).

The majority of cells in the dorsal LGN in fact have receptive fields in both eyes, although they have previously been considered monocular (109). In addition to the well known excitatory input from the dominant eye, cells in all layers of the dorsal LGN receive mostly weak inhibition from related receptive fields in the opposite retina. The inhibition from the nondominant eye may be postsynaptic (120). The same suggestion was given for surround inhibition in LGN (117).

Recently, cortical receptive fields were mapped in both cats and monkeys without anesthetics. Noda et al (87) used patterns of stripes projected onto a screen in front of awake cats. As in the anesthetized cat, diffuse illumination had little influence upon cortical neurons, but nearly all neurons responded to stimulation by some sort of visual contrast. Contrary to the result in anesthetized animals, responses to stationary stimuli did not adapt. The response could be maintained, however, by continuous small saccadic eye movements which are reduced or absent in anesthetized and paralyzed preparations. The cells in the visual cortex were also remarkably silent in the absence of patterned stimuli in waking cats. Normally when an alert animal (or human) is looking around, he sees patterns. In such a situation the activity of the visual cortical neurons apparently remains high, but it is greatly reduced when the eyes are closed or there is a uniform surface in front of the animal's gaze. The reduction of input to the visual cortex may then trigger the alpha rhythm (70).

In the awake cat, all cortical cells which responded either to moving stripes or to motionless gratings were under some influence from both eyes (88) but contralateral dominance was five times more frequent than ipsilateral.

In a series of papers on the visual cortical cells of behaving monkeys Wurtz (135–137) confirmed many of Hubel & Wiesel's findings on anesthetized monkeys (52). To be able to study the role of eye movements and stimulus movements, Wurtz trained monkeys to fix their eyes at a point on a tangent screen. The monkeys were rewarded with juice for responding to dimming of the light. Among 169 striate cortical units studied in detail, Wurtz found 13% with circular receptive fields, 60% with simple fields, 13% with more complex fields, and 14% with unclassified line shaped fields. In the anethetized monkey's striate cortex Hubel & Wiesel found the majority of cells (60%) to be complex. The complete mapping of the receptive field properties requires good cooperation between the unanesthetized monkey and the experimenter. In anesthetized and paralyzed animals, eye movements do not interfere with receptive field mapping and more time can be used per cell. Thus the difference in the proportions of simple to complex cells between anesthetized and awake monkey striate cortex may reflect these differences.

In the awake monkey as in the awake cat, nonadaptive responses to stationary stimuli are common (135). Wurtz discusses the possible role of small oscillating eye movements in shifting the stimulus in and out of the receptive field and thus maintaining the responses. When the images are stabilized on the human retina clear vision of an object fades within several seconds. Conceivably, maintenance of cortical responses by small eye movements may be necessary for maintained vision.

Other cells apparently are activated only by rapidly moving stimuli. Such cells adapt rapidly to stationary stimuli and many are selective to the direction of stimulus movement.

In studying the role of eye movements in cortical responses, Wurtz found that a neuron giving an excitatory response to stationary stimuli could during rapid eye movements give an excitatory response or no response or be suppressed. However, these cortical neurons did not respond when the eye movement was performed across a white homogeneous field, but required a patterned input. During the eye movements it appeared that the neurons did not discriminate differences in stimulus form with precision equal to that for stimuli presented when the eye was stationary. During eye movements the most vigorous responses were given by neurons with circular or simple receptive fields. This finding may relate to the psychophysical observations on man that a stimulus may be detected with decreased resolution of detail during a rapid eye movement. Those neurons that reversed their excitatory response to suppression during eye movement might provide some indication of the occurrence of rapid eye movements. When these responses are compared with responses of the same neurons to object movement over the receptive field with similar angular velocity, all neurons respond as they do during eye movements. Thus for the cortical neurons the response appears the same for stimulus movement as for eye movement. Wurtz concluded that since there is no difference between these two movement responses there is no evidence for a corollary discharge to any station of the afferent pathway or to the levels of the striate cortex.

It is an interesting possibility that the shape of receptive fields could vary when alteration in the weight of different synaptic inputs occurs (48). Bear et al (7) mapped quantitatively the contours of the receptive fields of neurons in the cat's striate cortex. Whereas the concentric receptive fields in LGN were stable under all anesthesia and EEG conditions, many visual cortex receptive fields were unstable in the presence of low voltage fast EEG activity and became stabilized under barbiturate anesthesia.

Dynamic changes in the visual receptive fields in a few neurons were observed in the human striate cortex during surgery for epilepsy (76). When an attentive subject focused at a screen which was then moved further away from him the angular receptive field size and position changed. It was suggested that the dynamic changes in the receptive fields that accompany changes in viewing distance could relate to the psychological phenomenon of perceived size constancy of objects of similar size at different distances from the observer. For elucidation of this possibility more systematic observations on unanesthetized trained animals would be needed.

Studies on further processing of visual information in the cat have dealt with the Clare-Bishop area and the middle suprasylvian gyrus. In the lateral suprasylvian gyrus (Clare-Bishop area) the neurons are reminiscent of those in areas 7, 18 and 19 (53). The receptive fields are larger than, but otherwise not different from, the complex and lower order hypercomplex cells in occipital areas. This area is topographically arranged and cells with common receptive field orientation are grouped together. Contralateral eye dominance is more common but is found mainly in cells with peripheral fields. In the anterior portion of the middle suprasylvian gyrus (22), neurons are sensitive to stimulus movement and to direction of stimulus movement and less sensitive to stimulus orientation. These responses are relayed through visual cortices in both hemispheres. Cells in this area might, by virtue of these properties, participate in the regulation of eye and head movements.

Several microphysiological studies have concentrated on visually activated regions in the primate temporal lobe. A histologically distinct, topographically organized visual area was found adjacent and rostral to area 19 in the middle temporal gyrus of the owl monkey (2). In the superior temporal sulcus of the rhesus monkey, cells are sensitive to visual movement, and most respond best to stimulus movements in a particular direction. This area appears arranged in columns for receptive field location and preferred direction of stimulus movement. Some properties of these neurons resemble those of cells in the superior colliculus and pulvinar (23, 140). In the temporal cortex, visually responsive cells have large receptive fields which always include the foveal region. Colored stimuli and black silhouettes are important for activation of units, some of which show very complex properties, e.g. responding optimally to the silhouette of the monkey hand when the fingers point upward in the same way as they would if the monkey inspected his own hand. The projection to this area could in part be from the pulvinar where receptive fields also cover the fovea (39). In the pulvinar, movement sensitive units react better to bars and edges than to punctate stimuli (134). These units probably function in the detection of changes in the velocity or direction of moving stimuli. Eye movements in darkness also activated cells in the LGN (58).

Important work on afferent mechanisms and eye movement control has recently been done on the cells in the superior colliculus. Wurtz & Goldberg (138) recorded single neuron responses from the superior colliculi of monkeys trained to move their eyes. They found visual receptive fields for neurons in the upper layers of the colliculus. In the deeper layers several cells were related to eye movements and discharged 100–150 msec before an eye movement in a particular direction. These cells had no visual receptive fields and discharged before saccades in darkness as well as in light, but poorly so with slow pursuit movements.

In another series of papers Wurtz & Goldberg (33a, 33b, 138a, 138b) indicated that, in addition to the visually activated cells in upper layers and the movement related cells in intermediate layers of the colliculus, there exist two transitional cell types. One of these discharges independently either in response to a visual stimulus or before an eye movement; the other cell type shows an enhancement of its response to a visual stimulus when the monkey attends to that stimulus prior to making a saccade toward it. By making lesions with the recording microelectrode, these authors demonstrated a considerable increase in the latency for a saccade to a spot of light which fell in the area

where the destroyed cells had their receptive fields. No deficit in the accuracy
of the saccades was noted, however. On the basis of these experiments the
authors suggested that the superior colliculus participates in the shifting of
attention and gaze toward a visual target, but it only does so by speeding up
the proper eye movements to roughly the region of the target. The fine eye
movements involved in the pursuit and foveation mechanisms would be a
function of other circuits. This interpretation of the role of the superior colliculus is different from that of Schiller & Koerner (110), although much of
the data of the two groups are similar.

Schiller & Koerner (110) mapped the receptive fields of superior colliculus neurons through one immobilized eye and studied the relation of cellular
discharges to the movements of the other eye. As the example shown in Figure
1 indicates, the discharge of neurons in the deeper layers of the superior colliculus was specific in terms of both the direction and the size of eye movements. The discharge was, however, independent of the initial position of the
eye in the orbit. Such a neuron typically had a receptive field in that area of
the visual field toward which the fovea was directed as a result of a saccade
associated with a discharge in that neuron. Cells with receptive fields very
close to the center of the fovea discharged both prior to small saccades and
during smooth pursuit. The discharge of these neurons preceded a saccade
which moved the fovea toward the object on the receptive field. Thus these
neurons appear to participate in the correction of retinal target errors during
tracking by producing a discharge when the gaze is moving away from a target. This discharge then serves to bring the target back on the receptive field.

Although it may sound optimistic, on the basis of the considerable amount
of new knowledge on higher visual mechanisms the stage now appears set for
rapid advancement in the elucidation of the neural mechanisms that relate
vision to behavior. One may assume that in the coming years microphysiological work on unanesthetized animals will broaden our understanding of
the dynamic control mechanisms involved in visual orientation and the role
of sensory input in gross electrical activity, sleep mechanisms, and attention.
The forthcoming literature in this field should be exciting.

OLFACTION AND TASTE

Much of the earlier work on olfaction was performed with pure chemical
or electrical stimuli which are not in the realm of everyday experience. Conceivably, use of chemically more complex but behaviorally significant natural
odorous stimuli could lead to an increased understanding of the afferent mechanisms of olfaction (21). A promising example is given by Macrides &
Chorover (73) who demonstrated, in the male deermouse olfactory bulb,
cellular responses to the scent of an estrous female, and, in the hamster pup,
differences in responses to its own litter bedding compared with unfamiliar
litter bedding.

The connections of the olfactory afferents with the limbic system are well

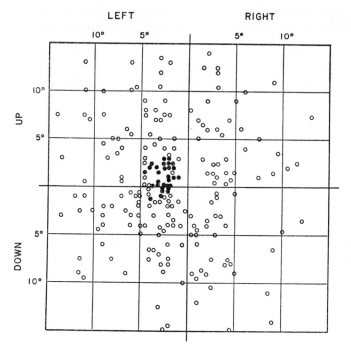

FIGURE 1. Saccades associated with unit response in a superior colliculus cell. Each mark represents the size and direction of a saccade from any initial position (the zero crossing). Direction and size of saccade is shown in degrees within quadrants designated left, right, up, and down. Solid discs show saccades which were preceded by unit activity whereas open circles represent saccades not associated with unit activity. When the visual receptive fields of such units were mapped through the other eye they would cover the same region as the black discs. Reproduced from (110) through the courtesy of P. H. Schiller and with the permission of the American Physiological Society.

established. In the awake squirrel monkey MacLean et al (139) used electrical stimulation of the olfactory bulb and the septum to study cellular responses in the hippocampus. Cells in the hippocampus did not discharge propagating action potentials in response to electrical stimulation of the olfactory bulb although they did respond so to electrical stimulation of the septum. Hippocampal cells responded only with local synaptic EPSPs to olfactory bulb stimulation. This study demonstrated the importance of synaptic convergence for the olfactory activation of the limbic neurons. One converging synaptic system is derived from the internal connections of the limbic system related to emotional behavior, hunger, sex, etc. The afferent sensory system, which transmits responses evoked by external stimuli impinging on the receptors, also converges. Probably only a proper combination of the two inputs can lead to propagating activity in the limbic system and thus to the behavioral consequences.

In another study (3) the same group could find no significant alteration of cellular activity in the rostral cingulate cortex evoked by behaviorally non-significant photic, auditory, and somatic stimulation, although neuronal and slow wave responses to stimulation of the vagus nerve were recorded. Considering the large amount of work needed for proper study of cells in awake, behaving animals, it would seem desirable that the remarkable series of experiments on the olfactory and limbic systems of awake squirrel monkeys (3, 119, 139) be directed to the study of neuronal responses to behaviorally meaningful changes in the environment. During evolutionary development, the synaptic connections in the monkey's limbic system have not developed to respond to artificially generated stimuli of electrical, photic, or auditory nature. Recordings of neuronal responses to behaviorally significant odorous stimuli (73) or to stimuli related to orientation in the environment (92) might well increase far more our understanding of the functional role of activity in various parts of the limbic system.

Few significant works on the taste pathways have been published during this review period. A new discovery was the combined anatomical and physiological demonstration of an afferent taste pathway to pontine parabrachial nuclei (91); the further projection is to the contralateral thalamus (30, 90, 91) and lateral frontal lobe (30). In the awake squirrel monkey, gustatory responses have been recorded in a few neurons in the frontal operculum where units also responded to mechanical stimulation of the oral cavity (119). In spite of these investigations the function of the cortex in taste remains to be demonstrated. Norgren's studies (89, 90), which attempt to correlate the neuronal activity in the hypothalamus with various gustatory stimuli in the awake rat, appear promising for behavioral analysis. Responses to sweet and bitter stimuli were spatially separated and, moreover, the regions responding to the sweet taste of sucrose maintained selfstimulation more often than other areas. In the future a systematic study of the connections of the taste afferents to the hypothalamic eating, drinking, and reward areas could be highly significant for the clarification of the basic mechanisms of emotional behavior.

VESTIBULAR SYSTEM

In the moving animal the vestibular input is used in reflex motor coordination to provide the sensory basis for compensatory muscle movements that keep the head position stable. This system is so intricately bound with kinesthetic afferents and motor control that its role as a sensory system is often less obvious. In the same way that the vestibular input aids motor control in the moving animal it also supports the function of the visual, auditory, and somesthetic systems in keeping the perceptual world stable in spite of continuous changes in the positions of the receptors. For the behavioral significance of the afferent mechanisms, studies of the higher order mechanisms of vestibular function appear to have more explanatory value than do those on the peripheral first and second order vestibular afferent neurons (29, 32, 33, 79, 80), although such studies, of course, are important in their own right for understanding of the function of the semicircular canals.

The cortical projection of the vestibular system was established as a distinct cytoarchitectural area next to, but outside, the face region in Brodmann's area 2 in the rhesus monkey (112). In this area single neurons respond to both vestibular and proprioceptive somatosensory stimuli. Moreover, the vestibular cortex differs from other modality-pure primary receiving areas, for within it neurons appear to integrate information from the semicircular canals with that from joints or muscles. Two types of neurons are found in this area: those responding to vestibular stimulation and joint rotation, and those responding to vestibular and muscle stimuli. The best activation was often observed in response to a specific combination of head and joint positions. This area would thus appear to be of behavioral significance for the position sense of different body parts in the field of gravity.

Some years ago, Wiersma, studying the visually activated nerve fibers of crayfish, found neurons that changed their visual receptive fields on the retina with rotation of the animal's body (132e). He showed that the receptors in the statocyst exercise an inhibitory effect on these "space-constant" fibers, blocking selectively excitation in that part of the visual receptive field which remains below the horizontal plane when the animal is rotated around its body axis.

More recently, observations of similar dynamic changes in visual receptive fields have been reported in the cat (33, 48, 61a). Jung (61a) first described experiments by Denney & Adorjani (19) for determining the orientation of longitudinal receptive fields of visual cortex neurons in the cat as a function of head tilt. Horn & Hill (48) found that during body tilt the retinal receptive fields of some visual cortex cells changed their orientation so that the optimal orientation of visual stimuli, projected on a tangent screen in front of the animal, remained roughly the same as before the tilt. This finding suggests that the vestibular influence selectively modifies the afferent synaptic input to the visual cortex. In a sample of 33 thoroughly studied visual cortex cells Denney & Adorjani (19) found several neurons that exhibited a compensatory change in the orientation of the retinal receptive fields after head tilt. There were many cells, however, which did not show this property, and some cells even changed the orientation of their receptive fields toward the same direction with the head tilt, resulting in a change that overshot the amount of head tilt.

The possibility that the psychological phenomena of constancy of orientation of visually perceived lines with head tilt could be explained by vestibular synaptic mechanisms appears attractive. However, more systematic studies on this convergent interaction are needed to determine its frequency in a population of cortical neurons and to shed light on the synaptic mechanism responsible for the receptive field change.

The above studies indicate that vestibular influences are integrated with visual and kinesthetic information without reaching a specific cortical projection site. Vestibular influences may also be shown in the future to be important in auditory localization mechanisms which compensate for changes in ear position.

AUDITION

When the behavioral significance of the work is assessed, the advances made during this review period in the study of the auditory system do not seem very significant. However, preliminary reports from several laboratories give the impression that this may be a tranquil moment that precedes new, potentially promising experiments on the auditory system of alert behaving animals. The following notes should be taken as a preview to the kinds of investigations that will be appearing in the coming years.

Miller et al (81a) made several interesting observations on the activity of auditory cortical neurons of the monkey as a function of the behavior of the animal. With positive reinforcement, rhesus monkeys were trained to release a response key rapidly at the onset of an acoustic stimulus. During the performance of this simple reaction time task approximately 150 single cells were examined in seven unanesthetized monkeys. The firing frequency of most cells studied was much higher during the performance of the task than when the animal received the same acoustic stimulus while not performing the task. In animals not trained in the task it was difficult to consistently activate cortical cells with repetitive clicks, noise bursts, or tonal stimulation. In these animals most cells exhibited a maintained responsiveness only to nonrepetitive acoustic stimulation, with the probability of response quickly decreasing during the first four to ten stimulus presentations. No similar decrease in response probability was observed in cells studied in monkeys trained to perform in the reaction time task. In trained animals the cellular responses to repetitive stimulation were also consistent during the nonperforming condition, and did not show the variability seen in untrained animals. Such stability of responses appeared as a long term effect of training. It will take more experiments to clarify the mechanism by which such effects are brought about, but it is significant that cellular responses in the auditory cortex show behavior that parallels the animal's attention and training.

Another interesting observation was reported by Morrell (81b) who studied the auditory input to cells in the visual cortex. In paralyzed, unanesthetized cats in all visual cortex cells activated by auditory stimuli (70 cells of 169 studied), the determining factor for auditory responsiveness was the location of the sound source. In the experiments the loudspeaker that delivered the acoustical stimuli was mounted behind a cheese cloth tangent screen used for mapping of the visual receptive fields. Such an arrangement revealed that the responses to acoustic stimulation were elicited from the same location where the visual receptive fields were. Whereas the visual receptive fields were sharply limited in all directions the auditory fields were limited only in the horizontal direction subtending large vertical angels. This finding emphasizes the importance of interaural delays and intensity differences as a basis for the localization mechanism. Moreover, the auditory responses were independent of the type of sound used as a stimulus. When the loudspeaker was optimally placed, cell discharge was obtained equally well with clicks, pure tone pulses, and noise bursts. Morrell proposed that a spatial organization of acoustic receptive fields in the visual cortex cells might serve to alert the visual system of an event occurring at a particular distance from the fovea and thus allow the oculomotor system to bring the area into direct foveal alignment. In an unrestrained, behaving animal it would be interesting to know what happens to the auditory receptive fields of visual cortex neurons when the eyes move but the head remains stable. If the acoustic receptive fields remain in the same position in relation to the animal's head when the visual receptive fields move, then the arrangement of the auditory receptive fields is in the auditory space rather than in the visual space.

In a study on the cat superior colliculus Wickelgren (132d) has emphasized the importance of spatial interactions between auditory and visual effective stimuli. In paralyzed unanesthetized cats, 57 cells of 98 studied in the deeper layers of the superior colliculus responded both to acoustic and to visual stimuli. Acoustically responsive cells responded well to complex sounds; the hissing sound of an air hose was particularly effective. Most cells responded only to moving visual and auditory stimuli and were directionally selective for both modalities. For both modalities the horizontal component of the preferred direction was always toward the periphery of the contralateral side. Wickelgren suggested that such direction selective units might function in the superior colliculus to provide information that enables the animal to track visually a moving stimulus regardless of the modality with which that stimulus first impinges upon the animal.

These examples emphasize the importance of the spatial localization functions of the auditory system (131). On the neuronal level, Brugge et al (12) showed marked differences in the discharge rates of some auditory cortex cells in the cat when interaural time and intensity of stimuli were varied; this has subsequently been confirmed (6). A thorough review of the sound source localization mechanisms was recently published (25).

Less clear are the attempts to find correlations between the complexity of the stimulus sound and responses of auditory cortical cells (1). In the awake squirrel monkey cingulate cortex (119) and auditory cortex (113) some cells have been found that respond to species specific vocalizations. In such experiments, however, it is important to prove for each cell studied that the responses to complex stimuli are not a simple product of continuous excitation arising when the complex sound sweeps irregularly back and forth across the response area of a narrowly tuned neuron.

Another important aspect of the function of the auditory system is the role of the efferent system. Nieder & Nieder (84–86) showed that crossed olivocochlear bundle stimulation enhanced gross neural responses from the cochlea for clicks presented in the presence of noise. They suggested that the response of low threshold afferents is blocked by crossed efferent stimulation making them available for response to higher level stimulation. Several different kinds of experiments have suggested the existence of inhibitory mechanisms in the cochlea and some of these are likely to be associated with the functions of the crossed olivocochlear bundle. For instance Rose et al (104) suggested a sensitivity control mechanism in the cochlea because they showed that an auditory nerve fiber remains sensitive to the waveform of the stimulus when the stimulus exceeds the sound pressure level which elicits a saturation discharge rate. In a round table discussion on auditory physiology the role of the efferent system remained quite open (17); studies on unanesthetized animals with chronic recording methods would conceivably be useful in the clarification of the function of the efferent system, since its function may be partially blocked in anesthetized preparations. That there are differences between alert and anethetized cats in the function of lower auditory conters was shown by Bock et al (9), who demonstrated in the inferior colliculus of alert cats much broader response areas (up to four to six octaves) than are seen in anethetized animals.

In conclusion, some interesting new observations have been made on the auditory system. The important areas where advances will be made in the near future appear to be the higher mechanisms for spatial localization of sound and for the analysis of complex sounds, the function of the efferent system, and mechanisms related to attention.

SOMESTHESIA

Muscle afferents.—In the cat the projection of muscle spindle afferents to the cerebral cortex has been shown to go through the medullary nucleus Z (69). This nucleus, located in the cat medulla just rostrally to the gracile nucleus close to the lateral recess of fourth ventricle, was previously considered a subnucleus in the vestibular complex. In chloralose anesthetized cats, Landgren & Silfvenius showed that the afferents to nucleus Z from muscle spindles travel in the dorsolateral fascicle of the spinal cord. The spinal course of the group I muscle afferents from the hind limb appears identical to that of the dorsal spinocerebellar tract. This projection is illustrated in Figure 2, as sketched by Silfvenius (115). From nucleus Z the path crosses over to fourth order cells in the VPL of the contralateral thalamus. The latencies of thalamic focal potentials suggest monosynaptic activation of VPL cells by group I hind limb medullothalamic fibers (68). In parallel anatomical work it was shown that degenerating axons from nucleus Z pass ventromedially in the medial lemniscus and terminate rostrally in the dorsolateral portions of the VPL and the nucleus ventralis lateralis (*VL*) (10). Cerebellectomy does not influence these thalamic potentials (115). Cortical neurons that respond to volleys in

CEREBRAL CORTEX

MEDIAL   DORSAL

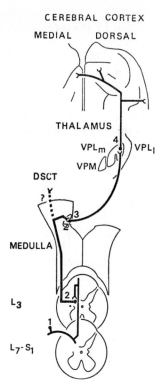

FIGURE 2. Diagram of the ascending pathway from group I muscle afferents of cat's hind limb as sketched by Silfvenius (115). The projection is indicated passing through the dorsal columns, dorsolateral fascicle, medullary nucleus Z to the contralateral VPL and the cortical projection zones. Reproduced with the permission of the author and the publisher, the Medical Faculty of Umeå University.

muscle nerves, located around the postcruciate dimple (106) and in the anterior suprasylvian sulcus in perinsular area 2 (116), are also excited by low threshold cutaneous afferents.

In the monkey, the study of the muscle projection to the cortex has further emphasized the functional significance of cytoarchitectural subdivisions of sensory areas. In that species Powell & Mountcastle (101) first indicated that the region between the postcentral koniocortex and the precentral agranular cortex (area 3a) receives a heavy projection from deep tissues. Recently Phillips, Powell & Wiesendanger (97) studied this projection in detail in the arm area of the lightly anesthetized baboon. Evoked responses to volleys in the deep radial nerve of the deep palmar branch of the ulnar nerve were clustered in area 3a, where 143 cells were studied which responded to electrical stimulation of low threshold muscle afferents. Although areas 1, 3b, and 4 were also frequently penetrated by microelectrodes, muscle responses were not seen. Lesions in the dorsolateral funiculus at C 3–4 did not change the responses but lesions in the dorsal columns completely abolished the cortical responses in area 3a. Thus it appears that the dorsolateral fascicle carries the muscle information in the cat (69), but in the monkey the dorsal columns mediate these impulses.

None of the neurons of area 3a could be identified as a corticospinal neuron. The authors also noted that strong microstimulation in area 3a through the recording electrode failed to evoke responses at another microelectrode in area 4 used for microstimulation of a low threshold hand muscle site in area 4. Thus, any functional linkage between areas 3a and 4 would appear to be complex. Evarts (28) showed that in monkeys rewarded for making learned displacement of the wrist, the outputs of motor cortex neurons and of muscle force are increased if the displacement is resisted by an external load. If the brain recruits α- and γ-motoneurons together [Granit's "alpha-gamma linkage" (37)], resisting the movement should cause increased signalling from the muscle spindles. This would lead to increased input from the primary endings and, on a reflex basis, to increased motoneuron firing and muscle force. The simplest afferent limb would be provided by a three-neuron pathway from the spindles to the pyramidal neurons. As a result of this work this hypothesis was rejected. The reasons for rejecting the three-neuron ascending path to motor cortex pyramidal cells was that no unitary spikes or focal potentials were seen in area 4 in response to muscle nerve stimulation although such stimuli readily activated cells in the adjacent Brodmann's area 3a. An alternative solution suggested by the authors is that an excitatory signal for increased force output is computed in the cerebellum or elsewhere when the wrist is held in the proper position against an increased resistance. Konorski & Tarnecki (66, 124) have shown that cerebellar Purkinje cells fire for certain joint positions.

More direct tests of the afferent link of a transcortical control loop can now be made in conscious humans with percutaneous microelectrode recording. Vallbo (125) studied 63 muscle spindle afferents in conscious healthy humans by manually introducing a tungsten microelectrode into the median nerve and searching for clearly localized slowly adapting receptors in deep structures. When such receptors were found, the subject was asked to make voluntary isometric contractions of hand or finger muscles. Previous work in anesthetized baboons (64) indicated that electrical stimulation of motor cortex may either increase or decrease fusimotor activity. Vallbo found that the majority of muscle spindle afferents did respond with a sustained increase of the discharge during voluntary contraction. However, such a response was only seen when a contraction of sufficient intensity was produced in that particular part of the muscle where the spindle was located. If this condition was not met, many fibers failed to show increased discharge during voluntary contraction. Considering the unloading effect of the contraction, increased muscle spindle activity is strong evidence for fusimotor activity. This result is consonant with the notion that alpha-gamma linkage is a pronounced feature in voluntary motor acts.

In anesthetized and decerebrate animals an increase in the fusimotor activity often precedes the skeletomotor activity [for references see (38)]; this suggests that the fusimotor system controls the contraction through the spindle reflex arc. Studying the time relation between the onset of skeletomotor activity and the onset of acceleration in 31 single muscle spindle afferents during voluntary contraction, Vallbo (126) found that the spindle acceleration regularly started after the onset of the skeletomotor contraction as revealed by electromyography. The α- and γ-motoneurones of the same muscle are known to be located close to each other in the ventral horns (13) and can be simultaneously activated from supraspinal structures. The latency between skeletomotor contraction and spindle acceleration was 10–50 msec and often more (126). This latency was of the same order of magnitude as the difference in conduction times from the spinal cord to the recording points. Thus, the outflow from the spinal cord is synchronously initiated in the fusimotor and skeletomotor neurones. This anatomical and functional alpha-gamma linkage would thus not serve as a servo loop in the initiation of movement. Voluntary contractions were, however, initiated without the support of an increased spindle afferent discharge. Findings were the same for both slow and fast contractions. Vallbo concluded that the initiation of the skeletomotor contraction is not the result of the reflex action of the spindle afferents on the alpha-motoneurons, as would be the case if the muscle activity were totally controlled by the length servo principle. Nor is the function of the fusimotor system to provide preparatory adjustment of the strength of the skeletomotor contraction.

On the basis of psychophysical observations, Goodwin et al (34–36) reiterated the classical view that muscle receptors contribute to kinesthesia together with joint receptors. When they vibrated a subject's muscle tendon he had the illusion that the corresponding joint had moved, just as if the muscle had been stretched. When a blindfolded subject's biceps tendon was vibrated the subject made large systematic errors in indicating with his other arm the perceived position of the vibrated arm. Local anesthesia, by ringblock, of the index finger produced a total anesthesia of that finger but the innervation of the muscles moving the finger was preserved intact. Awareness of passive movements persisted in both finger joints when the movements were rapid. Discrimination of various movements was easier with tensed than relaxed muscles. Even with anoxic anesthesia of the whole hand the kinesthesia was preserved. After this procedure the subject did not feel lateral movements of the finger joints but could still discriminate extension and flexion mediated by the long muscles of the forearm. These findings indicate a kinesthetic role for the muscle receptors together with the joint receptors.

Pain.—After combined shock-escape and food-reward training in the monkey (128), lesions of the contralateral column elevated pain thresholds, as expected. However, ipsilateral dorsal column lesions decreased the somatic motor response to pain as revealed by higher latencies and lower forces of escape responses. Moreover, ipsilateral lesions in the dorsolateral column produced hyperesthesia, i.e. reduced escape latencies, and increased escape forces without affecting thresholds. These results suggest that the pain information carried in the lateral columns is sharpened by the dorsal columns and attenuated by the dorsolateral columns.

In the bulbar reticular formation of the awake cat, cells respond with increasing discharge when electrical stimulation of a cutaneous nerve is elevated to levels that elicit escape behavior. These neurons discharge vigorously in response to noxious somatic stimuli and are not activated by other modalities. That these units participate in pain mechanisms is suggested by the fact that cats respond with escape behavior to electrical microstimulation through the recording electrode (14). Neurons in the ventral reticular nucleus of the rat's medulla are responsive to nociceptive stimulation with excitation or inhibition (8). Mayer et al (77) abolished responsiveness to intense pain in rats by electrical stimulation of several mesencephalic and diencephalic sites that also supported self-stimulation. The peripheral field of analgesia was usually restricted to one body half or quadrant.

Although we know very little of the function of the pain system, surgical lesions aimed at relieving intractable pain are often successful. Elucidation of the function of pain receptors, pain pathways, and central mechanisms of pain and analgesia continues to be one of the major challenges for workers in the somesthetic system.

Temperature.—Kenshalo & Brearley (11, 62) tested the behavioral and electrophysiological sensitivity of the cat's upper lip to warm and cool stimuli. With avoidance conditioning, warm thresholds as small as 1°C and cool thresholds of 5°C were obtained. Warm thresholds increased when the background skin temperature was low and cool thresholds increased when the background skin temperature was high, with the turning point at 33°C. In electrophysiological experiments, similar stimuli were applied and integrated activity in few-fiber preparations of the infraorbital nerve was measured. Transient cooling resulted in increased activity and transient warming in decreased activity.

In a way the results of these electrophysiological experiments appear paradoxical. Whereas cold thresholds increase at high adapting temperatures, the electrophysiological responses to equal transient cold stimuli also increase at high adapting temperatures. One would think that with increasing responsiveness the thresholds would decrease. However, it has been demonstrated by Iggo (54a) that in integrated recordings from several fibers in mixed nerves the dominating results can be derived from mechanoreceptors activated by thermal stimuli instead of from thermoreceptors. Because the mechanoreceptor fibers are larger in diameter and have faster response rates than the thermoreceptive afferents, their activity can mask entirely the activity of the latter. Therefore, the results of Kenshalo & Brearley (62) on few-fiber preparations can be considered equivocal until the results have been confirmed with single fiber recordings.

In the behaving animal, thermal receptors are bound up with both thermal sensations and thermoregulation. In the study of thermal afferents the possibility of centrifugal control of sensitivity through efferent sympathetic nerves has been largely ignored. Probably for all the functions of the anterolateral system—temperature, pain, itch, and tickle—the centrifugal control is important, and for the clarification of the function of the anterolateral system, recordings of the efferent discharges should also be made. Preliminary observations of Hagbarth et al (40) in conscious human subjects with percutaneously inserted microelectrodes indicate that the efferent sympathetic activity provoked by cooling is correlated with the temperature change. This technique might be valuable in the study of the anterolateral system.

Darian-Smith & Dykes (18) studied the cold sensitive delta-afferents in the monkey hand and made psychophysical experiments with similar stimuli on humans. Upon transient cooling from a fixed background temperature, the subjective magnitude estimations were linearly related to temperature change and so were the numbers of impulses per response (or per time unit) in afferent fibers. Such a close correlation between the response magnitude in peripheral fibers of the monkey and the human perception of sensory magnitude suggests that humans perceive cold by a similar set of cold receptors.

Warm-response C fibers have also been described in the primate by Hensel & Iggo (45). One of the current central questions in the perception of warmth, to be clarified with combined psychophysical and neurophysiological experiments, is the roles that the myelinated A-delta cold fibers play as compared with those of the nonmyelinated warm-sensitive C fibers.

Pressure sense.—An interesting cutaneous receptor is the touch corpuscle or the Haarscheibe of Pinkus. This receptor, also called type I slowly adapting cutaneous afferent or tactile pad receptor, is capable of well graded responses to cutaneous pressure (55, 130). However, Pinkus, in his original description (98), pointed out that these receptors in human skin do not give rise to any conspicuous sensation. This negative finding was recently confirmed by Harrington & Merzenich (42), who could not arouse any definite sensation by punctate stimuli delivered under microscopic observation onto these domes in the upper arm of human observers. Such responses were readily appreciated when delivered to adjacent areas of skin.

Petit & Burgess (96) showed with antidromic cervical dorsal column stimulation that these tactile pad receptors do not project into the dorsal columns in the cat. On the other hand, with microelectrode recording Whitsel et al (132a, 132b) demonstrated that fibers are resorted in the squirrel monkey dorsal columns so that at the cervical level only skin fibers are seen in the fasciculus gracilis. Mann et al (75) provided evidence that the tactile pad input is relayed in the dorsal spinocerebellar tract and possibly in the spinocervical tract. Cortical evoked responses can be recorded in response to stimuli confined to these receptors (56, 74); when conditioned to respond to stimuli applied to single receptors pads, cats displayed greater sensitivity on these spots than on adjacent skin (122). Because of these species differences, the role of the tactile pad receptor currently remains obscure.

Harrington & Merzenich concluded that the human pressure receptors in hairy skin are the type II slowly adapting receptors identified histologically in the cat by Chambers & Iggo (15). These receptors in the monkey are sensitive to skin stretch and react to degrees of indentation or elevation of the skin with a remarkable correspondence to the human stimulus response relation in pressure sense as studied in the classical psychophysical experiments of von Frey.

In studies on the mechanoreceptive afferents in human glabrous skin, receptors have been described which are similar to those described in monkeys (41, 63). However, it has been claimed that there is a greater number of slowly adapting fibers in humans than in monkeys (63) but a study with more material and similar stimuli in both species should be performed to confirm this difference.

Skin vibration.—In a comparative study on vibratory sensibility in monkeys and humans, Mountcastle et al (82) established sensory detection thresholds and reaction times to cutaneous vibration at various frequencies with careful psychophysical techniques. The monkey thresholds, measured at the 50% correct detection level of psychometric functions, appeared very similar to human thresholds when measured on the glabrous skin of hands and fingers in both species. In both species sine wave amplitude thresholds were high at low frequencies, with the lowest threshold at 200–250 Hz. At this best frequency humans are probably slightly more sensitive than monkeys. Interestingly enough, reaction times were also identical for the two species in a vibration detection task. At threshold they were 400–500 msec and at higher stimulus amplitudes they dropped asymptotically to 300–350 msec. Thus it can be inferred that not only are the properties of vibration sensitive receptors identical in humans and monkeys, but also the cerebral decision making process works with identical speed in both species.

Having established the monkey vibration thresholds, Mountcastle et al recorded from primary afferents for an accurate comparison of receptor function with psychophysical thresholds in the monkey. The results confirm previous results based on a cross-species assumption (121). At low frequency vibration, cutaneous afferents are recruited at amplitudes comparable with psychophysical thresholds, and at high frequency the thresholds of the subcutaneous Pacinian corpuscles correspond to the monkey psychophysical thresholds.

Slowly adapting receptors have not been considered as important in vibratory sensibility (81, 121). However, with suitable stimulus arrangement even they may produce periodically tuned responses to vibration as was shown by Tapper et al (123). The tactile pad receptors reviewed above were studied with a vibrating bimorph without surface displacement, and one-to-one frequency following was observed up to 400 Hz. However, the thresholds for one-to-one firing at 400 Hz were quite high. The authors suggest that these pad receptors are uniquely suitable for detection of mites and parasites walking with minimal displacement on the skin.

In magnitude estimation tasks on skin vibration, a close to linear relationship is found between vibration amplitude and perceived intensity (81, 121, 127). Yet, contrary to other modalities so investigated, the number of impulses per unit time evoked by vibrating stimuli is not a function of stimulus amplitude in single primary afferent fibers (121). Due to the one-to-one tuning to stimulus sine wave, the number of impulses per second replicates the stimulus frequency and not its amplitude. Increasing vibration amplitudes recruit fibers with receptive fields further away from the vibrating point on skin by virtue of the surface waves spreading from the stimulus site. At the stimulus site, individual afferent fibers increase their responses from no activity to one-to-one following and with higher amplitudes sometimes to two-to-one and rarely to three-to-one firing. On the other hand the thresholds of all fibers are not identical and fibers with higher thresholds are successively recruited by increasing stimulus amplitude. Johnson (59) measured the one-to-one thresholds of a representative sample of afferent fibers and found that these are log-normally distributed with stimulus amplitude and that the amplitude of skin vibration is attenuated in proportion to the square of distance from the stimulus site. From these facts Johnson computed the numbers of fibers recruited by various amplitudes of sine wave and also the total number of impulses fired by all active afferent fibers per unit time in response to a vibratory stimulus. His findings indicated that both the number of fibers recruited and the total number of impulses fired by those afferents are linearly related to the stimulus amplitude. From these results it is not possible to conclude which of these two forms of code is the one for stimulus magnitude in vibration. Both explain well the psychophysically established linear relationship between vibration amplitude and subjective magnitude. It is important in this connection that, although the rate of discharge in individual fibers is likely to contribute to perceived sensory magnitude, it is possible in this case to explain sensory magnitude solely on the basis of the size of the activated peripheral population.

Telencephalic mechanisms.—In a review article Wall (129) has summarized evidence that indicates the significance of the dorsal column system in active exploration. The effectiveness of lesions in the dorsal columns was evaluated by Dobry & Casey (20) both on behavioral and on cortical neuronal activity. Only very close to total dorsal column destruction detectably altered cortical sensory function and impaired behavioral discriminative capacity. For significant results in behavioral lesion work it is important that the lesions be complete to the extent planned. Another contribution to the behavioral study of the function of the sensory cortex comes from Schwartzman & Semmes (111). They studied with a graduated series of nylon filaments bent against the palm the effects of ablations of SI and SII on the tactile thresholds in monkeys. Monkeys subjected to removal of the SI hand area contralateral to the tested palm showed only transient or no deficits; others with complete ablations of SI and SII showed only slight losses. The authors mentioned that this lesion, which produced no residual loss in tactile sensitivity when tested passively, produced a severe impairment when tested by manual discrimination tasks that required active palpation by the monkey subject—even when the objects to be discriminated were grossly different. On the other hand, monkeys with lesions in the motor or premotor hand areas learned the active discrimination tasks with normal facility, and furthermore, monkeys with lesions of the sensory hand area showed no clear-cut deficiency in exploring the stimuli that might have explained their difficulty in learning to disciminate them.

Schwartzman & Semmes (111) mentioned another study in preparation by Porter in which it was shown that monkeys with nearly complete ablations of contralateral SI and bilateral SII manifested no impairment of the ability to discriminate fine temperature differences between objects even though this ability was tested in a situation that required active manual palpation. The negative findings after precentral lesions suggest that the sensory-motor exploratory process does not involve an interaction between sensory and motor cortical areas but instead is entirely governed by the postcentral sensory cortex. The role of the postcentral efferent fibers would thus seem important in the function of this region.

In two recent works the functional organization of the primary somesthetic cortex was reinvestigated. Whitsel et al (132) confirmed a modality segregation of input to SI, so that muscle afferents are represented anteriorly on the gyrus in area 3a, the cutaneous slowly and quickly adapting afferents in area 3b, and the joint afferents posteriorly. They proposed that the dermatomal afferents in the dorsal roots fan out according to modality in anterio-posteriorly oriented columns to produce this cortical modality distribution.

According to Paul et al (94) the hand is separately and fully represented in area 3b, with fingertips down in the sulcus, and in area 1 with a similar distribution—the fingertips anteriorly and the proximal parts posteriorly on the gyrus. After section and regeneration of hand nerves somewhat different changes in the projection to these two areas are seen. The representation in area 3 remains modality pure and cells with multiple receptive fields are rare, whereas in area 1 multiple receptive fields and mixing of modalities (93) are common.

The discovery of separate somatotopic maps in the hand area of areas 3 and 1 is of some interest since anatomically the projections to these areas are not identical (60). The projection from VPL to area 3 of SI is very heavy and composed of thick fibers, while that to areas 1 and 2 is lighter and made up of thin fibers. A separate short latency projection from the thalamic ventro-basal nucleus to the parietal association area in cats has been demonstrated (99) using physiological methods.

The functional organization of the cellular responses in the somesthetic cortex (101) may be simpler than in the visual cortex (51). This would not be surprising since the number of synaptic stations preceding the cortex is less in the somesthetic pathway than in the visual. The ease of activation by natural stimuli in area 3 in experimental situations is comparable to that of driving ganglion cells in the retina or cells in the LGN. However, occasionally more complex cells are also seen in the primary sensory cortex. A small number of directionally selective cutaneous cells in SI were reported by Mountcastle et al (83); recently more such cells have been observed (54, 108, 113, 132c). Complex cells appear to be very rare or entirely absent in area 3 but less rare in area 2 (108, 113). As was originally shown by Powell & Mountcastle (101), area 2 receives much of its input from joint receptors. A convergence of information about limb position and joint movement with sensitivity to direction of cutaneous movement could be envisaged as useful to sensorimotor interaction. A hierarchical convergence from joint and cutaneous units to the parietal associative area 5 was in fact demonstrated by Sakata (108). Using chronically prepared paralyzed monkeys, Sakata showed that many cells in area 5 were excited by complex combinations of stimuli. A cell would for instance be activated only if the left shoulder and elbow joints were in a certain position and the right elbow was being flexed so that the right hand moved over the left shoulder from distal to proximal. If during this movement the right hand rubbed the skin of the shoulder the response was better than with pure joint excitation. Such complex cells could signal very specific posture and movement patterns automatically and thus rapidly aid purposeful motor behavior. Figure 3 shows an example of such a cell.

In some features these cells are reminiscent of visual cortex cells which have complex receptive fields and which are each sensitive to movement in a specific direction (50, 51). Whereas such complex cells are common within the visual cortex, it appears that within the somesthetic system they are rare in the primary area but more common in the associative area.

A similar conclusion was also made by Duffy & Burchfield (24) who showed convergence of excitation from many joints to single cells in monkey area 5, and suggested a hierarchical arrangement of input to this area from the primary somesthetic area. Jones & Powell (61) have demonstrated anatomically a projection from SI to area 5.

The finding by Hubel & Wiesel (50, 51) of complex cells inspired Konorski (65) to coin the term "gnostic units" in particular brain analyzer areas. This idea appears now to be substantiated also in the somesthetic sense. The observations of Schwartzman & Semmes (111) quoted above could now be combined with the demonstration by Sakata (108) of the "gnostic" units of somesthesia in area 5. With lesions in SI, part of the input to the parietal area is blocked and the complex units in this cortical somesthetic analyzer [in the Pavlovian terminology (95)] do not receive normal input. This defect renders these gnostic units useless and leads to an inability to recognize an object by a synthetic combination of its features as extracted by cutaneous and kinesthetic mechanosensory modalities. Although the subject

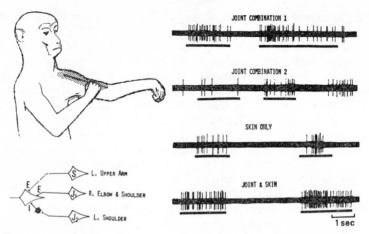

FIGURE 3. Recording from a cell in parietal associative area 5 by Sakata to show that the most effective stimulus is right elbow flexion when the left shoulder is in the indicated position and right arm is rubbing along the skin of left shoulder from distal to proximal (lowest record to right). Reproduced from (108) by permission of the author and the publisher, Georg Thieme Verlag.

is capable of performing the necessary exploratory movements with his intact motor system, in the absence of this somesthetic analyzer he is unable to synthesize a picture of what he is manipulating.

Concluding Remarks

Past studies on afferent mechanisms in behaving animals have largely been conducted with the methods of surgical ablation, electrical stimulation, and EEG recording. Whereas ablation experiments and related clinical knowledge have furnished negative information on the behavioral significance of the lack of a region, the use of the new microphysiological techniques in alert animals can now add the positive counterpart to this knowledge by revealing how cells in a region are activated during specified behavior. EEG techniques and electrical stimulation have often fallen short of indicating how the neural tissue functions because they involve synchronous activity in a large volume of tissue. Under normal circumstances such synchronous activation does not occur, although it is readily triggered with electrical stimulation, light flashes, and loud clicks. The handicap of microphysiological recording is that variations in the function of individual cells necessitate the study of several hundreds of cells for firm conclusions—a time consuming process with a difficult technique. Although this method has its drawbacks, it nevertheless appears capable of yielding gradually a deeper understanding of the function of the alert brain.

The era of evoked potential and electrical stimulation produced important results: the delineation of specific sensory and motor cortical regions under deep barbiturate anesthesia. On the other hand, during the facilitatory influence of chloralose anesthesia volleys of activity were also evoked in polysensory regions, which appear silent under barbiturate anesthesia. In the alert animal the associative, "silent" areas are not silent but function with vigor and can be studied in relation to the animal's normal behavior. From such studies new knowledge will arise in areas such as the polysensory afferent mechanisms and effects of sleep and waking, emotion, motivation, attention, and learning on the sensory systems. It is yet too early for an appraisal of significant results in these new fields but, hopefully, the reader has been aroused to follow the literature that will be appearing on these topics in the coming years.

LITERATURE CITED

1. Abeles, M., Goldstein, M. H., Jr. 1972. Responses of single units in the primary auditory cortex of the cat to tones and to tone pairs. *Brain Res.* 42:337–52
2. Allman, J. M., Kaas, J. H. 1971. A representation of the visual field in the caudal third of the middle temporal gyrus of the owl monkey. *Brain Res.* 31:85–105
3. Bachman, D. S., MacLean, P. D. 1971. Unit analysis of inputs to cingulate cortex in awake, sitting squirrel monkeys I. Exteroceptive systems. *Int. J. Neuroscience* 1:109–12
5. Baldwin, B. A., Siegel, J., Yates, J. O. 1971. A method for recording unit neural activity in unanesthetized sheep and goats. *Physiol. Behav.* 7:935–38
6. Barrett, T. W. 1972. Effects on the Q value of tuning curves and post-stimulus time histograms of cat auditory cortex neurons. *Exp. Neurol.* 34:484–96
7. Bear, D. M., Sasaki, H., Ervin, F. R. 1971. Sequential change in receptive fields of striate neurons in dark adapted cats. *Exp. Brain Res.* 13:256–72
8. Benjamin, R. M. 1970. Single neurons in the rat medulla responsive to nociceptive stimulation. *Brain Res.* 24:525–29
9. Bock, G. R., Webster, W. R., Aitkin, L. M. 1972. Discharge patterns of single units in inferior colliculus of the alert cat. *J. Neurophysiol.* 35:265–77
10. Boivie, J., Grant, G., Silfvenius, H. 1970. A projection from the nucleus Z to the ventral nuclear complex of the thalamus in the cat. *Acta Physiol. Scand.* 79:11A
11. Brearley, E. A., Kenshalo, D. R. 1970. Behavioral measurements of the sensitivity of cat's upper lip to warm and cool stimuli. *J. Comp. Physiol. Psychol.* 70:1–4
12. Brugge, J. F., Aitkin, L. M., Dubrovsky, N. A., Anderson, D. J. 1969. Sensitivity of single neurons in auditory cortex of cat to binaural tonal stimulation: Effects of varying interaural time and intensity. *J. Neurophysiol.* 32:1005–24
13. Bryan, R. N., Trevino, D. L., Willis, W. D. 1972. Evidence for a common location of alpha and gamma motoneurons. *Brain Res.* 38:193–96
14. Casey, K. L. 1971. Somatosensory responses of bulboreticular units in awake cat: Relation to escape-producing stimuli. *Science* 173:77–80
15. Chambers, M. R., Iggo, A. 1967. Slowly-adapting cutaneous mechanoreceptors. *J. Physiol. London* 192:26–27P
16. Cleland, B. G., Dubin, M. W., Levick, W. 1971. Sustained and transient neurons in the cat's retina and lateral geniculate nucleus. *J. Physiol. London* 217:473–96
17. Dallos, P. 1972. Discussion to the round table on auditory physiology. *Audiology* 11:73–76

18. Darian-Smith, I., Dykes, R. W. 1971. Peripheral neural mechanism of thermal sensation. In *Oral-Facial Sensory and Motor Mechanisms*, ed. R. Dubner, Y. Kawamura, 7–21. New York: Appleton

19. Denney, D., Adorjani, C. 1972. Orientation specificity of visual neurons after head tilt. *Exp. Brain Res.* 14:312–17

20. Dobry, P. J. K., Casey, K. L. 1970. Behavioural discriminative capacity and cortical unit responses in cats with dorsal column lesions. *Physiologist* 13: 180

21. Doving, K. B. 1970. Experiments in olfaction. In *Ciba Foundation Symposium on Taste and Smell in Vertebrates*, ed. G. E. W. Wolstenholme, J. Knight, 197–225. London: Churchill

22. Dow, B. M., Dubner, R. 1971. Single-unit responses to moving visual stimuli in middle suprasylvian gyrus of the cat. *J. Neurophysiol.* 34:47–55

23. Dubner, R., Zeki, S. M. 1971. Response properties and receptive fields of cells in an anatomically defined region of the superior temporal sulcus in the monkey. *Brain Res.* 35:528–32

24. Duffy, F. H., Burchfield, J. L. 1971. Somatosensory system: Organizational hierarchy from single units in monkey area 5. *Science* 172:273–75

25. Erulkar, S. D. 1972. Comparative aspects of spatial localization of sound. *Physiol. Rev.* 52:237–360

26. Evarts, E. V. 1966. Methods for recording activity of individual neurons in moving animals. In *Methods in Medical Research*, ed. R. F. Rushmer, 241–50. Chicago: Yearb. Med.

27. Evarts, E. V. 1968. A technique for recording activity of subcortical neurons in moving animals. *Electroencephalogr. Clin. Neurophysiol.* 24:83–86

28. Evarts, E. V. 1968. Relation of pyramidal tract activity to force exerted during voluntary movement. *J. Neurophysiol.* 31: 14–27

29. Fernández, C., Goldberg, J. M. 1971. Physiology of peripheral neurons innervating semicircular canals of the squirrel monkey. II. Response to sinusoidal stimulation and dynamics of peripheral vestibular system. *J. Neurophysiol.* 34:661–75

30. Ganchrow, D., Erickson, R. P. 1972. Thalamocortical relations in gustation. *Brain Res.* 36: 289–305

31. Gasanov, U. G., Vanetsian, G. L. 1971. Method of chronic investigation of unit activity in alert and anaesthetized cats. *Zh. Vyssh. Nerv. Deyatel. im. I. P. Pavlova* 21:820–26

32. Goldberg, J. M., Fernández, C. 1971. Physiology of peripheral neurons innervating semicircular canals of the squirrel monkey. I. Resting discharge and response to constant angular accelerations. *J. Neurophysiol.* 34: 635–60

33. Goldberg, J. M. Fernández, C. 1971. Physiology of peripheral innervating semicircular canals of the squirrel monkey. III. Variations among units in their discharge properties. *J. Neurophysiol.* 34:676–83

33a. Goldberg, M. E., Wurtz, R. H. 1972. Activity of superior colliculus in behaving monkey. I. Visual receptive fields of single neurons. *J. Neurophysiol.* 35: 542–59

33b. Goldberg, M. E., Wurtz, R. H. 1972. Activity of superior colliculus in behaving monkey. II. Effect of attention on neuronal responses. *J. Neurophysiol.* 35: 560–74

34. Goodwin, G. M., McCloskey, D. I., Matthews, P. B. C. 1972. The persistence of appreciable kinesthesia after paralysing joint afferents but preserving muscle afferents. *Brain Res.* 37:326–29

35. Goodwin, G. M., McCloskey, D. I., Matthews, P. B. C. 1972. A systematic distortion of position sense produced by muscle vibration. *J. Physiol. London* 221:8–9P

36. Goodwin, G. M., McCloskey, D. I., Matthews, P. B. C. 1972. Proprioceptive illusions induced by muscle vibration: Contribution by muscle spindles to perception? *Science* 175:1382–84

37. Granit, R. 1955. *Receptors and Sensory Perception*. New Ha-

ven:Yale Univ. Press

38. Granit, R. 1970. *The Basis of Motor Control*. New York:Academic

39. Gross, C. G., Rocha-Miranda, C. E., Bender, D. B. 1972. Visual properties of neurons in inferotemporal cortex of the macaque. *J. Neurophysiol.* 35:96–111

40. Hagbarth, K.-E., Hallin, R. G., Hongell, A., Torebjörk, H. E., Wallin, B. G. 1972. General characteristics of sympathetic activity in human skin nerves. *Acta Physiol. Scand.* 84:164–76

41. Hagbarth, K.-E., Hongell, A., Hallin, R. G., Torebjörk, H. E., 1970. Afferent impulses in median nerve fascicles evoked by tactile stimuli of the human hand. *Brain Res.* 24:423–42

42. Harrington, T., Merzenich, M. M. 1970. Neural coding in the sense of touch: Human sensations of skin indentation compared with the responses of slowly adapting mechanoreceptive afferents innervating the hairy skin of monkeys. *Exp. Brain Res.* 10:251–64

43. Hayward, J. N., Fairchild, M. D., Stuart, D. G., Deemer, J. A. 1964. A stereotaxic platform for microelectrode studies in chronic animals. *Electroencephalogr. Clin. Neurophysiol.* 16:522–24

45. Hensel, H., Iggo, A. 1971. Analysis of cutaneous warm and cold fibres in primates. *Pfluegers Arch.* 329:1–8

46. Hobson, J. A. 1972. A method of head restraint for cats. *Electroencephalogr. Clin. Neurophysiol.* 32:443–44

47. Hoffmann, K.-P., Stone, J. 1971. Conduction velocity of afferents to cat visual cortex: a correlation with cortical receptive field properties. *Brain Res.* 32:460–66

48. Horn, G., Hill, R. M. 1969. Modification of receptive fields of cells in the visual cortex occurring spontaneously and associated with bodily tilt. *Nature* 221:186–88

49. Hubel, D. H. 1959. Single unit activity in striate cortex of unrestrained cats. *J. Physiol. London* 147:226–38

50. Hubel, D. H., Wiesel, T. N. 1962. Receptive fields, binocular interaction and functional architecture in the cat's visual cortex. *J. Physiol. London* 160:106–54

51. Hubel, D. H., Wiesel, T. N. 1965. Receptive fields and functional architecture in two non-striate visual areas (18 and 19) of the cat. *J. Neurophysiol.* 28:229–89

52. Hubel, D. H., Wiesel, T. N. 1968. Receptive fields and functional architecture of monkey striate cortex. *J. Physiol. London* 195:215–43

53. Hubel, D. H., Wiesel, T. N. 1969. Visual area of the lateral suprasylvian gyrus (Clare-Bishop area) of the cat. *J. Physiol. London* 202:251–60

54. Hyvärinen, J., Poranen, A., Jokinen, Y., Näätänen, R., Linnankoski, I. 1973. Observations on unit activity in the primary somesthetic cortex of behaving monkeys. In *The Somatosensory System*, ed. H. H. Kornhuber. Stuttgart, Germany: Georg Thieme. In press

54a. Iggo, A. 1969. Cutaneous thermoreceptors in primates and subprimates. *J. Physiol. London* 200:403–30

55. Iggo, A., Muir, A. R. 1969. The structure and function of a slowly adapting touch corpuscle in hairy skin. *J. Physiol. London* 200:763–96

56. Iggo, A., Ramsey, R. L. 1971. Cortical projection of the type I slowly adapting cutaneous afferent units. *J. Physiol. London* 217:46–47P

57. Jasper, H. H., Bertrand, G. 1966. Thalamic units involved in somatic sensation and voluntary and involuntary movements in man. In *The Thalamus*, ed. D. P. Purpura, 365–90. New York: Columbia Univ. Press

58. Jeannerod, M., Putkonen, P. T. S. 1971. Lateral geniculate unit activity and eye movements: Saccade-locked changes in dark and in light. *Exp. Brain Res.* 13:533–46

59. Johnson, K. 1970. The mechanoreceptive population response to vibratory stimulus. Thesis, Johns Hopkins University

60. Jones, E. G., Powell, T. P. S.

1970. Connexions of the somatic sensory cortex of the rhesus monkeys. III. Thalamic connexions. *Brain* 93:37–53

61. Jones, E. G., Powell, T. P. S. 1970. An anatomical study of converging sensory pathways within the cerebral cortex of the monkey. *Brain* 93:793–820

61a. Jung, R. 1968. Optisch-vestibuläre Regulation der Augenbewegungen, des Bewegungssehens und der Vertikal-Horizontal-Wahrnehmung; Ein Beitrag zur optischvestibulären, optisch-oculomotorischen und optischgravizeptorischen Integration. In *Brain and Mind Problems,* ed. R. Vizoli, 185–226. Rome: Il Pensiero Scientifico

62. Kenshalo, D. R., Brearley, E. A. 1970. Electrophysiological measurements of the sensitivity of cat's upper lip to warm and cool stimuli. *J. Comp. Physiol. Psychol.* 70:5–14

63. Knibestöl, M. Vallbo, Å. B. 1970. Single unit analysis of mechanoreceptor activity from the human glabrous skin. *Acta Physiol. Scand.* 80:178–95

64. Koeze, T. H., Phillips, C. G., Sheridan, J. D. 1968. Thresholds of cortical activation of muscle spindles and alpha motoneurones of the baboon's hand. *J. Physiol. London* 195: 419–49

65. Konorski, J. 1967. *Integrative Activity of the Brain.* Chicago: Univ. Chicago Press

66. Konorski, J., Tarnecki, R. 1970. Purkinje cells in cerebellum: their responses to postural stimuli in cats. *Proc. Nat. Acad. Sci. USA* 65:892–97

67. Lamarre, Y., Joffroy, A. J., Filion, M., Bouchoux, R. 1970. A stereotaxic method for repeated sessions of central unit recording in the paralyzed or moving animal. *Rev. Can. Biol.* 29: 371–76

68. Landgren, S., Silfvenius, H. 1970. The projection of group I muscle afferents from the hindlimb to the contralateral thalamus of the cat. *Acta Physiol. Scand.* 79:10A

69. Landgren, S., Silfvenius, H. 1971. Nucleus Z, the medullary relay in the projection path to the cerebral cortex of group I muscle afferents from the cat's hind limb. *J. Physiol. London* 218: 551–71

70. Lehtonen, J. B., Lehtinen, I. 1972. Alpha rhythm and uniform visual field in man. *Electroencephalogr. Clin. Neurophysiol.* 32: 139–47

71. Li, C. L., Friauf, W., Cohen, G., Tew, J. M., Jr. 1965. A method of recording single cell discharges in the cerebral cortex of man. *Electroencephalogr. Clin. Neurophysiol.* 18:187–90

72. MacLean, P. D. 1967. A chronically fixed stereotaxic device for intracerebral exploration with macro- and micro-electrodes. *Electroencephalogr. Clin. Neurophysiol.* 22:180–82

73. Macrides, F., Chorover, S. L. 1971. Olfactory bulb units: Activity correlated with inhalation cycles and odor quality. *Science* 175:84–87

74. Mann, M. D., Kasprzak, H., Hiltz, F. L., Tapper, D. N. 1972. Activity in single cutaneous afferents: Spinal pathways and cortical evoked potentials. *Brain Res.* 39:61–70

75. Mann, M. D., Kasprzak, H., Tapper, D. N. 1971. Ascending dorsolateral pathways relaying type 1 afferent activity. *Brain Res.* 27:176–78

76. Marg, E., Adams, J. E. 1970. Evidence for a neurological zoom system in vision from angular changes in some receptive fields of single neurons with changes in fixation distance in the human visual cortex. *Experientia* 26:270–71

77. Mayer, D. J., Wolfle, T. L., Akil, H., Carder, B., Liebeskind, J. C., 1971. Analgesia from electrical stimulation in the brainstem of the rat. *Science* 174:1351–54

78. McIlwain, J. T. 1972. Central vision: Visual cortex and superior colliculus. *Ann. Rev. Physiol.* 34:291–314

79. Melvill Jones, G., Milsum, J. H. 1970. Characteristics of neural transmission from the semicircular canal to the vestibular nuclei of cats. *J. Physiol. London* 209:295–316

80. Melvill Jones, G., Milsum, J. H. 1971. Frequency-response anal-

ysis of central vestibular unit activity resulting from rotational stimulation of the semicircular canals. *J. Physiol. London* 219: 191–215

81. Merzenich, M. M., Harrington, T. 1969. The sense of flutter-vibration evoked by stimulation of the hairy skin of primates: Comparison of human sensory capacity with the responses of mechanoreceptive afferents innervating the hairy skin of monkeys. *Exp. Brain Res.* 9: 236–60

81a. Miller, J. M. et al 1972. Single cell activity in the auditory cortex of rhesus monkeys: Behavioral dependency. *Science* 177:449–51

81b. Morrell, F. 1972. Visual system's view of acoustic space. *Nature* 238:44–46

82. Mountcastle, V. B., LaMotte, R. H., Carli, G. 1972. Detection thresholds for stimuli in humans and monkeys: Comparison with threshold events in mechanoreceptive afferent nerve fibers innervating the monkey hand. *J. Neurophysiol.* 35:122–36

83. Mountcastle, V. B., Talbot, W. H., Sakata, H., Hyvärinen, J. 1969. Cortical neuronal mechanisms in flutter-vibration studied in unanesthetized monkeys. Neuronal periodicity and frequency discrimination. *J. Neurophysiol.* 32:452–84

84. Nieder, P. C., Nieder, I. 1970. Crossed olivocochlear bundle: Electrical stimulation enhances masked neural responses to loud clicks. *Brain Res.* 21:135–37

85. Nieder, P., Nieder, I. 1970. Antimasking effect of crossed olivocochlear bundle stimulation with loud clicks in guinea pig. *Exp. Neurol.* 28:179–88

86. Nieder, P., Nieder, I. 1970. Stimulation of efferent olivocochlear bundle causes release from low level masking. *Nature* 227: 184–85

87. Noda, H., Freeman, R. B., Jr., Gies, B., Creutzfeldt, O. D. 1971. Neuronal responses in the visual cortex of awake cats to stationary and moving targets. *Exp. Brain Res.* 12:389–405

88. Noda, H., Creutzfeldt, O. D., Freeman, R. B., Jr. 1971. Binocular interaction in the visual cortex of awake cats. *Exp. Brain Res.* 12:406–21

89. Norgren, R. 1970. Gustatory responses in the hypothalamus. *Brain Res.* 21:63–77

90. Norgren, R. 1970. Behavioral correlates of the thalamic gustatory area. *Brain Res.* 22:221–30

91. Norgren, R., Leonard, C. M. 1971. Taste pathways in rat brainstem. *Science* 173:1136–39

92. O'Keefe, J., Dostrovsky, J. 1971. The hippocampus as a spatial map. Preliminary evidence from unit activity in the freely-moving rat. *Brain Res.* 34:171–75

93. Paul, R. L., Goodman, H., Merzenich, M. 1972. Alterations in mechanoreceptor input to Brodmann's areas 1 and 3 of the postcentral hand area of Macaca mulatta after nerve section and regeneration. *Brain Res.* 39:1–19

94. Paul, R. L., Merzenich, M., Goodman, H. 1972. Representation of slowly and rapidly adapting cutaneous mechanoreceptors of the hand in Brodmann's areas 3 and 1 of Macaca mulatta. *Brain Res.* 36:229–49

95. Pavlov, I. P. 1965. *Psychopathology and Psychiatry*, ed. Y. Popov, L. Rokhlin. Moscow:Foreign Languages Publ.

96. Petit, D., Burgess, P. R. 1968. Dorsal column projection of receptors in cat hairy skin supplied by myelinated fibers. *J. Neurophysiol.* 31:849–55

97. Phillips, C. G., Powell, T. P. S., Wiesendanger, M. 1971. Projection from low-threshold muscle afferents of hand and forearm to area 3a of baboon's cortex. *J. Physiol. London.* 217: 419–46

98. Pinkus, F. 1905. Über Hautsinnesorgane neben dem menschlichen Haar (Haarscheiben) und ihre vergleihend-anatomische Bedeutung. *Arch. Mikrosk. Anat.* 65:121–79

99. Poliakova, A. G. 1972. Origin of the early component of the evoked response in the association cortex of the cat. *Electroen-*

cephalogr. Clin. Neurophysiol.
32:129–38

100. Porter, R., Lewis, M. McD., Linklater, G. F. 1971. A headpiece for recording discharges of neurons in unrestrained monkeys. *Electroencephalogr. Clin. Neurophysiol.* 30:91–93

101. Powell, T. P. S., Mountcastle, V. B. 1959. Some aspects of the functional organization of the cortex of the postcentral gyrus of the monkey: a correlation of findings obtained in a single unit analysis with cytoarchitecture. *Bull. Johns Hopkins Hosp.* 105:133–62

102. Rettig, G. M. 1971. A head-holding device for repeated microelectrode studies in monkeys during operant responding. *Electroencephalogr. Clin. Neurophysiol.* 30:462–64

103. Rodieck, R. W. 1971. Central nervous system: afferent mechanisms. *Ann. Rev. Physiol.* 33:203–40

104. Rose, J. E., Anderson, D. J., Hind, J. E., Brugge, J. F. 1971. Some effects of stimulus intensity on response of auditory nerve fibers in the squirrel monkey. *J. Neurophysiol.* 34:685–99

106. Rosen, I, Asanuma, H. 1971. Receptive fields of group I activated cells in the cerebral cortex examined by natural stimulation. *Fed. Proc.* 30:664

107. Rushton, W. A. H. 1972. Review Lecture. Pigments and signals in colour vision. *J. Physiol. London* 220:1–31P

108. Sakata, H. 1973. Somatosensory responses of neurons in the parietal association area (area 5) in monkeys. In *The Somatosensory System*, ed. H. H. Kornhuber. Stuttgart: Georg Thieme. In press

109. Sanderson, K. J., Bishop, P. O., Darian-Smith, I. 1971. The properties of the binocular receptive fields of lateral geniculate neurons. *Exp. Brain Res.* 13:178–207

110. Schiller, P. H., Koerner, F. 1971. Discharge characteristics of single units in superior colliculus of the alert rhesus monkey. *J. Neurophysiol.* 34:920–36

111. Schwartzman, R. J., Semmes, J. 1971. The sensory cortex and tactile sensitivity. *Exp. Neurol.* 33:147–58

112. Schwarz, D. W. F., Fredrickson, J. M. 1971. Rhesus monkey vestibular cortex: a bimodal primary projection field. *Science* 172:280–81

113. Schwarz, D. W. F., Fredrickson, J. M. 1971. Tactile direction sensitivity of area 2 oral neurons in the rhesus monkey cortex. *Brain Res.* 27:397–401

114. Siegel, J., Lineberry, C. G. 1971. A method for recording single unit activity from unanesthetized chronic cats. *Physiol. Behav.* 6:607–08

115. Silfvenius, H. 1972. Projections to the cat cerebral cortex from fore- and hind limb group I muscle afferents. *Umeå Univ. Med. Diss.*, No. 4

116. Silfvenius, H. 1972. Properties of cortical group I neurones located in the lower bank of the anterior suprasylvian sulcus of the cat. *Acta Physiol. Scand.* 84:555–76

117. Singer, W., Pöppel, E., Creutzfeldt, O. 1972. Inhibitory interaction in the cat's lateral geniculate nucleus. *Exp. Brain Res.* 14:210–26

118. Stone, J., Hoffmann, K.-P. 1971. Conduction velocity as a parameter in the organisation of the afferent relay in the cat's lateral geniculate nucleus. *Brain Res.* 32:454–59

119. Sudakov, K, MacLean, P. D., Reeves, A., Marino, R. 1971. Unit study of exteroceptive inputs to claustrocortex in awake, sitting, squirrel monkey. *Brain Res.* 28:19–34

120. Suzuki, H., Takahashi, M. 1970. Organization of lateral geniculate neurons in binocular inhibition. *Brain Res.* 23:261–64

121. Talbot, W. H., Darian-Smith, I, Kornhuber, H. H., Mountcastle, V. B. 1968. The sense of flutter-vibration: comparison of the human capacity with response patterns of mechanoreceptive afferents from the monkey hand. *J. Neurophysiol.* 31:301–34

122. Tapper, D. N. 1970. Behavioral evaluation of the tactile pad receptor system in hairy skin of the cat. *Exp. Neurol.* 26:447–59

123. Tapper, D. N., Galera-Carcia, C., Brown, P. B. 1972. Sinusoidal mechanical stimulation of the tactile pad receptor: tuning curves. *Brain Res.* 36:223–27

124. Tarnecki, R., Konorski, J. 1970. Patterns of responses of Purkinje cells in cats to passive displacements of limbs, squeezing and touching. *Acta Neurobiol. Exp.* 30:95–119

125. Vallbo, Å. B. 1970. Discharge patterns in human muscle spindle afferents during isometric voluntary contractions. *Acta Physiol. Scand.* 80:552–66

126. Vallbo, Å. B. 1971. Muscle spindle response at the onset of isometric voluntary contractions in man. Time difference between fusimotor and skeletomotor effects. *J. Physiol. London* 218:405–31

127. Verrillo, R. T., Fraioli, A. J., Smith, R. L. 1969. Sensation magnitude of vibrotactile stimuli. *Percept. Psychophys.* 6:366–72

128. Vierck, C. J., Jr., Hamilton, D. M., Thornby, J. I. 1971. Pain reactivity of monkeys after lesions to the dorsal and lateral columns of the spinal cord. *Exp. Brain Res.* 13:140–58

129. Wall, P. D. 1970. The sensory and motor role of impulses travelling in the dorsal columns towards cerebral cortex. *Brain* 93:505–24

130. Werner, G., Mountcastle, V. B. 1965. Neural activity in mechanoreceptive cutaneous afferents: Stimulus-response relations, Weber functions, and information transmission. *J. Neurophysiol.* 28:359–97

131. Whitfield, I. C. 1971. Mechanisms of sound localization. *Nature* 233:95–97

132. Whitsel, B. L., Dreyer, D. A., Roppolo, J. R. 1971. Determinants of body representation in postcentral gyrus of Macaques. *J. Neurophysiol.* 34:1018–34

132a. Whitsel, B. L., Petrucelli, L. M., Sapiro, G. 1969. Modality representation in the lumbar and cervical fasciculus gracilis of squirrel monkeys. *Brain Res.* 15:67–78

132b. Whitsel, B. L., Petrucelli, L. M., Sapiro, G., Ha, H. 1970. Fiber sorting in the fasciculus gracilis of squirrel monkeys. *Exp. Neurol.* 29:227–42

132c. Whitsel, B. L., Roppolo, J. R., Werner, G. 1972. Cortical information processing of stimulus motion on primate skin. *J. Neurophysiol.* 35:691–717

132d. Wickelgren, B. 1971. Superior colliculus: Some receptive field properties of bimodally responsive cells. *Science* 173:69–72

132e. Wiersma, C. A. G., Yamaguchi, T. 1967. Integration of visual stimuli by the crayfish central nervous system. *J. Exp. Biol.* 47:409–31

133. Wollberg, Z., Newman, J. D. 1971. Auditory cortex of squirrel monkey: Response patterns of single cells to species-specific vocalizations. *Science* 175:212–14

134. Wright, M. J. 1971. Responsiveness to visual stimuli of single neurones in the pulvinar and lateral posterior nuclei of the cat's thalamus. *J. Physiol. London* 219:32–33P

135. Wurtz, R. H. 1969. Visual receptive fields of striate cortex neurons in awake monkeys. *J. Neurophysiol.* 32:727–42

136. Wurtz, R. H. 1969. Response of striate cortex neurons to stimuli during rapid eye movements in the monkey. *J. Neurophysiol.* 32:975–86

137. Wurtz, R. H. 1969. Comparison of effects of eye movements and stimulus movements on striate cortex neurons of the monkey. *J. Neurophysiol.* 32:987–94

138. Wurtz, R. H., Goldberg, M. E. 1971. Superior colliculus cell responses related to eye movements in awake monkeys. *Science* 171:82–84

138a. Wurtz, R. H., Goldberg, M. E. 1972. Activity of superior colliculus in behaving monkey. III. Cells discharging before eye movements. *J. Neurophysiol.* 35:575–86

138b. Wurtz, R. H., Goldberg, M. E. 1972. Activity of superior colliculus in behaving monkey. IV. Effects of lesions on eye movements. *J. Neurophysiol.* 35:587–96

139. Yokota, T., Reeves, A. G. Mac-

Lean, P. D., 1970. Differential effects of septal and olfactory volleys on intracellular responses of hippocampal neurons in awake, sitting monkeys. *J. Neurophysiol.* 33:96–107

140. Zeki, S. M. 1971. Convergent input from the striate cortex (area 17) to the cortex of the superior temporal sulcus in the rhesus monkey. *Brain Res.* 28: 338–40

Ann. Rev. Physiol. 1973. 35:273–304

BIOCHEMICAL PHYSIOLOGY OF CENTRAL SYNAPSES[1]

1097

Ross J. Baldessarini[2]

Laboratory of Neuropharmacology, Department of Psychiatry
Massachusetts General Hospital and Harvard Medical School
Boston, Massachusetts

Manfred Karobath

Department of Experimental Psychiatry
Psychiatrische Universitätsklinik
University of Vienna, Austria

The complexity and relative inaccessibility of the central nervous system have greatly impeded the study of synaptic physiology. However, in recent years a fruitful approach to the problem has been to apply methods of chemical and pharmacological analysis. The present review is almost exclusively limited to biochemical studies of synaptic function in the mammalian CNS. It is not a comprehensive review of this vast topic, but rather an attempt to highlight important current approaches and trends. Previous reviewers have dealt with many aspects of synaptic biochemistry and pharmacology (9, 64, 66, 68, 73, 80, 92, 95, 103, 121, 142, 158, 163, 173). The topics reviewed in the present paper include general metabolism of synapses and the more specialized presynaptic metabolism of neurotransmitters as well as their postsynaptic actions.

METABOLISM OF SYNAPSES

In general, neurons in the CNS are separated by a system of clefts about 150 Å in width, except at highly specialized points of contact, the synapses. These structures have several consistent morphologic features, including specialized thickenings of the adjacent cell membranes, large numbers of small membrane-enclosed vesicles, and usually mitochondria in what is presumed

[1] Partially supported by U.S. Public Health Service (NIMH) Grant MH-16674–02.

[2] Recipient of Research Scientist Career Development Award, Type II, National Institute of Mental Health: KO2-MH-74370.

to be the presynaptic side of the synapse (24, 72). It is generally agreed that transmission of impulses from one neuron to another occurs unidirectionally across these adjacent cell membranes and over a finite period of time by release of specific small molecules from the presynaptic site to alter the state of membrane polarization of a postsynaptic cell. Since thousands of synaptic contacts converge upon each of the millions of central neurons, and since each neuron in turn projects thousands of terminals upon other cells, it is clear that neuronal interactions are extraordinarily complex. Despite this complexity, several approaches have been made to obtain some degree of anatomical specificity of tissue for biochemical analysis. One approach includes studies of relatively simple nervous systems of lower organisms or of the mammalian peripheral nervous system. In both cases the mechanisms of synaptic transmission involved bear at least some similarity to those in the mammalian CNS. In the mammalian CNS, various levels of dissection have been used, including regional fragmentation into classical neuroanatomical structures, slicing a given structure into different layers, and microdissection to isolate individual cells. Alternatively, homogenates of brain can be fractionated by centrifugation techniques to prepare cellular (83, 179) or subcellular fractions (55, 120, 204). One of the fractions which has been studied very intensively consists mainly of isolated nerve ending particles (synaptosomes) (55, 204). They appear to represent the synaptic complex, which has broken off and resealed to form discrete morphologically identifiable units, enclosed by cell membranes, which retain many of the constituents and metabolic activities of neuronal cytoplasm. Other biochemical features of synapses may also provide some degree of specificity to observations. They include high-affinity transport processes and specifically localized enzyme activities. Furthermore, selective "marking" or labeling of molecules to facilitate their isolation, the inhibition of specific reactions, or the selective destruction of specific types of nerve endings by drugs have also been employed and will be discussed.

Several investigations of the general metabolism of the synaptic complex, including studies of energy metabolism, have been made. These have focused on synaptosomes and reveal high rates of respiration, including glycolysis and oxidative phosphorylation leading to production of lactate, ATP, and phosphocreatine; the synaptosomes also convert glucose to amino acids (51). Provided that synaptosomes are incubated in "physiological" media, their rates of respiration resemble those of more intact tissue, such as brain slices. Rates of oxygen consumption in such preparations are increased by electrical impulses or by high external concentrations of K^+ and may represent a metabolic response to membrane depolarization (51). The activity of the ATPase stimulated by Na^+ and K^+, which is part of the enzyme system responsible for the transport of Na^+ outward and K^+ inward across cell membranes, is extraordinarily high in brain tissue, and the highest specific activities of this enzyme have been found associated with synaptosomal membranes (6). Accordingly, intact synaptosomes accumulate K^+ (59) and extrude Na^+ (126) by a temperature-sensitive and time-dependent process. Uptake of K$^+$ is optimally stimulated by extracellular [Na$^+$] of 50–60 mM and saturated by external [K$^+$] of 10 mM (59). As has been found in whole cells, ouabain and metabolic poisons such as cyanide and p-dinitrophenol interfere with the maintainence of gradients of Na$^+$ and K$^+$. About 95% of internal K$^+$ can exchange with exogenous K$^+$ (202), and very little of the internal K$^+$ is reported to remain associated with synaptic membranes; in contrast, as much as 80% of intrasynaptosomal Na$^+$ was retained after prolonged exposure of the synaptosomes to a hypotonic medium, and therefore may be more firmly bound to plasma membranes, synaptic vesicles, or mitochondria (126). As in other tissues, there seems to be a mechanism for the exclusion of Ca^{2+} from synaptosomes. This mechanism requires extracellular Na$^+$ and is sensitive to ouabain (23). There is evidence that internal Ca^{2+} may be sequestered, perhaps by mitochondria, which are known to accumulate Ca^{2+} (23). During membrane depolarization at nerve terminals, conditions should be such that Ca^{2+} entry would be facilitated; its entry may be an early step in the process of transmitter release (173).

Some studies on the entry of substrates of important intracellular pathways have also been undertaken. Most of these have been limited to amino acids and choline (77). In striking contrast to in vitro studies with brain slices (111), the accumulation of amino acids by synaptosomes (13, 71) occurs at a rapid rate and is linear for about five minutes, while slices accumulate linearly for an hour or more. This difference is probably largely due to geometric factors: in synaptosomes entry occurs into relatively finely divided particles with a high surface-to-volume ratio held in suspension, while penetration of labeled amino acids into brain slices occurs slowly through a complex tissue through multiple compartments. Studies on the uptake of L-tryptophan by synaptosomes indicated a saturable carrier-mediated transport and counter-transport mechanism, half-saturated by substrate concentrations (K_t) on the order of mM (71), which was not Na$^+$-dependent and was relatively insensitive to ouabain; similar results were obtained with L-methionine (13). This type of "low-affinity" (high K_t) uptake occurs with most amino acids and is probably an important means of supplying them locally for synaptic metabolism. Alternative mechanisms for supplying amino acids might include proteolysis since lysosomes and protein hydrolysis have been described in nerve terminals (69) and axoplasmic flow could provide a readily available source of "excess" protein.

In addition to the general nonspecific uptake of amino acids, several of them are taken up into nerve endings by more specific "high-affinity" (low K_t) uptake processes. Thus, the proposed neurotransmitter amino acids, γ-aminobutyric acid (*GABA*) (134), glycine (104, 128), L-glutamate (128), L-aspartate (128), and perhaps taurine (50) and choline (56) (the precursor of acetylcholine) are reported to have apparent K_t values of 10 to 50 μM with synaptosomes. At least for GABA, the "high-affinity" uptake may be Na$^+$-dependent (134), although Na$^+$ is also reported to facilitate nonspecific binding of GABA to synaptic membranes (191). The high-affinity transport of the putative transmitter amino acids more closely resembles that of cate-cholamines than the nonspecific transport of amino acids, and it may represent a means of inactivating neurotransmitter substances following their release. The high-affinity uptake of amino acids has facilitated radioautographic localization in specific nerve endings (57, 87, 151) and shows promise of permitting the development of subcellular fractionation methods to separate specifically labeled subpopulations of synaptosomes for biochemical study (187).

Another area which received a great deal of attention is the origin of protein molecules at nerve endings. It is known that the metabolism of protein in brain is vigorous, and half-lives of protein in synaptosomes as in whole brain average about 2–3 weeks (146). There is a long held view that nerve ending proteins are synthesized in the region of the perikaryon and transported to more distal portions of the neuron by means of axoplasmic transport. Both rapid (up to 400 mm/day) and slow (about 0.4 mm/day) rates of longitudinal axoplasmic transport of protein have been observed in the CNS (123, 136). The slow component appears to include both soluble and particulate proteins, while the fast component involves particulate material predominantly. For example, in the brain, mitochondria appear to move along axons at slow rates of transport (15), while pituitary hormones stored in vesicles leave the hypothalamus by very rapid transport (100). In peripheral neurons at least, vesicles, including catecholamine storage particles (127), as well as the catecholamine synthesizing enzyme dopamine-β-hydroxylase, but not tyrosine hydroxylase (66), appear to be transported rapidly. The mechanisms and the driving force for these phenomena are still poorly characterized, although there is some evidence that the rapid axonal transport of protein is dependent on oxygen (157), and it has been shown that the fast movement of acetylcholinesterase can be blocked by colchicine, a drug known to depolymerize intra-axonal microtubular proteins (106, 115). Rapid axonal transport of protein does not appear to depend on continuing protein synthesis at the nerve cell body (136).

In addition to the transport of preformed protein and organelles synthesized in perikarya, there is accumulating evidence that macromolecules can also be synthesized locally in nerve terminals. Synaptosomal fractions of brain incubated in vitro incorporate labeled amino acids (7, 8, 29) or monosaccharides (29, 61) into protein, glycoprotein, and glycolipids. In these experiments, evidence was presented to rule out significant contributions to protein synthesis by contaminating bacteria or by microsomal membranes, including the lack of an inhibitory effect of ribonuclease. On the other hand, radioautographic analyses of synaptosomal preparations after incubation with radioactive amino acids suggest that only about half of the amino-acid incorporation occurred in structures with typical morphologic characteristics of synaptosomes (45). Other properties of protein synthesis by synaptosomal fractions include the following (7, 8): in addition to the lack of sensitivity to ribonuclease treatment, synaptosomal protein synthesis does not depend on exogenous ATP; it is interrupted completely by hypo-osmotic shock, and proceeds in simple isotonic buffer solutions with only a single labeled amino acid added. While Na^+ in the presence of high $[K^+]$ or high $[K^+]$ alone stimulated protein synthesis, the basis of ionic effects in such experiments is difficult to elucidate, since the complex interrelationships between precursor uptake, membrane properties, ATP generation, and ion concentrations have only been partially studied and are not understood. Incorporation of leucine was markedly inhibited by cycloheximide, which inhibits protein synthesis in mammalian cells, and by puromycin, a general inhibitor of ribosomal protein synthesis, but only to a small extent by chloramphenicol, which inhibits bacterial and mitochondrial protein synthesis; these pharmacologic findings are evidence against a major contribution of mitochondria to protein synthesis by synaptosomal fractions. In general, the preceding observations make it clear that isolated nerve endings exhibit many of the features of protein synthesis observed with intact cells. About 80% of the labeled products in such experiments was found to be associated with membranes. Recently evidence has been presented that membrane fragments prepared from lysed synaptosomes synthesize protein (67). ATP, GTP, Mg^{2+}, and supernatant enzyme factors for protein synthesis prepared from whole synaptosomes were required, and metabolic inhibitors had no effect. In contrast to intact synaptosomes, K^+ stimulated protein synthesis (optimum, 120 mM), and at concentrations above 100 mM, Na^+ inhibited synthesis in this "cell"-free system. Cycloheximide, puromycin, and phosphate ion inhibited protein synthesis, but chloramphenicol had no effect. The distribution of the synaptosomal membrane products on polyacrylamide gels differed from the product of brain microsomal protein synthesis. The localization of protein synthesis to nerve endings raises several questions about the role of the membrane products of this synthesis in synaptic physiology and about the means of maintaining and regulating a localized system of protein synthesis remote from the cell body.

SPECIALIZED METABOLISM OF SYNAPSES

In recent years a long and growing list of candidate neurotransmitter substances has accumulated (Figure 1). Their consideration has usually depended first on the detection and chemical isolation first in brain, and then in nerve ending fractions, of substances with the ability to alter the electrical or contractile responses of nerve or muscle cells. There are usually found to be mechanisms for the presynaptic synthesis and storage of such molecules. They are released by nerve depolarization and mechanisms exist for their efficient inactivation. The candidates include several small molecules, most of which are amines or amino acids, and in addition a group of polypeptides, "substance P." Evidence partially supports such a function for acetylcholine and the catecholamines, norepinephrine, and dopamine. There is also good evidence for GABA and glutamate being transmitters in the brain and for glycine in the spinal cord, and some evidence for serotonin in the brain and spinal cord. Although the evidence is less impressive, histamine may also be a transmitter in the brain. For other candidates the support is generally less persua-

PROPOSED CENTRAL NEUROTRANSMITTERS

COMPOUND	STRUCTURE	SYNTHESIS	INACTIVATION
ACETYLCHOLINE (ACh)	$H_3C\ \overset{\overset{O}{\|\|}}{C}-O-(CH_2)_2\overset{+}{N}(CH_3)_3$	Choline acetylation	● Hydrolysis by acetylcholinesterase (AChE)
NOREPINEPHRINE (NE)	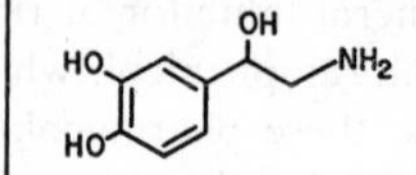 (structure)	Dopamine-β-hydroxylation	● Reuptake ● Oxidative deamination by monoamine-oxidase (MAO) ● 3-O-Methylation by catechol-o-methyl transferase (COMT)
DOPAMINE (DA)	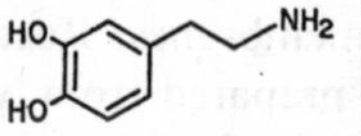 (structure)	Tyrosine hydroxylation, DOPA decarboxylation	● Reuptake ● MAO ● COMT
SEROTONIN (5HT)	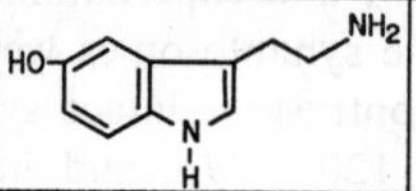 (structure)	Tryptophan hydroxylation, 5-OH-Tryptophan decarboxylation	● Reuptake ● MAO
HISTAMINE	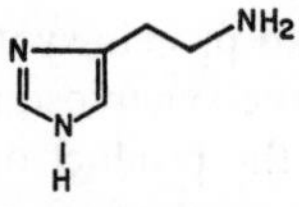 (structure)	Histidine decarboxylation	● N-methylation by histamine-N-methyl transferase (HNMT) ● Oxidative deamination (MAO?)
EXCITATORY AMINO ACIDS e.g. Glutamate, Aspartate	$CH_2\,(CH_2)_n\ CH\,NH_2$ $\|\qquad\qquad\|$ $COOH\qquad COOH$ $n=0-1$	—	● Reuptake
INHIBITORY AMINO ACIDS e.g. γ-Amino-butyrate (GABA)	$CH_2\,(CH_2)_n\ NH_2$ $\|$ $COOH$ $n=0-4$	GABA by glutamate decarboxylation	● Reuptake ● GABA: transamination and oxidation to succinate
SUBSTANCE P	Polypeptide, MW~1400	—	● Proteases (?)
PROSTAGLANDINS (? Post-synaptic)	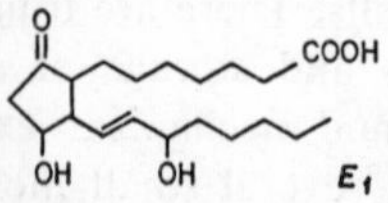 (structure) E_1	From fatty acids via phospholipases (?)	—

FIGURE 1. Proposed neurotransmitters of the CNS. Reproduced from Mountcastle & Baldessarini (147) by permission of the publisher, C. V. Mosby Co.

sive. The problem of identifying biochemical mediators of synaptic transmission in the brain has been discussed at some length elsewhere (147, 158). The presynaptic and postsynaptic metabolism of the most throughly studied of these substances will be considered.

PRESYNAPTIC METABOLISM OF SYNAPTIC TRANSMITTERS

Acetylcholine (ACh).—Much of the work supporting the candidacy of ACh as a neurotransmitter in the CNS has been reviewed previously (80, 147, 158, 163). ACh has long been known to occur in isolated nerve endings; recent experiments with techniques allowing the quantitative isotonic disruption of synaptosomes confirm that about half of the ACh in nerve endings is firmly bound in vesicles and that the remainder is in the cytoplasm (192). In studies in which ACh was synthesized by brain in vitro (169) or in vivo (36) from labeled choline, very little labeled ACh could be recovered from synaptic vesicle fractions. Since at least half of endogenous ACh remains associated with similar vesicular preparations, the lack of such association of newly synthesized labeled ACh implies either that newly synthesized ACh enter vesicles very slowly or that it is more sensitive than endogenous ACh to dissociation from vesicles during the preparative procedures currently employed. On the other hand, rapid binding of exogenous ACh by synaptic vesicles isolated from cerebral cortex in a non-ionic medium has been observed, and ACh so bound was resistant to the action of acetylcholinesterase (75). Vesicular storage probably represents a means of protecting ACh synthesized in the nerve ending. In contrast to the storage of other amine transmitters, almost nothing is known about the molecular mechanisms involved in the vesicular storage of ACh.

Choline acetyltransferase is known to occur in central nerve endings. It is a strongly cationic enzyme which adsorbs to negatively charged particles; this property might account for reports of the association of the enzyme with microsomal particles when tissues were prepared in media with low salt concentrations (63). In vivo, choline acetyltransferase is most probably a cytoplasmic enzyme. It behaves on Sephadex columns as a globular protein of mol wt 65,000 (162). Choline and acetyl coenzyme-A, the cosubstrates of this enzyme do not cause substrate inhibition, and although coenzyme-A can compete with its acetyl-charged congener (K_i = 16 μM) (162), it is unlikely that this competition could provide a means of regulating ACh synthesis since acetyl coenzyme-A is mainly required for several other reactions. The detailed mechanisms of choline acetylation have been further studied recently (165). ACh itself inhibits choline acetylation very slightly (IC_{50} = 200 mM) without competing with either cosubstrate (162). Thus product inhibition is also unlikely to occur during production of ACh, although some mass action inhibitory effect of ACh upon its own synthesis might occur. Nevertheless, if the concept of sequestration of ACh into vesicular stores (55, 163, 184, 192, 204) is valid, and since intracellular acetylcholinesterase

(184) is likely to hydrolyze unprotected ACh extremely rapidly, it seems improbable that free cytoplasmic ACh is present physiologically at the high levels required for appreciable inhibition of choline acetyltransferase by mass action. If it were to be shown that the acetyltransferase is a vesicular enzyme, inhibition by mass action of high vesicular concentrations of ACh might occur. An alternative possibility is that modulation of the synthesis of ACh, if it occurs at all, might involve the availability of choline. Choline acetyltransferase is probably saturable by concentrations of choline greater than mM (reported values of K_m for choline vary, but are about 0.8 mM); the average reported values for free choline in brain are only 0.1–0.3 mM (44), and large doses of choline can increase levels of ACh (21). Thus, it is likely that the enzyme is not fully saturated with the substrate choline under physiological conditions. While choline is probably not synthesized in brain (5), it can be made available by uptake into nerve endings from an extracellular location (56) or by the hydrolysis of ACh or of phospholipids (5). The importance of choline accumulation for the synthesis of ACh has been shown in peripheral cholinergic neurons, and hemicholinium-3, a competitive inhibitor of choline uptake (K_i = 40–60 μM), decreases the synthesis of ACh (161) and depletes ACh in the brain (172). The K_t of uptake of choline has been estimated variously from 0.05 to 0.23 mM (56, 161, 176); furthermore, locally high concentrations of choline are likely to occur in the synaptic cleft during synaptic activity and upon hydrolysis of ACh by acetylcholinesterase. Thus it is highly likely that the uptake of choline provides a means of reutilizing substrate to form new molecules of ACh, and it may also be a means of regulating synthesis of ACh. Choline acetyltransferase is highly specific for choline and analogs of choline have been tried as possible inhibitors of the enzyme with limited success.

The general unavailability of potent and specific inhibitors of choline acetyltransferase and the toxicity of the potent acetylcholinesterase inhibitors have limited attempts to study the physiological role of ACh in the CNS by altering its metabolism. Another difficulty is the lack of methods to delineate precisely central cholinergic pathways (80). Histochemical methods for acetylcholinesterase demonstrate its rather diffuse distribution throughout the CNS (80, 184). Furthermore, there are no specific and sufficiently sensitive histochemical reactions for ACh which are suitable for use in mammalian brain tissue. Newer histochemical methods for choline acetyltransferase (110) may provide a more specific means of localizing cholinergic cells.

Amino acids proposed as neurotransmitters.—Studies which strongly suggest that several amino acids are neurotransmitters in submammalian species, as well as electrophysiologic observations in the mammalian CNS of potent effects of microiontophoretically applied amino acids, contribute to the growing impression that amino acids may act as neurotransmitters in the mammalian nervous system (48, 80, 103, 121, 158, 170). Greatest interest has been directed to several neutral amino acids including GABA, glycine, taurine, and alanine, which have inhibitory effects when applied to central neurons, and to several acidic amino acids, notably glutamate and aspartate, which have potent widespread excitatory effects. Such pharmacological effects occur in a way which corresponds very crudely to the endogenous gross regional distribution of each amino acid (16, 103, 121, 170). In the CNS glutamic acid is decarboxylated irreversibly by the enzyme glutamic acid decarboxylase to GABA. While only small amounts of GABA are found in peripheral tissues, levels in brain are very high and even surpass those of ACh. The pathway α-ketoglutarate $\rightarrow$ glutamate $\rightarrow$ GABA $\rightarrow$ succinic semialdehyde $\rightarrow$ succinate—sometimes referred to as the "GABA shunt"—describes the close connection of the metabolism of GABA with the tricarboxylic acid cycle. The final enzymatic step can be localized in brain histochemically (185). Only minor alternative pathways of GABA have been described, and GABA is not incorporated into protein. It is not known whether synthesis is regulated in response to altered rates of utilization of GABA. However, long term increases in GABA levels in developing avian brain have been shown to lead to a reversible decrease in the synthesis of glutamic acid decarboxylase (189).

Glutamic acid decarboxylase, a soluble enzyme, (170) and a similar enzyme which produces taurine from cysteinesulfinate (2) have been found in nerve endings. The subcellular distribution of several endogenous and labeled amino acids has also been studied (2, 97, 167, 191) and up to 40% of GABA was found in particulate fractions of brain homogenates. The significance of these findings is unclear, however; unlike ACh, amino acids are not found in vesicular fractions (132, 167) and extensive redistribution of GABA has been reported to occur with current fractionation techniques (191). Similar examinations with many amino acids, including GABA and several others proposed to function as neurotransmitters, failed to reveal any specific subcellular distribution (2, 132, 167). Since free amino acids occur throughout the cytoplasm of most cells and they participate in many metabolic activities, it may not be reasonable to expect to find a specific synaptic localization, although selected small pools of certain amino acids might be involved in synaptic transmission.

There are only a limited number of means by which synapses utilizing an amino acid as a transmitter could provide the spatial and functional specificity required for local synaptic function. Since for most amino acids selective synthesis in particular neurons does not occur, other mechanisms must be used. The two most likely ones are selective release and the presence of specific postsynaptic receptors. Two means of providing for selective release would be either a "gating" mechanism or the sequestration of transmitter molecules at particular nerve terminals in locally high concentrations. Although there is presently no evidence for vesicular storage of amino acids, concentrative accumulation of certain amino acids by high-affinity transport at nerve endings does occur and might provide a mechanism of such sequestration.

This high affinity transport of certain amino acids shows regional specificity. For example, the uptake of glycine by high affinity transport is reported to be specific to the spinal cord (128), while the uptake as well as the release of glutamate is most vigorous in the cortex (78). In the retina, the uptake of GABA, particularly into horizontal cells, was stimulated by light (122). The high-affinity transport for GABA and several other amino acids has enabled radioautographic studies to be made (57, 87, 151) which showed differential accumulation of radioactive amino acids in particular cell layers. Not all terminals upon a given neuron were labeled and some labeling of nonneuronal elements also occurred. The radioautographic demonstration of stratified localization of GABA in certain tissues appears to correlate well with the distribution of GABA and glutamic acid decarboxylase activity (170).

Aromatic amines: a general discussion.—In contrast to most of the amino acid transmitters, the catecholamines (CAs) and serotonin (5-hydroxytryptamine, 5HT) are synthesized by specific enzymes localized to certain neurons in discrete neuronal systems. Ring-hydroxylation of an aromatic amino acid precursor is the first, most specific, and rate-limiting step in their synthesis, and is followed by immediate decarboxylation by a relatively nonspecific and very active L-aromatic amino acid decarboxylase. Relatively specific inhibitors of the hydroxylation of tyrosine (α-methyl-*p*-tyrosine) (145) and tryptophan (*p*-chlorophenylalanine) (113) exist. In norepinephrine (*NE*)-containing neurons a second nonspecific side-chain hydroxylation occurs at the β-carbon atom. Other aromatic amines are known to occur in the CNS; they include *p*-tyramine (131), octopamine (143), histamine (73), and unidentified indoleamines (22). The nonspecific L-aromatic amino acid decarboxylase responsible for the synthesis of CAs and 5HT provides the only known route of synthesis for tyramine and octopamine in the brain. It is not known whether these substances are formed in discrete neurons or if they are merely coproducts of the synthesis of other aromatic amines. There is evidence that histidine can be decarboxylated to histamine by an enzyme specific for histidine (73, 194).

Sensitive histochemical methods have permitted the examination of CAs and 5HT at the cellular level. These methods have made possible the description of amine-containing neuronal systems and firmly support the conclusion that these amines are highly concentrated at neuronal terminal varicosities (64). Subcellular distribution studies of the CNS reveal that these amines occur predominantly in synaptosomes and are further localized to synaptic vesicles (55, 204). Storage of CAs in intracellular vesicles and granules has been studied more intensively in peripheral tissues (66, 74, 112, 186) where, for example it appears that NE is stored in adrenal medullary granules as a complex with phosphorylated nucleotides, including ATP and Mg^{2+} in the presence of protein molecules called chromogranins, as well as dopamine-β-hydroxylase (112). Amines have been found to aggregate in vitro with several phosphonucleotides, particularly ATP (164), and the high molecular weight complexes so formed are disaggregated by high concentrations of divalent cations and by drugs such as reserpine and tyramine which interfere with the storage of amines in nerve endings (19).

The physiological importance of the high-affinity transport of catecholamines is well established in peripheral tissues and appears to terminate the actions of many neurotransmitters in the CNS (95). This process has been utilized to label endogenous stores of CAs in vivo by intraventricular injection of the amine to circumvent the blood-brain barrier (68), and has been studied in vitro with brain slices and synaptosomal preparations (14, 187, 197, 203). Thus the accumulation of several aromatic amines is temperature dependent and is inhibited by ouabain, by lack of Na^+, and by tricyclic antidepressant drugs, cocaine, reserpine, and several "anticholinergic" drugs used in the treatment of Parkinson's disease. It has been proposed that amine transport may be secondary to the provision of a $[Na^+]$ gradient across the neuronal membrane by the Na^+-pump associated with ATP-ase (197, 203). Regional differences in the uptake of CAs exist; the greatest accumulations occur in the corpus striatum in which the highest density of CA-containing nerve terminals occurs (187). Kinetic analysis revealed differences between the striatum, an area richest in dopamine (DA), and other areas where the predominant CA is NE (187). Uptake into DA-containing neurons, in which the endogenous CA is not β-hydroxylated, was not stereospecific at the β-carbon; it had high affinity for DA ($K_t = 0.08$ μM) but lower and equal affinities for d- and l-NE ($K_t = 1.6$ μM). In contrast, uptake into neurons in which the predominant CA is l-NE showed some stereospecificity (K_t for l- and d-NE, respectively, was 0.3 and 1.1 μM). 5HT was accumulated by a similar mechanism ($K_t = 0.2$ μM), but was also taken up by another less specific process ($K_t = 8.0$ μM) (187), possibly into CA-containing neurons (95, 187). While such uptake processes occur in isolated nerve endings (43), it is not certain whether similar transport normally occurs at other portions of the neuronal surface or in glia. Uptake of various transmitter substances into preparations enriched in glial cells was reported, although a small but critical contamination of the preparation by synaptosomes was not excluded (83). Due to the uniquely dense localization of vesicles, presumably used for storage of amines at presynaptic terminals, uptake there may be strongly favored. Present methods do not permit quantitative evaluation of the separate contributions of uptake at the plasma membrane and into the storage vesicles.

The vigorous uptake of CAs made it possible to destroy CA-containing neurons selectively, but partially by the action of accumulated 6-hydroxydopamine (198), a drug which produces "chemical sympathectomy" in peripheral adrenergic neurons (76). An hydroxylated indoleamine ("6-hydroxyserotonin") has been reported recently to produce an analogous selective destruction of central 5HT-containing neurons (17). Such selective destruction of specific neural systems offers a unique opportunity for future investigations of the functions of amine-containing neurons.

Several attempts have been made to estimate rates of turnover of amines in the CNS. Various methods give the impression that half-times of turnover are several minutes for histamine (177, 193), less than an hour for 5HT (125), and several hours for NE (152, 195). One difficulty in interpreting such estimates of overall rates of synthesis or of the disappearance of neurotransmitters in the CNS is that regional differences in turnover probably occur. For example, there appears to be an inverse relationship between turnover rates and endogenous content of NE in various parts of the brain (96); furthermore, spontaneous daily rhythms which involve up to fourfold changes in NE content occur in separate areas of the CNS and are strikingly asynchronous (168). It is also highly improbable that rates of turnover are equal throughout the cell, and evidence for differences in turnover between cell bodies and terminals has been obtained in the peripheral sympathetic nervous system (144). Even within nerve terminals, more than one compartment of transmitter molecules might exist, since newly synthesized NE (195) or DA (20) is released preferentially. Also, the presence of an efficient system for reuptake which recaptures within milliseconds most but not all of NE released at physiological rates of stimulation indicates that a transmitter molecule can be used many times before it is metabolized (34, 81, 95). Thus, estimates of the turnover rates or lifetimes of such molecules may not reveal rates of their physiological functions. Nevertheless, some indirect relationships must exist, as changes in rates of turnover of transmitter molecules have been observed in grossly differing states in intact animals, particularly during stress in contrast to hibernation (12, 200).

Catecholamines (CAs).—Tyrosine hydroxylation is the rate-limiting step in the synthesis of CAs, although the activity of pteridine reductase or the levels of the required reduced pteridine cofactor may be the important rate-limiting factors (149). Tyrosine hydroxylase occurs in brain and has been found in synaptosomal fractions (137). Although its intracellular localization is unsettled, association of this enzyme with synaptic vesicles has been reported (60). This claim is based on the finding that among subcellular fractions the vesicle fraction had the highest specific enzyme activity, although the enzyme activity in this fraction accounted for only 17% of the total. Tyrosine hydroxylase is a mixed function oxygenase which catalyzes the conversion of L-tyrosine to L-dopa and utilizes a tetrahydropteridine as cofactor. Recently the catalytic properties of partially purified tyrosine hydroxylase from beef adrenal medulla have been reexamined with tetrahydrobiopterin as cofactor, and the affinities of substrates and cofactor were found to be very different from those observed in earlier studies with another synthetic cofactor (181). Thus, in contrast to earlier findings, phenylalanine and tyrosine were hydroxylated at comparable rates in the presence of tetrahydrobiopterin. Furthermore, severe substrate inhibition by tyrosine, but not phenylalanine at concentrations only 2–3 times above K_m for tyrosine was observed. Synaptosomes prepared from brain catalyzed the biosynthesis of catechol compounds with an endogenous pteridine cofactor (107, 137), possibly tetrahydrobiopterin. Such nerve-ending preparations from several species formed catechol compounds from phenylalanine as well as tyrosine at comparable rates utilizing only the natural endogenous cofactor (109).

In recent years a great deal of attention has been given to possible ways of regulating the synthesis of amine transmitters. It has become apparent that the rate of CA synthesis varies with the degree of neuronal activity. An initial concept was that catechol products might inhibit tyrosine hydroxylase (188); this form of negative feedback is believed to occur by an interaction between catechols and the pteridine cofactor (149). In support of this idea, it has been found that exogenous CAs taken up from an incubation medium led to inhibition of tyrosine hydroxylation in synaptosomes (107) or cortical slices (79), and that disinhibition of synthesis of CAs was observed following release of CAs by elevated [K+] (79). The mechanism of product-inhibition is believed to depend on the level of catechols in the presence of the pteridine cofactor of tyrosine hydroxylase in the nerve ending. A variety of factors may alter these levels of products, including changes in neuronal activity produced by local or peripheral stimulation, and the effects of a variety of drugs acting to alter levels of catechols either locally or more indirectly by altering neuronal activity (3, 102, 200). Since the availability of the pteridine cofactor to tyrosine hydroxylase appears to be responsible for the short-term regulation of CA-synthesis, it is remarkable that almost nothing is known about its extract structure, concentration and regeneration, most likely by a soluble pteridine reductase (149), in central or peripheral adrenergic neurons although an enzyme which reduces oxidized pteridines in the brain has been described (148). In addition to this rapidly acting mechanism of modulating the rate of tyrosine hydroxylation, a second slower mechanism may also operate under extended and drastic demands placed on adrenergic neurons. Certain drugs and environmental stresses which deplete transmitter stores or decrease their synaptic effects appear to increase tyrosine hydroxylase, possibly by increased synthesis of new enzyme molecules, while other drugs which increase the availability of CAs at the synapse appear to produce an opposite change in levels of tyrosine hydroxylase (49, 178, 196).

A new assay has allowed the examination in brain of dopamine-β-hydroxylase, the final enzyme required for the synthesis of NE and octopamine (46). This enzyme is concentrated in noradrenergic nerve endings and appears to have a similar low affinity of substrate ($K_m = 0.9$ mM) and cofactor requirements as described previously for the adrenal medulla. The brain contains potent unidentified inhibitors of the enzyme which are inactivated by Cu^{2+}. An inhibitor of this enzyme in peripheral tissues has been partially characterized (41). The possible physiological importance of such inhibitors in regulating NE synthesis is unknown. The observation that amounts of exogenous L-dopa capable of producing large increases in levels of DA in brain, produce little or no increase in NE (37) suggests that β-hydroxylation might be a second limiting step in the synthesis of NE. There are several potent inhibitory drugs which block this enzyme (4, 84).

Serotonin (5HT).—This indoleamine and perhaps other indoleamines are found in central neurons (22, 118). The cell bodies of origin of 5HT-containing neurons are almost all located in the brain stem raphe nuclei (118). Central nerve terminals contain tryptophan 5-mono-oxygenase (117), a rate-limiting enzyme in the synthesis of 5HT which resembles tyrosine hydroxylase in its cofactor requirements (94). In contrast to tyrosine, however, tryptophan does not saturate the hydroxylase in vivo and synthesis of 5HT is dependent on tryptophan concentrations (70). By analogy to the regulation of CA-synthesis, control of tryptophan hydroxylation has been suggested. An inverse relationship between accumulation of 5HT from labeled tryptophan and endogenous 5HT levels was observed in vivo after inhibition of mono-amine oxidase (*MAO*) (129). On the other hand, it has not been possible to demonstrate such a mechanism in vitro with partially isolated nerve endings (108). Since synthesis of 5HT is dependent on tryptophan concentration in the CNS, regulation of the levels of this precursor could secondarily exert control on the entire synthetic pathway (70, 129). Maintenance of relatively steady levels of any amine in the CNS could be provided if rates of synthesis are in excess of the amounts of transmitter required for functional needs and if the excess is metabolized by intraneuronal MAO. This may occur since increased synthesis of 5HT by loading doses of tryptophan is followed by only small increases of 5HT but by large increases of 5-hydroxyindoleacetic acid (*5HIAA*) (70). If the assumption is valid that some amine transmitter substances including 5HT are synthesized at rates in excess of release onto the postsynaptic receptor, then this phenomenon would further support the conclusion that estimates of rates of "turnover" do not reflect the rates of utilization of a molecule as a transmitter (70).

Histamine.—This imidazoleamine which reacts as a diamine exists in the brain in extremely low concentrations (73). While much of the histamine in the median eminence and the neurohypophysis occurs in mast cells, there appears to be appreciable histamine in hypothalamic cells, including neurons, in several mammalian species, with consistently low levels throughout the remainder of the CNS (73). Recently methodological ambiguities in the assay of diamines in the brain have been resolved (73), and a new highly sensitive and specific assay has greatly facilitated the study of histamine (193, 194). Histamine is found in isolated nerve endings, and its redistribution during tissue fractionation, including binding to microsomal membranes, may account (119) for earlier reports of a unique histamine-containing fraction of small nerve-ending particles, although this has been disputed (139). There is evidence that histamine is synthesized from histidine by a specific decarboxylase which differs from aromatic amino acid decarboxylase in its sensitivity to inhibitors (177, 194). Since the K_m of the decarboxylase for histidine is greater than normal tissue levels of the substrate, synthesis of histamine can be increased by high doses of L-histidine (177, 193). Most of histamine in brains of several species appears to be 3-N-ring-methylated to form

"1,4"-methylhistamine, which is a substrate for MAO (73), and is converted to 1,4-methylimidazoleacetic acid, the major urinary metabolite of histamine (73, 175). With the possible exception of the rat brain, most mammalian brains do not have an amine oxidase specific for histamine so that the major pathway of histamine is ring-N-methylation (73, 175). There is no evidence for a high-affinity uptake for histamine and perhaps as a consequence, exogenous labeled histamine does not mix selectively with endogenous histamine in central neurons in vivo (119). Since imidazoleacetic acid has neuropharmacological activity in crustaceans and mammals (133) the possibility exists that metabolites of histamine may have important physiologic functions.

Polypeptides.—In addition to amino acids and amines, polypeptides have also been considered to be physiologically important neurosecretory substances. One group of such substances, known since the 1930s to have extraordinarily potent smooth-muscle-constricting and vasodilatory effects, is called "substance P" and has been partially characterized chemically (207). This material appears to be a group of similar polypeptides of molecular weight about 1400 which have many pharmacological and chemical similarities to the smaller kinins (91, 207). Recently, the amino acid sequence of one such 11-amino acid peptide from hypothalamus has been determined and the peptide has been synthesized (38). These peptides occur in the brain with an uneven regional distribution; the highest concentrations are in the substantia nigra (over 1500 $\mu g/g$ tissue), hypothalamus, and other subcortical centers (207). Substances P appear not to occur in glia but have been found in nerve ending particles; in addition, microsomal fractions contain a protease capable of inactivating substances P (91, 207). Such polypeptides are released from the cerebral cortex at rates that increase during peripheral sensory stimulation (180). They produce sedation and hypotension in the intact animal (10) and may release ACh at the cortex (207). As yet there is no known specific antagonist to their actions. Studies of this material have been limited because "substance P" is a complex and unstable mixture of compounds which are difficult to prepare in pure form. Although more work needs to be done on the biochemistry of these substances, it is interesting to note the apparent similarity between these peptides and the octapeptide neurosecretions of the neurohypophysis and to the polypeptide releasing-factors which affect the anterior pituitary hormones. The posterior pituitary hormones, similar to neurotransmitters are formed in neurons, stored in vesicles at neuronal terminals, and released by depolarization along with larger proteins (neurophysins) by a process which requires Ca^{2+} (174).

Release and inactivation of transmitter substances.—One line of evidence that implies that ACh and NE are neurotransmitters is their release at peripheral nerve terminals by stimulation or depolarization of preterminal axons. In the CNS, however, it is virtually impossible to design physiological experiments comparable to the use of an isolated perfused organ preparation with stimulation of a single nerve. Nevertheless, several attempts have been made to observe release of transmitter substances from intact animal brain. Most often the techniques employed have involved the collection of fluid bathing tissue in small cups placed on the cortex (101, 141) or on subcortical structures, following local removal of cortex (20) or by perfusing limited areas of the brain with small invasive cannulae (138), or by perfusing the cerebral ventricular system (160, 199). Such experiments have shown spontaneous efflux as well as increases in release of several amines and amino acids evoked by depolarizing stimuli. Recently several attempts have been made to correlate the rate of appearance of putative transmitters in locally superfusing fluid, with functional states or with activity in specific pathways. Thus, central stimulant drugs such as amphetamine have been shown to increase the rate of appearance of previously accumulated labeled NE (35); it is also reported that DA locally synthesized from labeled tyrosine can be released from the caudate nucleus by stimulant drugs (20) or by electrical stimulation of the substantia nigra (199). Electrical stimulation of cells in the raphe nuclei also led to increased formation of 5HIAA in the forebrain (1). Local efflux of endogenous ACh appeared from the auditory cortex during stimulation of the medial geniculate (82) and endogenous GABA was released from the visual cortex during electrophysiologically monitored inhibitory events (98). Furthermore, evidence has been presented that cerebellar stimulation increased the appearance of GABA in the fourth ventricle, possibly mediated by a Purkinje cell-vestibular nucleus pathway (155). Labeled DA also was released from the superfused retina in response to flashes of light (114).

Another approach to studying the release of transmitter substances has been the use of slices of brain tissue superfused in vitro and stimulated by electrical fields or high [K$^+$] (11, 111). In such experiments it has usually been necessary to measure the efflux of radioactively labeled transmitter molecules either previously taken up per se (11, 50, 78, 90, 105, 111) or formed from labeled precursors (111, 153). The availability of very sensitive assays has also permitted studies of the release of endogenous ACh (30) and histamine (194) from slices. Electrically evoked release from synaptosomes is technically difficult to achieve, although some selective release of amino acids thought to be involved in neurotransmission has been observed after prolonged electrical stimulation of synaptosomes (31, 51). Elevation of [K$^+$] of the suspending media resulted in augmentation of the rates of efflux of aromatic amines from synaptosomes (27). These in vitro studies demonstrated that presumed neurotransmitter substances can be released from CNS tissue by brief mild electrical stimuli or by depolarizing concentrations of K$^+$ by a process that requires Ca^{2+}. Several lines of evidence support the conclusion that most of the released material came from nerve endings. These include localization of the released molecules by electron microscopic radioautography, by subcellular distribution, by release of substances formed in nerve endings from precursors, and by interference with release by drugs which selectively block the transport and storage of transmitters or produce destruction of nerve endings (11, 105, 111, 153). Nevertheless, a general limitation of many experiments of this type is that some exogenous labeled molecules probably enter nerve endings in which they are not normally stored. In most reported studies, release of substances has been contrasted to the failure to release compounds for which there is negligible or only weak concentrative accumulation into cells (e.g. urea, inulin, water, amphetamine, or amino acids with low-affinity uptake), and which, therefore, might not be expected to be released.

Substances which have been shown to be released by the application of depolarizing stimuli to neuronal tissue are apparently all concentrated at nerve endings by high affinity transport (some amino acids) or local synthesis and storage (ACh) or both (CAs and 5HT). Thus descriptively, release appears to represent the redistribution of substances previously highly accumulated intracellularly, and it might occur with almost any substance so accumulated, whether or not it acts postsynaptically as a neurotransmitter. The general characteristics of those substances known to be released are that they can be rapidly accumulated locally in nerve endings to concentrations many times those of surrounding tissues or incubating media and accumulation usually appears to be dependent on the maintenance of physiological polarization of the cell membrane by Na^+ transport. One possibility then is that the "release" of some neurotransmitters may merely represent transient lapses in their accumulation during the shifts of cation concentrations which presumably mark the invasion of action potentials into nerve terminals. If more complex chemical events intervene between depolarization and the release of neurotransmitter molecules from central nerve terminals, they have not yet been described. Promising concepts may, however, emerge from studies of peripheral neurons. For example, when peripheral sympathetic nerves to the spleen (186, 201) or adrenal (112) are stimulated, release of CAs is accompanied by simultaneous release of other vesicular contents such as ATP, chromogranin proteins, and dopamine-β-hydroxylase by a process requiring Ca^{2+}. These observations support the concept that release of CAs from peripheral adrenergic neurons occurs from vesicular storage particles (66). The release of neurohormones from hypophysial nerve endings from storage particles along with neurophysin proteins by a process which requires Ca^{2+} (174) and the efflux of soluble proteins with ACh from cerebral synaptic vesicles (135) suggest that similar processes might occur at other central nerve terminals during release of neurotransmitters.

With the possible exceptions of ACh, for which uptake of uncertain physiologic importance has been reported (124, 176), and histamine, the actions of most proposed neurotransmitter substances are likely to be terminated by reuptake into presynaptic terminals. It is also possible that uptake into other cells such as glia might contribute to the inactivation of released transmitters (83, 87). If the concept of rapid reuptake is valid, then enzymatic modifications of transmitter molecules would probably play only lesser and secondary roles in physiological inactivation of released transmitters. This view is consistent with the observation that none of the enzymes involved in the degradative metabolism of transmitter amines or amino acids, with the exception of acetylcholinesterase, is found in pre- or postsynaptic neuronal membranes; GABA-transaminase and MAO are mitochondrial enzymes, and catechol-O-methyltransferase (COMT) is a ubiquitous soluble enzyme (68, 99, 170). These enzymes seem to function as scavengers of excess transmitter molecules which are not stored or reutilized for transmission, and inhibition of these enzymes results in increased levels of transmitters (68, 170).

It has recently become clear that in the CNS, reduction of the aldehyde products of MAO is more extensive than in peripheral organs (32), and a NADPH-linked aldehyde reductase, specific for aromatic aldehydes, has been characterized in brain (190). The removal of deaminated products from the CNS appears to involve transport from the CSF probably at the choroid plexus, by a process inhibited by probenecid (40). While it is known that the deaminated products of amines are to a great extent excreted as conjugates of glucuronide or sulfate, it has also been pointed out that sulfate conjugation of the amine 5HT can occur in brain (85). The physiological importance of this pathway as a means of inactivating 5HT is unknown, but it might become significant following the inhibition of deamination by drugs.

POSTSYNAPTIC BIOCHEMICAL ACTIONS OF SYNAPTIC TRANSMITTERS

Support for the possible role of several substances as central neurotransmitters has been gained by the use of microiontophoretic application of the substances to a very small area while simultaneously recording electrical responses of a subjacent neuron through another micropipette (25, 47, 48, 80, 116, 154, 156, 158). A common experience in general surveys of the actions of such highly biologically active substances was that either variable depolarizing or hyperpolarizing effects were obtained with the same substance (e.g. CAs and 5HT), or that a single molecule produced similar effects in many regions, with little apparent correlation to its endogenous distribution or suspected local functions (e.g. amino acids). Since such experiments represent pharmacological studies of the actions of potent substances which may or may not be applied to their physiological post-synaptic sites of action, these results are understandable. Recent iontophoretic experiments have concentrated on correlating pharmacological responses with the findings of regional neurochemistry in systems which are relatively well characterized cytoarchitecturally and electrophysiologically. Thus, for example, several studies have concentrated on the inhibitory inputs to the cerebellar Purkinje cells (206), to the descending outputs of cerebellar cells to the vestibular nuclei of the brainstem (156), to inhibitory effects on ventral spinal motoneurons (47), or to inhibitory effects on specific cells of the olfactory bulb (154). Generally, these attempts to specify probable local synaptic actions have been most successful with the inhibitory amino acids GABA and glycine.

Developmental studies of the rat cerebellum suggest that the responses of Purkinje cells to iontophoretically applied putative neurotransmitters resemble those of the adult CNS even at a time prior to the onset of synaptogenesis and in this system at least, postsynaptic "receptors" may be determined by intrinsic properties of the receptive neurons (205). It has not yet been directly demonstrated that topographical specification of receptivity to neurotransmitters occurs in the CNS on neuronal surfaces following the formation of synaptic contacts. Such events probably do occur since denervation in peripheral cholinergic or adrenergic systems leads to the phenomenon of "post-denervation supersensitivity." The observed increases in responsiveness of denervated tissues to applied neurotransmitter substances may be due to several factors, including not only an increased amount of "receptor" at the myoneural junction (140), and possibly in sympathetically denervated tissues (33), but also loss of inactivation mechanisms such as reuptake of NE (33).

In its most general form, the pharmacological concept of "receptor" postulates a specific chemical interaction between a "drug" or hormone molecule and specific sites in tissue, leading to a pharmacological action. In a more specific form, the concept of "receptor" for neurotransmitters usually postulates an initial interaction between a transmitter molecule and macromolecules of the postsynaptic neuronal plasma membrane, leading to the effects of the transmitter (65). Many attempts have been made to isolate and identify receptor molecules for neurotransmitters. These have usually involved the use of radioactively labeled agonists or antagonists of a neurotransmitter to bind to and thus specifically mark the tissue receptor sites for isolation (28, 52, 54, 58, 140, 150). When small molecules presumed to react with adrenergic or cholinergic receptors were used in such studies, binding to several subcellular fractions was observed and led to conflicting identifications of the macromolecular binding sites. This approach is limited by problems of specificity of the molecular interactions involved. Since the specificity of such interactions should vary directly with the size and complexity of the marker molecule, the use of labeled small molecules should increase the chance for nonspecific binding at sites other than the postsynaptic receptor. These sites might include pre- or postsynaptic "carriers" and enzymes involved in the transport and metabolism of the neurotransmitter as well as less specific interactions based on charge and lipid solubility. One approach to these problems has been to utilize specialized tissues containing a high density of receptor sites, such as the electric organs of certain species (39, 54, 58); unfortunately this approach is not possible with the mammalian CNS. Recently the irreversible binding of radioactively labeled α-bungarotoxin, a polypeptide constituent (mol wt 8000) of a snake venom which blocks neuromuscular cholinergic transmission, has been used to isolate a pure bungarotoxin-receptor complex from electric organ and skeletal muscle (140) as well as guinea pig cerebral cortex (28). The purified cerebral receptor complex appeared to be a protein and the estimated molecular weight of the complex was 94,000. The isolated material was devoid of activity of cholinesterase or several other enzymes. Selective interference with the binding of bungarotoxin by ACh, d-tubocurarine and gallamine, but not by atropine, suggested that the isolated material was of a nicotinic nature. If one molecule of the toxin is bound to one molecule of receptor, then guinea pig cerebral cortex contains a surprisingly large quantity of receptor: $17.5 \ nM$, or about 1.5 mg of nicotinic receptor per gram of wet tissue, assuming a molecular weight of 86,000 (28). Other physiologic and pharmacologic studies have suggested that cortical cholinergic receptors are either muscarinic or of intermediate types without clearly muscarinic or nicotonic features (158). The chemical nature of receptors of other proposed neurotransmitters is not known, although there is some evidence that adrenergic receptors do not behave pharmacologically as either α or β receptors as described in peripheral tissues (26, 158).

The postsynaptic actions of neurotransmitters in the CNS are not understood at a biochemical level. However, adenosine-3',5'-cyclic monophosphate (cAMP), believed to be involved in mediating the effects of various hormones and neurotransmitters in peripheral target tissues (171), may also have some importance in the CNS. Adenylcyclase (53), a phosphodiesterase specific for cAMP (53, 62), and a cAMP-dependent protein kinase (130) occur in mammalian brain and are found in high specific activities in synaptosomal or microsomal fractions. The activity of adenylcyclase in brain is the highest known of all mammalian tissues (53). The activity of 3,5-nucleotide phosphodiesterase has been localized by a cytochemical method postsynaptically at nerve endings (62). Furthermore, synthesis of cAMP in brain is stimulated by various substances, noteably depolarizing agents such as K^+ and veratridine, putative neurotransmitters such as NE, 5HT, and histamine, as well as adenosine (171, 182). This chemically induced stimulation of the synthesis of cAMP by adenyl cyclase can be prevented by a variety of drugs believed to be receptor-blocking agents in the periphery (171). However, there are great variations in responses to chemicals by the adenylcyclase system in slices or minces of brain prepared from different brain regions, different species or at various stages of development (171). The interpretation of these experiments is further complicated by the heterogeneity of the brain tissue used, since simultaneous responses of neural and glial cells are probably included (42). Of several approaches to reducing the complexity of tissues in such experiments, the use of subcellular fractionation techniques has not been very successful, since sensitivity of adenyl cyclase to putative neurotransmitters is almost lost by homogenization of most areas of the CNS (171). Another approach has been to use tissue cultures of single cell types, such as astrocytoma cells (42). It is also possible to use microiontophoretic techniques to study specific neurons in the intact brain. This latter approach has led to the suggestion that the inhibitory effect of NE upon Purkinje cells of the cerebellum may be mediated by cAMP, potentiated by theophylline, which inhibits the hydrolysis of cAMP by phosphodiesterase, and inhibited by prostaglandins E_1 and E_2 (183).

Several of the prostaglandins, a group of fatty acid derivatives, occur in the CNS, in the order of concentrations about $\mu g/g$ wet tissue (18). They do not seem to be associated with any specific cell fraction (89). Speculations about them include their possible role as neurotransmitters or in modifying postsynaptic effects of transmitters. Spontaneous and evoked release of prostaglandin-like substances at the cerebral cortex (166) and into the cerebral ventricles (88) have been reported. While small intraventricular doses of prostaglandins can have central depressant effects, the forms which are pharmacologically active do not necessarily correspond to the endogenous prostaglandins (93). Their effects when iontophoretically applied are complex and variable (86). The prostaglandins continue to be released even from sympathetically denervated peripheral tissues or following direct application of exogeneous NE and ACh (18, 159), and they can interfere with the effects of NE on Purkinje cells (159, 183). These and similar findings have led to the hypothesis that prostaglandins may be local postsynaptic tissue hormones involved in regulating the actions of transmitters, particularly since they can form rapidly from fatty acids, liberated by membrane phospholipases. Speculations about their mode of action include relations to the actions of cAMP and to the movement and binding of Ca^{2+} (18, 159).

SUMMARY AND CONCLUSIONS

Recent contributions to the biochemical physiology of central synapses were reviewed. A major problem for the field is to provide some degree of anatomical specificity in extremely complex tissue. Much attention has been given to the biochemistry of isolated nerve endings, or synaptosomes, which behave as miniature cells and resemble brain slices in their general metabolism. They are also able to synthesize protein locally, although the means for regulation of protein synthesis remote from the perikaryon is unknown. Similar to intact neurons, isolated nerve endings can also accumulate, store, and synthesize putative neurotransmitter molecules. Newer histochemical methods for enzymes involved in the metabolism of suspected neurotransmitters promise to complement the previously available fluorescence histochemical methods used to map systems of neurons containing specific biogenic amines. The somewhat restrictive models of synaptic transmission based on adrenergic and cholinergic transmission in the periphery are rapidly expanding as many new substances are considered as candidate neurotransmitters. Most of these are amino acids, amines, or small polypeptides.

An extremely important feature of nerve terminals is their ability to take up and store transmitter molecules by very efficient high-affinity transport processes. These processes are likely to be more important than enzymatic degradation to inactivate released transmitter molecules at most noncholinergic synapses. The uptake processes also provide relative anatomical specificity in the use of radioactively labeled transmitter molecules to study metabolism, or as markers to isolate nerve endings by ultracentrifugation and to localize transmitters by radioautography; in addition they permit the selective accumulation of toxic substances which lead to the destruction of specific nerve endings. One possibility is that the release of some neurotransmitters may represent a lapse in the uptake and accumulation process during membrane depolarization.

The synthesis of neurotransmitters seems to be very responsive to immediate and prolonged changes in functional demands upon synaptic transmission. It is unclear whether the short-term means of regulation of catecholamine synthesis by end-product inhibition at the rate-limiting enzyme occurs for other amines. The availability of cofactors and of substrates may also be important in the regulation of the synthesis of neurotransmitters. Measurements of overall turnover of transmitters in the whole brain are of little use in evaluating physiological rates of utilization of transmitters at specific synapses.

The relatively specific interactions between binding sites of neurotransmitters and large marker molecules such as [³H]α-bungarotoxin for cholinergic synapses has facilitated tentative attempts to isolate postsynaptic "receptors," but the use of smaller agonists or antagonists of transmitters is likely to provide less specific interactions. The postsynaptic biochemical events at central synapses are poorly understood, although there is some evidence to suggest that prostaglandins and cyclic AMP may be involved.

LITERATURE CITED

1. Aghajanian, G. K., Rosecrans, J. A., Sheard, M. H. 1967. Serotonin: release in the forebrain by stimulation of midbrain raphe. *Science* 156:402–3
2. Agrawall, H. C., Davison, A. N., Kaczmarek, L. K. 1971. Subcellular distribution of taurine and cysteinesulfinate decarboxylase in developing rat brain. *Biochem. J.* 122:759–63
3. Andén, N.-E., Corrodi, H., Fuxe, K., Ungerstedt, U. 1972. Importance of nervous impulse flow for the neuroleptic induced increase in amine turnover in central dopamine neurons. *Eur. J. Pharmacol.* 15:193–99
4. Andén, N.-E., Fuxe, K. 1971. A new dopamine-β-hydroxylase inhibitor: effects on the noradrenaline concentration and on the action of L-dopa on the spinal cord. *Brit. J. Pharmacol.* 43:747–56.
5. Ansell, G. B., Spanner, S. 1971. Studies on the origin of choline in the brain of the rat. *Biochem. J.* 122:741–50
6. Ata, A., Abdel-Latif, A. A., Smith, J. P., Hedrick, N. 1970. Adenosinetriphosphatase and nucleotide metabolism in synaptosomes of rat brain. *J. Neurochem.* 17:391–401
7. Austin, L., Morgan, I. G., Bray, J. J. 1970. The biosynthesis of proteins within axons and synaptosomes. In *Protein Metabolism of the Nervous System,* ed. A Lajtha, 271–89. New York: Plenum
8. Autillio, L. A., Appel, S. H., Pettis, P., Gambetti, P. L. 1968. Biochemical studies of synapses *in vitro*: I. Protein synthesis. *Biochemistry* 7:2615–22
9. Axelsson, J. 1971. Catecholamine functions. *Ann. Rev. Physiol.* 33:1–30
10. Baile, C. A., Meinardi, H. 1967. Action of substance P on the central nervous system of a goat. *Brit. J. Pharmacol.* 30:302–6
11. Baldessarini, R. J. 1971. Release of aromatic amines from brain tissues of the rat *in vitro*. *J. Neurochem.* 18:2509–18
12. Baldessarini, R. J. 1972. Biogenic

amines and behavior. *Ann. Rev. Med.* 23:343–54
13. Baldessarini, R. J., Karobath, M. 1972. Effects of L-dopa and L-3-0-methyldopa on uptake of [³H]L-methionine by synaptosomes. *Neuropharmacology* 11: In press
14. Baldessarini, R. J., Vogt, M. 1971. The uptake and subcellular distribution of aromatic amines in the brain of the rat. *J. Neurochem.* 18:2519–33
15. Barondes, S. H. 1968. Incorporation of radioactive glucosamine into macromolecules at nerve endings. *J. Neurochem.* 15: 699–706
16. Battistin, L., Grynbaum, A., Lajtha, A. 1969. Distribution and uptake of amino acids in various regions of the cat brain *in vitro*. *J. Neurochem.* 16: 1459–68
17. Baumgarten, H. G., Lachenmayer, L. 1972. Chemically induced degeneration of indoleamine-containing nerve terminals in rat brain. *Brain Res.* 38:228–32
18. Bergström, S., Carlson, L. A., Weeks, J. R. 1968. The prostaglandins: a family of biologically active lipids. *Pharmacol. Rev.* 29:1–48
19. Berneis, K. H., Pletscher, A., Da Prada, M. 1970. Phase separation in solutions of noradrenaline and adenosine triphosphate: influence of bivalent cations and drugs. *Brit. J. Pharmacol.* 39:382–89
20. Besson, M.-J., Cheramy, A., Feltz, P., Glowinski, J. 1971. Dopamine: spontaneous and drug induced release from the caudate nucleus in the cat. *Brain Res.* 32:407–24
21. Bhatnagar, S. P., MacIntosh, F. C. 1967. Effects of quarternary bases and inorganic cations on acetylcholine synthesis in nervous tissue. *Can. J. Physiol. Pharmacol.* 45:249–68
22. Björklund, A., Falck, B., Stenesi, U. 1971. Classification of monoamine neurones in the rat mesencephalon: distribution of a new monoamine neurone system. *Brain Res.* 32:269–85
23. Blaustein, M. P., Wiesmann, W. P.

1970. Effect of sodium ions on calcium movements in isolated synaptic terminals. *Proc. Nat. Acad. Sci. USA.* 66:664–71

24. Bloom, F. E. 1970. The fine structural localization of biogenic monomines in nervous tissue. *Int. Rev. Neurobiol.* 13:27–66

25. Bloom, F. E., Hoffer, B. J., Siggins, G. R., Barker, J. L., Nicoll, R. A. 1972. Effects of serotonin on central neurons: microiontophoretic administration. *Fed. Proc.* 31:97–106

26. Boakes, R. J., Bradley, P. B., Brookes, N., Candy, J. M., Wolstencroft, J. H. 1969. Effects of noradrenaline and its analogues on brainstem neurones. *J. Physiol. London* 201:20–21P

27. Bogdanski, D. F., Tissari, A., Brodie, B. B. 1968. Role of sodium, potassium, ouabain and reserpine in uptake, storage and metabolism of biogenic amines in synaptosomes. *Life Sci.* 7:419–28

28. Bosmann, H. B. 1972. Acetylcholine receptor. *J. Biol. Chem.* 247:130–45

29. Bosmann, H. B., Hemsworth, B. A. 1970. Intraneural mitochondria: incorporation of amino acids and monosaccharides into macromolecules by isolated synaptosomes and synaptosomal mitochondria. *J. Biol. Chem.* 245: 363–71

30. Bowers, M. B., Jr. 1967. Factors influencing maintenance and release of acetylcholine in rat cortical brain slices. *Int. J. Neuropharmacol.* 6:399–403

31. Bradford, H. F. 1969. Metabolic response of synaptosomes to electrical stimulation: release of amino acids. *Brain Res.* 19: 239–47

32. Breese, G. R., Chase, T. N., Kopin, I. J. 1969. Metabolism of some phenylethylamines and their β-hydroxylated analogs in brain. *J. Pharmacol. Exp. Ther.* 165:9–13

33. Brimijoin, S., Pluchino, S., Trendelenburg, U. 1970. On the mechanism of super-sensitivity to norepinephrine in the denervated cat spleen. *J. Pharmacol. Exp. Ther.* 175:503–13

34. Brown, G. L. 1965. The Croonian Lecture, 1964. The release and fate of the transmitter liberated by adrenergic nerves. *Proc. Roy. Soc. B.* 162:1–19

35. Carr, L. A., Moore, K. E. 1970. Release of norepinephrine and normetanephrine from cat brain by central nervous system stimulants *Biochem. Pharmacol.* 19:2671–75

36. Chakrin, L. W., Whittaker, V. P. 1969. The subcellular distribution of [N-Me-³H]-acetylcholine synthesized in brain *in vivo. Biochem. J.* 113:97–107

37. Chalmers, J., Baldessarini, R. J., Wurtman, R. J. 1971. Effects of L-dopa on norepinephrine metabolism in the brain. *Proc. Nat. Acad. Sci. USA* 68:662–66

38. Chang, M. M., Leeman, S. E., Niall, H. D. 1971. Amino acid sequence of substance P. *Nature, New Biol.* 232:86–87

39. Changeux, J.-P., Kasai, N., Lee, C. Y. 1970. Use of a snake venom toxin to characterize the cholinergic receptor protein. *Proc. Nat. Acad. Sci. USA* 67: 1241–47

40. Chase, T. N., Katz, R. I., Kopin, I. J. 1970. Effect of diazepam on fate of intracisternally injected serotonin-C¹⁴. *Neuropharmacology* 9:103–8

41. Chubb, I. W., Preston, B. N., Austin, L. 1969. Partial characterization of a naturally occurring inhibitor of dopamine-β-hydroxylase. *Biochem. J.* 111:243–44

42. Clark, R. B., Perkins, J. P. 1971. Regulation of adenosine 3′:5′-cyclic monophosphate concentration in cultured human astrocytoma cells by catecholamines and histamine. *Proc. Nat. Acad. Sci. USA* 68:2757–60

43. Colburn, R. W., Goodwin, F. K., Murphy, D. L., Bunney, W. E., Jr., Davis, J. M. 1968. Quantitative studies of norepinephrine uptake by synaptosomes. *Biochem. Pharmacol.* 17:957–64

44. Collier, B., Poon, P., Salehoghaddam, S. 1972. The formation of choline and of acetylcholine by brain *in vitro. J. Neurochem.* 19:51–60

45. Cotman, C. W., Taylor, D. A. 1971. Autoradiographic analysis

of protein synthesis in synaptosomal fractions. *Brain Res.* 29: 366–72

46. Coyle, J. T., Axelrod, J. 1972. Dopamine-β-hydroxylase in the rat brain: developmental characteristics. *J. Neurochem.* 19: 449–59

47. Curtis, D. R., Duggan, A. W., Johnston, G. A. R. 1970. Inactivation of extracellularly administered amino acids in the feline spinal cord. *Exp. Brain Res.* 10:447–62

48. Curtis, D. R., Feliz, D. 1971. The effect of bicuculline upon synaptic inhibition in the cerebral and cerebellar cortices of the cat. *Brain Res.* 34:301–21

49. Dairman, W., Udenfriend, S. 1971. Decrease in adrenal tyrosine hydroxylase and increase in norepinephrine synthesis in rats given L-dopa. *Science* 171: 1022–24

50. Davison, A. N., Kaczmarek, L. K. 1971. Taurine—a possible neurotransmitter? *Nature* 234: 107–8

51. De Belleroche, J. S., Bradford, H. F. 1972. Metabolism of beds of mammalian cortical synaptosomes: response to depolarizing influences. *J. Neurochem.* 19: 585–602

52. De Robertis, E. 1971. Molecular biology of synaptic receptors. *Science* 171:963–71

53. De Robertis, E., Rodriguez de Lores Arnaiz, G., Alberici, M., Butcher, R. W., Sutherland, E. W. 1967. Subcellular distribution of adenylcyclase and cyclic phosphodiesterase in rat brain cortex. *J. Biol. Chem.* 242: 3487–93

54. De Robertis, E., Lunt, G. S., LaTorre, J. L. 1971. Multiple binding sites for acetylcholine in a proteolipid from electric tissue. *Mol. Pharmacol.* 7:97–103

55. De Robertis, E., Rodriguez de Lores Arnaiz, G. 1969. Structural components of the synaptic region. In *Handbook of Neurochemistry, Vol. II*, ed. A. Lajtha, 365–92. New York: Plenum

56. Diamond, I., Kennedy, E. P. 1969. Carrier-mediated transport of choline into synaptic nerve endings. *J. Biol. Chem.* 244:3258–63

57. Ehinger, B., Falck, B. 1971. Autoradiography of some suspected neurotransmitter substances: GABA, glycine, glutamic acid, histamine, dopamine and L-dopa. *Brain Res.* 33:157–72

58. Eldefrawi, M. E., Eldefrawi, A. T., O'Brien, R. C. 1971. Binding of five cholinergic ligands to housefly brain and torpedo electroplax. *Mol. Pharmacol.* 7:104–10

59. Escueta, A. V., Appel, S. H. 1969. Biochemical studies of synapses in vitro. II. Potassium Transport. *Biochemistry* 8:725–33

60. Fahn, S., Rodman, J. S., Coté, L. J. 1969. Association of tyrosine hydroxylase with synaptic vesicles in bovine cuadate nucleus. *J. Neurochem.* 16: 1293–1300

61. Festoff, B. W., Appel, S. H., Day, E. 1971. Incorporation of [14C] glucosamine into synaptosomes in vitro. *J. Neurochem.* 18: 1871–86

62. Florendo, N. T., Barrnett, R. J., Greengard, P. 1971. Cyclic 3′,-5′nucleotide phosphodiesterase: cytochemical localization in cerebral cortex. *Science* 173: 745–47

63. Fonnum, F. 1968. Choline acetyltransferase binding to and release from membranes. *Biochem. J.* 109:389–98

64. Fuxe, K., Hökfelt, T., Ungerstedt, U. 1970. Morphological and functional aspects of central monoamine neurons. *Int. Rev. Neurobiol.* 13:93–126

65. Garland, J. T., Durell, J. 1970. Chemical mechanisms of transmitter-receptor interaction. *Int. Rev. Neurobiol.* 13:159–80

66. Geffen, L. B., Livett, B. G. 1971. Synaptic vesicles in sympathetic neurons. *Physiol. Rev.* 51:98–157

67. Gilbert, J. 1972. Evidence for protein synthesis in synaptosomal membranes. *J. Biol. Chem.* 247: 6541–50

68. Glowinski, J., Baldessarini, R. J. 1966. Metabolism of norepinephrine in the central nervous system. *Pharmacol. Rev.* 18: 1201–38

69. Gordon, M. K., Bensch, K. G.,

Deanin, G. G., Gordon, M. W. 1968. Histochemical and biochemical study of synaptic lysosomes. *Nature* 217:523–27

70. Grahame-Smith, D. G. 1971. Studies *in vivo* on the relationship between brain tryptophan, brain 5HT synthesis and hyperactivity in rats treated with a monoamine oxidase inhibitor and L-tryptophan. *J. Neurochem.* 18:1053–66

71. Grahame-Smith, D. G., Parfitt, A. G. 1970. Tryptophan transport across the synaptosomal membrane. *J. Neurochem.* 17:1939–53

72. Gray, E. G., Willis, R. A. 1970. On synaptic vesicles, complex vesicles and dense projections. *Brain Res.* 24:149–68

73. Green, J. P. 1970. Histamine. In *Handbook of Neurochemistry*, Vol. *IV*, ed. A. Lajtha, 221–50. New York:Plenum

74. Goetz, U., Da Prada, M., Pletscher, A. 1971. Adenine, guanine- and uridine-5'-phosphonucleotides in blood platelets and storage organelles of various species. *J. Pharmacol. Exp. Ther.* 178:210–15

75. Guth, P. S. 1969. Acetylcholine binding by isolated synaptic vesicles *in vitro*. *Nature* 224:384–85

76. Haeusler, G., Haefely, W., Thoenen, H. 1969. Chemical sympathectomy of the cat with 6-hydroxydopamine. *J. Pharmacol. Exp. Ther.* 170:50–61

77. Haga, T. 1971. Synthesis and release of [C14]acetylcholine in synaptosomes. *J. Neurochem.* 18:781–98

78. Hammerstad, J. P., Murray, J. E., Cutler, R. W. P. 1971. Efflux of amino acid neurotransmitters from rat spinal cord slices. II. Factors influencing the electrically induced efflux of [14C] glycine and [3H]GABA. *Brain Res.* 35:337–55

79. Harris, J. E., Roth, R. H. 1971. Potassium-induced acceleration of catecholamine biosynthesis in brain slices. *Mol. Pharmacol.* 7:593–604

80. Hebb, C. 1970. CNS at the cellular level: identity of transmitter agents. *Ann. Rev. Physiol.* 32:165–92

81. Hedqvist, P., Stajärne, L. 1969. The relative role of recapture and of de novo synthesis for the maintenance of neurotransmitter homeostasis in noradrenergic nerves. *Acta Physiol. Scand.* 76:270–83

82. Hemsworth, B. A., Mitchell, J. F. 1969. The characteristics of acetylcholine release mechanisms in the auditory cortex. *Brit. J. Pharmacol* 36:161–70

83. Henn, F. A., Hamberger, A. 1971. Glial cell function: uptake of transmitter substances. *Proc. Nat. Acad. Sci. USA* 68:2686–90

84. Hidaka, H. 1971. Fusaric (5-butylpicolinic) acid, an inhibitor of dopamine-β-hydroxylase, affects serotonin and noradrenaline. *Nature* 231:54–55

85. Hidaka, H., Nagatsu, T., Yagi, K., 1969. Occurrence of a serotonin sulfotransferase in the brain. *J. Neurochem.* 16:783–85

86. Hoffer, B. J., Siggins, G. R., Bloom, F. E. 1969. Prostaglandins E1 and E2 antagonize norepinephrine effects on cerebellar Purkinje cells: microiontophoretic study. *Science* 166:1418–20

87. Hökfelt, T., Ljungdahl, Å. 1971. Light and electron microscopic autoradiography on spinal cord slices after incubation with labeled glycine. *Brain Res.* 32:189–94

88. Holmes, S. W. 1970. The spontaneous release of prostaglandins into the cerebral ventricles of the dog and the effect of external factors on this release. *Brit. J. Pharmacol.* 38:653–58

89. Hopkin, J. M., Horton, E. W., Whittaker, V. P. 1968. Prostaglandin content of particulate and supernatant factions of rabbit brain homogenates. *Nature* 217:71–2

90. Hopkin, J. M., Neal, M. J. 1970. The release of 14C-glycine from electrically stimulated rat spinal cord slices. *Brit. J. Pharmacol.* 4:136–37P

91. Hori, S. 1968. The presence of a bradykinin-like polypeptide, kinin releasing and destroying activity in brain. *Jap. J. Physiol.* 18:772–87

92. Hornykiewicz, O. 1966. Dopamine (3-hydroxy-tyramine) and brain

function. *Pharmacol. Rev.* 18: 925–64

93. Horton, E. W., Main, J. H. M. 1967. Further observations on the central nervous actions of prostaglandins F$_{2a}$ and E$_1$. *Brit. J. Pharmacol. Chemother.* 30: 568–81

94. Ichiyama, A., Nakamura, S., Nishizuka, Y., Hayaishi, O. 1970. Enzymic studies on the biosynthesis of serotonin in mammalian brain. *J. Biol. Chem.* 245:1699–1709

95. Iversen, L. L. 1971. Role of transmitter uptake mechanisms in synaptic neurotransmission. *Brit. J. Pharmacol.* 41:571–91

96. Iversen, L. L., Glowinski, J. 1966. Regional studies of catecholamines in the rat brain II. Rate of turnover of catecholamines in various brain regions. *J. Neurochem.* 13:671–82

97. Iversen, L. L., Johnston, G. A. R. 1971. GABA uptake in rat central nervous system: comparison of uptake in slices and homogenates and the effects of some inhibitors. *J. Neurochem.* 18:1939–50

98. Iversen, L. L., Mitchell, J. F., Srinivasan, V. 1971. The release of γ-aminobutyric acid during inhibition in the cat visual cortex. *J. Physiol. London* 212:519–34

99. Jarrott, B. 1971. Occurrence and properties of catechol-O-methyl transferase in adrenergic neurons. *J. Neurochem.* 18:17–27

100. Jasinski, A., Gorbman, A., Hara, T. J. 1966. Rate of movement and redistribution of stainable neurosecretory granules in hypothalamic neurons. *Science* 154:776–78

101. Jasper, H. H., Koyama, I. 1969. Rate of release of amino acids from the cerebral cortex in the cat as affected by brainstem and thalamic stimulation. *Can. J. Physiol. Pharmacol.* 47:889–905

102. Javoy, F., Hamon, M., Glowinski, J. 1970. Disposition of newly synthesized amines in cell bodies and terminals of central catecholaminergic neurons. *Eur. J. Pharmacol.* 10:178–88

103. Johnson, J. L. 1972. Glutamic acid as a synaptic transmitter in the nervous system. A Review. *Brain Res.* 37:1–19

104. Johnston, G. A. R., Iversen, L. L. 1971. Glycine uptake in rat central neurons system slices and homogenates: evidence for different uptake systems in spinal coral and cerebral cortex. *J. Neurochem.* 18:1951–61

105. Johnston, G. A. R., Mitchell, J. F. 1971. The effect of bicuculline, metrazol, picrotoxin and strychnine on the release of [³H]GABA from rat brain slices. *J. Neurochem.* 18: 2441–46

106. Karlsson, J-O., Sjöstrand, J. 1969. The effect of colchicine on the axonal transport of protein in the optic nerve and tract of the rabbit. *Brain Res.* 13:617–19

107. Karobath, M. 1971. Catecholamines and the hydroxylation of tyrosine in synaptosomes isolated from rat brain. *Proc. Nat. Acad. Sci. USA* 68:2370–73

108. Karobath, M. 1972. Serotonin synthesis with rat brain synaptosomes. *Biochem. Pharmacol.* 21:1253–63

109. Karobath, M., Baldessarini, R. J. 1972. Formation of catechol compounds from phenylalanine and tyrosine with isolated nerve endings. *Nature, New Biol.* 236:206–8

110. Kasa, P., Morris, D. 1972. Inhibition of choline acetyltransferase and its histochemical localization. *J. Neurochem.* 19:1299–1304

111. Katz, R. I., Chase, T. N. 1970. Neurohumoral mechanisms in the brain slice. *Advan. Pharmacol. Chemother.* 8:1–30

112. Kirshner, N., Kirshner, A. G. 1971. Chromagranin A, dopamine β-hydroxylase and secretion from the adrenal medulla. *Phil. Trans. Roy. Soc. London B* 261:279–89

113. Koe, B. K., Weissman, A. 1966. p-chlorophenylalanine: a specific depletor of brain serotonin. *J. Pharmacol. Exp. Ther.* 154: 499–516

114. Kramer, S. G. 1971. Dopamine: a retinal neurotransmitter. *Invest. Ophthalmol.* 10:438–52

115. Kreutzenberg, G. W. 1969. Neuronal dynamics and axonal flow, IV. Blockage of intra-ax-

onal enzyme transport by colchicine. *Proc. Nat. Acad. Sci. USA* 62:722–28

116. Krnjevic, K., Schwartz, S. 1967. Some properties of unresponsive cells in the cerebral cortex. *Exp. Brain Res.* 3:306–19

117. Kuhar, M. J., Roth, R. H., Aghajanian, G. K. 1971. Selective reduction of tryptophan hydroxylase activity in rat forebrain after midbrain raphe lesions. *Brain Res.* 35:167–76

118. Kuhar, M. J., Roth, R. H., Aghajanian, G. K. 1972. Synaptosomes from forebrains of rats with midbrain raphe lesions: selective reduction of serotonin uptake. *J. Pharmacol. Exp. Ther.* 181:36–45

119. Kuhar, M. J., Taylor, K. M., Snyder, S. H. 1971. The subcellular localization of histamine and histamine methyltransferase in rat brain. *J. Neurochem.* 18:1515–27

120. Lagercrantz, H., Pertoft, H. 1972. Separation of catecholamine storing synaptosomes in colloidal silica density gradients. *J. Neurochem.* 19:811–23

121. Lajtha, A., Ed. 1970. *Handbook of Neurochemistry, Vol. IV, Control Mechanisms in the Central Nervous System.* New York: Plenum

122. Lam, D. M. K., Steinman, L., 1971. The uptake of [^{3}H]-γ-aminobutyric acid in the goldfish retina. *Proc. Nat. Acad. Sci. USA* 68:2777–81

123. Lasek, R. 1968. Axoplasmic transport in cat dorsal root ganglion cells: as studied with [^{3}H]L-leucine. *Brain Res.* 7:36–77

124. Liang, C. C., Quastel, J. H. 1969. Uptake of acetylcholine in rat brain cortex slices. *Biochem. Pharmacol.* 18:1169–85

125. Lin, R. C., Costa, E., Neff, N. H., Wang, C. T., Ngai, S. H. 1969. *In vivo* measurement of 5-hydroxytryptamine turnover rate in the rat brain from the conversion of C^{14}-tryptophan to C^{14}-5-hydroxytryptamine. *J. Pharmacol. Exp. Ther.* 170:232–38

126. Ling, C.-M., Abdel-Latif, A. A. 1968. Studies on sodium transport in rat brain nerve ending particles. *J. Neurochem.* 15:721–29

127. Livett, B. G., Geffen, L. B., Austin, L. 1968. Axoplasmic transport of C^{14}-noradrenaline and protein in splenic nerves. *Nature* 217:278–79

128. Loban, W. J., Snyder, S. H. 1971. Unique high affinity uptake systems for glycine, glutamine and aspartic acids in central nervous tissue of the rat. *Nature* 234:297–99

129. Macon, J. B., Sokoloff, L., Glowinski, J. 1971. Feedback control of rat brain 5-hydroxytryptamine synthesis. *J. Neurochem.* 18:321–31

130. Maeno, H., Johnson, E. M., Greengard, P. 1971. Subcellular distribution of adenosine 3′-5′-monophosphate-dependent protein kinase in rat brain. *J. Biol. Chem.* 246:134–42

131. Majer, J. R., Boulton, A. A. 1970. Absolute, unambiguous ultramicroanalysis of metabolites present in complex biological extracts. *Nature* 225:658–60

132. Mangan, J. L., Whittaker, V. P. 1966. The distribution of free amino acids in subcellular fractions of guinea pig brain. *Biochem. J.* 98:128–37

133. Marcus, R. J., Winters, W. D., Roberts, E., Simonsen, D. G. 1971. Neuropharmacological studies of imidazole-4-acetic acid actions in the mouse and rat. *Neuropharmacology* 10:203–15

134. Martin, D. L., Smith, A. A., III 1972. Ions and the transport of gamma-aminobutyric acid by synaptosomes. *J. Neurochem.* 19:841–55

135. Matsuda, T., Saito, K., Katsuki, S., Hata, F., Yoshida, H. 1971. Studies on soluble proteins released from the synaptic vesicles of rat brain cortex. *J. Neurochem.* 18:713–19

136. McEwen, B., Grafstein, B. 1968. Fast and slow components in axonal transport of protein. *J. Cell. Biol.* 38:494–508

137. McGeer, P. L., Bagchi, S. P., McGeer, E. G. 1965. Subcellular localization of tyrosine hydroxylase in beef caudate nucleus. *Life Sci.* 4:1859–67

138. McLennan, A. 1964. The release

of acetylcholine and 3-hydroxytyramine from the caudate nucleus. *J. Physiol. London* 174: 152–61

139. Michaelson, I. A., Smithson, H. R. 1971. Relative redistribution of [³H]histamine and [¹⁴C]spermidine in homogenates of dog brain. *Biochem. Pharmacol.* 20: 2091–94

140. Miledi, R., Potter, L. T. 1971. Acetylcholine receptors in muscle fibers. *Nature* 233:599–603

141. Mitchell, J. F. 1963. The spontaneous and evoked release of acetylcholine from the cerebral cortex. *J. Physiol. London* 165: 98–116

142. Molinoff, P. B., Axelrod, J. 1971. Biochemistry of catecholamines. *Ann. Rev. Biochem* 540:465–500

143. Molinoff, P. B., Axelrod, J. 1972. Distribution and turnover of octopamine in tissues. *J. Neurochem.* 19:157–63

144. Moore, K. E., Bhatnagar, R. K. 1972. Regulation of norepinephrine contents in neuronal cell bodies and terminals during and after cessation of preganglionic stimulation. *J. Pharmacol. Exp. Ther.* 180:265–76

145. Moore, K. E., Dominic, J. A. 1971. Tyrosine hydroxylase inhibitors. *Fed. Proc.* 30:859–70

146. Morris, S. J., Ralston, H. J., III, Shooter, E. M. 1971. Studies on the turnover of mouse brain synaptosomal protein. *J. Neurochem.* 18:2279–90

147. Mountcastle, V. B., Baldessarini, R. J. 1973. Synaptic transmission. In *Medical Physiology,* ed. V. B. Mountcastle, chapter 6. St. Louis: Mosby In press

148. Musacchio, J. M., Craviso, G. L., Wurzburger, R. J. 1972. Dihydropteridine reductase in the rat brain. *Life Sci. (Part II)* 11:267–76

149. Musacchio, J. M., D'Angelo, G. L., McQueen, C. A. 1971. Dihydropteridine reductase: implication on the regulation of catecholamine biosynthesis. *Proc. Nat. Acad. Sci. USA* 68:2087–91

150. Namba, T., Grob, D. 1967. Ribonucleoprotein in human skeletal muscle with affinity for d-tubo-

curarine and acetylcholine. *Biochem. Pharmacol.* 16:1135–38

151. Neal, M. J., Iversen, L. L. 1972. Autoradiographic localization of ³H-GABA in rat retina. *Nature* 235:217–18

152. Neff, N. H., Ngai, S. H., Wang, C. T., Costa, E. 1969. Calculation of the rate of catecholamine synthesis from the rate of conversion of tyrosine-¹⁴C to catecholamines. *Mol. Pharmacol.* 5:90–99

153. Ng, K. Y., Chase, T. N., Colburn, R. W., Kopin, I. J. 1971. Dopamine: stimulation-induced rerelease from central neurons. *Science* 172:487–89

154. Nicoll, R. A. 1971. Pharmacological evidence for GABA as the transmitter in granule cell inhibition in the olfactory bulb. *Brain Res.* 35:137–49

155. Obata, K., Takeda, K. 1969. Release of γ-aminobutyric acid into the fourth ventricle induced by stimulation of the cat's cerebellum. *J. Neurochem.* 16:1043–47

156. Obata, K., Takeda, K., Shinozaki, H. 1970. Further study on pharmacological properties of the cerebellar-induced inhibition of Deiters neurones. *Exp. Brain Res.* 11:327–42

157. Ochs, S., Ranish, N. 1970. Metabolic dependence of fast axoplasmic transport in nerve. *Science* 167:878–79

158. Phyllis, J. W. 1970. *The Pharmacology of Synapses.* Oxford: Pergamon

159. Pickles, V. R. 1967. The prostaglandins. *Biol. Rev.* 42:614–52

160. Portig, P. J., Vogt, M. 1969. Release into the cerebral ventricles of substances with possible transmitter function in the caudate nucleus. *J. Physiol. London* 204:687–715

161. Potter, L. T. 1970. Synthesis, storage and release of [¹⁴C] acetylcholine in isolated rat diaphragm muscles. *J. Physiol. London* 206:145–66

162. Potter, L. T., Glover, V. A. S. 1971. Metabolism of Amino Acids and Amines. In *Methods in Enzymology, Vol. XVII B,* ed. S. P. Colowick, N. O. Ka-

plan, 798–801. New York:Academic

163. Pradhan, S. N., Dutta, S. N. 1971. Central cholinergic mechanisms and behavior. *Int. Rev. Neurobiol.* 14:173–231

164. Rajan, K. S., Davis, J. M., Colburn, R. W., Jarke, F. H. 1972. Metal chelates in the storage and transport of neurotransmitters:formation of mixed ligand chelates of Mg^{2+}-ATP with biogenic amines. *J. Neurochem.* 19:1099–1116

165. Rama Sastry, B. V., Henderson, G. I. 1972. Kinetic mechanisms of human placental choline acetyltransferase. *Biochem. Pharmacol.* 21:787–802

166. Ramwell, P. W., Shaw, J. E. 1966. The spontaneous and evoked release of prostaglandins from the cerebral cortex of anaesthetized cats. *Am. J. Physiol.* 211:125–34

167. Rassin, D. K. 1972. Amino acids as putative transmitters: failure to bind to synaptic vesicles of guinea pig cerebral cortex. *J. Neurochem.* 19:139–48

168. Reis, D. J., Weinbren, M., Corvelli, A. 1968. A circadian rhythm of norepinephrine regionally in cat brain. *J. Pharmacol. Exp. Ther.* 164:135–45

169. Richter, J. A., Marchbanks, R. M. 1971. Isolation of [³H]acetylcholine pools by subcellular fractionation of cerebral cortex slices incubated with [³H]-choline. *J. Neurochem.* 18:705–12

170. Roberts, E., Kuriyama, K. 1968. Biochemical physiological correlations in studies of the γ-aminobutyric acid system. *Brain Res.* 8:1–35

171. Robison, G. A., Butcher, R. W., Sutherland, E. W. 1971. *Cyclic AMP.* New York:Academic

172. Rodriguez de Lores Arnaiz, G., Zieher, L. M., De Robertis, E. 1970. Neurochemical and structural studies on the mechanism of action of hemicholinium-3 in central cholinergic synapses. *J. Neurochem.* 17:221–29

173. Rubin, R. P. 1970. The role of calcium in the release of neurotransmitter substances and hormones. *Pharmacol. Rev.* 22:389–428

174. Sachs, H. 1970. Neurosecretion. In *Handbook of Neurochemistry, Vol. IV,* ed. A. Lajtha, 373–428. New York:Plenum

175. Schayer, R. W., Reilly, M. A. 1970. *In vivo* formation and catabolism of [¹⁴C]histamine in mouse brain. *J. Neurochem.* 17:1649–55

176. Schuberth, J., Sundwall, A. 1967. Effects of some drugs on the uptake of acetylcholine in cortex slices of mouse brain. *J. Neurochem.* 14:807–12

177. Schwartz, J. C., Lampart, C., Rose, C. 1972. Histamine formation in rat brain *in vivo:* effects of histidine loads. *J. Neurochem.* 19:801–10

178. Segal, D. S., Sullivan, J. L., III, Kuczenski, R. T., Mandell, A. J. 1971. Effects of long-term reserpine treatment on brain tyrosine hydroxylase and behavioral activity. *Science* 173:847–49

179. Sellinger, O. Z., Azcurra, J. M., Johnson, D. E., Ohlsson, W. G., Lodin, Z. 1971. Independence of protein synthesis and drug uptake in nerve cell bodies and glial cells isolated by a new technique. *Nature, New Biol.* 230:253–56

180. Shaw, J. E., Ramwell, P. W. 1968. Release of a substance P polypeptide from the cerebral cortex. *Am. J. Physiol.* 215:261–67

181. Shiman, R., Akino, M., Kaufman, S. 1971. Solubilization and partial purification of tyrosine hydroxylase from bovine adrenal medulla. *J. Biol. Chem.* 246:1330–40

182. Shimizu, H., Daly, J. W. 1972. Effect of depolarizing agents on accumulation of cyclic adenosine 3'-5'-monophosphate in cerebral cortical slices. *Eur. J. Pharmacol.* 17:240–52

183. Siggins, G. R., Hoffer, B. J., Bloom, F. E. 1971. Studies on norepinephrine containing afferents to Purkinje cells of rat cerebellum III. Evidence for mediation of norepinephrine effects by cyclic 3'-5'-adenosine monophosphate. *Brain Res.* 25:535–55

184. Silver, A. 1967. Cholinesterases of

the central nervous system with special reference to the cerebellum. *Int. Rev. Neurobiol.* 10: 57–109

185. Sims, K. L., Weitsen, H. A., Bloom, F. E. 1971. Histochemical localization of brain succinic semialdehyde dehydrogenase—a γ-aminobutyric acid degradative enzyme. *J. Histochem. Cytochem.* 19:405–15

186. Smith, A. D., De Potter, W. P., Moerman, E. J., De Schaepdryver, A. F. 1970. Release of dopamine β-hydroxylase and chromagranin A upon stimulation of the splenic nerve. *Tissue & Cell* 2:547–68

187. Snyder, S. H., Kuhar, M. J., Green, A. I., Coyle, J. T., Shaskan, E. G. 1970. Uptake and subcellular localization of neurotransmitters in the brain. *Int. Rev. Neurobiol.* 13:127–58

188. Spector, S., Gordon, R., Sjoerdsma, A., Udenfriend, S. 1967. End product inhibition of tyrosine hydroxylase as a possible mechanism for regulation of norepinephrine synthesis. *Mol. Pharmacol.* 3:549–55

189. Sze, P. Y., Kuriyama, K., Haber, B., Roberts, E. 1971. Effects of GABA on L-glutamic acid decarboxylase activities in chick embryo brain. *Brain Res.* 26: 121–30

190. Tabakoff, B., Erwin, V. G. 1970. Purification and characterization of a reduced nicotinamide adenine dinucleotide phosphate-lined aldehyde reductase from brain. *J. Biol. Chem.* 245: 3263–68

191. Tachiki, K. H., DeFeudis, F. V., Aprison, M. H. 1972. Studies on the subcellular distribution of γ-aminobutyric acid in slices of rat cerebral cortex. *Brain Res.* 36:215–17

192. Takeno, K., Nishjo, A., Yanagiya, I. 1969. Bound acetylcholine in the nerve ending particles. *J. Neurochem.* 16:47–52

193. Taylor, K. M., Snyder, S. H. 1972. Dynamics of the regulation of histamine levels in mouse brain. *J. Neurochem.* 19:341–54

194. Taylor, K. M., Snyder, S. H. 1972. Isotopic microassay of histamine, histidine, histidine decarboxylase and histamine meth-

yltransferase in brain tissue. *J. Neurochem.* 19:1343–58

195. Thoa, N. B., Johnson, D. G., Kopin, I. J. 1971. Selective release of newly synthesized norepinephrine in the guinea pig vas deferens during hypogastric nerve stimulation. *Eur. J. Pharmacol.* 15:29–35

196. Thoenen, H., Mueller, R. A., Axelrod, J. 1970. Phase difference in the induction of tyrosine hydroxylase in cell body and nerve terminals of sympathetic neurones. *Proc. Nat. Acad. Sci. USA.* 65:58–62

197. Tissari, A. H., Schönhöfer, P. S., Bogdanski, D. F., Brodie, B. B. 1969. Mechanism of biogenic amine transport II. *Mol. Pharmacol.* 5:593–604

198. Uretsky, N. J., Iversen, L. L. 1970. Effects of 6-hydroxydopamine on catecholamine containing neurones in the rat brain. *J. Neurochem.* 17:269–78

199. Von Voigtlander, P. F., Moore, K. E. 1971. The release of H³-dopamine from cat brain following electrical stimulation of the substantia nigra and caudate nucleus. *Neuropharmacology* 10:733–41

200. Weiner, N. 1970. Regulation of norepinephrine biosynthesis. *Ann. Rev. Pharmacol.* 10:273–90

201. Weinshilboum, R. M., Thoa, N. B., Johnson, D. G., Kopin, I. J., Axelrod, J. 1971. Proportional release of norepinephrine and dopamine-β-hydroxylase from sympathetic nerves. *Science* 174:1349–51

202. Weinstein, H., Kuriyama, K. 1970. Retention and exchange of potassium in a synaptosomal fraction of mouse brain. *J. Neurochem.* 17:493–501

203. White, T. D., Keen, P. 1971. Effects of inhibitors of $(Na^+ + K^+)$-dependent adenosine triphosphatase on the uptake of norepinephrine by synaptosomes. *Mol. Pharmacol.* 7: 40–45

204. Whittaker, V. P. 1969. The synaptosome. In *Handbook of Neurochemistry*, *Vol. II*, ed. A. Lajtha, 327–64. New York: Plenum

205. Woodward, D. J., Hoffer, B. J., Siggins, G. R., Bloom, F. E. 1971. The ontogenetic development of synaptic junctions, synaptic activation and responsiveness to neurotransmitter substances in rat cerebellar Purkinje cells. *Brain Res.* 34:73–97

206. Woodward, D. J., Hoffer, B. J., Siggins, G. R., Oliver, A. P. 1971. Inhibition of Purkinje cells in the frog cerebellum. II. Evidence for GABA as the inhibitory transmitter. *Brain Res.* 33:91–100

207. Zetler, G. 1970. Biologically active peptides (Substance P). In *Handbook of Neurochemistry, Vol. IV,* ed. A. Lajtha, 135–48. New York:Plenum

Ann. Rev. Physiol. 1973. 35:305–328

COMPARATIVE PHYSIOLOGY: PINEAL GLAND[1] 1098

RUSSEL J. REITER[2]

Department of Anatomy, The University of Texas Medical School at San Antonio, San Antonio, Texas

INTRODUCTION

There are several extra-hypothalamic areas that have a rather profound influence on the neuroendocrine axis. Included in this group are the amygdaloid nuclei, the hippocampus, the reticular formation and the epithalamo-epiphyseal complex. Additionally, exteroceptive factors such as sight, olfaction, audition and touch serve to modulate pituitary function. The means by which these systems affect the hypothalamo-hypophyseal axis are diverse, frequently intriguing and in general, rather poorly understood. The present review will consider the influence that one of these systems, namely the pineal gland and its constituents, exerts on the brain and on the neuroendocrine axis. In particular, the presentation will concentrate on the physiologic importance of the pineal influence on gonadotropins and on brain chemistry and electrical activity. Besides these influences, the pineal gland also regulates the secretion of other trophic hormones from the adenohypophysis; the literature on these actions has been reviewed elsewhere (52, 67, 72, 77, 107).

During the first half of this century, while endocrine physiology was in its formative years, the pineal gland was widely neglected primarily because it seemed to be completely expendable as a life-sustaining organ. Although this is, in a sense, true, nevertheless, the pineal may not be without significant effects on the survival of some species. Thus, the pineal gland may play an important role in synchronizing pregnancy and birth with the season (spring) maximally conducive to survival of the young, e.g., in the hamster (76, 82, 83).

About 15 years ago research on the pineal gland came to a veritable impasse. A new direction or approach was needed to liberate the pineal from the vestigiality complex it had acquired. The discovery of a potential pineal hormone (48) and the demonstration of a relationship between ambient lighting and the biosynthetic activity of the pineal parenchyma (65, 108)

[1] Investigations by the author were supported by research grants HD-02937 and HD-06523.

[2] The author is a recipient of a USPHS Career Development Award, HD-42398.

305

provided the impetus for the subsequent burgeoning number of investigations of this oft-time baffling organ. Since this time remarkable advances have been made in elucidating the endocrine functions of the pineal. Despite the astonishing progress, some authors have persisted in perpetuating an image of the pineal gland which characterizes it as an unknown organ. One author recently stated his opinions simultaneously in three different languages (90–92). It is hoped that the present review will help to counterbalance such reports.

PINEAL GLAND AND THE CONTROL OF PITUITARY GONADOTROPINS

Unfortunately, pinealectomy is a notoriously unreliable means of illustrating the gonad-inhibiting activity of the pineal gland. In addition to characteristically producing only a slightly accelerated rate of gonadal growth (41, 58, 75, 76), pineal extirpation in some instances has undetectable effects on the reproductive system (42, 104). Such equivocal data do not muster support for the pineal gland as an important organ of internal secretion. The sequelae of pineal removal are as varied among avian (68) as among mammalian species (82).

Failure of pineal removal to provoke profound changes in the rate of maturation of the sexual organs could usually be explained on the basis of inappropriate light:dark schedules used by the investigators. I have been especially persistent in criticizing the maintenance of normally burrow-dwelling nocturnal species in "long days" (12–16 hours of light per 24 hours) and then expecting pineal ablation to alter reproductive physiology (75, 76). It is my opinion that under such experimental conditions all animals are effectively "pinealectomized" since photic information is known to be inhibitory to pineal function (39, 41, 45, 107).

On the contrary, if the antigonadotropic potential of the pineal gland is stimulated by restricting the animals' exposure to light, the growth of the reproductive organs is affected accordingly. In no species is this more apparent than in the golden hamster. Hoffman & Reiter (36) found that if sexually mature hamsters were placed in an environment which allowed one hour of light per day, the testes suffered severe atrophic changes within 4 to 6 weeks. Under these conditions histological involution of the reproductive organs was as obvious as the decremental changes in the size of the gonads and adnexae. Proof that this alteration in growth was a consequence of a hyperactive pineal gland was demonstrated by the fact that dark-maintained hamsters that had been pinealectomized failed to exhibit reproductive regression. Planometric measurements also showed that in dark-exposed hamsters the pinealocyte nuclei were larger than those of hamsters kept in 16 hours of light per day. This was taken as further evidence that darkness augmented the metabolism of the pineal gland. Later it was shown that absence of light exaggerates the concentration of the melatonin forming enzyme, hydroxyindole-O-methyltransferase, in the hamster pineal (7). Shortly thereafter it was demonstrated that bilateral superior cervical ganglionectomy rendered the pineal incapable of inducing gonadal involution in hamsters deprived of light (69, 78). Sympathetically denervated pineal glands are unable to respond to changes in environmental lighting since the information about the photoperiod gets to the pineal by way of the peripheral autonomic nervous system (9, 10, 45, 106). Subsequent studies in the hamster on the interrelationships among photoperiodic information, pineal activity, and reproductive physiology have proven this animal to be especially valuable for demonstrating the endocrine capability of the pineal (76, 82). Unfortunately, the specific pineal antigonadotropic substance in this species has not yet been identified unequivocally.

In rats as well, curtailing the amount of light to which the animals were exposed stimulated the enzymatic machinery of the pineal gland (43, 44, 108). On this basis it was predicted and shown that blinding immature rats would retard the maturation of their sexual organs. Indeed, depriving rats of light before puberty delayed pubertal onset and gonadal maturation only in those animals which had not been pinealectomized (70).

There are a number of conditions which sensitize the hypothalamo-pituitary-gonadal axis of rats to the pineal influence. These have been designated "potentiating factors" and include anosmia, early postnatal androgen treatment, and qualitative and quantitative nutritional factors (77, 83, 99). The mechanisms by which these conditions predispose the neuroendocrine axis to the suppressive influence of the pineal are unclear. The most likely explanation is that they modify hypothalamic neurons which are directly or indirectly responsible for the release or synthesis of the gonadotropins. Based on the enzymatic activity (43, 83) and the melatonin content (86) of the pineal gland, neither anosmia nor sterilization with androgens altered the ability of the rat pineal to form gonad inhibiting hormone. However, this inference is based on the assumption that melatonin is the essential pineal antigonadotropic substance—a point which is currently under considerable debate (15, 57).

Every conceivable means has been used to administer pineal substances, especially N-acetyl-5-methoxytryptamine (melatonin), in an attempt to prove the endocrine capability of the organ and to identify the pineal hormone. Characteristically, the administration of melatonin produces rather modest effects on the reproductive organs (82, 98, 107), but occasionally the changes are quite dramatic (84, 102, 103). Undoubtedly, some investigators have been reluctant to classify melatonin as a hormone because of the variable and minimal response it may yield. Nevertheless, it seems well established that it possesses antigonadotropic capability. Polypeptides of pineal origin are potent inhibitors of reproduction and, therefore, must also be considered potential pineal hormones (14, 15, 57).

Pineal gland and luteinizing hormone.—There is little evidence to indicate that the pineal gland or its principles normally determine the synthesis or release of specific pituitary gonadotropins. Moreover, the experiments designed to test this possibility have not always yielded unequivocal or reproducible results. Nevertheless, it is increasingly obvious that the pineal exerts some control over individual gonadotropins.

Pituitary LH levels have been measured in pinealectomized rats. According to Fraschini & Martini (28), removal of the pineal gland from young adult male rats resulted in a conspicuous and highly significant enhancement of the pituitary LH content. This elevation of LH content appeared within only 12 days after pineal ablation, and the increase was nearly equivalent to that following castration, a very potent stimulus for enhanced LH synthesis and release. Few other investigators have been fortunate enough to observe changes in pituitary LH levels, especially of this magnitude, after short term pinealectomy.

After the daily injection of melatonin (100 μg/day), Adams and his colleagues (1) reported an increased pituitary LH content in maturing female rats. The authors interpreted this to mean that the indoleamine acted at the level of the gonadotropins to curtail LH release. These results could not be duplicated in growing male rats, where the daily injection of 300 μg melatonin for 30 days stymied reproductive organ growth, while pituitary LH levels were unaffected.

Inconsistent results such as these forced Fraschini and co-workers (28) to approach the problem somewhat differently. Adult male castrated rats were gonadectomized to stimulate the production and storage of LH in the anterior pituitary. By means of cannulae, various pineal-derived indoles were then placed into several central nervous system areas believed to govern gonadotropin metabolism (29). When deposited into the median eminence, both melatonin and 5-hydroxytryptophol significantly retarded the accumulation of LH in the pituitary. 5-Methoxytryptophol and serotonin proved to be ineffective at this site. When placed into the midbrain reticular formation, only serotonin failed to prevent the rise in adenohypophyseal LH. Implants of any type directly into the pituitary gland did not influence the rate of accumulation of LH. Fraschini et al (29) concluded that the median eminence and the reticular formation contain receptors which are responsive to changes in the concentration of pineal indoles. These data are of interest but open an important question concerning the mode of secretion by the pineal gland which has not been resolved. If the pineal releases its hormones into the ventricular fluid, the results of Fraschini and co-workers may be directly applicable to what happens normally, since in neither instance (i.e., after central implantation or after secretion into the cerebrospinal fluid) would the compounds have to cross the blood-brain barrier to reach the reticular formation neurons that were responsive to the hormones. Conversely, a systemic vascular route of secretion of the pineal principles necessitates a transport of the hormones across the blood-brain barrier. Whether in fact each of these substances have ready access to the brain from the vascular system has not been satisfactorily established.

Kamberi and associates (37) provided the best evidence to date that melatonin is capable of acting directly or via an intermediary cell on the re-

TABLE 1. Inhibition of ovulation by peripherally administered melatonin in immature rats treated with PMS

Treatment	N	Number that ovulated (%)	Number of ova per ovulating rat
20 I.U. PMS +diluent	21	19 (91)	31.6±2.5[a]
20 I.U. PMS +1.5 mg melatonin	20	9 (45)	28.5±3.1

[a] Means ±standard errors

leasing factor neurons of the brain. The infusion of melatonin (2 μg/min for 30 min) directly into a cannulated stalk portal vessel, the blood of which drains into the sinusoids of the anterior pituitary, did not affect the concentration of LH in the peripheral serum. Its administration via the ventricular route caused a marked, albeit transitory, reduction in serum LH. Indeed, LH fell to undetectable levels after intraventricular injection of 50 μg of melatonin. The blood levels of the gonadotropin returned to normal within 2 hours. From these results it appears that melatonin has the ability to inhibit the release of luteinizing hormone releasing factor into the primary portal plexus.

In immature rats ovulation induced by pregnant mare's serum (*PMS*) has been used to demonstrate the suppressive influence of melatonin on gonadotropin release (49, 79). If the indoleamine is given at the approximate time of endogenous LH release (approximately 54 to 58 hr after PMS administration), about one-half of the animals do not ovulate in response to PMS. For example, the melatonin given to the rats listed in Table 1 was injected in three 500 μg doses each at 54, 55 and 56 hr after PMS administration. The essential feature appears to be that the melatonin be given at about the time the pituitary would normally secrete the gonadotropin to cause the necessary serum LH surge. When serum LH levels were measured by radioimmunoassay in PMS-treated rats, melatonin prevented the rise of LH which would normally cause the shedding of the ova (84). In other words, melatonin acted at the level of the anterior pituitary or the brain and not at the level of the ovary.

In adult rats the situation appears to be slightly different. Collu and colleagues (19) reported that the intraventricular administration, but not the subcutaneous injection, of melatonin restricted spontaneous ovulation in normally cycling rats. Again the melatonin had to be given near the "critical period" of LH release to be effective. Collu et al (19) offered four possible explanations for their results and also concluded that the findings support the hypothesis that the physiological route of secretion of melatonin is through the cerebrospinal fluid. As noted earlier, this latter idea is intriguing but, for the reasons summarized by Kappers (40), it is far from proven.

Pineal gland and follicle stimulating hormone.—The central mechanisms governing the control of FSH secretion by the adenohypophysis have been studied in great detail. The release of this hormone depends upon a releasing factor which enters the blood vascular system within the primary portal plexus of the median eminence. The specific site of production of the FSH releasing factor is still under investigation. As with LH, one means by which the pineal gland probably influences FSH secretion is by an action at some central nervous system locus.

One experimental model that has been rather widely used in investigating the role of the pineal gland in controlling FSH is compensatory ovarian hypertrophy (*COH*) after unilateral ovariectomy. Benson and colleagues (16) were able to detect, using a modified Steelman-Pohley bioassay, a transient rise in serum FSH after unilateral overiectomy in rats. Although this is not proof that only an elevation in FSH is responsible for compensatory growth of the ovary, it suggests that the hormone is involved in the response. The daily administration of melatonin restricted the degree of COH in rats and prevented the associated elevation in serum FSH (96).

The degree of ovarian enlargement at 10 days after unilateral ovariectomy is uniformally about 60% for the Swiss-Webster and CD-1 strains of mice. A single 100 μg dose of melatonin, injected intraperitoneally at the time of unilateral ovariectomy, retarded significantly the growth of the remaining ovary (100). A dose-response curve was established by administering progressively smaller doses of melatonin, (101). About 12.5 μg of melatonin was the minimal effective dose which caused a significant retardation of COH. The largest amount utilized, i.e., 100 μg, reduced enlargement of the remaining ovary by at least 50% when the hypertrophy is measured 9 to 10 days after unilateral ovariectomy. It is noteworthy that only a single injection of melatonin was needed to prevent maximal enlargement of the contralateral ovary. However, the melatonin must be injected either at the time of unilateral ovariectomy or within 24 hours of the operation (102). If administered later it did not block the compensatory hypertrophic response. Likewise, repeated injections of 100 μg doses of melatonin on successive days after removal of one ovary was no more effective than a single injection (87). Longer term studies revealed that a single injection of melatonin merely delayed, rather than prevented, COH. By 30 days postoperatively the remaining ovaries of melatonin-treated mice reached the size of those in control animals (87).

Vaughan et al (103) have done a comprehensive study in which the ability of each of the pineal indoles to block compensatory ovarian enlargement in mice was compared. When measured 10 days after unilateral ovariectomy, N-acetylserotonin, 5-hydroxytryptophol, and 5-methoxytryptophol, along with melatonin, were effective inhibitors of COH. On the other hand, 5-hydroxytryptophan, 5-hydroxytryptamine (serotonin), 6-hydroxymelatonin, 5-hydroxyindole acetic acid, and 5-methoxyindole acetic acid were all without a significant depressant action on induced gonadal growth following unilateral ovariectomy. All compounds were given intraperitoneally as 100 μg doses at the time of unilateral ovariectomy. In the same report, the ability of a melatonin-free, ninhydrin-positive extract of bovine pineal tissue was tested for its influence on COH. A 0.2 ml dose of the extract (equivalent to 2 g wet pineal tissue) was as effective as 100 μg of melatonin in restricting the enlargement of the remaining ovary (103).

The results of Vaughan and co-workers (103) using a melatonin-free pineal extract are similar to those obtained by another group of workers. Benson, Matthews & Rodin (14, 15, 51) isolated a small polypeptide in the 500 to 1000 molecular weight range which also restricts COH in mice. Evidence for the specific anti-FSH activity of such partially purified polypeptides came from the laboratories of Ebels & Moszkowska (26, 57, 59). The polypeptides bear especially close watching as important pineal antigonadotropic substances.

In rats, if one ovary is removed from animals that have been previously blinded, COH is partially blocked unless the animals are also pinealectomized (97). The rise in serum FSH which follows unilateral castration is also depressed by bilateral orbital enucleation (24). The absence of photic information is, of course, a primary stimulus for increased pineal synthetic, and presumably, secretory activity (9, 45, 108).

More direct evidence implicating the pineal gland in the control of FSH has also been obtained. Under conditions where the pineal was theoretically maximally stimulated and the gonads were infantile, the serum FSH levels measured by radioimmunoassay were significantly lower than in pinealectomized control rats (83). After daily injections of 300 μg of melatonin from the 21st to the 51st day of age, the pituitary content of FSH in male rats was substantially decreased (23). Moreover, a parallel retardation in the growth of the testes was observed.

Simple pinealectomy led to approximately a threefold rise in the pituitary concentration of FSH in young adult male rats (28). Only 12 days was required for this change to occur. The response was not as great as that following bilateral gonadectomy but, nevertheless, it was an unexpectedly large rise considering the slight reproductive changes which follow pineal ablation. According to Fraschini & Martini (28), the effects of pinealectomy on FSH levels are not mediated by melatonin. Based on the results of experiments utilizing the central nervous system implantation of pineal indoles, they concluded that 5-methoxytryptophol and serotonin are responsible for the antagonistic action of the pineal on FSH accumulation in the pituitary. When mixed with cocoa butter and placed into the median eminence, both of these compounds prevented the rise in hypophyseal FSH levels normally associated with gonadectomy. On the basis of these data and those mentioned earlier, Fraschini & Martini (27, 28) described two distinctly separate channels by which the pineal exerts control over the anterior pituitary gonadotropins.

They believe that 5-methoxytryptophol and serotonin are the pineal envoys exclusively responsible for the control of FSH secretion and that the pineal substances, melatonin and 5-hydroxytryptophol, are normally concerned with the regulation of LH (27, 28). This scheme is by no means accepted by all investigators working in the field, however.

The most obvious conflict with this theory is the work of Kamberi et al (38). With the aid of sophisticated surgical techniques and a specific radio-immunoassay they showed that intraventricular injection of small quantities of melatonin depressed, by 50%, FSH titers in blood recovered from a peripheral artery. When the indoleamine was infused into the anterior pituitary by way of a cannulated portal vessel, the peripheral concentration of FSH was unchanged. Kamberi and associates (38) speculated that melatonin controlled the discharge of the hypothalamic releasing factor normally concerned with FSH. Under similar experimental conditions, serotonin also depressed FSH levels in the serum, presumably by a similar mechanism.

Pineal gland and proclactin.—Pineal-prolactin interrelationships have been investigated in relatively few studies. It can be inferred from several investigations that blind rats are deficient in prolactin and milk production (18, 73) and that this effect may be a consequence of an activated pineal gland (73).

Female rats, pinealectomized at 21 days of age, developed mammary tissue at the normal rate, judging from the mammotrophic index (54). The mammotropic index relies on morphological criteria for an assessment of mammary gland maturation. A subsequent study by the same group showed that removal of the pineal gland was associated with a modest (13%) decrease in milk yield during the second half of the nursing period (62). By the time the young were weaned, however, milk production was comparable in pinealectomized and sham-operated mother rats. These findings were essentially confirmed by Mizuno & Sensui (55).

Prolactin has an essential role in the maintenance of lactation in the rabbit so it seemed to be an ideal animal in which to check the influence of melatonin on milk yield. Deposition of melatonin by means of stainless steel cannulae, into the median eminence of New Zealand white rabbits, caused a mild and persistent lowering of milk yield (93). Since this effect was induced by several other compounds as well, the authors inferred that the reduction in prolactin secretion was either due to a nonspecific mechanism or secondary to a depression in food intake. At any rate, the investigators were not convinced that melatonin had a distinct influence on prolactin release.

In contrast, Kamberi et al (38) reported a correlation between prolactin release and pineal activity, when melatonin was injected either into the cerebral ventricles or into a cannulated portal vessel. Prolactin measurements after the intraventricular administration of melatonin indicated that the indoleamine depressed the discharge of prolactin inhibiting factor and thereby increased prolactin titers in the peripheral blood. The change was appreciably more dramatic than with FSH in that serum prolactin concentration increased threefold after melatonin was placed into the cerebrospinal fluid.

More recently, Donofrio & Reiter (25) reported diminished levels of prolactin in the pituitary glands of female rats rendered blind and anosmic shortly after weaning and killed 10 weeks later. This obvious trend was reversed if the dual sensory deprived rats were pinealectomized. Due to the amount of variation within the various groups, differences in plasma prolactin titers could not be verified. There is at least one obvious reason why Kamberi et al (38) were able to show significant differences in serum prolactin levels; they had the advantage of collecting serial blood samples from their animals and thus, each rat served as its own control. The results of our work and that of Kamberi et al are apparently in conflict, but in view of the differences in experimental designs, it is difficult to decipher the meaning of the two experiments relative to each other. One experiment was chronic and the other acute; one tested the effect of pinealectomy and the other of melatonin administration. It seems too early to speculate on the primary role of the pineal in prolactin release and milk production. It seems safe to say, however, they are related in some important manner.

PINEAL GLAND AND SEASONAL REPRODUCTIVE RHYTHMS

I have long contended that one of the most important functions of the pineal gland may be to control or modulate seasonal reproductive rhythms in photosensitive animals (71, 82). To a degree, probably all animals fall into this category. Certainly, the pivotal position of the pineal in photo-periodically-mediated gonadal responses has been amply demonstrated (72, 76, 107). There are, however, effects of continuous light on the reproductive system that are not mediated via the pineal gland. The best example of this is constant estrus induced by continual light exposure. On the other hand, all of the effects of darkness on genital functions seem to involve the pineal gland as an intermediary.

Almost all natural populations of animals show some degree of seasonality with regard to reproduction. These variations occur in animals living not only in the boreal and temperate zones but in the tropics as well. The most potentially powerful impeller of these seasonal rhythms is the length of the photoperiod since it is the most consistently reproducible factor in the natural environment. This does not mean, however, that light:dark schedules are the only cause of fluctuations in sexual competence. Some species which populate arid regions may breed immediately following a rainfall; these are referred to as opportunistic breeders and are in the minority. Nutritional and temperature fluctuations may also serve to trigger reproductive cycles (60). Regardless of the specific factors which impel such rhythms, one major consequence of placing wild species in the laboratory is to spread the breeding cycle throughout the year. Under laboratory environments where photoperiodic, nutritional, and temperature conditions are held constant, the importance of the pineal is probably obviated since the pineal surely functions as a sensor of changes in the environment. Hence, it should not be surprising that testing pineal function under the finely regulated environmental conditions of the laboratory have provided us with such few answers to the pineal problem.

The importance of seasonality in reproduction lies in the fact that the progeny are born and nurtured during a season that is maximally conducive to their survival. The spring of the year most frequently meets all these requirements and thus parturition invariably occurs, in natural populations, at this time. However, the duration of pregnancy varies considerably among species. Thus, breeding and insemination may occur during any season. Because of the various mating times, animals employ a number of means to ensure parturition in the spring, e.g., long or short gestation periods and delayed implantation. These phenomena all may be directly or indirectly regulated by the photoperiod and the pineal gland.

In the laboratory, the superimposition of light and temperature changes may induce periods of reproductive quiescence similar to that seen in animals in their natural habitat (71, 76). The hamster is an example of a species where this phenomenon may be readily tested. Even under controlled laboratory conditions the reproductive organs of this species exhibit a propensity to decline functionally during the winter months. Interestingly, this reduction in sexual competence could be negated by increasing the photoperiod length to which the animals were exposed (20, 22). This undoubtedly was an effect mediated by the pineal gland since it was obviated by additional light. When hamsters were maintained under short photoperiods in the laboratory, i.e., 1 to 2 hr of light per day, the gonads of both sexes completely degenerated (35). Proof that this was a pineal-mediated response was provided by the observation that pinealectomy prevented the dark-induced gonadal involution (36).

The feature which convinced Hoffman et al that the pineal may be related to seasonal reproductive rhythms was the observation that the sexual organs of hamsters that were forced to degenerate under the influence of an activated pineal gland did not remain permanently quiescent (35, 71). Rather, after about 25 weeks of darkness the gonads spontaneously recrudesced and became grossly, microscopically, and functionally mature even though the animals were still confined to darkness (71, 74). Either after this period of stimulation the gonads became refractory to the pineal influence or the pineal temporarily lost its antigonadotropic capability (74).

What is especially enticing about this observation is that the duration of sexual dormancy (approximately 20 weeks) under these circumstances is equivalent in length to the period of reproductive quiescence these animals experience under field conditions. Therefore, the reproductive cycle which hamsters exhibit in the field may have been duplicated in the laboratory by simulating the photoperiodic conditions these animals are exposed to in the wild. Recall that hamsters enter underground burrows, and hence complete darkness, in the fall of the year and hibernate in the absence of light until the following spring. The pineal gland must be intact in order for gonadal regression to ensue during darkness (71).

The spontaneous regeneration of the gonads after long term exposure to the dark may also be reminiscent of the regrowth of the sexual organs of burrow dwelling hamsters as spring approaches. This regrowth comes about even though the animals are still hibernating (95). The importance of the pineal in the survival of the species thus becomes apparent. With decreasing photoperiodic length (due to naturally shortening days in the autumn or progressively more time spent in burrows) the pineal gland induces gonadal involution and the animals enter hibernation. The regressed gonads offer two important advantages. It prevents the animals from breeding and delivering young at a time (winter) which would not be ideal for survival. Secondly, a necessary prerequisite for hibernation is that the reproductive system be suppressed (34). As spring approaches the restraining influence which the pineal exerts on the neuroendocrine axis is lifted, by mechanisms not completely understood, and the regeneration of the gonads follows (74). When the hamsters exit from their burrows in the early spring they are sexually competent and breed almost immediately. The young are thus born shortly thereafter at the optimal time of the year. Hamsters may have additional litters during the summer months but about the time of the autumnal equinox the photoperiodic length becomes shortened to a point where the pineal is again activated and the gonads involute. The animals then enter hibernation, their reproductive cycle complete, having been synchronized with the season by the photoperiod acting by way of the pineal gland. Some experimental data indicate that during the summer months the hypothalamo-pituitary-gonadal axis may in fact be refractory to the pineal gland, even if it is stimulated by light deprivation (74). The sensitivity of the brain to the pineal may also change with the season of the year. These interactions are summarized in Figure 1.

Support for the theory in which the pineal is the primary organ for synchronizing insemination, pregnancy, parturition, and nurturing of the young with the annual cycle of vegetation, etc., has come from studies in which hamsters were maintained under natural environmental conditions. For example, Czyba and associates (21) observed that the winter decline in fertility in male hamsters which was a normal sequel of shortening photoperiods was prevented by removal of the pineal gland. In a more complete but as yet unpublished experiment, I extended these findings to show that the genital apparatus of male hamsters exposed to uncontrolled environmental photoperiodic and temperature conditions experienced gonadal regression if their pineal gland is intact, whereas pinealectomized controls remained sexually competent throughout the year. These findings lend credence to the suggested importance of the pineal gland to the survival of the species.

The reproductive cycle of another photoperiodically sensitive species, the

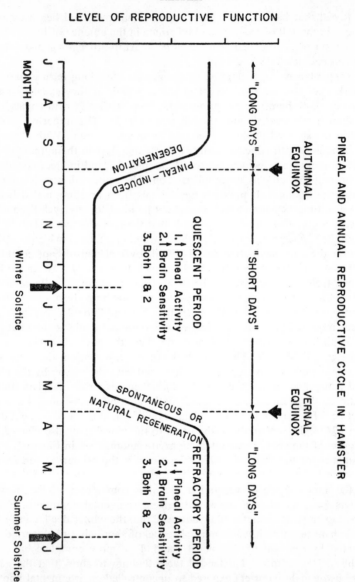

FIGURE 1. Theoretical role of the pineal gland in seasonal reproductive phenomena in the golden hamster. During the winter months ("short days"), reproductive organ growth is held in check by an increased pineal activity and probably by an increased sensitivity of the brain to pineal substances. During the "long day" period (summer), the neuroendocrine-gonadal axis may be refractory to the pineal influence.

ferret, has been investigated relative to the influence of lighting conditions and the pineal gland (31, 32). Pinealectomy does not prevent the occurrence of the anestrous interval in this species but it does significantly influence the onset of estrus. Pinealectomized, sham-operated, and unoperated female ferrets were exposed to natural daylight and the results analyzed. In the first spring all of the animals came into estrus at about the same time and this was followed by the usual anestrous interval. In the second spring, however, the onset of estrus in the three groups differed markedly. Whereas both the sham-operated and unoperated control ferrets came into heat again in the spring, none of the pinealectomized ferrets showed evidence of estrus until the fall, about 20 to 30 weeks later than normal. Pinealectomy did not alter the duration of the estrous period, however. The data again show, as in the hamster, that the pineal gland is inextricably linked with synchronizing the ferret's estrus with the appropriate season. This nexus is readily apparent when the animals are kept under natural daylight. It seems somewhat contradictory that in neither the hamster nor the ferret does melatonin have any suppressive influence on reproduction, yet, they are both very sensitive to the influence of the pineal (31, 76).

Investigations into the role of the pineal gland in annual reproductive rhythm in other classes of animals have been sparse. Barfuss & Ellis (12) recently published the results of a rather complete study from which they concluded that in the house sparrow (*Passer domesticus*), the activity of the pineal is not related to the seasonal cycle of testicular development.

PINEAL-BRAIN INTERACTIONS

Pineal gland and electrical activity of the brain.—One of the initial findings supporting the supposition that one of the main functions of the pineal gland is to modulate neural activity was provided by the work of Roldan and associates (89). They observed changes in the electrical activity of various regions of cat brain following intravenous administration of unrefined extracts of bovine pineal. Using bipolar stainless steel electrodes implanted under stereotaxic control, they recorded an augmentation of the frequency and the voltage of the electrical activity of the paraventricular and periventricular nuclei within 5 sec after the administration of the extracts. This activation reportedly spread to other nuclear groups in the brain and 5 min following the injections the tracings returned to normal. Roldan & Anton-Tay (88) later investigated the influence of pineal extracts on the convulsive activity of cats. Somewhat surprisingly, the extracts had a potent suppressive effect on seizures which were electrically elicited in the cerebral cortex. The depressant action of the pineal preparations appeared within 15 to 45 min after its administration and persisted for about 9 hr. In the same study, the authors found that the electrical activity of a number of subcortical nuclear groups changed from high amplitude slow frequency rhythms to a pattern of faster low voltage activity in response to the injection of the pineal extracts.

Removal of the pineal gland also permanently alters neural electrical activity in several species. In 1965 Bindoni & Rizzo (17), recording from chronically implanted electrodes, noted convulsive patterns of activity in the dorsal hippocampal neurons of pinealectomized rabbits after contralateral homotypical stimulation. Such increases in the voltage of interhippocampal potentials could not be elicited in rabbits with intact pineal glands. The neuronal hyperexcitability and the convulsive patterns of activity in the hippocampi are of special interest to me because of the seizures associated with pinealectomy in the rat. These data are discussed later in this paper.

Changes in the electrical activity of the brain following pineal ablation are not restricted to the rabbit. In rats, Nir et al (61) found that surgical removal of the pineal gland altered the EEG pattern of cortical activity recorded from the dura mater. So that each animal could serve as its own control, the following protocol was used: electrical recordings were taken from rats and they were then pinealectomized; after a 2 to 3 week recuperative period EEG's were again recorded. The authors found what they identified as seizure-like discharges after pinealectomy. The electrical recordings from the cortex of these animals showed intermittent general paraoxysmal outbursts of slow waves with high amplitudes of centrocephalic origin. They postulated that the electrical changes, which are indicative of alertness, may account for the endocrine aberrations which become manifested in pinealectomized rats. In a subsequent study, the same workers (13) observed that the effects of lethal doses of sodium pentobarbitone were delayed in pinealectomized rats. This observation also may be explicable in terms of the increased excitatory level of the central nervous system in rats lacking the pineal gland. In a brief report, Milcu & Demetrescu (53) claimed that crude bovine pineal extracts changed the electrical activity of the human brain as well.

The successful use of melatonin to combat the symptoms of epilepsy and Parkinsonism has recently been reported by Anton-Tay and associates (4, 5). A single dose of melatonin, ranging from 0.25 to 1.25 mg/kg, was followed by a generalized deactivation of the electrophysiological pattern in at least two patients suffering from temporal lobe epilepsy. Following this acute treatment, there was a slowing of the electroencephalographic rhythm, an increase in rapid eye movement sleep, and, most significantly, a rise of the convulsive threshold. These changes were not accompanied by deterioration of brain function. In the two Parkinsonian patients, where the treatment with melatonin was chronic, the authors reported a notable improvement during the second week of administration (4). The subjects expressed a general feeling of well being along with an obvious improvement in the performance of routine tasks. One nonambulatory patient was able to walk after three weeks of treatment. There was a remission of rigidity and tremor in both patients. When a placebo was substituted for the melatonin, the Parkinsonian subjects deteriorated within two weeks (5). The mechanisms whereby melatonin causes improvement in these clinical situations is far from clear. However, the authors surmise that it may be due to the ability of melatonin to alter neurotransmitter balance within the central nervous system. Melatonin reportedly has some influence on central neurotransmitter synthesis and sleep mechanisms in experimental animals (2, 3).

Pineal gland and brain constitutents.—The hypothalamic concentration of gamma-aminobutyric acid (*GABA*) doubled after the intraperitoneal injection of 50 μg/kg of melatonin into rabbits (2); there was also a statistically significant rise in the concentration of this compound in the cerebral cortex. The level of serotonin, an indoleamine found in nerve endings throughout the brain but whose cell bodies are located primarily in the midbrain, fluctuates in response to melatonin administration as well (3). The temporal sequence of the alterations in serotonin concentration changes according to what brain regions are examined. The sum of the changes, however, indicates that melatonin may cause a release of serotonin at the axonal endings, followed by an augmented synthesis of the monoamine in the midbrain.

The action of melatonin on GABA and serotonin ostensibly is mediated by its stimulatory influence on pyridoxal kinase (6). Pyridoxal kinase serves to catalyze the formation of pyridoxal phosphate, which is a prosthetic group of the enzyme aromatic-L-amino acid decarboxylase where it is a requirement for the formation of both GABA and serotonin. Pyridoxal kinase activity in the brain increases twofold after the intraperitoneal injection of 200 μg of melatonin to rats. Within 6 hr the concentration of the enzyme returns to pre-injection levels. Melatonin seems to cause the de novo synthesis of the enzyme since its stimulatory effect is blocked by actinomycin.

Relevant to a discussion of pineal-brain interactions is the observation that melatonin induces sleep. Unrestrained adult cats slept for 2 hr after the bilateral deposition of crystalline melatonin (15–30 μg) into the preoptic area (50). During the period of sleep there was an obvious synchronization in the EEG cortical leads with a marked increased amplitude and a slowing of the electrical activity in the subcortical structures. Barchas and colleagues (11) and Hishikawa and associates (33) confirmed this finding by showing that the intravenous injection of melatonin into chicks, whose blood brain barrier is relatively undeveloped, caused sleep of about 30 to 45 min duration. The sedative action of melatonin on the central nervous system is also apparent from studies where melatonin was given in conjunction with a barbiturate. There was a 50% increase in the sleeping time of mice after they received a combination of hexobarbital and melatonin (11). In rats, melatonin prolonged pentobarbital-induced sleep by 15 to 45%, depending upon the amount of the indole injected (28). Considering that serotonin has been experimentally linked with sleep phenomena, melatonin may facilitate barbiturate-induced sleep through the activation of serotonin-dependent pathways. In fact, Koella (46) suggested that normal sleep processes may involve the "leakage" of serotonin from the pineal gland directly into the posterior aspect of the third ventricle. He theorized that after its release into the ventricular system, the pineal serotonin then flows into the fourth ventricle along with the cerebrospinal fluid and exerts its hypersynchronizing effect via the area postrema, nucleus tractus solitarii, and upper brain stem. This proposal obviously requires careful scrutiny.

The actions of melatonin on the brain are consistent with the observation that a radioactive form of the compound is taken up by the brain, particularly when it is injected directly into the ventricular system (8).

Probably even more basic evidence implicating the pineal gland in the control of brain metabolism is a finding that Quay (66) reported in 1965. In a series of studies designed to examine the significance of the pineal organ in controlling body electrolytes, Quay observed that rats lacking the pineal glands were unable to maintain cerebral potassium levels during sodium deficiency. Despite the potential importance of this work, it has not been seriously pursued since then. In view of the importance of sodium and potassium balance in maintaining the excitability of nerve cell membranes, it is imperative that these data, although initially well documented, be confirmed before we can venture speculations on their real meaning.

Pineal gland and seizure activity.—Since pinealectomy enhances the electrical activity of the brain, it may not have been surprising to find that, under special circumstances removal of the pineal induces violent convulsive seizures in rats. Although I have done several thousand surgical pinealectomies during the past five years, I have never seen a rat or hamster exhibit seizure activity following this procedure alone. Recently, however, we found that if previously thyro-parathyroidectomized immature male rats were subjected to pineal ablation, a large percentage of the animals convulsed within 8 hr (85). The onset of the convulsions usually fell between 3 and 5 hr after pineal removal, and the seizures were characterized initially by hypermobility and tonic contractions of the extremities. This was followed by an intensive seizure of both the trunk and limb musculature. After repeated convulsions some of the animals died, usually during a seizure, from asphyxiation. A subsequent investigation revealed that the prerequisites for the seizures were merely parathyroidectomy (rather than thyroparathyroidectomy) followed by pinealectomy (80). A large number of ancillary experiments have been done to attempt to prove that the seizures were, in fact, related to surgical removal of the pineal gland. Interestingly, if the pineal gland of parathyroidectomized rats is denervated by superior cervical ganglionectomy or by transection of the nervi conarii, the seizures do not ensue (80). An intact pineal innervation has been found to be essential for pineal function in several other experimental conditions (77, 78, 107). Brains of rats that had experienced several convulsions contained less norepinephrine than those of nonconvulsing controls, while serotonin and dopamine levels remained unchanged (80,

81). The seizures were inhibited temporarily by a single injection of diazepam or chlordiazepoxide (20 or 50 mg/kg) given at the time of pineal removal, but diphenylhydantoin had no ameliorative effects on the convulsive activity (81). Although removal of the parathyroid gland caused a drop in serum calcium levels, this may not be a predisposing factor for the convulsions.

Comment.—The previously discussed findings seem to leave little doubt that the pineal gland and its indoleamines have an influence on biosynthetic and electrical parameters of brain function. The electrical changes probably merely reflect the underlying alterations in the release and formation of neurochemicals. These nonendocrine effects may ultimately be responsible for the associated neuroendocrine consequences of pineal manipulation, i.e., the changes in the activity of the pituitary-regulated endocrine glands may, in fact, be secondary to modifications produced in the hypothalamus or in extrahypothalamic neurons whose axons eventually connect to releasing factor cells in the medial basal hypothalamus. For example, it is well known that serotonin concentrations determine the functioning of the neuroendocrine axis (30) and that the amount of this monoamine in the brain is altered by melatonin (3, 105). In certain experimental situations, pinealectomy is followed by a decrease in central norepinephrine content (80); this catecholamine also exerts an influence on the neuroendocrine system (47). Although a definitive effect of the pineal on dopamine has not yet been established, it has also not been investigated sufficiently aggressively to preclude a pineal-dopamine interaction.

The relationship put forth by Koella (46) between pineal serotonin and normal sleep patterns is worthy of investigation; however, it requires at least one process that is still in the realm of theory. Essential to the proposal is that serotonin from the pineal gland gain access to the ventricular system by way of the pineal recess. The idea that the pineal releases its hormones into the cerebrospinal fluid has, of course, been mentioned by a number of workers (8, 94) but this possibility is far from established. In fact, based on detail anatomical descriptions of the epithalamus, Kappers (40) has strenuously denied the possibility of a direct route of secretion in adult animals. This is an important problem which must be resolved before the mechanism of action of the pineal on both nonendocrine and endocrine functions can be understood.

The observation that seizures follow removal of the pineal from parathyroidectomized rats opens a new area of research. These findings emphasize the potential importance of the pineal in maintaining brain homeostasis. The convulsions seem to involve norepinephrine (80) and possibly sodium and potassium fluxes as well (66). The effect is consistent with the now well-documented finding that melatonin has powerful sedative and hypnotic effects on the brain of animals (11, 33, 50) and anticonvulsant action in humans (4,

5). Thus pinealectomy, which removes a source of melatonin, would predictably cause hyperexcitability of the central nervous system, which it apparently does.

CONCLUDING REMARKS

The nexus between the pineal gland and the gonadotropins is well established and in general, appears to be of an inhibitory nature. This statement is made with the realization that a facilitatory influence of the pineal on reproduction has also been proposed and certainly must not be disregarded. The data, however, remain scanty.

There have been no hypothalamic inhibiting factors identified which control LH and FSH synthesis and secretion by the anterior pituitary gland. Perhaps the pineal gland functions as a counterpart to the releasing factor system by providing the inhibitory principles necessary for the fine regulation of the pituitary gonadotropins. In this regard, the pineal polypeptides which exhibit antigonadotropic activity may be of particular interest since the releasing factors also are combinations of amino acids. The evidence for the existence of the inhibitory polypeptides comes from their discovery in extracts of the pineal gland (15, 26, 59). Based on their disappearance from the urine of pinealectomized rats (63), they are also assumed to be secreted by the pineal. Thus, the indoleamines, which initially captured most of the attention of scientists working in the field, must now be considered in conjunction with another family of pineal compounds.

The impact of the pineal gland on sexual physiology is most easily seen when animals are exposed to artificially shortened days or to natural daylight. Surprisingly, these observations were made almost a decade after Quay (64) and Mogler (56) noted seasonal changes in the morphological characteristics of the pinealocytes of white-footed mice and golden hamsters, respectively. Investigators should use natural photoperiodic conditions (or reduced photoperiodic length in the laboratory situation) when attempting to demonstrate the potential of the pineal gland relative to the other endocrine organs. The exposure of nocturnal rodents to light:dark schedules routinely used in animal facilities where the duration of artificial light is 12 to 16 hr per day may severely bias or completely negate any pineal effect. At least relative to reproduction, pinealectomizing rodents that experience long days may be analogous to ovariectomizing animals that have been previously hypophysectomized. In either case the consequences of the operations, i.e., pinealectomy or ovariectomy, are hardly detectable. However, it is incorrect to conclude from this that the organs are functionless.

Basic to the understanding of the endocrine system is a working knowledge of the neural-endocrine axis. Considering that the pineal gland has now been shown to influence brain constituents and possibly synaptic transmission, it is likely that it may control the peripheral organs of internal secretion by a mechanism which involves central indoleamine and catecholamine concentrations or turn over. Certainly, each of these transmitter substances has a great deal to do with the functioning of the hypothalamo-hypophyseal system.

Among scientists, if not among fiction writers, the pineal gland has finally come out of the realm of the occult. The pineal is now known to be an inextricable part of that closely knit congeries of servomechanisms referred to as the endocrine system. Anyone who would deny this would be in error.

LITERATURE CITED

1. Adams, W. C., Wan, L., Sohler, A. 1965. Effect of melatonin on anterior pituitary luteinizing hormone. *J. Endocrinol.* 31: 295–96
2. Anton-Tay, F. 1971. Pineal-brain relationships. *The Pineal Gland,* ed. G. E. W. Wolstenholme, J. Knight, 213–27. London: Churchill
3. Anton-Tay, F., Chou, C., Anton, S., Wurtman, R. J. 1968. Brain serotonin concentration: elevation following intraperitoneal administration of melatonin. *Science* 162:277–78
4. Anton-Tay, F., Diaz, J. L., Fernández-Guardiola, A. 1971. On the effect of melatonin upon human brain. Its possible therapeutic implications. *Life Sci. (Part I)* 10:841–50
5. Anton-Tay, F., Fernández-Guardiola, A. 1973. Changes in human brain activity after melatonin administration. *Pineal Gland: Biochemistry and Physiology,* ed. D. C. Klein. New York:Raven. In press
6. Anton-Tay, F., Sepulveda, J., González, S. 1970. Increase of brain pyridoxal phosphokinase activity following melatonin administration. *Life Sci. (Part II)* 9:1283–88
7. Anton-Tay, F., Wurtman, R. J. 1968. Stimulation of hydroxy-indole-O-methyl-transferase activity in hamster pineal gland by blinding or continuous darkness. *Endocrinology* 82:1245–1246
8. Anton-Tay, F., Wurtman, R. J. 1969. Regional uptake of ³H-melatonin from blood or cerebrospinal fluid by rat brain. *Nature* 221:474–75
9. Axelrod, J. 1970. The pineal gland. *Endeavor* 29:144–48
10. Axelrod, J. 1970. Comparative biochemistry of the pineal gland. *Am. Zool.* 10:259–67
11. Barchas, J., Da Costa, F., Spector, S. 1967. Acute pharmacology of melatonin. *Nature* 214:919–20
12. Barfuss, D. W., Ellis, L. D. 1971. Seasonal cycles in melatonin synthesis by the pineal gland as related to testicular function in

the house sparrow (*Passer domesticus*). *Gen. Comp. Endocrinol.* 17:183–93
13. Behroozi, K., Assael, M., Ivriani, I., Nir, I. 1970. Electrocortical reactions on pinealectomized and intact rats to lethal doses of pentobarbital. *Neuropharmocology* 9:219–22
14. Benson, B., Matthews, M. J., Rodin, A. E. 1971. A melatonin-free extract of bovine pineal with antigonadotropic activity. *Life Sci.* (Part I) 10:607–12
15. Benson, B., Matthews, M. J., Rodin, A. E. 1972. Studies on a non-melatonin pineal antigonadotrophin. *Acta Endocrinol.* 69:257–66
16. Benson, B., Sorrentino, S., Evans, J. S. 1969. Increase in serum FSH following unilateral ovariectomy in the rat. *Endocrinology* 84:369–74
17. Bindoni, M., Rizzo, R. 1965. Hippocampal evoked potentials and convulsive activity after electrolytic lesions of the pineal body, in chronic experiments on rabbits. *Arch. Sci. Biol.* 49: 223–33
18. Browman, L. G. 1971. Microphthalamia, prolactin and fertility in rats. *J. Reprod. Fert.* 24: 353–60
19. Collu, R., Fraschini, F., Martini, L. 1971. Blockade of ovulation by melatonin. *Experientia* 27: 844–45
20. Cusick, F. J., Cole, H. 1959. An improved method of breeding golden hamsters. *Tex. Rep. Biol. Med.* 17:201–4
21. Czyba, J. C., Girod, C., Durand, N. 1964. Sur l'antagonisme épiphyso-hypophysaire et les variations saisonieres de la spermatogénése chez le hamster doré (*Mesocricetus auratus*). *Compt. Rend. Soc. Biol.* 158: 742–45
22. Deansley, R. 1938. The reproductive cycle of the golden hamster, *Cricetus auratus. Proc. Zool. Soc. London* 108:31–37
23. Debeljuk, L., Feder, V. M., Paulucci, O. A. 1970. Effect of treatment with melatonin on the pituitary-testicular axis of the

male rat. *J. Reprod. Fert.* 21: 363–64

24. Dickson, K., Benson, B., Tate, G., Jr. 1971. The effect of blinding and pinealectomy in unilaterally ovariectomized rats. *Acta Endocrinol.* 66:177–82

25. Donofrio, R. J., Reiter, R. J. 1972. Depressed pituitary prolactin levels in blinded anosmic female rats: role of the pineal gland. *J. Reprod. Fert.* In press

26. Ebels, I. 1967. Etude chimique des extraits épiphysaires fractionnés. *Biol. Med.* 56:395–402

27. Fraschini, F. 1969. The pineal gland and the control of LH and FSH secretion. *Progress in Endocrinology*, ed. C. Gual, 637–44. Amsterdam:Excerpta Medica

28. Fraschini, F., Martini, L. 1970. Rhythmic phenomena and pineal principles. *The Hypothalamus*, ed. L. Martini, M. Motta, F. Fraschini, 529–49. New York:Academic

29. Fraschini, F., Mess, B., Piva, F., Martini, L. 1968. Brain receptors sensitive to indole compounds: function in control luteinizing hormone secretion. *Science* 159:1104–5

30. Fuxe, K., Hökfelt, T. 1970. Central monoaminergic systems and hypothalamic function. *The Hypothalamus*, ed. L. Martini, M. Motta, F. Fraschini, 123–38. New York:Academic

31. Herbert, J. 1971. The role of the pineal gland in the control by light of the reproductive cycle of the ferret. *The Pineal Gland*, ed. G. E. W. Wolstenholme, J. Knight, 303–27. London: Churchill

32. Herbert, J. 1972. Initial observations on pinealectomized ferrets kept for long periods in either daylight or artificial illumination. *J. Endocrinol.* In press

33. Hishikawa, Y., Cramer, H., Kuhlo, W. 1969. Natural and melatonin-induced sleep in young chickens—a behavioral and electrographic study. *Exp. Brain Res.* 7:84–94

34. Hoffman, R. A. 1964. Speculations on the regulation of hibernation. *Ann. Acad. Sci. Fenn., Ser. A 4, Biol.* 17:202–16

35. Hoffman, R. A., Hester, R. J., Townes, C. 1965. Effect of light and temperature on the endocrine system of the golden hamster (*Mesocricetus auratus,* Waterhouse). *Comp. Biochem. Physiol.* 15:525–33

36. Hoffman, R. A., Reiter, R. J. 1965. Pineal gland: influence on gonads of male hamsters. *Science* 148:1609–11

37. Kamberi, I. A., Mical, R. S., Porter, J. C. 1970. Effect of anterior pituitary perfusion and intraventricular injection of catecholamines and indoleamines on LH release. *Endocrinology* 87:1–12

38. Kamberi, I. A., Mical, R. S., Porter, J. C. 1971. Effects of melatonin and serotonin on the release of FSH and prolactin. *Endocrinology* 88:1288–93

39. Kappers, J. A. 1969. The mammalian pineal organ. *J. Neuro-Visc. Rel.* Suppl. 9:140–84

40. Kappers, J. A. 1971. The pineal organ: an introduction. *The Pineal Gland*, ed. G. E. W. Wolstenholme, J. Knight, 3–34. London:Churchill

41. Kappers, J. A. 1971. Regulation of the reproductive system by the pineal gland and its dependence on light. *J. Neuro-Visc. Rel.,* Suppl. 10:141–52

42. Kincl, F. A., Benagiano, G. 1967. The failure of the pineal gland removal in neonatal animals to influence reproduction. *Acta Endocrinol.* 54:189–92

43. Klein, D. C., Reiter, R. J., Weller, J. L. 1971. Pineal N-acetyltransferase activity in blinded and anosmic male rats. *Endocrinology* 89:1020–23

44. Klein, D. C., Weller, J. L. 1970. Indole metabolism in the pineal gland: a circadian rhythm in N-acetyltransferase. *Science* 169: 1093–95

45. Klein, D. C., Weller, J. L., Moore, R. Y. 1971. Melatonin metabolism: neural regulation of pineal serotonin: acetyl coenzyme A N-acetyltransferase activity. *Proc. Nat. Acad. Sci. USA* 68: 3107–10

46. Koella, W. P. 1969. Serotonin and sleep. *Exp. Med. Surg.* 27:157–68

47. Kordon, C., Glowinski, J. 1970. Role of brain catecholamines in the control of anterior pituitary functions. *Neurochemical As-*

pects of Hypothalamic Function, ed. L. Martini, J. Meites, 85–100. New York:Academic

48. Lerner, A. B., Case, J. D., Takahashi, Y., Lee, T. H., Mori, W. 1958. Isolation of melatonin, the pineal factor that lightens melanocytes. *J. Am. Chem. Soc.* 80:2587

49. Longenecker, D. E., Gallo, D. G. 1971. The inhibition of PMSG-induced ovulation in immature rats by melatonin. *Proc. Soc. Exp. Biol. Med.* 137:623–25

50. Marczynski, T. J., Yamaguchi, N., Ling, G. M., Grodzinska, L. 1964. Sleep induced by the administration of melatonin (5-methyoxy-N-acetyltryptamine) to the hypothalamus in unrestrained cats. *Experientia* 20:435–36

51. Matthews, M. J., Benson, B., Rodin, A. E. 1971. Antigonadotropic activity in a melatonin-free extract of human pineal glands. *Life Sci. (Part I)* 10:1375–79

52. Mess, B. 1968. Endocrine and neurochemical aspects of pineal function. *Int. Rev. Neurobiol.* 11:171–98

53. Milcu, St. M., Demetrescu, M. 1963. Decrease of alpha rhythm irradiation in the anterior leads following pineal extract administration. *Electroencephalogr. Clin. Neurophysiol.* 15:535

54. Mishkinsky, J., Nir, I., Lajtos, Z. K., Sulman, F. G. 1966. Mammary development in pinealectomized rats. *J. Endocrinol.* 36:215–16

55. Mizuno, H., Sensui, N. 1970. Lack of effects of melatonin administration and pinealectomy on the milk ejection response in the rat. *Endocrinol. Jap.* 17:417–20

56. Mogler, R. K. H. 1958. Das Endokrinesystem des syrichen Goldhamster unter Berücksichtigung des Natürlichen und Experimentellen Winterschläf. *Z. Morph. Oekol. Tiere*, 47:267–308

57. Moszkowska, A., Ebels, I. 1970. Rôlemodulateur de l'épiphyse sur la fonction gonadotrope hypophysaire. *Neuroendocrinologie*, ed. J. Benoit, C. Kordon, 235–47. Paris:Centre National de la Recherche Scientifique

58. Moszkowska, A., Ebels, I. 1971. The influence of the pineal body on the gonadotropic function of the hypophysis. *J. Neuro-Visc. Rel.*, Suppl. 10:160–76

59. Moszkowska, A., Kordon, C., Ebels, I. 1971. Biochemical fractions and mechanisms involved in the pineal modulation of pituitary gonadotropin release. *The Pineal Gland*, ed. G. E. W. Wolstenholme, J. Knight, 241–258. London: Churchill

60. Negus, N. C., Berger, P. J. 1972. Environmental factors and reproductive processes in mammalian populations. *Biology of Reproduction: Basic and Clinical Studies*, ed. J. T. Velardo, B. Kasprow. Mexico City: Bay Publ. In press

61. Nir, I., Behroozi, K., Assael, M., Ivriani, I., Sulman, F. G. 1969. Changes in the electrical activity of the brain following pinealectomy. *Neuroendocrinology* 4:122–27

62. Nir, I., Mishkinsky, J., Eshchar, N., Sulman, F. G. 1968. Effect of pinealectomy on milk yield in rats. *J. Endocrinol.* 42:161–62

63. Ota, M., Hsieh, K. S., Obara, K. 1971. Absence of gonadotropin-inhibiting substance in the urine of pinealctomized rats. *Endocrinology* 88:816–20

64. Quay, W. B. 1956. Volumetric and cytologic variation in the pineal body of *Peromyscus leucopus* (rodentia) with respect to sex, captivity and day-length. *J. Morphol.* 98:471–95

65. Quay, W. B. 1963. Circadian rhythm in rat pineal serotonin and its modification by estrous cycle and photoperiod. *Gen. Comp. Endocrinol.* 3:473–79

66. Quay, W. B. 1965. Experimental evidence for pineal participation in homeostasis of brain composition. *Progr. Brain Res.* 10:646–53

67. Quay, W. B. 1970. Endocrine effects of the mammalian pineal. *Am. Zool.* 10:237–46

68. Ralph, C. L. 1970. Structure and alleged functions of avian pineals. *Am. Zool.* 10:217–35

69. Reiter, R. J. 1967. The effect of

pineal grafts, pinealectomy and denervation of the pineal gland on the reproductive organs of male hamsters. *Neuroendocrinology* 2:138–46

70. Reiter, R. J. 1968. The pineal gland and gonadal development in male rats and hamsters. *Fert. Steril.* 19:1009–17

71. Reiter, R. J. 1969. Pineal function in long term blinded male and female hamsters. *Gen. Comp. Endocrinol.* 12:460–68

72. Reiter, R. J. 1971. Physiologic role of the pineal gland. *The Action of Hormones*, ed. P. P. Foa, 283–314. Springfield: Thomas

73. Reiter, R. J. 1972. Effects of the pineal gland on reproductive organ growth and fertility in dual sensory deprived female rats. *Endocrinol. Exp.* 6:3–10

74. Reiter, R. J. 1972. Evidence for refractoriness of the pituitary-gonadal axis to the pineal gland in golden hamsters and its possible implications in annual reproductive rhythms. *Anat. Rec.* 173:365–372

75. Reiter, R. J. 1972. Pineal control of reproductive biology. *Biology of Reproduction: Basic and Clinical Studies*, ed. J. T. Velardo, B. Kasprow. Mexico City: Bay Publ. In press

76. Reiter, R. J. 1972. Pineal. *Reproductive Biology*, ed. H. Balin, S. Glasser, 71–114. Amsterdam: Excerpta Medica

77. Reiter, R. J., Fraschini, F. 1969. Endocrine aspects of the mammalian pineal gland: a review. *Neuroendocrinology* 5:219–55

78. Reiter, R. J., Hester, R. J. 1965. Interrelationships of the pineal gland, the superior cervical ganglia and the photoperiod in the regulation of the endocrine systems of hamsters. *Endocrinology* 79:1168–70

79. Reiter, R. J., Monaco, L., Donofrio, R. J. 1969. The influence of the pineal gland and its constituents on PMS-induced ovulation in immature rats. *Am. Zool.* 9:1087

80. Reiter, R. J., Morgan, W. W. 1972. Attempts to characterize the convulsive response of parathyroidectomized rats to pineal gland removal. *Physiol. Behav.*

In press

81. Reiter, R. J., Morgan, W. W., Talbot, J. A. 1972. Pineal interaction with the brain: evidence from thyroparathyroidectomized rats. *Fed. Proc.* 31:221

82. Reiter, R. J., Sorrentino, S., Jr. 1970. Reproductive effects of the mammalian pineal. *Am. Zool.* 10:247–58

83. Reiter, R. J., Sorrentino, S., Jr. 1971. Factors influential in determing the gonad-inhibiting activity of the pineal gland. *The Pineal Gland*, ed. G. E. W. Wolstenholme, J. Knight, 329–44. London:Churchill

84. Reiter, R. J., Sorrentino, S., Jr. 1971. Ihibition of luteinizing hormone release and ovulation in PMS-treated rats by peripherally administered melatonin. *Contraception* 4:385–92

85. Reiter, R. J., Sorrentino, S., Jr., Hoffman, R. A. 1972. Muscular spasms and death in thyroparathyroidectomized rats subjected to pinealectomy. *Life Sci. (Part I)* 11:123–33

86. Reiter, R. J. et al 1971. Some endocrine effects of blinding and anosmia in adult male rats with observations on pineal melatonin. *Endocrinology* 88:895–900

87. Reiter, R. J., Vaughan, M. K., Vaughan, G. M. 1972. Melatonin action on the time course of compensatory ovarian hypertrophy in the Swiss-Webster mouse. *Int. J. Fert.* 17:59–62

88. Roldan, E., Anton-Tay, F. 1968. EEG and convulsive threshold changes produced by pineal extract administration. *Brain Res.* 11:238–45

89. Roldan, E., Anton-Tay, F., Escobar, A. 1964. Studies on the pineal gland. IV. The effect of pineal extract on the electroencephalogram. *Biol. Inst. Estud. Méd. Biol.* 22:145–56

90. Schneider, J. J. 1971. L'epifisi, questa sconosciuta. *Minerva Med.* 63:2615–16

91. Schneider, J. J. 1971. L'épiphyse, celte méconnue. *Cah. Med.* (Paris) 12:555–56

92. Schneider, J. J. 1971. Die Unbekannte Epiphyse. *Münch. Med. Woch.* 113:1266–67

93. Shani (Mishkinsky), J., Knaggs, G. S., Tindal, J. S. 1971. The

effect of noradrenaline, dopamine, 5-hydroxytryptamine and melatonin on milk yield and composition in the rabbit. *J. Endocrinol.* 50:543–44

94. Sheridan, M. N., Reiter, R. J., Jacobs, J. J. 1969. An interesting anatomical relationship between the hamster pineal gland and the ventricular system of the brain. *J. Endocrinol.* 45:131–32

95. Smit-Vis, J. H., Akkerman-Bellaart, M. A. 1967. Spermiogenesis in hibernating golden hamsters. *Experientia* 23:844–45

96. Sorrentino, S., Jr. 1968. Antigonadotropic effects of melatonin in intact and unilaterally ovariectomized rats. *Anat. Rec.* 160:432

97. Sorrentino, S., Jr., Benson, B. 1970. Effects of blinding and pinealectomy on the reproductive organs of adult male and female rats. *Gen. Comp. Endocrinol.* 15:242–46

98. Sorrentino, S., Jr., Reiter, R. J., Schalch, D. S. 1971. Hypotrophic reproductive organs and normal growth in male rats treated with melatonin. *J. Endocrinol.* 51:213–14

99. Sorrentino, S., Jr., Reiter, R. J., Schalch, D. S. 1971. Interactions of the pineal gland, blinding, and underfeeding on reproductive organ size and radioimmunoassayable growth hormone. *Neuroendocrinology* 7:105–15

100. Vaughan, M. K., Benson, B., Norris, J. T. 1970. Inhibition of compensatory ovarian hypertrophy in mice by 5-hydroxytryptamine and melatonin. *J. Endocrinol.* 47:397–398

101. Vaughan, M. K., Benson, B., Norris, J. T., Vaughan, G. M. 1971. Inhibition of compensatory ovarian hypertrophy in mice by melatonin, 5-hydroxytryptamine and pineal powder. *J. Endocrinol.* 50:171–75

102. Vaughan, M. K., Reiter, R. J., Vaughan, G. M. 1971. Effect of delaying melatonin injections on the inhibition of compensatory ovarian hypertrophy in mice. *J. Endocrinol.* 51:787–88

103. Vaughan, M. K., Reiter, R. J., Vaughan, G. M., Bigelow, L., Altschule, M. D. 1972. Inhibition of compensatory ovarian hypertrophy in the mouse and vole: a comparison of Altschule's pineal extract, pineal indoles, vasopressin and oxytocin. *Gen. Comp. Endocrinol.* 18:372–77

104. Wragg, L. 1967. Effects of pinealectomy in the newborn female rat. *Am. J. Anat.* 120:391–402

105. Wurtman, R. J. 1969. Control of the mammalian pineal by light and sympathetic nerves. *Progress in Endocrinology*, ed. C. Gual, 627–30. Amsterdam: Excerpta Medica

106. Wurtman, R. J., Axelrod, J., Fischer, J. E. 1964. Melatonin synthesis in the pineal gland: effect of light mediated by the sympathetic nervous system. *Science* 143:1328–30

107. Wurtman, R. J., Axelrod, J., Kelly, D. E. 1968. *The Pineal.* New York:Academic. 199 pp.

108. Wurtman, R. J., Axelrod, J., Phillips, L. S. 1963. Melatonin synthesis in the pineal gland: control by light. *Science* 142:1071–73

Ann. Rev. Physiol. 1973. 35:329–356

NEUROLOGICAL SUBSTRATES OF AGGRESSIVE BEHAVIOR[1]

CARMINE D. CLEMENTE AND MICHAEL H. CHASE

Departments of Anatomy and Physiology and the Brain Research Institute
UCLA School of Medicine, Los Angeles

INTRODUCTION

Stalking attack, defensive reactions, flight, cooperative interactions between members of a species in a fight, display of the "killer" instinct, and predation are but some of the overt agonistic behaviors recognized among various animal species, including man. Ethologists frequently distinguish between interspecific hunting behavior, predation, which generally is used by animals to satisfy a physiologic need such as hunger, and intraspecific social aggression, or fighting behavior, which may be more related to an emotional gratification and which frequently does not result in death of the participants. Eibl-Eibesfeldt (56), however, has noted that in some instances hunting behavior among predators is not especially related to hunger satisfaction.

It appears evident that specific neural mechanisms underlie aggressive behavior since an animal's pattern of activity can be changed from quiescent to savage or from savage to docile by electrical stimulation of specific brain sites. That such transformations may take place regardless of the environmental milieu and that they cannot be conditioned indicate the existence of so-called innate determined patterns of agonistic behavior. On the other hand, stimulation of other brain sites may also lead to aggressive reactions which are situation-dependent and which can easily and quickly be conditioned. The neural mechanisms underlying these latter patterns seem not predetermined, but appear dependent upon preceding, current, and predicted environmental experience.

In this review the neural substrates of specific aggressive behaviors will be examined.[2] Our objectives will be to define patterns of agonistic behavior, to

---

[1] Most of the articles and books cited in this review were published between 1960 and 1972. Earlier works are included only when they are of special relevance.

[2] For coverage of the broader social, biological, and pharmacological aspects of aggression the reader is referred to a number of reviews (55, 62, 80, 94, 95, 105, 175, 185, 186, 190) and monographs (24, 36, 38, 65, 110, 118, 159).

describe those brain structures whose excitation or destruction modify these behaviors, and to differentiate induced stereotypic patterns from those which can be altered by environmental conditions. The central nervous system of the cat has perhaps been investigated more thoroughly by neurophysiological methods than that of any other species. For this reason, our definitions will be focused more on this animal than on other species. It is recognized that an animal's behavior is dependent on that species' particular motor responses and capabilities (a cat can hardly flap his feathers and fly away). Expected analogous behaviors related to aggression in many species, however, have been described, as have the homologous brain centers and neural circuits.

On the basis of somatomotor and visceromotor responses, aggression in animals is manifested by three basic behaviors: attack, defense, and flight. In this review the terms agonistic behavior and aggressive reactions will be used at times to denote in a more general sense these basic behaviors. Attack, defense, and flight have all been induced by brain stimulation in the cat. Of these, stalking attack (sometimes termed prey-killing) is accompanied by relatively few affective patterns (65, 67, 91, 107, 108, 191, 192). Vocalization, piloerection, and pupillary dilatation are minimal, if present at all. The predominant pattern in the cat is akin to predatory behavior, i.e. the body is lowered, the neck extended, the ears are out but not flattened, and movements appear well controlled (147). When an appropriate object or animal is within the immediate environment, it is approached on a direct line, seized in the animal's jaws and bitten rhythmically and repetitively (86, 111, 146). In contrast, the attack or fighting behavior which one sees when a cat is combating an equal is accompanied by salivation, pupillary dilatation, piloerection, flattened ears, hissing, urination, and intense motor activity. This behavior probably reflects a combination of the components of attack, defense, and flight and has been designated affective attack or simply as attack (191).

Defensive behavior in the cat is characterized by crouching with the head retracted and the ears flattened. It is accompanied by growling, pupillary dilatation, and piloerection (31, 74, 78, 91, 108, 182). This behavior can easily be elicited by brain stimulation and may possibly serve as an initial alerting reaction from which the cat either displays further defensive activities or, alternatively, from which flight or attack may commence.

When a cat flees, its pupils dilate, its respiratory rate increases, and there may be hissing, slight piloerection (30, 31, 108, 151, 182), urination, or defecation (151). Generally it appears that the motor responses during flight behavior are typically associated with fear reactions which occur in conjunction with the frantic locomotor activity of flight (73, 91).

Comparable agonistic patterns have been observed in other animals. As an example, spontaneous or centrally elicited attack in the opossum, *Didelphis virginiana,* is initially characterized by a fixed gaze and a deliberate approach with the neck extended. Biting of the aggressor's object is followed, as in the cat, by rhythmic masticatory movements. Defensive behavior in this animal consists of growling with an open mouth and swinging of the head and shoulders from side to side (148). In the ring dove, *Streptopelia risoria*, spontaneous or centrally elicited attack consists of wing-flapping and pecking. This is accompanied by retraction of the head and extension of the feathers, apparently serving to increase the effectiveness of the attack behavior. The ring dove's defensive posture is characterized by "puffing up" and wing-raising (thereby expanding the body surface area) and by fending and slapping (73). Such activity patterns in these species have led behaviorists to conclude that these reactions are analogous to those described for the cat (73, 110, 148). Stimulation of homologous brain sites in these species results in behaviors comparable to those described for carnivores, subhuman primates, and even man.

Although decortication in mammals is known to result in lowered thresholds for rage induction (16, 17, 19), this increased aggressiveness is probably due to the removal of inhibitory influences over subcortical mechanisms responsible for the integration of agonistic behavior. Since aggressive behavior is, in fact, observable in the decorticate animal, it is obvious that the cerebral cortex is not essential for the overt expression of this behavior. Of the central neural structures, the hypothalamus, amygdala, midbrain, and septum have most frequently been implicated in the elaboration of agonistic patterns and in behaviors related to attack, defense, and flight.

HYPOTHALAMUS

Kaada (91) has surveyed the different agonistic behaviors resulting from electrical stimulation of the medial and lateral hypothalamus. By eliminating those studies in which there is insufficient description to permit categorization of behavior into attack, defense, or flight, and those which lack histological data, remarkably consistent and relatively simple patterns of aggressive reactions have been observed based upon the excitation of discrete hypothalamic loci. These studies indicate that there exists in the cat a topographical organization in the hypothalamus for the behaviors of attack, defense, and flight. The region from which attack behavior can be induced is located laterally, defensive behavior can be induced ventromedially, and flight behavior dorsally (30, 81, 91, 147, 150, 151, 162, 171). These zones extend the length of the hypothalamus, although responses can be induced quite readily at the anterior-posterior level of the ventromedial nucleus.

Attack and quiet stalking (prey-killing) activity with directed biting in the cat is induced primarily by stimulation of the lateral and dorsomedial hypothalamic areas, generally within a plane 2 to 3 mm from the midline and extending 2 to 5 mm below the horizontal zero coordinate (53, 63, 86, 127, 146, 147, 165). There appears to be no distinct anatomical nucleus or functional subdivision of the hypothalamus located within these boundaries which may be linked specifically to this behavior.

The "defense zone" is located principally within the ventromedial portion of the anterior, middle, and posterior nuclei. This zone parallels the course of the fornix as it passes through the anterior and middle hypothalamus and overlaps the ventromedial nucleus (76, 81). Along the lateral boundary of this zone, between it and the prey-killing zone, lie sites from which affective attack may be elicited (127, 191). It could be judged that this represents a mixture of the two responses of prey-killing and defense, although it might also be a unique behavior with a distinct structural basis.

Flight reactions result from stimulation of points in the dorsal hypothalamus extending from the anterior through the posterior hypothalamus, 1 to 3 mm lateral to the third ventricle (67, 150, 151, 199). This behavior may be induced principally by stimulation near or within the dorsomedial nucleus. This site is dorsal to those eliciting defense behavior and medial to those eliciting attack.

Other species exhibit a topographic organization similar to that described for the cat. In the monkey the effect of electrical stimulation of the hypothalamus has been investigated principally by Delgado (43–47). His results, and those of others (149) indicate that the simian behaviors of attack, defense, and flight are analogous to those in the cat. In certain of these studies a detailed description of the sites of stimulation is lacking, but from the information that is available, the responsible hypothalamic loci are homologous to those in the cat. An excellent study on the behavioral responses following brain stimulation in the opossum has been reported (148). Attack, defense, and flight behaviors in this animal were comparable to those described in the cat and monkey, as were hypothalamic loci from which they could be induced. In the ring dove (73), as in the chicken (139) and pigeon (5, 6), agonistic behaviors have also been elicited by hypothalamic stimulation.

Although a number of studies exist relating the effects of hypothalamic lesions to agonistic behavior in general, these are not as well-documented as those dealing with hypothalamic stimulation. There is much evidence indicating that lesions in the caudal hypothalamic nuclei result in a decreased level of arousal and a tendency toward somnolence and catelepsy (75, 87, 141). No marked changes in alimentary or affective behavior have been specifically observed following destruction of the anterior hypothalamic nuclei, Ganser's commissure, suprachiasmatic nucleus, supraoptic nucleus, fornix, perifornical area, or dorsomedial nucleus (195). Effective modifications in aggressive behavior, however, have been produced by destruction of hypothalamic sites involving the ventromedial nucleus (*VMH*) and its adjacent structures. Thus, the behavior of cats with either large or punctate lesions of VMH has been described as savage, with the added commentary that these animals attacked observers in a vicious, aggressive manner, biting and clawing when attempts were made to pet them or when other innocuous stimuli were applied (195). Additionally, there was a tendency to use teeth or claws in escaping painful stimuli (120). Most animals also presented voracious appetites and "attacked" their food. Such animals were less likely to exhibit savage behavior immediately prior to being fed, especially if their meal was in sight, indicating a possible interrelationship between attack behavior and the alimentary process.[3]

In some animals the irritable savage behavior manifested itself immediately after the operation, but more usually it developed gradually over a period of weeks. Neither flight nor defensive attitudes were displayed with any degree of consistency in these animals; rather, there was the singular behavior of attack, which was the basis for the term "savage" used by Wheatley (195). The anatomical data which he presented indicated that the flight zone as well as the defense zone were destroyed in these savage animals, whereas, the attack zone, lying lateral to the ventromedial nucleus of the hypothalamus, was not injured. Aggressiveness resulting from ventromedial nucleus lesions is not abated by bilateral amygdaloid lesions (102). Such aggressive animals show impairment of avoidance learning in comparison to controls (120).

Unanswered by these studies is the question of how stimulation and destruction of the same structure (VMH) can apparently yield a similar behavioral response. Denervation supersensitivity has been mentioned (91) as an explanation, since the lateral hypothalamic area normally is in functional relationship to the ventromedial nucleus and thus if the ventromedial region is destroyed, neurons in the lateral sites become extremely sensitive to circulating neurohumors or synaptic activity. This explanation is based upon concepts which Cannon & Rosenbleuth (34) formulated regarding the development of increased reactivity of denervated structures to chemical agents. The gradual development of rage phenomena in some of the ventromedial animals might support this idea. Unfortunately, it does not explain the immediate development of rage in some animals, nor the fact that when rage develops slowly in others, the aggressiveness lasts for years (beyond the time accountable by the concept of supersensitivity). The deposition of metallic ions through the use of metal electrodes in the production of ventromedial lesions has been proposed as resulting in irritative lesions (144). It is reasoned that the resulting effect is a stimulation of ventrolateral hypothalamus (140).

Another hypothesis which has been forwarded is that the lateral hypothalamic attack center is under inhibitory control by the ventromedial defense zone which, if destroyed, allows attack behavior to proceed unchecked. This explanation seems more plausible since it is apparent that the different patterns of agonistic behavior (attack, defense, and flight) are dependent upon the functional integrity of distinct loci and when these loci are destroyed, the specific behaviors disappear. It might be predicted that defensive behavior would be lost following ventromedial nuclear destruction, but that flight and attack would remain, whereas after lateral lesions defense and flight would

[3] Intracranial tumors and other pathological conditions involving the hypothalamus or other limbic structures in man lead to the development of aggressive behavior comparable to that seen in animals (116, 142, 154).

remain, but attack would no longer be present, etc. Thus, stimulation of VMH would initiate defensive reactions and lesions here would lead to a disappearance of this behavior, perhaps even with an augmentation of attack or flight. Consistent with this concept is the fact that a number of the correlated physiological parameters of attack, defense, and flight vary in a manner unique to the specific behavior. For example, piloerection occurs during defense but not during stalking attack. Thus, if piloerection is represented in regions separate from the defensive site, it must be postulated that defensive reactions and piloerection are functionally integrated. Complementary reactions could then be expressed simultaneously while other inappropriate reactions are suppressed. In this regard, stimulation of the defensive zone would suppress changes in physiological parameters compatible with attack but facilitate those processes common to both states.

Experiments reporting the results of simultaneously stimulating two hypothalamic sites support this latter concept (31). The sites were either two which yielded defense reactions, two which induced flight, or one which resulted in flight and the other defense. When either two defense or two flight points were stimulated, the evoked reactions summated, i.e. a more complete reaction occurred at a reduced latency. When stimulation of a defense point was coupled with excitation of a flight point, the resulting activity appeared to represent a combination of inhibition or facilitation of the individual elements of the behavioral pattern. In general, those behavioral elements which were common to both patterns summated in effect, while antithetical responses were reduced.

Similar concepts may be considered with respect to other behaviors. Food consummatory behavior can be elicited by stimulation of the lateral hypothalamus (LH). This behavior can be observed to the point of hyperphagia when the ventromedial aphagia zone is destroyed. Inhibitory connections from VMH to LH may be the functional basis for the increase in food intake following VMH lesions and for the decrease in food consumption which occurs after LH lesions (173). If this information is extended to include agonistic behaviors, the following statements seem justified: (a) eating and attack are complementary, (b) defense (or flight) and food consumption antithetical, (c) stimulation of VMH leads to aphagia and defensive activities, and (d) lesions of VMH lead to hyperphagia and an increased attack behavior.

Although it is not definitely established that the hypothalamus is the prime center for the integration and elaboration of agonistic behavior, much of the evidence to date points toward this conclusion. An interesting study, however, was published by Ellison & Flynn (57). Integrated patterns of aggressive behavior persisted when the hypothalamus was functionally isolated from the rest of the brain. Visually directed and environmentally appropriate aggressive behaviors were not completely dependent upon the functional integrity of hypothalamic centers. Ellison (personal communication) has suggested that the hypothalamus may not be essential for the elaboration of all aspects of agonistic behavior, although when present and functional in the intact animal, it is the principal site for the integration of attack, defense, and flight behavior. Although spontaneous reactions were absent in their hypothalamic cats, these authors stated that "a very normal-appearing attack with a concomitant autonomic and skeletal display could be elicited in each of these animals by a pinch to the tail or flank" (57). The attack was visually directed and lasted as long as the nociceptive stimulus was applied. This pattern was similar to the stimulus time-locked attack described by Wasman & Flynn (191), i.e. the attack response was totally under stimulus control in that the attack behavior ceased precisely with the termination of the stimulus. Since attack was the most prominent aggressive behavior observed in animals with the isolated hypothalamic islands, it must be assumed that sites other than the hypothalamic attack zone can also initiate this behavioral pattern. In most instances these other brain regions elicit their agonistic behaviors through hypothalamic relays, but this may not be the case if Ellison & Flynn's studies can be confirmed. With regard to agonistic behavior, the hypothalamus is intimately related to the amygdala, the midbrain, and the septum.

Amygdala

The amygdala, situated within the pyriform lobe in the cat and found in the rostromedial aspect of the temporal lobe in primates, is composed of a number of nuclei which have traditionally been divided into a phylogenetically older corticomedial group and newer basolateral complex. The principal efferent projections of the amygdala are the stria terminalis from the corticomedial nuclei and the ventral amygdalofugal path which emerges mainly from the basolateral nuclear group. Through these connections the amygdala is in functional relationship with the hypothalamus, preoptic region, septum, and thalamus. Additionally, other efferent amygdaloid fibers join with the stria medullaris and the medial forebrain bundle and become a part of Nauta's limbic system-midbrain circuit (132, 133).

The electrical activity of the amygdala is influenced by a variety of interoceptive and exteroceptive stimuli, for it receives information, either directly or indirectly, concerning practically all sensory modalities as well as information from a variety of brain structures (50, 68, 112). It is therefore not surprising that the amygdaloid nuclei are involved in the elaboration of certain reactions related to aggression. Although the literature relating the amygdala to aggression is more confusing than that relating the hypothalamus to aggression, the following statements tend to be generally supportable from stimulation and lesion experiments: (a) electrical stimulation of the amygdala can give rise to both flight and defensive reactions, but not to attack behavior; (b) the two principal "efferent" amygdaloid pathways, the stria terminalis and the ventral amygdalofugal path, contain significant numbers of afferent fibers; (c) these paths not only relay to hypothalamic centers which themselves elicit agonistic reactions upon stimulation, but they also carry information from the hypothalamus; (d) amygdaloid-induced aggressive behavior can be abolished by relatively discrete lesions in the hypothalamus or midbrain; and (e) although lowered thresholds for rage have been observed in some animals following bilateral amygdaloid lesions, the most consistent social-affective changes seen resulting from such lesions have been placidity, docility, and tameness.

There appears to be agreement that separate and anatomically differentiable systems exist within the amygdala for flight (fear) and for defense (rage). Inconsistencies, however, also are found. While both Hunsperger & Fernandez de Molina (61) and Ursin & Kaada (183, 184) indicated that the central, lateral, and basal nuclei are involved with attention-defensive-flight responses, they also disagreed, since the former group believed these patterns to be dependent upon the functional integrity of the medial nucleus while the latter group did not implicate this structure with these functions. Further, although the studies both of Hilton & Zybrozyna (79) and of Fernandez de Molina & Hunsperger (60, 61) indicated that the stria terminalis is involved in defense reactions, the former stressed its afferent connections to the amygdala, while the latter pointed out the importance of its efferent fibers to the hypothalamus with regard to the defensive reaction. One point which has been confirmed in most studies and appears not to be controversial is the fact that stalking attack behavior cannot be induced by electrical stimulation of amygdaloid nuclei nor does it arise subsequent to their destruction.

The papers of Ursin & Kaada (91, 182–184) describing circumscribed stimulation and lesion experiments will now be examined more thoroughly, and the extent to which their findings are supported or contradicted by other investigators will be analyzed. The most common initial response which Ursin & Kaada and others have observed from amygdaloid stimulation was attention; this involved a cessation of ongoing spontaneous movement, attitudinal changes in the direction of alertness, orienting reactions, and desynchronization of electrocortical activity (92, 93, 114, 160, 171, 184). This response occurred upon stimulation of the basolateral amygdala and sites extending through the region of the central nucleus into the region of the internal capsule (92, 184). The medial extension of the responsive area coincided with the ventral amygdalofugal pathway. Stimulation of the medial nucleus and the medial division of the basal nucleus did not give rise to this response. About one half of the responses which yielded the attention reaction at low levels of excitation culminated in either flight or defense with higher intensities of stimulation (184). Additionally, Ursin & Kaada described two separate zones within the amygdaloid complex involved in the elaboration of aggressive behavior (92, 184); one was related to flight and the other to defense. Flight responses were evoked by stimulation of a band of tissue extending from the rostral portion of the lateral nucleus through the central nucleus and into the region of the internal capsule; lesions of this zone selectively reduced flight behavior. Defense reactions were elicited by stimulation of the caudal part of the lateral nucleus and from the lateral part of the basal nucleus; lesions in this region reduced defensive behavior (183, 184). These zones are situated somewhat parallel to each other and overlap in the region of the central nucleus.

Hilton & Zbrozyna (79) found that defense reactions were elicitable from the magnocellular portion of the basal nucleus as well as from the stria terminalis. These results essentially support those of Ursin & Kaada. Stimulation of these same sites, however, at increased intensities, would initiate behavior patterns more akin to flight behavior, such as "running wildly round the observation cage, jumping up the walls and urination" (79). Bearing in mind the concept of separate differentiable systems in the amygdala for defense and flight proposed by Ursin & Kaada, the study of Hilton & Zbrozyna demonstrated both defense and flight behaviors resulting from stimulation of the same site but at different intensities. No attempt was made by the latter authors to determine whether more discrete excitation with finer electrodes would yield responses which were independent of stimulus intensity.

Fernandez de Molina & Hunsperger (60) reported that defense and flight behavior could be elicited from the dorsomedial parts of the amygdala and from the stria terminalis with results somewhat similar to the previous studies of MacLean & Delgado (113) and Magnus & Lammers (114). Wood (196, 197) induced "fear" and "anger" from stimulation of the basal and central nuclei, while Shealy & Peele (160) obtained "rage" from sites located in the medial and central areas. Thus, Hunsperger & Fernandez de Molina (60, 61, 81) concluded that the basal, medial, and central nuclei were the areas involved in defensive behavior, whereas Ursin & Kaada did not implicate the medial nucleus, but did additionally include the lateral nucleus. The work of Wood (196, 197) and that of Shealy & Peele (160) also involved the medial nucleus.

Hernandez-Peon et al (74) induced both rage and flight by chemically stimulating, with acetylcholine, the basal regions of the amygdala. Attack behavior was not induced. Electrical stimulation of amygdaloid structures in human patients has also led to their experiencing subjective feelings of fear and rage (37, 42, 59, 170).

It is well established that bilateral lesions of the amygdaloid nuclei or temporal lobe in man, monkeys, cats, lynx, dogs, rats, and agouti result in behavioral placidity (22, 68, 72, 98, 101, 103, 104, 124, 135, 136, 138, 156, 157, 189, 193, 198). Amygdalotomy performed in epileptic patients displaying uncontrollable violence has resulted in some beneficial regression of aggressive behavior (77, 130). The lesion sites in most of these studies tend to support the localization of flight and defense zones established by stimulation studies. Increased rage reactions, however, have also been reported (18, 72, 167) following amygdalectomy. This behavior has been observed to develop gradually over a period of weeks (18, 71). Wood (196) reported an increase in aggressiveness in cats after small electrolytic lesions were placed in the basal and central nuclei. He also reported that stimulation of these nuclei in animals without lesions induced fear or rage and proposed that the central and lateral nuclei "balance one another in their influence on emotional reactions. . . ." It is interesting that either stimulation or destruction of the same nuclear groups (basal and central) gave rise to aggressive behavior, a pattern similar to that obtained from the ventromedial nucleus of the hypothalamus. It is possible that within the amygdaloid complex, as proposed for internuclear hypothalamic relationships, there exist reciprocal inhibitory and excitatory influences based upon mutually exclusive functions.

Another explanation has been offered to resolve the contrasting behaviors reported by different investigators following amygdaloid lesions, for placidity and rage clearly cannot occur together. The possible development of epileptogenic foci resulting in amygdaloid defense or flight zone discharges was suggested as a possible cause of the rage responses following lesions (72) since (a) the amygdala and ventral hippocampus have very low thresholds for seizure discharges; (b) the observed rage responses develop gradually after a latency of weeks or even months; and (c) Green et al (72) have observed that cats with amygdaloid lesions displaying postoperative rage all developed epileptic seizures, thereby suggesting that the savage behavior was due to focal discharge at the periphery of the lesions.

The concept that a differentiated anatomical system within the brain controls aggressive behavior is supported by the finding that aggressive reactions induced by stimulation of the amygdala may be blocked by an ipsilateral lesion at the hypothalamic or midbrain level (61). The effectiveness of such unilateral lesions points to the probability that aggressive behaviors are elaborated by a rather circumscribed pathway instead of through many diffuse nuclear groups and fiber systems. According to Fernandez de Molina & Hunsperger (61) amygdaloid-induced aggressive behaviors are mediated via the stria terminalis to preoptic-hypothalamic and midbrain sites and presumably then to brain stem and spinal final common paths for the visceral and somatic motor expression of behavior.

There is controversy regarding the efferent path from the amygdala subserving aggressive behavior. Since stimulation along the course of the stria terminalis was reported to lead to defensive reactions, it was suggested that amygdaloid-elicited behaviors were mediated along this path (60, 61). It has been demonstrated, however, that the stria terminalis also contains afferent fibers (8, 40, 134). Further, Hilton & Zbrozyna (79) found that neither unilateral nor bilateral lesions of the stria abolished defensive reactions induced by stimulation of the amygdala. On the other hand, placing lesions in the ventral amygdalofugal path did eliminate defensive reactions in some experiments (79, 184, 200), but not in others (60, 84). Thus, at this stage no certain conclusion can be made about which efferent amygdaloid path is necessary for defensive reactions elicited by amygdaloid stimulation or whether both major pathways transmit this type of information to the hypothalamus.

Résumé of amygdaloid-hypothalamic interaction.—The functional relationships between the amygdala and hypothalamus have been examined thoroughly. Subthreshold stimulation of the basolateral amygdaloid complex facilitates flight behavior induced by hypothalamic stimulation, as evidenced by a reduction in the latency for the onset of the behavior. Electrophysiological data have shown both a suppression and an enhancement of hypothalamic activity dependent on the site of amygdaloid stimulation (18, 51, 52, 69, 155, 172). Basolateral amygdaloid stimulation increases hypothalamic excitability while corticomedial stimulation suppresses the activity of hypothalamic ventromedial neurons (51, 52).

The functional dichotomy of amygdalo-hypothalamic pathways has even been studied in the behavioral situation (53, 54). Stimulation of the amygdala was carried out at low current levels so that no overt motor activity was induced. This level of amygdaloid stimulation was then combined with the excitation of the lateral hypothalamus which, by itself, led to attack behavior. Combined stimulation of the two structures reduced the attack response. The effective amygdaloid sites for behavioral suppression were in the medial portion of the lateral nucleus and the magnocellular portion of the basal nucleus. A facilitatory effect was observed upon the stimulation of the dorsolateral portion of the lateral nucleus. It appears that the dorsal amygdaloid efferent path, the stria terminalis, exerts an inhibitory action on ventromedial neurons, whereas the ventral amygdalofugal path exerts an initial excitatory action followed by inhibition of ventromedial cells (54).

Magnus & Lammers (114) suggested that amygdaloid-induced aggressive reactions are mediated by hypothalamic structures. Similar defensive reactions are elicited by stimulation of either the amygdala or the hypothalamus, although the amygdaloid-induced reactions develop gradually and last beyond the period of stimulation, while those of hypothalamic origin occur fully developed at the onset of stimulation and cease quite abruptly with its termination (79, 113). The best support for the concept of hypothalamic mediation of amygdaloid aggression comes from the experiments dealing with lesions of amygdalofugal pathways to the hypothalamus as well as from the reports of the loss of amygdaloid-induced reactions following hypothalamic lesions. Conversely, amygdaloid lesions were ineffective in modifying hypothalamically induced defense or flight (60, 61).

MIDBRAIN

There has been general agreement for a long period of time that rage reactions, albeit of a fragmentary nature and uncoordinated in direction or purpose, occur in animals in which all structures rostral to the midbrain have been ablated (21, 96, 197). Therefore, in addition to containing zones which receive fibers of passage from higher centers implicated in aggressive behaviors, the midbrain may also be responsible for integrating some aspects of these behaviors.

Destruction of the central gray region of the midbrain has reduced pain-fear-escape reactions in many behavioral situations and in a number of species. Liebman et al (109) found that central gray lesions reduced normal expressions of fear in rats, concluding that "mesencephalic central gray matter, and in particular its ventrolateral aspect, is critical to the normal expression of fear." Their findings and interpretations are consistent with the observation that cats with central gray lesions did not exhibit normal defensive reactions to dogs (82). Lesions placed in central gray sites where prior electrical stimulation had induced coordinated rage left the animals in a state of passivity and reduced affect.

Two carefully executed studies have compared the effects of lesions of mesencephalic fiber tracts with the destruction of specific nuclear groups in cats (117, 168). The data of these studies somewhat contradict each other. Malliani et al (117) initially decorticated their animals and then made bilateral lesions in the following midbrain sites: (a) the medial lemnisci and adjacent lateral spinothalamic tracts, (b) the reticulo-diencephalic pathway which "likely represents the anatomical substrate of the activating reticular system," (c) the ascending component of the dorsal longitudinal fasciculus, and (d) the mesencephalic mammillary peduncle. They concluded that "only severe encroachment upon the medial and lateral reticular formation can abolish spontaneous and peripherally evoked behavior . . ." and that the medial lemnisci, lateral spinothalamic tracts, central periaqueductal gray, mammillary peduncles, dorsal longitudinal fasciculus, the ventral tegmental region, as well as the interpeduncular region and the medial reticular formation more rostrally at the midcollicular level, were not involved in rage reactions. Only lesions which destroyed both the medial and lateral portions of the reticular formation in the midbrain abolished spontaneous and evoked rage behavior.

The study by Sprague et al (168) reported that large bilateral lesions in the lateral part of the rostral midbrain, which spared the reticular formation, medial pathways, and central gray, but interrupted the classical sensory and corticomesencephalic pathways, resulted in a "reduction of both somatic and autonomic signs of affective behavior" (see also 70). In contrast, these animals were hyperactive and displayed marked exploratory activity. Sprague et al also observed hypoactivity in animals with large, bilateral medial lesions, as did Mallianni et al, but noted that they could be easily aroused and, when aroused, were capable of displaying pleasure as well as rage responses. They concurred that the medial systems were important in the regulation of a general level of excitability, but only in a nonspecific fashion insofar as behavioral responses were concerned.

Sprague et al (168), along with Fernandez de Molina & Hunsperger (61), proposed that the midbrain was an area involved with the integration of behavior and not simply the site of passage or relay for fiber systems from above. In support of this concept, these authors pointed out that many of the symptoms of lemniscal cats occurred following lesions or stimulation of other midbrain structures, such as the central gray and adjacent tegmentum (1, 41, 81, 97, 115, 163), indicating to them a widespread integrative activity of extensive regions of the midbrain. Whether the reticular formation is essential for the genesis of aggressive reactions or whether the lemniscal system must be present for the expression of this behavior is still unresolved. Since affective responses were obtained in brainstem-transected animals in which only the caudal brainstem was intact, it seems possible that the mechanisms responsible for the maintenance of some aspects of aggressive reactions are present at or below this level of the neuraxis (17, 96).

Electrical stimulation studies have also implicated the central gray and the tegmental reticular formation in aggressive reactions. The central gray surrounds the aqueduct of Sylvius and is composed of dorsal, lateral, and ventral portions. It is traversed principally by the dorsal longitudinal fasciculus; ventrolaterally lies the tegmentum, which includes the mesencephalic reticular formation. One site from which rage or affective-defense responses have been obtained is a region of the central gray in the rostral midbrain extending from the trochlear complex to the posterior commissure (81, 82, 84). The response had elements of both defense and attack, defensive behaviors being observed at low levels of stimulation while directed attack occurred at higher levels (82). Somewhat later (83) these behaviors were redefined as threat and flight, with threat evokable from the central portion of the responsive region described above, and flight obtained by stimulating the surrounding peripheral regions (83). The elicitation of affective-defense and flight from the dorsal tegmentum (82) has been confirmed (161).

Defense and attack have also been obtained by stimulation of the periaqueductal gray in the rostral midbrain beneath the superior colliculus, whereas stimulation of the caudal mesencephalon resulted only in fragmented components of flight rather than the integrated patterns elicited more rostrally (164). Hissing and growling have been obtained by either electrical or chemical (carbachol) stimulation of the midbrain periaqueductal gray (20). No aggressive responses were obtained by Skultety (164) from any region outside the periaqueductal gray at the level of the caudal mesencephalon, and contrary to Hunsperger's findings (81, 82, 84), integrated flight was not obtained either from mesencephalic central gray or from the regions surrounding it at this level of the lower midbrain.

Discrepancies between Skultety's and Hunsperger's reports might be accounted for by differences in both the parameters of stimulation and in the experimental chambers. Definition of responses may also be involved. Skultety stated that flight as defined by Hunsperger was unobtainable from periaqueductal gray stimulation although, in fact, the elements of flight described by Skultety from the caudal region seemed to us to be much the same as those reported by Hunsperger. Nakao et al (128, 129) examined escape behavior by stimulating points in and around the central gray, allowing the animals to "switch off" the stimulation. Positive points were obtained in the middle and caudal central gray, lateral and ventral to the aqueduct of Sylvius. These authors observed a fear-flight response from the same posterior central gray region from which Skultety obtained fragmented flight reactions (164).

Other investigators also reported responses similar to "sham rage" (106), "attack" (161), and "fear-like" reactions (48, 152) following midline stimulation. Liebman et al (109) even postulated that the central gray of the mesencephalon is specifically responsible for the integration of fear and for its accompanying behavioral patterns and, in fact, flight responses have been observed by many investigators (49, 81, 122, 164, 166, 188).

Defensive reactions observed in monkeys following midbrain central gray stimulation were hypothesized to be due to pain subsequent to the activation of sensory paths (41, 44). In man, stimulation of the midbrain results in the induction of fear and pain (131, 143, 166). Because of these reports, Kaada (91) believed that midbrain participation in the integration of defensive behavior still remains to be shown. Since the relationship of pain to aggressive reactions is outside the scope of this review, the reader is referred to recent articles which examine this question (4, 9–15, 44, 48, 64, 85, 126, 137, 177–181). Generally, these reports indicate that painful stimuli can induce specific behaviors of attack, defense, and flight, depending upon the pattern and place of stimulation and the modes of reaction available to the animal.

SEPTUM

Brady & Nauta (27) were the first to report that circumscribed lesions of the septum in rats resulted in the development of aggressive, savage behavior. Such animals attack objects thrust toward them, are dangerous to handle, and show startle and flight behavior patterns. In many studies utilizing a variety of testing paradigms, increased aggressiveness following septal lesions has been confirmed not only in rats (4, 7, 26, 32, 33, 35, 99, 158, 174, 176, 194), but in cats as well (23, 121, 123, 167). It is interesting that the increased aggressiveness following septal destruction occurs immediately, but gradually declines over a period of days or weeks, whereas the aggressiveness observed following ventromedial hypothalamic lesions arises only after a period of days and increases with the passage of time, often requiring weeks to develop to its fullest extent (195). Almost all of the component elements of aggression such as hyperexcitability, attack, flight, biting, defense postures, and vocalization are characteristics of the septal syndrome. This behavior is, therefore, difficult to classify in terms of attack, defense, or flight, and it has been suggested that removal of the septum results in a general disinhibition of hypothalamic mechanisms, so that they function unchecked by septal inhibitory control (91). The aggressiveness resulting from septal lesions can be reversed to tameness immediately by making lesions in the amygdala (100).

As might be expected from the results of lesions, electrical stimulation of the septal region produces a marked suppression of both somatomotor and visceromotor activity (28, 89, 90); septal stimulation also increases the latency for the onset of hypothalamically induced attack (162) as does electrical stimulation more ventral to the septal region in the diagonal band of Broca (88). These basal forebrain structures are capable of suppressing behavior even to the extent of inducing sleep (39, 169). Stimulation of one of the septal efferent paths, the medial forebrain bundle, reduces fear or rage reactions induced by hypothalamic stimulation (58, 91). Septal stimulation in the monkey has also resulted in a general reduction in aggressive behavior (153).

Résumé of mesencephalic and septal interaction with the hypothalamus.— Rage reactions can be elicited by midbrain stimulation. Sheard & Flynn (161) found that stimulation of the midbrain reticular formation at levels which produced only slight alerting reactions facilitated hypothalamically induced attack when both structures were stimulated simultaneously. Midbrain-induced defensive reactions were not modified by bilateral coagulation of the hypothalamic defense zones (81, 82), whereas midbrain coagulation did reduce hypothalamically induced flight (81), presumably through the destruction of some of the efferent hypothalamic paths. The pons and medulla exert both facilitatory and inhibitory influences on diencephalic sham rage (25). Unit recordings from cells in the midbrain central gray in a chronically prepared cat showed responses with action potentials only during fighting behavior and not when the animal was at rest (2). The septum influences aggressive behavior principally through its interaction with the hypothalamus and midbrain, for there are few direct connections between the septum and the amygdala (40, 66).

THE CONDITIONING OF AGGRESSIVE BEHAVIOR

Can patterns of aggressive behavior which are induced by electrical stimulation of the brain be conditioned? This question is of interest because such conditioning may allow the behavioral physiologist to determine whether stimulation is inducing a behavior which has meaning or significance to the animal, or whether stimulation induces a more simple direct motor response without affect or cognition. Masserman (119) believed that the hypothalamus mediated only the motor and endocrine expression of affective states and not their emotional or subjective foundation. He attempted to condition, in the classical sense, hypothalamically induced rage behavior in cats. Hypothalamic stimulation was preceded by indifferent sensory cues such as light, sound, or a puff of air. In most of his animals (eighteen) no evidence of a conditioned response was obtained. In some of his cats (six) transient startle responses and pupillary dilation occurred in response to the sensory stimuli following 80 to 160 conditioning trials. One qualification to Masserman's negative results should be pointed out. The behavior he elicited as the unconditioned response by stimulation of the hypothalamus consisted of explosive, nondirected, stimulus-bound behavior independent of the environment. The cats exhibited a mixed pattern of response including growling, ear retraction, salivation, piloerection, and striking with their claws. Masserman did not specify the site of stimulation other than that it was hypothalamic, and the pattern of the unconditioned response indicated the probable simultaneous stimulation of all three hypothalamic zones involved in attack, flight, and defense.

More recent attempts to condition hypothalamically induced behavior have met with varying degrees of success (29, 187). Wada & Matsuda (187), stimulating the hypothalamus at sites from which flight reactions have been obtained (150, 191), designed their experiments to determine whether cats could learn either to escape or to avoid stimulation. The animals rapidly learned to terminate hypothalamic stimulation by pushing a plate. However, they did not learn to push a plate or move to a safe compartment in response to a bell (conditioned stimulus) which had been repeatedly paired with hypothalamic stimulation. Thus, escape behavior was conditionable while avoidance behavior was not, although some "anticipatory" avoidance behavior was noted in response to the conditioned stimulus, results similar to those of Masserman (119). Brown & Cohen (29), stimulating in approximately the same hypothalamic site, found that their cats would learn to traverse a runway in order to avoid hypothalamic stimulation and also traverse a runway to obtain hypothalamic stimulation. They proposed that a lateral hypothalamic stimulus may act as a drive-arousing mechanism to produce both avoidance and approach learning in the same cat. According to these authors, the tasks which the animals performed were accomplished because hypothalamic stimulation induced an "excitatory state" which could be conditioned to a tone and served to motivate the cats.

Nakao (127, 129) successfully conditioned flight reactions induced by hypothalamic stimulation. Conditioning trials consisted of an auditory cue from a buzzer followed by hypothalamic stimulation in or near the dorsolateral nucleus. A conditioned response developed which did not correspond exactly to the unconditioned response but did consist of (a) interruption of ongoing activities, (b) pupillary dilation, and (c) walking or running. In another experiment, nociceptive stimulation induced an avoidance response which was successfully transferred to hypothalamic stimulation. The animals also learned to avoid a compartment or food which was associated with hypothalamic stimulation. Roberts (145) found that cats would learn to escape from hypothalamic stimulation which induced a flight response, but could not learn to avoid it. His sites of stimulation, however, were located more posteriorly in the hypothalamus than the more rostral sites used by Nakao which, upon stimulation, have been described as inducing "pure" flight responses.

Attempts to condition attack behavior induced by hypothalamic stimulation have not proved especially successful. Nakao (127), using the hypothalamic zone from which several investigators have elicited attack behavior (53, 146, 191), was able to show a conditioned response which consisted of trembling, crouching, retraction, pupillary dilation, running, and jumping.

The conditioned behavior was quite different from the unconditioned attack reaction. Adams & Flynn (3) found that transfer in a shock-avoidance situation occurred only in conjunction with hypothalamically induced flight, but not attack. Hypothalamically induced attack may possess motivational properties. Roberts & Kiess (147) were able to demonstrate that cats, stimulated in the region described for inducing stalking attack, would consistently pick the limb of a Y maze which contained a rat, even though stimulation was not contingent upon the animals' choice of either limb of the maze. When placed in this situation without hypothalamic stimulation, no limb traversal or attack occurred. Thus, although stimulation was effective in motivating a learned response, it did not lead to a conditioned reaction.

Pure defensive responses have not been examined in conditioning studies. It would appear, however, from the description of the anatomical sites of stimulation used and from the animals' resultant behavior, that some aspects of the defense reaction have been involved in many of the experiments in which flight or attack reactions were examined.

In many experiments it has been demonstrated that peripherally applied nociceptive stimuli lead to aggressive patterns of behavior (4, 9, 48, 64, 125, 137, 178, 180, 181). Attack, for example, was observed following the application of electrical shock to the feet of cats (181). Adams & Flynn (3) sought to determine whether cats which had learned to escape an electrical shock by jumping onto a stool would perform a similar response during hypothalamic stimulation. This study was primarily oriented toward determining whether nociceptive stimulus-induced attack was functionally linked to attack elicited by hypothalamic stimulation. They examined two types of attack behavior which were induced by hypothalamic stimulation; both patterns of attack were directed and consisted of biting or striking an anesthetized rat. One attack pattern was accompanied by vocalization, piloerection ear retraction, and other affective signs, while the other pattern was similar to stalking attack, consisting of none of the foregoing display, but rather "discernible primarily because the cat bit the rat, usually at the back of its neck." Stimulation of sites that induced attack plus vocalization and display led to the behavior which had been conditioned to the exteroceptive stimulus. The stalking pattern of attack did not transfer to the conditioned response associated with electrical shock to the feet. The authors concluded that the brain systems controlling attack associated with display and vocalization are independent but closely related to those involved with peripherally elicited attack, while the neural mechanisms involved with quiet biting attack are separate and do not overlap with the central neural processes mediating affective attack or nociceptively induced attack.

Rather clear-cut results were obtained in similar studies using, as the unconditioned stimulus, midbrain stimulation within or near the periaqueductal gray (188). Six out of seven cats which displayed fearlike or escape behavior in response to midbrain stimulation successfully learned to escape central stimulation. Of the six animals which learned to escape midbrain stimulation, four also learned an avoidance task. In this same study none of the cats learned the avoidance paradigm when hypothalamic stimulation was the unconditioned stimulus and flight behavior the unconditioned response. Roberts (145) obtained both escape and avoidance conditioning with stimulation of the medial lemniscus in the midbrain. The unconditioned stimulus was described as an "alarm" reaction and consisted of a general heightened activity interspersed with periods of pauses and crouching.

Ross et al (152) were able to condition responses evoked by electrical stimulation of the midbrain reticular formation, the central gray, and the stratum profundum of the superior colliculus. Utilizing an auditory cue as the conditioned stimulus, they were able to demonstrate conditioned responses in trace and avoidance paradigms. Moreover, all of the attendant epiphenomena, such as differentiation, reinforcement, and extinction were observed. These results indicate that flight behavior of midbrain origin can easily be conditioned whether it occurs as the result of excitation of primary sensory systems (48) or of regions related to the integration of behavior (152).

The participation of pain as a possible basis for the relative ease of learning with mesencephalic stimulation cannot be excluded, since the periaqueductal gray has been linked to the brain mechanisms responsible for the integration of pain sensations. In fact, flight behavior has been easily conditioned when it was induced by stimulation of midbrain sites which have been directly implicated in the transmission and integration of pain (48).

SUMMARY

The central neural structures involved in aggressive reactions appear to be functionally and anatomically interrelated. The hypothalamus is the focal structure in the elaboration of agonistic behavioral patterns since its destruction disrupts both spontaneous and induced aggression. The amygdala exerts its influence on aggressive reactions principally by modulating the activity of the hypothalamus, while the septum appears to inhibit agonistic patterns by suppressing aggressive behavior of both amygdaloid and hypothalamic origin. The midbrain serves principally as a relay for information descending from above, but seems to possess some integrative capabilities as well.

The evidence indicates that certain of the component behaviors of centrally induced aggressive reactions can be conditioned and presumably have some subjective meaning to the animal. The responses induced by hypothalamic stimulation, when they are explosive, purposeless, undirected and stimulus-bound, do not seem to be conditionable and likely represent strictly motor responses. Cats can be at least partially conditioned to escape and to avoid behaviors of attack, defense, and flight which are produced by excitation of certain hypothalamic sites. Midbrain-induced flight is more easily conditioned. It may be that each of the behaviors of aggression could be conditioned if "pure" responses of attack, defense, or flight could be obtained and the appropriate experimental design utilized.

ACKNOWLEDGMENT

The authors wish to thank the Brain Information Service at UCLA, which is supported under Contract NIH-NINDS-70-2063, for assistance in obtaining many of the citations used in this review.

LITERATURE CITED

1. Adametz, J., O'Leary, J. L. 1959. Experimental mutism resulting from periaqueductal lesions in cats. *Neurology* 9:636–42
2. Adams, D. 1968. Cells relating to fighting behavior recorded from midbrain central gray neuropil of cat. *Science* 159:894–96
3. Adams, D., Flynn, J. P. 1966. Transfer of an escape response from tail shock to brain-stimulated attack behavior. *J. Exp. Anal. Behav.* 9:401–8
4. Ahmad, S. S., Harvey, J. A. 1968. Long-term effects of septal lesions and social experience on shock-elicited fighting in rats. *J. Comp. Physiol. Psychol.* 66:596–602
5. Akerman, B. 1966. Behavioural effects of electrical stimulation in the forebrain of the pigeon. I. Reproductive behaviour. *Behavior* 26:323–38
6. Akerman, B. 1966. Behavioural effects of electrical stimulation in the forebrain of the pigeon. II. Protective behaviour. *Behavior* 26:339–50
7. Allikmets, L. K., Ditrikh, M. E. 1965. Effects of lesions in limbic system on emotional reactions and conditioned reflexes in rats. *Fed. Proc. Transl. Suppl.* 24:1003–7
8. Alphen, H. A. Van 1969. The anterior commissure of the rabbit. *Acta Anat. Basel* 74: Suppl. 57, 9–111
9. Azrin, N. H., Hake, D. F., Hutchinson, R. R. 1965. Elicitation of aggression by a physical blow. *J. Exp. Anal. Behav.* 8:55–57
10. Azrin, N. H., Hutchinson, R. R., Hake, D. F. 1963. Pain induced fighting in the squirrel monkey. *J. Exp. Anal. Behav.* 6:620
11. Azrin, N. H., Hutchinson, R. R., Hake, D. F. 1966. Extinction induced aggression. *J. Exp. Anal. Behav.* 9:191–204
12. Azrin, N. H., Hutchinson, R. R., McLaughlin, R. 1965. The opportunity for aggression as an operant reinforcer during aversive stimulation. *J. Exp. Anal. Behav.* 8:171–80
13. Azrin, N. H., Hutchinson, R. R., Sallery, R. D. 1964. Pain-aggression toward inanimate objects. *J. Exp. Anal. Behav.* 7: 223–28
14. Azrin, N. H., Rubin, H. B., Hutchinson, R. R. 1968. Biting attack by rats in response to aversive shock. *J. Exp. Anal. Behav.* 11:633–39
15. Azrin, N. H., Ulrich, R. E., Hutchinson, R. R., Norman, D. G. 1964. Effect of shock duration on shock-induced fighting. *J. Exp. Anal. Behav.* 7:9–11
16. Bard, P. 1928. A diencephalic mechanism for the expression of rage with special reference to the sympathetic nervous system. *Am. J. Physiol.* 84:490–515
17. Bard, P. 1939. Central nervous mechanisms for emotional behavior patterns in animals. *Res. Publ. Assoc. Res. Nerv. Ment. Dis.* 19:190–218
18. Bard, P., Mountcastle, V. B. 1948. Some forebrain mechanisms involved in expression of rage with special reference to suppression of angry behavior. *Res. Publ. Assoc. Res. Nerv. Ment. Dis.* 27:362–404
19. Bard, P., Rioch, D. 1937. A study of four cats deprived of neocortex and additional portions of the forebrain. *Bull. Johns Hopkins Hosp.* 60:73–147
20. Baxter, B. L. 1968. Elicitation of emotional behavior by electrical or chemical stimulation applied to the same loci in cat mesencephalon. *Exp. Neurol.* 21:1–10
21. Bazett, H. C., Penfield, W. G. 1922. A study of the Sherrington decerebrate animal in the chronic as well as the acute condition. *Brain* 45:185–265
22. Ben-Ishay, D., Welner, A. 1969. Sensitivity to experimental hypertension and aggressive reactions in rats. *Proc. Soc. Exp. Biol. Med.* 132:1170–73
23. Bergquist, E. H., 1970. Output pathways of hypothalamic mechanisms for sexual, aggressive, and other motivated behaviors in opossum. *J. Comp. Physiol. Psychol.* 70:389–98
24. Berkowitz, L. 1962. *Aggression: A Social Psychological Analysis.* New York: McGraw-Hill. 361 pp.

25. Bizzi, E., Malliani, A., Apelbaum, J., Zanchetti, A. 1963. Excitation and inhibition of sham rage behavior by lower brain stem stimulation. *Arch. Ital. Biol.* 101:614–31

26. Blanchard, R. J., Blanchard, D. C. 1968. Limbic lesions and reflexive fighting. *J. Comp. Physiol. Psychol.* 66:603–5

27. Brady, J. V., Nauta, W. J. H. 1953. Subcortical mechanisms in emotional behavior: affective changes following septal forebrain lesions in the albino rat. *J. Comp. Physiol. Psychol.* 46:339–46

28. Bromley, D. V., Holdstock, T. L. 1969. Effects of septal stimulation on heart rate in vagotomized rats. *Physiol. Behav.* 4:399–401

29. Brown, G. W., Cohen, B. D., 1959. Avoidance and approach learning motivated by stimulation of identical hypothalamic loci. *Am. J. Physiol.* 197:153–57

30. Brown, J. L., Hunsperger, R. W., Rosvold, H. E. 1969. Defense, attack, and flight elicited by electrical stimulation of the hypothalamus of the cat. *Exp. Brain Res.* 8:113–29

31. Brown, J. L., Hunsperger, R. W., Rosvold, H. E. 1969. Interaction of defense and flight reactions produced by simultaneous stimulation at two points in the hypothalamus of the cat. *Exp. Brain Res.* 8:130–49

32. Bunnell, B. N., Bemporad, J. R., Flesher, C. K. 1966. Septal forebrain lesions and social dominance behavior in the hooded rat. *Psychon. Sci.* 6:207–8

33. Bunnell, B. N., Smith, M. H. 1966. Septal lesions and aggressiveness in the cotton rat, *Sigmodon hispidus. Psychon. Sci.* 9:443–44

34. Cannon, W. B., Rosenbleuth, A. 1949. *The Supersensitivity of Denervated Structures.* New York: Macmillan. 245 pp.

35. Carey, R. J. 1968. A further localization of inhibitory deficits resulting from septal ablation. *Physiol. Behav.* 3:645–49

36. Carthy, J. D., Ebling, F. J., Eds. 1964. *The Natural History of Aggression. Institute of Biology Symposia* 14. London: Academic. 159 pp.

37. Chapman, W. P. et al 1954. Physiological evidence concerning the importance of the amygdaloid nuclear region in the integration of circulatory function and emotion in man. *Science* 120:949–50

38. Clemente, C. D., Lindsley, D. B., Eds. 1967. *Aggression and Defense. Neural Mechanisms and Social Patterns. UCLA Forum Med. Sci.* 7. Los Angeles: Univ. Calif. Press. 361 pp.

39. Clemente, C. D., Sterman, M. B. 1967. Basal forebrain mechanisms for internal inhibition and sleep. *Res. Publ. Ass. Res. Nerv. Ment. Dis.* 45:127–47

40. Cowan, W. M., Raisman, G., Powell, T. P. S. 1965. The connexions of the amygdala. *J. Neurol. Neurosurg. Psychiat.* 28:137–51

41. Delgado, J. M. R. 1955. Cerebral structures involved in transmission and elaboration of noxious stimulation. *J. Neurophysiol.* 18:261–75

42. Delgado, J. M. R. 1960. Emotional behavior in animals and humans. *Psychiat. Res. Rep.* 12:259–66

43. Delgado, J. M. R. 1966. Aggressive behavior evoked by radio stimulation in monkey colonies. *Am. Zool.* 6:669–81

44. Delgado, J. M. R. 1967. Social rank and radio-stimulated aggressiveness in monkeys. *J. Nerv. Ment. Dis.* 144:383–90

45. Delgado, J. M. R. 1969. Offensive-defensive behavior in free monkeys and chimpanzees induced by radio stimulation of the brain. In *Aggressive Behavior*, ed. S. Garattini, E. B. Sigg, 109–19. New York: Wiley. 387 pp.

46. Delgado, J. M. R. et al 1968. Intracerebral radio stimulation and recording in completely free patients. *J. Nerv. Ment. Dis.* 147:329–40

47. Delgado, J. M. R., Mir, D. 1969. Fragmental organization of emotional behavior in the monkey brain. *Ann. NY Acad. Sci.* 159:731–51

48. Delgado, J. M. R., Roberts, W. W., Miller, N. E. 1954. Learning motivated by electrical stimulation

of the brain stem. *Am. J. Physiol.* 179:587–93

49. Delgado, J .M. R., Rosvold, H. E., Looney, E. 1956. Evoking conditioned fear by electrical stimulation of subcortical structures in the monkey brain. *J. Comp. Physiol. Psychol.* 49:373–80

50. Dell, P., Olson, R. 1951. Projections "secondaires" mésencéphaliques, diencéphaliques et amygdaliennes des afferences viscérales vagales. *Compt. Rend. Soc. Biol.* 145:1088–1091

51. Dreifuss, J. J. 1972. Effect of electrical stimulation of the amygdaloid complex on the ventromedial hypothalamus. In *The Neurobiology of the Amygdala,* ed. B. E. Eleftheriou, 295–317. New York: Plenum. 819 pp.

52. Dreifuss, J. J., Murphy, J. T., Gloor, P. 1968. Contrasting effects of two identified amygdaloid efferent pathways on single hypothalamic neurons. *J. Neurophysiol.* 31:237–248

53. Egger, M. D., Flynn, J. P. 1963. Effects of electrical stimulation of the amygdala on hypothalamically elicited attack behavior in cats. *J. Neurophysiol.* 26:705–720

54. Egger, M. D., Flynn, J. P. 1967. Further studies on the effects of amygdaloid stimulation and ablation on hypothalamically elicited attack behavior in cats. In *Structure and Function of the Limbic System,* ed. W. R. Adey, T. Tokizane, *Progr. Brain Res.* 27:165–82. Amsterdam: Elsevier. 489 pp.

55. Eibl-Eibesfeldt, I. 1961. The fighting behavior of animals. *Sci. Am.* 205(6):112–22

56. Eibl-Eibesfeldt, I. 1967. Ontogenetic and maturational studies of aggressive behavior. In *Aggression and Defense: Neural Mechanisms and Social Patterns,* ed. C. D. Clemente, D. B. Lindsley. *UCLA Forum Med. Sci.* 7:57–94. Los Angeles: Univ. Calif. Press. 361 pp.

57. Ellison, G. D., Flynn, J. P. 1968. Organized aggressive behavior in cats after surgical isolation of the hypothalamus. *Arch. Ital. Biol.* 106:1–20

58. Endroczi, E., Koranyi, L. 1969. Integration of emotional reactions in the brain stem, diencephalic and limbic system. In *Aggressive Behavior,* ed. S. Garattini, E. B. Sigg, 132–40. New York: Wiley. 387 pp.

59. Feindel, W. 1961. Response patterns elicited from the amygdala and deep temporoinsular cortex. In *Electrical Stimulation of the Brain,* ed. D. E. Sheer, 519–33. Austin: Univ. Texas Press. 641 pp.

60. Fernandez de Molina, A., Hunsperger, R. W. Central representation of affective reactions in forebrain and brainstem: Electrical stimulation of amygdala, stria terminalis, and adjacent structures. *J. Physiol. London* 145:251–69

61. Fernandez de Molina, A., Hunsperger, R. W. 1962. Organization of the subcortical system governing defense and flight reactions in the cat. *J. Physiol. London* 160:200–13

62. Feshbach, S. 1964. The function of aggression and regulation of aggressive drive. *Psychol. Rev.* 71:257–72

63. Flynn, J. P. 1969. Neural aspects of attack behavior in cats. *Ann. NY Acad. Sci.* 159:1008–12

64. Galef, B. G., Jr. 1970. Target novelty elicits and directs shock associated aggression in wild rats. *J. Comp. Physiol. Psychol.* 71:87–91

65. Garattini, S., Sigg, E. B., Eds. 1969. *Aggressive Behavior.* New York: Wiley. 387 pp.

66. Genton, C. 1969. Etude, par la technique de Nauta, des dégenérescences consecutives à une lesion electrolytique de la region septale chez le mulot sylvestre (*Apodemus sylvaticus*). *Brain Res.* 14:1–23

67. Gloor, P. 1955. Electrophysiological studies on the connections of the amygdaloid nucleus in the cat. Part I: The neuronal organization of the amygdaloid projection system. Part II: The electrophysiological properties of the amygdaloid projection system. *Electroencephalogr. Clin. Neurophysiol.* 7:223–64

68. Gloor, P. 1960. Amygdala. In *Handbook of Physiology: Section I. Neurophysiology,* ed. J. Field, H. W. Magoun, V. E.

Hall, Vol. 2:1395–1420. Washington, DC: Am. Physiol. Soc. 2013 pp.

69. Glusman, M., Roizin, L. 1960. Role of the hypothalamus in the organization of agonistic behavior in the cat. *Trans. Am. Neurol. Assoc.* 85:177–79

70. Glusman, M., Won, W., Burdock, E. I., Ransohoff, J. 1962. Effects of midbrain lesions on "savage" behavior induced by hypothalamic lesions in the cat. *Trans. Am. Neurol. Assoc.* 86:216–18

71. Goddard, G. V. 1964. Functions of the amygdala. *Psychol. Bull.* 62:89–109

72. Green, J. D., Clemente, C. D., de Groot, J. 1957. Rhinencephalic lesions and behavior in cats. *J. Comp. Neurol.* 108:505–36

73. Harwood, D., Vowles, D. M. 1967. Defensive behaviour and the aftereffects of brain stimulation in the ring dove (*Streptopelia risoria*). *Neuropsychologia* 5:345–66

74. Hernandez-Peon, R., O'Flaherty, J. J., Mazzuchelli-O'Flaherty, A. L. 1967. Sleep and other behavioral effects induced by acetylcholine stimulation of basal temporal cortex and striate structures. *Brain Res.* 4:243–67

75. Hess, W. R. 1954. *The Diencephalon*. New York: Grune & Stratton. 79 pp.

76. Hess, W. R., Brügger, M. 1943. Das subkorticale Zentrum der affektiven Abwehrreaktion. *Acta Helv. Physiol. Pharmacol.* 1:33–52

77. Heimberger, R. R., Whitlock, C. C., Kalsbeck, J. E. 1966. Stereotaxic amygdalotomy. *J. Am. Med. Assoc.* 198:741–45

78. Hilton, S. M. 1965. Hypothalamic control of the cardiovascular responses in fear and rage. *Sci. Basis Med.* 217–38. London: Athlon. 334 pp.

79. Hilton, S. M., Zbrozyna, A. W. 1963. Amygdaloid region for defense reactions and its afferent pathway to the brain stem. *J. Physiol. London* 165:160–73

80. Hinde, R. A. 1969. The bases of aggression in animals. *J. Psychosom. Res.* 13:213–19

81. Hunsperger, R. W. 1956. Affektreaktionen auf elektrische Reizung im Hirnstamm der Katze.

Acta Helv. Physiol. Pharmacol. 14:70–92

82. Hunsperger, R. W. 1956. Role of substantia grisea centralis mesencephali in electrically induced rage reaction. In *Progress in Neurobiology*, ed. J. A. Kappers, 289–94. New York: Elsevier. 384 pp.

83. Hunsperger, R. W., Brown, J. L., Rosvold, H. E. 1964. Combined stimulation in areas governing threat and flight behavior in the brain stem of the cat. In *Topics in Basic Neurobiology*, ed. W. Bargmann, J. P. Schade. *Progr. Brain Res.* 6:191–97. Amsterdam: Elsevier. 249 pp.

84. Hunsperger, R. W., Bucher, V. M. 1967. Affective behavior produced by electrical stimulation in the forebrain and brain stem of the cat. In *Structure and Function of the Limbic System*, ed. W. R. Adey, T. Tokizane. *Progr. Brain Res.* 27:103–27. Amsterdam: Elsevier. 489 pp.

85. Hutchinson, R. R., Azrin, N. H., Renfrew, J. W. 1968. Effects of shock intensity and duration on the frequency of biting attack by squirrel monkeys. *J. Exp. Anal. Behav.* 11:83–88

86. Hutchinson, R. R., Renfrew, J. W. 1966. Stalking attack and eating behaviors elicited from the same sites in the hypothalamus. *J. Comp. Physiol. Psychol.* 61:360–67

87. Ingram, W. R., Barris, R. W., Ranson, S. W. 1936. Catalepsy: an experimental study. *Arch. Neurol. Psychiat.* 35:1175–97

88. Inselman, B. R., Flynn, J. P. 1972. Modulatory effects of preoptic stimulation on hypothalamically-elicited attack in cats. *Brain Res.* 42:73–87

89. Kaada, B. R. 1951. Somato-motor, autonomic and electrocorticographic responses to electrical stimulation of "rhinencephalic" and other structures in primates, cat and dog. *Acta Physiol. Scand.* 24:Suppl. 83.

90. Kaada, B. R. 1960. Cingulate, posterior orbital, anterior insular, and temporal pole cortex. In *Handbook of Physiology: Section I. Neurophysiology*, ed. J. Field, H. W. Magoun, V. E. Hall, Vol. 2:1345–72. Washing-

ton, DC: Am. Physiol. Soc. 2013 pp.

91. Kaada, B. R. 1967. Brain mechanisms related to aggressive behavior. In *Aggression and Defense: Neural Mechanisms and Social Patterns*, ed. C. D. Clemente, D. B. Lindsley. *UCLA Forum Med. Sci.* 7:95–133. Los Angeles: Univ. of Calif. Press. 361 pp.

92. Kaada, B. R., Andersen, P., Jensen, J., Jr. 1954. Stimulation of the amygdaloid nuclear complex in unanesthetized cats. *Neurology* 4:48–64

93. Kaada, B. R., Ursin, H. 1957. Further localisation of behavioral responses elicited from the amygdala in unanesthetized cats. *Acta Physiol. Scand.* 42: Suppl. 145, 80–81

94. Kahn, M. W., Kirk, W. E. 1968. The concepts of aggression: a review and reformulation. *Psychol. Rec.* 18:559–73

95. Karli, P. 1968. Système limbique et processus de motivation. *J. Physiol. Paris* 60; Suppl. 1:3–148

96. Keller, A. D. 1932. Autonomic discharges elicited by physiological stimuli in midbrain preparations. *Am. J. Physiol.* 100:576–86

97. Kelly, A. H., Beaton, L. E., Magoun, H. W. 1946. A midbrain mechanism for faciovocal activity. *J. Neurophysiol.* 9:181–89

98. Kennard, M. A. 1957. Effect of temporal pole ablation on epileptic tendencies of monkeys. *Neurology* 7:404–14

99. King, F. A. 1958. Effects of septal and amygdaloid lesions on emotional behavior and conditioned avoidance responses in the rat. *J. Nerv. Ment. Dis.* 126:57–63

100. King, F. A., Meyer, P. M. 1958. Effects of amygdaloid lesions upon septal hyperemotionality in the rat. *Science* 128:655–56

101. Kling, A., Orbach, J., Schwarz, N., Towne, J. 1960. Injury to the limbic system and associated structures in cats. *Arch. Gen. Psychiat.* 3:391–420

102. Kling, A., Hutt, P. J. 1958. Effect of hypothalamic lesions on the amygdala syndrome in the cat.

Arch. Neurol. Psychiat. 79: 511–17

103. Klinger, J., Gloor, P. 1960. The connections of the amygdala and of the anterior temporal cortex in the human brain. *J. Comp. Neurol.* 115:333–69

104. Klüver, H., Bucy, P. C. 1939. Preliminary analysis of the functions of the temporal lobes in monkeys. *Arch. Neurol. Psychiat.* 42:979–1000

105. Krsiak, M., Steinberg, H. 1969. Psychopharmacological aspects of aggression: a review of the literature and some new experiments. *J. Psychosom. Res.* 13: 243–52

106. Kuroki, T. 1958. Arrest reaction elicited from the brain stem. *Folia Psychiat. Neurol. Jap.* 12: 317–40

107. Levinson, P. K., Flynn, J. P. 1965. The objects attacked by cats during stimulation of the hypothalamus. *Anim. Behav.* 13: 217–20

108. Leyhausen, P. 1956. *Verhaltensstudien an Katzen.* Berlin: Parey. 120 pp.

109. Liebman, J. M., Mayer, D. J., Liebeskind, J. C. 1970. Mesencephalic central gray lesions and fear-motivated behavior in rats. *Brain Res.* 23:353–70

110. Lorenz, K. 1966. *On Aggression* New York: Harcourt, Brace & World. 306 pp.

111. MacDonnell, M. F., Flynn, J. P. 1964. Attack elicited by stimulation of the thalamus of cats. *Science* 144:1249–50

112. Machne, X., Segundo, J. P. 1956. Unitary responses to afferent volleys in amygdaloid complex. *J. Neurophysiol.* 19:232–40

113. MacLean, P. D., Delgado, J. M. R. 1953. Electrical and chemical stimulation of fronto-temporal portion of limbic system in the waking animal. *Electroencephalogr. Clin. Neurophysiol.* 5:91–100

114. Magnus, O., Lammers, H. J. 1956. The amygdaloid-nuclear complex. *Folia Psychiat. Neurol. Neurochir. Neer.* 59:555–82

115. Magoun, H. W., Atlas, D., Ingersoll, E. H., Ranson, S. W. 1937. Associated facial, vocal and respiratory components of emotion: an experimental study. *J.*

Neurol. Psychopathol. 17:241–55

116. Malamud, N. 1967. Psychiatric disorders with intracranial tumors of the limbic system. *Arch. Neurol. Chicago* 17:113–23

117. Malliani, A., Bizzi, E., Apelbaum, J., Zanchetti, A. 1963. Ascending afferent mechanisms maintaining sham rage behavior in the acute thalamic cat. *Arch. Ital. Biol.* 101:632–47

118. Mark, V. H., Ervin, F. R. 1970. *Violence and the Brain.* New York. Harper & Row. 170 pp.

119. Masserman, J. H. 1941. Is the hypothalamus a center of emotion? *Psychosom. Med.* 3:3–25

120. McAdam, D. W., Kaelber, W. W. 1966. Differential impairment of avoidance learning in cats with ventromedial hypothalamic lesions. *Exp. Neurol.* 15:293–98

121. McCleary, R. A. 1961. Response specificity in the behavioral effects of limbic system lesions in the cat. *J. Comp. Physiol. Psychol.* 54:605–13

122. Monnier, M., Tissot, T. 1958. Correlated effects in behavior and electrical brain activity evoked by stimulation of the reticular system, thalamus and rhinencephalon in the conscious animal. In *Neurological Basis of Behavior,* ed. G. E. W. Wolstenholme, C. M. O'Conner, 105–20. London: Churchill. 400 pp.

123. Moore, R. Y. 1964. Effects of some rhinencephalic lesions on retention of conditioned avoidance behavior in cats. *J. Comp. Physiol. Psychol.* 57:65–71

124. Morgane, P. J., Kosman, A. J. 1957. Alterations in feline behaviour following bilateral amygdalectomy. *Nature* 180:598–600

125. Myer, J. S. 1968. Associative and temporal determinants of facilitation and inhibition of attack by pain. *J. Comp. Physiol. Psychol.* 66:17–21

126. Naka, K. I., Kido, R. 1962. Hypothalamic spike potentials recorded by chronically implanted tungsten microelectrodes. *Brain Res.* 5:422–24

127. Nakao, H. 1958. Emotional behavior produced by hypotha-lamic stimulation. *Am. J. Physiol.* 194:411–18

128. Nakao, H. 1967. Facilitation and inhibition in centrally induced switch-off behavior in cats. In *Structure and Function of the Limbic System,* ed. W. R. Adey, T. Tokizane. *Prog. Brain Res.* 27:128–43. Amsterdam: Elsevier. 489 pp.

129. Nakao, H., Yoshida, M., Sasaki, T. 1968. Midbrain central gray and switch-off behavior in cats. *Jap. J. Physiol.* 18:462–70

130. Narabayashi, H., Uno, M. 1966. Long range results of stereotaxic amygdalotomy for behavioral disorders. *Confin. Neurol.* 27:168–71

131. Nashold, B. S., Wilson, W. P., Slaughter, D. G. 1969. Sensations evoked by stimulation in the midbrain of man. *J. Neurosurg.* 30:14–24

132. Nauta, W. J. H. 1956. An experimental study of the fornix in the rat. *J. Comp. Neurol.* 104:247–72

133. Nauta, W. J. H. 1958. Hippocampal projections and related neural pathways to the midbrain in the cat. *Brain* 81:319–40

134. Nauta, W. J. H. 1961. Fibre degeneration following lesions of the amygdaloid complex in the monkey. *J. Anat.* 95:515–31

135. Pinto-Hamuy, T., Santibanez, G., Gonzales, C., Vicencio, E. 1957. Changes in behavior and visual discrimination performances after selective ablations of the temporal cortex. *J. Comp. Physiol. Psychol.* 50:379–85

136. Poirier, L. J. 1952. Anatomical and experimental studies on the temporal lobe of the macaque. *J. Comp. Neurol.* 96:209–48

137. Powell, D. A., Francis, J., Braman, M. J., Schneiderman, N. 1969. Frequency of attack in shock-elicited aggression as a function of the performance of individual rats. *J. Exp. Anal. Behav.* 12:817–23

138. Pribram, K. H., Bagshaw, M. 1953. Further analysis of the temporal lobe syndrome utilizing frontotemporal ablations. *J. Comp. Neurol.* 99:347–75

139. Putkonen, P. T. 1966. Attack elicited by forebrain and hypo-

thalamic stimulation in the chicken. *Experientia* 22:405-7

140. Rabin, B. M. 1968. Effect of lesions of the ventromedial hypothalamus on the electrical activitiy of the ventrolateral hypothalamus. *Electroencephalogr. Clin. Neurophysiol.* 25:344-50

141. Ranson, S. W. 1939. Somnolence caused by hypothalamic lesions in the monkey. *Arch. Neurol. Psychiat.* 41:1-23

142. Reeves, A. G., Plum, F. 1969. Hyperphagia, rage and dementia accompanying a ventromedial hypothalamic neoplasm. *Arch. Neurol. Chicago* 20:616-24

143. Reyes, V., Henny, G. C., Baird, H., Wycis, H. T., Spiegel, E. A. 1951. Localization of centripetal pathways of the human brain by recording of evoked potentials. *Trans. Am. Neurol. Assoc.* 76:246-48

144. Reynolds, R. W. 1965. An irritative hypothesis concerning the hypothalamic regulation of food intake. *Psychol. Rev.* 150:105-16

145. Roberts, W. W. 1958. Rapid escape learning motivated by hypothalamic stimulation in cats. *J. Comp. Physiol. Psychol.* 51:391-99

146. Roberts, W. W., Bergquist, E. H. 1968. Attack elicited by hypothalamic stimulation in cats raised in social isolation. *J. Comp. Physiol. Psychol.* 66:590-95

147. Roberts, W. W., Kiess, H. O. 1964. Motivational properties of hypothalamic aggression in cats. *J. Comp. Physiol. Psychol.* 58:187-93

148. Roberts, W. W., Steinberg, M. L., Means, L. W. 1967. Hypothalamic mechanisms for sexual, aggressive and other motivational behaviors in the opossum, *Didelphis virginiana. J. Comp. Physiol. Psychol.* 64:1-15

149. Robinson, B. W., Alexander, M., Bowne, G. 1969. Dominance reversal resulting from aggressive responses evoked by brain telestimulation. *Physiol. Behav.* 4:749-52

150. Romaniuk, A. 1965. Representation of aggression and flight reactions in the hypothalamus of

the cat. *Acta Biol. Exp. Warsaw* 25:177-86

151. Romaniuk, A. 1967. The role of the hypothalamus in defensive behavior. *Acta Biol. Exp. Warsaw* 27:339-43

152. Ross, N. et al 1965. Conditioning of midbrain behavioral responses. *Exp. Neurol.* 11:263-76

153. Rubinstein, E. H., Delgado, J. M. 1963. Inhibition induced by forebrain stimulation in the monkey. *Am. J. Physiol.* 205:941-48

154. Sano, K. 1962. Sedative neurosurgery, with special reference to postero-medial hypothalamotomy. *Neurol. Med-Chir.* 4:112-42

155. Sawa, M., Maruyama, N., Hanai, T., Kaji, S. 1959. Regulatory influence of amygdaloid nuclei upon the unitary activity in ventromedial nucleus of hypothalamus. *Folia Psychiat. Neurol. Jap.* 13:235-56

156. Schreiner, L., Kling, A. 1953. Behavioral changes following rhinencephalic injury in cat. *J. Neurophysiol.* 16:643-59

157. Schreiner, L., Kling, A. 1956. Rhinencephalon and behavior. *Am. J. Physiol.* 184:486-90

158. Schwartzbaum, J. S., Kellicutt, M. H., Spieth, T. M., Thompson, J. B. 1964. Effects of septal lesions in rats on response inhibition associated with food-reinforced behavior. *J. Comp. Physiol. Psychol.* 58:217-24

159. Scott, J. P. 1958. *Aggression.* Chicago: Univ. Chicago Press. 148 pp.

160. Shealy, C., Peele, J. 1957. Studies on amygdaloid nucleus of cat. *J. Neurophysiol.* 20:125-39

161. Sheard, M. H., Flynn, J. P. 1967. Facilitation of attack behavior by stimulation of the midbrain of cats. *Brain Res.* 4:324-33

162. Siegel, A., Skog, D. 1970. Effects of electrical stimulation of the septum upon attack behavior elicited from the hypothalamus in the cat. *Brain Res.* 23:371-80

163. Skultety, F. M. 1958. The behavioral effects of destructive lesions of the periaqueductal gray matter in adult cats. *J. Comp. Neurol.* 110:337-66

164. Skultety, F. M. 1963. Stimulation of periaqueductal gray and hypothalamus. *Arch. Neurol.* 8: 608–20

165. Smith, D. E., King, M. B., Hoebel, B. G. 1970. Lateral hypothalamic control of killing: evidence for a cholinoceptive mechanism. *Science* 167:900–1

166. Spiegel, E. A., Kletzkin, M., Szekely, E. G. 1954. Pain reactions upon stimulation of the tectum mesencephali. *J. Neuropathol. Exp. Neurol.* 13:212–20

167. Spiegel, E. A., Miller, H. R., Oppenheimer, M. J. 1940. Forebrain and rage reactions. *J. Neurophysiol.* 3:538–48

168. Sprague, J. M. et al 1963. A neuroanatomical and behavioral analysis of the syndromes resulting from midbrain lemniscal and reticular lesions in the cat. *Arch. Ital. Biol.* 101:225–95

169. Sterman, M. B., Clemente, C. D. 1962. Forebrain inhibitory mechanisms: sleep patterns induced by basal forebrain stimulation in the behaving cat. *Exp. Neurol.* 6:103–17

170. Stevens, J. R., Mark, V. H., Erwin, F., Pachero, P., Suematsu, K. 1969. Deep temporal stimulation in man. Long latency, long lasting psychological changes. *Arch. Neurol.* 21:157–69

171. Stokman, C. L. J., Glusman, M. 1970. Amygdaloid modulation of hypothalamic flight in cats. *J. Comp. Physiol. Psychol.* 71: 365–75

172. Sutin, J. 1963. An electrophysiological study of the hypothalamic ventromedial nucleus in the cat. *Electroencephalogr. Clin. Neurophysiol.* 15:786–95

173. Teitelbaum, P., Cheng, M. F., Rozin, P. 1969. Development of feeding parallels its recovery after hypothalamic damage. *J. Comp. Physiol. Psychol.* 67: 430–41

174. Thomas, G. J., Moore, R. Y., Harvey, J. A., Hunt, H. F. 1959. Relations between the behavioral syndrome produced by lesions in the septal region of the forebrain and maze learning of the rat. *J. Comp. Physiol. Psychol.* 52:527–32

175. Tinbergen, N. 1968. On war and peace in animals and man: an ethologist's approach to the biology of aggression. *Science* 160:1411–18

176. Turner, B. H. 1970. Neural structures involved in the rage syndrome of the rat. *J. Comp. Physiol. Psychol.* 71:103–13

177. Ulrich, R. E. 1966. Pain as a cause of aggression. *Am. Zool.* 6:643–61

178. Ulrich, R. E., Craine, W. H. 1964. Behavior persistence of shock-induced aggression. *Science* 143:971–73

179. Ulrich, R. E., Symannek, B. 1969. Pain as a stimulus for aggression. In *Aggressive Behavior,* ed. S. Garattini, E. B. Sigg, 56–69. New York: Wiley. 387 pp.

180. Ulrich, R. E., Wolfe, M., Dulaney, S. 1969. Punishment of shock-induced aggression. *J. Exp. Anal. Behav.* 12:1005–15

181. Ulrich, R. E., Wolff, P. C., Azrin, N. H. 1964. Shock as an elicitor of intra- and inter-species fighting behavior. *Anim. Behav.* 12: 14–5

182. Ursin, H. 1964. Flight and defense behavior in cats. *J. Comp. Physiol. Psychol.* 58:180–86

183. Ursin, H. 1965. The effect of amygdaloid lesions on flight and defense behavior in cats. *Exp. Neurol.* 11:61–79

184. Ursin, H., Kaada, B. R. 1960. Functional localization within the amygdaloid complex in the cat. *Electroencephalogr. Clin. Neurophysiol.* 12:1–20

185. Valzelli, L. 1967. Drugs and aggressiveness. *Advan. Pharmacol.* 5:79–108

186. Vernon, W. M. 1969. Animal aggression: review of research. *Genet. Psychol. Monogr.* 80, Part 1:3–28

187. Wada, J. A., Matsuda, M. 1970. Can hypothalamically induced escape behavior be conditioned? *Exp. Neurol.* 28:507–12

188. Wada, J. A., Matsuda, M., Jung, E., Hamm, A. E. 1970. Mesencephalically induced escape behavior and avoidance performance. *Exp. Neurol.* 29:215–20

189. Walker, A. E., Thomson, A. F., McQueen, J. D. 1953. Behavior and the temporal rhinencephalon in the monkey. *Bull. Johns Hopkins Hosp.* 93:65–93

190. Washburn, S. L. 1969. The origins of aggressive behavior. *Ment. Health Program Rep.* 3:255–72

191. Wasman, M., Flynn, J. P. 1962. Directed attack elicited from hypothalamus. *Arch. Neurol.* 6: 220–27

192. Wayner, M. J. 1970. A theoretical review: motor control functions of the lateral hypothalamus and adjunctive behavior. *Physiol. Behav.* 5:1319–25

193. Weiskrantz, L. 1956. Behavioral changes associated with ablation of the amygdaloid complex in monkeys. *J. Comp. Physiol. Psychol.* 49:381–91

194. Wetzel, A. B., Conner, R. L., Levine, S. 1967. Shock-induced fighting in septal-lesioned rats. *Psychon. Sci.* 9:133–34

195. Wheatley, M. D. 1944. The hypothalamus and affective behavior in cats: a study of the effects of experimental lesions, with anatomic correlations. *Arch. Neurol. Psychiat.* 52:296–316

196. Wood, C. D. Behavioral changes following discrete lesions of temporal lobe structures. *Neurology* 8:215–20

197. Wood, C. D., Schottelius, B., Frost, L. L., Baldwin, M. 1958. Localization within the amygdaloid complex of unanesthetized animals. *Neurology* 8: 477–80

198. Woods, J. W. 1956. Taming of the wild Norway rat by rhinencephalic lesions. *Nature* 178:869

199. Yasukochi, G. 1960. Emotional responses elicited by electrical stimulation of the hypothalamus in cat. *Folia Psychiat. Neurol. Jap.* 14:260–67

200. Zbrozyna, A. W. 1972. The organization of the defense reaction elicited from amygdala and its connections. In *The Neurobiology of the Amygdala,* ed. B. E. Eleftheriou, 597–606. New York: Plenum. 819 pp.

Ann. Rev. Physiol. 1973. 35:357–390

HYPOTHALAMIC CONTROL OF ADENOHYPOPHYSIAL SECRETIONS

Richard E. Blackwell

Department of Physiology, Baylor College of Medicine, Houston, Texas

Roger Guillemin

The Salk Institute, La Jolla, California

OPENING REMARKS

This chapter has no pretense at being an exhaustive review of all the literature published over the last few years pertinent to its title. To the contrary, we want to make clear that we have selected about one-fifth of what we collected in preparation of this review, to be included here. The basis for selection of the literature quoted here is simply explained in terms of our own interests or shortcomings. If what we say in this chapter or how we say it generates some argument, we feel that there will be none for the statement that the most important contributions over the last few years to the efforts at understanding the mechanisms involved in the physiological control of adenohypophysial functions by the hypothalamus reside in the characterization of two of the hypothalamic hypophysiotropic hormones, TRF and LRF. The recent characterization and total synthesis by this laboratory of a hypothalamic peptide that specifically inhibits the secretion of immunoreactive growth hormone, may have similar significance and implications as it would represent the first of the long-postulated hypothalamic hypophysiotropic inhibitory factors for adenohypophysial secretions.

We think it of interest that this review should discuss a large number of clinical reports of physiological significance, thus showing the wide impact in clinical medicine and clinical investigation of the elucidation of the structure of TRF and LRF and their availability in unlimited quantities by total synthesis. Once more, basic research will have contributed to the practice of medicine and the welfare of innumerable patients.

ABBREVIATIONS

We use the following abbreviations in the text as defined here:

ACTH = adrenocorticotropin
CRF = ACTH-releasing factor

FRF   = FSH-releasing factor
FSH   = follicle stimulating hormone
GH   = growth hormone or somatotropin
LH   = luteinizing hormone
LRF   = LH-releasing factor
MIF   = MSH-release inhibiting factor
MRF   = MSH-releasing factor
MSH   = melanocyte stimulating hormone
PIF   = PRL-release inhibiting factor
PRF   = PRL-releasing factor
PRL   = prolactin
PTU   = propylthiouracyl
SME   = stalk-median eminence (fragments of hypothalamus containing SME)
SRIF = somatotropin-release inhibiting factor
TRF   = TSH-releasing factor
TSH   = thyroid stimulating hormone or thyrotropin
T_3 = triiodothyronine
T_4 = thyroxine

Abbreviations for all amino acids are in accordance with the IUPAC-IUB Tentative rules on Biochemical Nomenclature (*Biochemistry* 5:1445, 1966, and 6:362, 1967) except for pGlu, pyroglutamic acid or 2-pyrrolidone-5-carboxylic acid. Other abbreviations used occasionally will be defined in the text.

CONTROL OF THE SECRETION OF LUTEINIZING HORMONE AND FOLLICLE STIMULATING HORMONE

Over the last ten years, considerable evidence has accumulated that indicates that the hypothalamus contains factors that control the secretion of the gonadotropins, LH and FSH. Evidence for the development of this concept has been presented recently by Everett (46), Yates et al (170), and Guillemin (60), and will not be dealt with in this review.

Attempts to isolate these hypothalamic factors reached fruition when Schally et al (129) and Amoss et al (2) reported obtaining near homogeneous luteinizing hormone releasing factor from porcine and ovine hypothalamic materials, respectively. Both research groups concluded that their isolation product had the amino acid composition Glu 1, His 1, Tyr 1, Ser 1, Gly 2, Leu 1, Arg 1, Pro 1, after 6N HCl hydrolysis, and both reported that their preparation released LH and FSH concomitantly. This confirmed the observation of White (164) that semipurified LRF would release both gonadotropins in vitro. In addition, Amoss et al (2, 3) proposed that the Glu moiety in LRF was the N-terminal residue in the form of pGlu based on studies with the highly specific enzyme pyrolidonyl-carboxylyl peptidase.

Shortly thereafter, Matsuo et al (98) determined the primary sequence of porcine LRF using a combined Edman-dansyl procedure coupled with a selective C-terminus tritiation method. The sequencing was performed on 200 nmoles of peptide and the structure of LRF was shown to be pGlu-His-Trp-Ser-Tyr-Gly-Leu-Arg-Pro-Gly-NH$_2$. Subsequently, Burgus et al (24, 25) determined that ovine LRF has also as its primary structure, pGlu-His-Trp-Ser-Tyr-Gly-Leu-Arg-Pro-Gly-NH$_2$. This structure was determined by analysis of two aliquots of 20 nmoles LRF each, using hydrolysis of the peptide with chymotrypsin or pyrolidone-carboxylyl peptidase followed by Edman-^{14}C-dansylation and mass spectrometry of the degradation products.

Monahan et al (101) described the total synthesis of the decapeptide by solid-phase methodology on a benzhydrylamine resin, showing identity of their synthetic product with native ovine LRF. Likewise, Matsuo et al (97) and later several other investigators have synthesized LRF. All these synthetic preparations were reported to release LH and FSH in vitro and in vivo at nanogram levels, thus confirming the structural studies on native LRF of porcine or ovine origins. Amoss et al (4) demonstrated that oral administration of LRF releases both LH and FSH. The oral activity of LRF (a polypeptide which is destroyed by peptic digestion) was best explained by considering the high specific activity of LRF (picomoles being sufficient to release LH upon reaching the pituitary cells); thus, following oral administration of a large amount of LRF (10 μg to 1 mg in the rats), enough will penetrate the blood stream through the gastric mucosa to produce a plasma concentration high enough to produce stimulation of secretion of LH and FSH. Subcutaneous or intravenous administration of LRF to pentobarbital treated golden hamsters (7) or Innovar treated rabbits (1) caused ovulation.

Synthetic LRF has been shown to be highly active in man; Yen et al (171) reported eightfold elevation of plasma LH levels within 20–30 min by injecting 150 μg LRF intravenously into normal adult males. This treatment caused a concomitant, but quantitatively smaller, rise in plasma FSH levels. Similar studies have been carried out by Kastin et al (76). Subsequently, Yen et al (172) have demonstrated that doses as small as 10 μg LRF can elicit a significant increase in plasma gonadotropin levels.

Such observations suggest that LRF alone may control both LH and FSH release in the normal state, a concept that is supported by reports that plasma LH and FSH levels vary in parallel during the menstrual cycle (30, 143), including the hormonal surge that occurs just prior to ovulation. Additional support comes from the observation that urinary LH and FSH fluctuations are similar during the menstrual cycle (126). Such clinical findings, combined with reports that purified or synthetic LRF can increase plasma LH and FSH levels when administered to various species, has led Schally and collaborators (131) to propose that the decapeptide LRF is the sole (hypothalamic) controller of the secretion of the two gonadotropins LH and FSH.

The two groups that have reported the isolation and characterization of LRF, have followed the molecule throughout the purification by an assay based on evidence for the stimulation of the secretion of LH. No careful study with specific assays for FSH has been reported in which the FSH releasing activity present in hypothalamic extract was followed specifically throughout a purification procedure. Therefore, the statement that the decapeptide LRF is the sole hypothalamic controller of the secretion of LH and FSH may be somewhat premature at present, although it may eventually be shown to be correct.

Pertinent to this question is the observation that all synthetic analogs of the decapeptide LRF studied so far have the same ratios of biological activity when related to LRF as a reference standard, in terms of their ability to release either LH or FSH (155). No synthetic peptide related to the decapeptide LRF has been observed in which secretory activity for LH would have been dissociated from secretory activity for FSH. Vale et al (152) have reported that several analogs of the decapeptide LRF with either a substitution (Gly^2-LRF) or a deletion (des-His^2-LRF) have antagonistic properties against LRF; in this case again, the antagonists inhibit the stimulating activity of LRF in terms of either LH or FSH.

Despite the overall similarity of LH and FSH secretory patterns in the normal physiological state, numerous dissociations of the secretion of these hormones have nonetheless been reported. For instance, it has been shown that LH, but not FSH, secretion is increased during rapid eye movement sleep (125). The data of Goebelsmann et al (54) indicate that during the menstrual cycle in women plasma LH concentrations at midcycle reach a maximum 1½ to 2 days before FSH concentrations do. Also, Stevens (141) has reported that FSH secretory peaks occur 2 or 3 times during the normal menstrual cycle whereas LH secretion peaks only once. Similar dissociations have been observed by Cargille et al (31); they reported a surge of FSH secretion during the follicular phase of the menstrual cycle with no apparent change in the secretion of LH.

Such dissociations in LH and FSH secretion may be due to the presence of a hypothalamic FRF. However, another variable may be responsible for the observed differences in the secretion of these two hormones, namely the time at which blood samples were taken from the test subjects. Atkinson et al (10) observed that when hourly blood samples were taken from chronically ovariectomized adult rhesus monkeys during a 24 hr period, random peaks of LH secretion were found in all cases. When blood samples were withdrawn at 10, 20, and 30 min intervals for 6–12 hr, Dierschke et al (43) observed a striking rhythmic pattern in plasma LH levels which had a period of approximately 1 hr (plasma growth hormone levels showed asynchronous patterns). The LH changes had an excursion of 40–92% of the mean hormone concentration. These periodic (circhoral) changes in plasma LH were not observed in normal monkeys.

Midgley & Jaffe (99) reported that serum LH and FSH concentrations are maintained by multiple pulses of variable magnitude in humans. The pulsatile pattern of LH secretion is particularly well defined during the ascending phase of the mid-cycle peak which occurs prior to ovulation. Similarly, plasma LH levels in normal men were found to undergo abrupt elevations periodically throughout the day (107). Such a phenomenon has been observed in a third species by Gay & Sheth (53) who found pulsatile LH and FSH secretory patterns in normal and castrated rats.

Bhattacharya et al (14) have been able to suppress the circhoral release of LH by administration of chlorpromazine, haloperidol, phentolamine, or phenoxybenzamine to ovariectomized rhesus monkeys. These treatments caused abrupt cessation of the pulsatile discharge of LH for several hours. The inhibition was terminated by an acute resumption of the circhoral pattern. When either propranolol or pentobarbital was given to the test subjects, no effect on LH secretion was observed. It was concluded that these pulsatile discharges of gonadotropins are the result of intermittent catecholaminergic signals which act on LRF secretory centers.

These studies seem to establish that the gonadotropins are secreted periodically in discrete packets. Therefore, one should take into account not only the difference in half-life of the gonadotropins but also the circhoral rhythm when attempting to draw conclusions about the hypothalamic control of LH and FSH secretion, and one must consider that these phenomena may explain the differences in LH and FSH secretory patterns.

Another factor which contributes to the differential release of LH and FSH is the balance of sex steroids in plasma and brain tissues. For instance, the circhoral release of LH may be interrupted acutely by a single intravenous injection of 17β-estradiol (168). In the same system, administration of progesterone was without effect on gonadotropin secretion. Such observations agree with the findings of Tsai & Yen (148) who demonstrated that constant infusion of 17β-estradiol in premenopausal women during the follicular phase of the menstrual cycle caused a rapid decline in plasma LH and FSH levels; the negative feedback reduced LH levels by 47% and FSH levels by 17%. Tsai & Yen (149) have also shown that treatment of normal women with ethinyl estradiol abolished the early rise of plasma gonadotropins during the follicular phase. It was reported that the negative feedback was greater for FSH than LH in that LH secretion rebounded rapidly whereas FSH levels remained depressed for up to 36 hr. These studies suggest that estrogens play a major role in the differential negative control of both LH and FSH secretion. Apparently, the time of exposure to the steroids, as well as the dose, is important in determining whether the estrogens exert a negative or positive effect on gonadotropin secretion. For instance, it has been shown that ethinyl estradiol treatment initially depresses LH and FSH plasma levels in normal women, then augments the release of both of these hormones (174). It is of interest that Yen & Tsai describe the positive feedback as being greater for LH than FSH, whereas Arimura & Schally (9) have reported that estrogen treatment of rats seems to augment the release of LH in response to administration of LRF; no data concerning FSH were presented in the latter report. However, Ying et al (173) have demonstrated that administration of a single dose of 17β-estradiol to 30-day old female rats significantly elevated both serum LH and FSH levels. These studies clearly indicate that estrogens are capable of exerting a major positive regulatory effect on gonadotropin secretion.

Estrogens are not alone in controlling gonadotropin release in the female;

Hilliard et al (66) have reported that administration of progesterone inhibits ovulation induced by injection of LRF. The work of Spies & Niswender (140) supports this finding; they showed that progesterone treatment blocks the preovulatory surge of LH and, subsequently, ovulation in rhesus monkeys. In addition, Caligaris et al (29) found that progesterone exerts a biphasic effect on gonadotropin secretion in the presence of estrogens.

It is not clear how the steroids might modify the differential release of the gonadotropins in response to stimulation by either LRF or LRF and FRF. One might postulate that these agents act on a common pituitary cell type, since Nakane (106) has reported that LH and FSH frequently are found in the same pituitary cell. Similar observations have been made by Phifer et al (115) using human pituitaries and highly specific antisera to LH and FSH; they utilized the immunoglobulin peroxidase bridge procedure to locate the gonadotropins in tissue sections. Using this method, they always found LH and FSH in the same cell, although in variable concentrations. Conversely, one might envision that the regulators of LH and FSH secretion act on separate cell types.

Whether the various steroids act on one or two pituitary cell types to affect LH and FSH secretion is not clear at present, though the evidence indicates that the sex steroids can affect gonadotropin secretion at the level of the pituitary (41, 161, 168). Besides the pituitary, the hypothalamus (102) and the amygdala (142) can concentrate estradiol. Therefore, the steroids probably exert some effect on LH and FSH secretion by acting either directly on the hypothalamic centers which are presumed to produce LRF or FRF or both, or indirectly by stimulating or inhibiting other areas of the brain, i.e., the amygdala, afferents to the ventral hypothalamus.

Considerable more work remains to be done to enable us to understand the interrelationship between LH and FSH, their hypothalamic releasing factor(s), and the major agents such as the steroids, which exert either/or positive and negative feedback control on these systems. Of major importance in understanding these relationships is the clarification of whether LRF is the sole hypothalamic controller of LH and FSH secretion and whether LH and FSH are produced by single or multiple pituitary cell types. Once these questions are answered, a more meaningful evaluation can be made of the role the steroids play in the regulation of gonadotropin secretion.

PHYSIOLOGY OF THE SECRETION OF GROWTH HORMONE

Attempts to determine the nature of the hypothalamic control of GH secretion have evoked considerable controversy. Schally et al (132) have isolated a material GH-RH from porcine hypothalamic extract which is reported to produce depletion of the content of (rat) pituitary gland in growth hormone as measured by the tibia-test bioassay. GH-RH is also reported to elevate plasma levels of growth hormone and to stimulate its secretion in vitro, in both cases according to the bioassay. Porcine GH-RH has the structure H·Val-His-Leu-Ser-Ala-Glu-Glu-Lys-Glu-Ala·OH (131a). This peptide was synthesized by Veber et al (158) who noted a striking similarity between the structure of GH-RH and that of the beta chain amino terminal sequence of porcine hemoglobin. Neither native nor synthetic GH-RH is active in releasing GH in a variety of normal animals or in man as measured by highly specific radioimmunoassays. This confirms the earlier observation of Knobil et al (84) that porcine GRF isolated using pituitary depletion methods failed to stimulate GH secretion when administered to normal rats or monkeys.

The discrepancy observed when comparing pituitary depletion methods with measurements of GH by radioimmunoassay has not been explained. Rodger et al (122) have questioned the validity of the pituitary depletion assay, since they obtained random results using this method while trying to locate a GRF active zone following gel filtration of hypothalamic extracts. Reassay of the zones showed random results whether the tibia-test or radioimmunoassay was used as a secondary test for GH. Similar evidence has been presented by Daughaday et al (40) who were unable to detect any change in pituitary GH content measured by radioimmunoassay following administration of either crude or purified GRF. Conversely, Muller et al (103) have reported that intracarotid injection of 350 ng of pure porcine GH-RH caused a depletion of pituitary GH content which was accompanied by an increase in plasma GH levels as determined by tibia-test.

Many investigators have used the tibia-test to measure changes in GH levels following administration of some GRF-like agent in vitro or in vivo. Recently, Corvol et al (38) have observed that the anterior pituitary contains a factor or factors that exert a strong mitogenic action on articular chondrocytes using secondary monolayer culture. The factor was present in the NIH preparations of TSH, LH, and FSH of ovine and bovine origin. Preparations of GH, PRL, and ACTH did not contain the active factor. The growth promoting factor does not seem to be one of the pituitary hormones since highly purified preparations do not possess the activity. Addition of the factor to cells grown in monolayer culture produces a linear growth response. Since nothing is known about the way in which such factors might be released from the pituitary or under what conditions, and what their role might be in the tibia-test bioassay of whole extracts of rat pituitary glands, it may be cautious to suggest that efforts at characterizing the hypothetical growth hormone releasing factor should be based on the measurement of GH by radioimmunoassay.

Despite the problems connected with the characterization of a GRF, various data suggest that it should be present in hypothalamic extract. Stimulation of the ventromedial hypothalamic nuclei and the median eminence in rats produces an increase in plasma GH levels measured by radioimmunoassay (13). Similar observations were made by Smith & Root (136) in monkeys.

GRF activity has been reported to be present in crude extracts of ovine hypothalamus based on measurements of GH by radioimmunoassays. Frohman et al (52) have observed increases in plasma GH levels measured by radioimmunoassay following intrapituitary injection of the crude test preparation. The change in plasma GH levels was about 5 ng/ml. This is not a large change compared to preinjection levels; however, the resting levels were high since the animals were pretreated with pentobarbital, a stimulus which clearly elevates plasma GH levels in rats (68). It is of interest that intrapituitary injection of the equivalent of one sheep hypothalamic fragment caused 1% depletion of pituitary GH content, a change which is comparable to that seen following electrical stimulation of the hypothalamus in the rat.

The most recent evidence for the existence of a GRF comes from Wilber et al (165). They reported the localization in filtration over G-25 Sephadex of GRF activity using extracts derived from rat and porcine hypothalami; GRF activity is determined by incubation of the preparation with rat hemipituitaries in vitro followed by radioimmunoassay of the change in GH concentrations of the medium. Following G-25 Sephadex chromatography, the GRF active zone was reported to show an elution volume closely related to that of TRF and LRF and considerably greater than that described by Schally et al (132) for GH-RH. It should be noted that Wilber et al added doses equivalent to 4 hypothalamic fragments/ml medium. This produced a response of 400% of control when using the most active fractions. In view of the large amounts of hypothalamic material that was added to the medium, it is hoped that the responses observed were not due to damaged pituitary cells.

SPECIES DIFFERENCE IN THE RELEASE OF GH

The rat has been the primary test object of investigators seeking to isolate the brain factor or factors which control GH secretion. Recently, Takahashi et al (144) have demonstrated that ether anesthesia, hypertonic glucose treatment, 2-deoxyglucose injection, insulin-induced hypoglycemia, and epinephrine treatment inhibit the levels of plasma GH in rats as measured by radioimmunoassay. This is unlike the response of man and primates who elevate plasma GH levels following insulin-induced hypoglycemia, arginine infusion, 2-deoxyglucose injection, exercise, fasting, cold stress, ether anesthesia, and surgery. On the other hand, cats do not alter plasma GH levels following insulin-induced hypoglycemia, fasting, intravenous glucose treatment, arginine infusion, or injection of sheep hypothalamic extract (86). Such data indicate that the GH release control mechanism is probably different in various species and it seems advisable to study the secretory patterns in more than one species when trying to isolate GRF or study the GH control system.

NEURAL CONTROL OF GH SECRETION

The way in which the various brain areas affect the ultimate secretion of GH is partially recognized. Halász et al (63) have demonstrated that partial or total deafferentation of the medial basal hypothalamus (MBH) does not result in a major alteration of plasma GH levels in the rat. Therefore, they concluded that the MBH produces and releases a hypothalamic factor which maintains GH secretion. Further, they have suggested that neural afferents to the MBH are not involved in maintaining basal pituitary GH secretion.

Brown et al (23) have reported that capture and ether stress increase plasma GH levels in the squirrel monkey. A lesion of either the anterior or posterior median eminence blocks the stress-induced rise in plasma GH. Also, a lesion of the inferior third of the mammillary bodies blocks the stress response. Conversely, they report that placement of lesions in the middle of the optic chiasm greatly enhances the secretion of GH in response to ether stress. These studies suggest that basal GH secretion is subject to both positive and negative neural control.

Visual input may also play a role in the control of GH secretion. Krieger & Glick (87) reported that blind subjects do not show a peak of plasma GH levels following the onset of sleep as is observed in otherwise normal individuals. The blind patients respond to insulin-induced hypoglycemia by elevating their plasma GH levels, thus indicating the potential to release the hormone. Similar results have been noted by Sorrentino et al (138) using the young rat. However, they report an enhanced inhibition of GH secretion when the animals are both blind and anosmic. Therefore, these studies imply that both visual and olfactory input affects the secretion of GH.

A critical factor in obtaining an understanding of how the nervous system controls the secretion of GH is the isolation and characterization of its hypothalamic messenger. Most of the literature infers that the messenger is a GRF. However, considering the frequently unexpected inhibition in plasma GH levels one can not exclude the existence and possible physiological role of SRIF in one or more species. The recent characterization and total synthesis of a peptide of ovine hypothalamic origin that specifically inhibits the secretion of immunoreactive growth hormone in vitro or in vivo (21) should allow a new means for investigating the hypothalamic control of growth hormone secretion.

CONTROL OF THE SECRETION OF PROLACTIN

The secretion of PRL in mammals, in contrast to that of all other anterior pituitary hormones, has for more than 15 years been presumed to be subject to some tonic inhibition by a hypothalamic PIF. This concept was formulated after early studies suggested that the pituitary releases increased amounts of PRL after transplantation to a site removed from the base of the brain or after placement of a lesion in the ventral hypothalamus (45, 64). Furthermore, it has been reported that when quartered rat pituitaries were placed in vitro, they secreted large amounts of PRL and that addition of acid extracts of rat hypothalamus to these pituitary fragments caused a decrease in PRL secretion when compared to controls (146). More recent studies (to be discussed below) have led to the concept of a possible double hypothalamic regulation for PRL secretion through the existence not only of a PIF but also of a PRL releasing factor, or PRF.

PIF AND PRL SECRETION

Much of the classical data concerning the secretion of PRL were obtained using modifications of the pigeon crop sac assay. Recently Raud & Odell (118) compared this method with a specific radioimmunoassay for bovine PRL. They found good correlation between these techniques when assaying purified PRL; however, in all cases, the bioassay gave higher PRL potencies than the radioimmunoassay when impure materials were studied. Further, studies using various fractions of bovine pituitary extract showed that the ACTH fraction gave positive reactions in the bioassay; subsequently, bioassay for purified ACTH suggested that ACTH was capable of stimulating the development of the crop sac epithelium in a linear fashion. In view of these findings, caution should be exercised in interpreting data which were obtained using the crop sac bioassay.

Using as endpoints specific radioimmunoassay methods for prolactin, several groups have been unable to demonstrate specific PIF activity in various extracts of rat, ovine, or porcine hypothalami, either in vitro or in vivo; in many of these studies extracts of brain cortex were as effective as extracts of hypothalamus to modify plasma prolactin levels. Using female rats bearing female pituitary transplants, we have been unable to lower plasma PRL levels 30, 60, and 120 min post-injection of up to 15 fragment equivalents of ovine hypothalamic extract. Similar data have been reported by Arimura et al (8) who found that intracarotid infusion in sheep of an extract of the SME of the pig caused an increase in plasma PRL levels in eight experiments and a decrease in two experiments; in the same series of experiments, in vitro studies using sheep or goat pituitaries showed that addition of porcine hypothalamic extract to the medium resulted in a decrease in PRL secretion during the first 2 hr of incubation followed by an increase during the next 2 hr (PRL measured by radioimmunoassay). Arimura (5) reported further that intracarotid or intravenous infusion of freshly prepared rat SME for 30 min into rats bearing pituitary transplants under the kidney capsule did not alter plasma PRL levels.

Kamberi et al (73) have observed that infusion of $\frac{1}{12}$, $\frac{1}{6}$, and $\frac{1}{2}$ fragment equivalents of rat hypothalamus into the hypophysial portal vessels of nembutal treated rats caused a significant decrease in plasma PRL levels and an increase in plasma LH and FSH levels, all hormones measured by radioimmunoassays; infusion of cerebrocortical extract equivalent in weight to $\frac{1}{2}$ a hypothalamic fragment did not affect the level of plasma PRL, LH, or FSH. Arimura et al (6) demonstrated that nembutal anesthesia increased PRL secretion in rats. Further, they showed that infusion of either 3 rat SME or the equivalent weight of cortical extract produced a significant decrease in plasma PRL levels. In another series of experiments in the same report (6), intracarotid infusion of the same extracts of SME or brain cortex was unable to decrease the levels of plasma PRL elevated by pretreatment of the rats with perphenazine. No explanation is available at the moment to reconcile the results of Kamberi et al (73) with those of Arimura et al (6) or of our own laboratory; no clear cut picture emerges from these studies.

Parsons & Nicoll (114) observed that addition of rat hypothalamic extract (3 hypothalamic equivalents/ml) to paired (rats, males) pituitaries in vitro caused a 30% to 40% decrease in PRL secretion, using disc electrophoresis and densitometry measurements of the prolactin secreted in the incubation medium. When using female (rat) anterior pituitaries, addition of one fragment equivalent of rat hypothalamic extract did not produce a significant decrease in PRL secretion when compared to controls treated with the equivalent of an extract of cerebral cortex. In another experiment, addition of three fragments equivalents of rat hypothalamic extract was reported to produce a significant decrease in PRL secretion when compared with controls not treated with cortical extract.

So far, we have found no change in PRL secretion in vitro using pituitary cells in culture (154) when doses of 0.01 to 1 fragment equivalents of either ovine or murine hypothalamic extracts are added to the incubation medium. Further, we have found that addition of doses greater than one fragment equivalent causes detachment of pituitary cells from the culture dishes, a phenomenon which is associated with random increases or decreases of PRL secretion and which may represent toxicity to the cells. Considering the large amount of extract that must be used by other investigators to induce a marginal decrease in PRL secretion in vitro, it is suggested that the changes seen in such experimental setups may not necessarily be of physiological significance. Further studies attempting to characterize the hypothetical PRF and PIF with in vitro methods will certainly benefit from (and probably require) very carefully controlled conditions which do not appear to have been met so far.

Chen et al (34) have reported that transplantation of one to four female pituitaries under the kidney capsule of hypophysectomized recipient rats resulted in plasma PRL levels (measured by radioimmunoassay) that were similar to, or greater than, those found in rats during estrus. Further, they observed that plasma PRL levels declined steadily over a period of 10 weeks. Administration of estradiol (1 μg/day $\times$ 5) at that time to these transplant-bearing animals increased considerably the level of plasma PRL. Chen et al suggested that transplantation of the pituitary resulted in a release of the gland from chronic inhibition by a hypothalamic PIF. Since it is known that PRL secretion varies during the estrus cycle, the levels being low during diestrus and high during proestrus and estrus, it is not impossible that the elevated plasma PRL levels found in some rats following transplantation may reflect the donors' stage of estrus prior to death and not necessarily a release from chronic inhibition; this point requires further investigation. Caution is also appropriate when interpreting PRL levels in absolute values as observed in rats bearing multiple pituitary transplants.

Welsch et al (163) have shown that passing a 2–3 mA direct current through steel electrodes placed bilaterally in the hypothalamus of rats for 7–

10 sec produces a lesion, bounded rostrally by the optic chiasma, caudally by the pituitary stalk, laterally 1 mm from the mid-line, and dorsally 0.5 mm from the ventral surface of the brain; in animals bearing such lesions, plasma PRL levels were significantly increased tenfold over the pre-operative levels (600 ng/ml) by 30 min post-lesion, declined to 150 ng/ml by 120 hr post-lesion, and remained at that elevated level for 5 months. Likewise, Arimura et al (6) observed a ten- to thirtyfold rise in plasma PRL levels in rats within 2 hr following surgical ablation of the medial hypothalamus. The plasma PRL levels in these animals remained elevated, though with considerable variations, up to 26 days after the lesion.

Such results would favor the concept that the long lasting elevated levels of plasma PRL are due to the release of the pituitary PRL-secretion from a hypothalamic PIF (see also 47). It is thus puzzling that in the same report (6), Arimura et al observed that intracarotid infusion of hypothalamic or cortical extract to these animals did not lower the elevated plasma PRL levels.

LRF AND PRL SECRETION

The chemical nature of the postulated hypothalamic PIF has not been elucidated; no one has isolated a PIF from hypothalamic extracts. A material that will inhibit depletion of pituitary PRL following nursing is said to be strongly retarded on G-25 Sephadex (42) and to overlap the zone of effluent containing LRF. Schally et al (130) have reported a partial separation of this material from LRF. Recently, Blackwell et al (16) have demonstrated that synthetic LRF will not affect PRL secretion in vitro at doses which cause near maximal release of LH and FSH; therefore, LRF does not appear to be PIF. We have also confirmed that injection of large doses of synthetic LRF in vivo (rat, sheep, humans) does not acutely elevate levels of plasma PRL. Therefore, LRF is not the postulated PRF.

Though LRF does not affect PRL secretion directly at the level of the pituitary, there is evidence that this hypothalamic factor may be involved in the regulation of PRL secretion indirectly via the sex steroids. Injection of 17β-estradiol into rats resulted in an increase in plasma PRL levels similar to that seen prior to ovulation (36). This finding correlates with the reports that plasma PRL levels are low during metestrus and high during proestrus and early estrus in sheep (119). Neill et al (110) have reported that administration of antiserum to estrogens during diestrus-2 in rats blocks the proestrus surge of PRL. Also, Freeman et al (51) have demonstrated that injection of anti-LH serum at 10 AM on the day of proestrus does not affect the proestrus surge of PRL. However, if anti-LH serum is administered at 10 AM on the day before proestrus, i.e. diestrus-2, the proestrus surge of PRL is inhibited and the incidence of uterine ballooning and ovulation is reduced.

These conclusions are also supported by the finding that ergocornine, an ergot alkaloid that inhibits lactation (134), has been shown to inhibit the rise in plasma PRL levels that is seen following injection of 17β-estradiol in rats (91). Wuttke et al (167) further reported that chronic injection of ergocornine or a single implant of this drug placed in the median eminence suppresses the fluctuations of both plasma PRL and LH during the estrus cycle. Also, injection of ergocornine early in the afternoon of proestrus inhibits the rise in plasma PRL which normally occurs later in the day; the proestrus surge of LH was not inhibited until a dose of 200 μg was given to the test animals.

One of the most important contributions to the physiology of the secretion of PRL is to be found in the very elegant studies of Freeman & Neill (50) who studied the pattern of PRL secretion during pseudopregnancy in the rat and observed that following induction of peudopregnancy by cervical stimulation, the levels of plasma PRL would remain low throughout the period of pseudopregnancy except for short surges of PRL secretion occurring regularly every night with a remarkably constant frequency. The maximal mean PRL value during these daily nocturnal surges ranged from 40-110 ng/ml, the surges alternating with periods in which the plasma PRL concentrations were not different from those of animals in diestrus. These regular peaks of secretion disappeared on the eleventh day (end of pseudopregnancy) to be replaced by a typical proestrus secretion pattern followed by resumption of the normal pattern of a 4 or 5 day rat cycle. In the same series of experiments corpus luteum regression, which begins on day 7 of pseudopregnancy as evidenced by a decline in progesterone secretion, was not associated with major decreases in PRL secretion. The nocturnal surges of PRL secretion were observed on day 11 at a time at which progesterone secretion had already decreased to the low levels observed during the estrus cycle. These observations are in agreement with the earlier conclusions of Rothchild (124) suggesting that the cause of luteal regression in the rat cannot be explained simply by the withdrawal of luteotropic support, i.e., prolactin secretion.

CATECHOLAMINES AND PRL SECRETION

Since catecholamines are found in high concentrations in the area of the median eminence (39), they have been studied by several groups as a possible PIF. MacLeod (93) has reported that $10^{-6}M$ norepinephrine caused a 70%–80% decrease in PRL secretion within 7 hr after being added to rat pituitary fragments surviving in vitro. Similar results were found by Birge et al (15) who observed that 0.5 μg norepinephrine/ml medium or 1.0 μg epinephrine/ml medium inhibited PRL secretion. Koch et al (85) reported that catecholamine treatment caused a biphasic secretion of PRL in vitro. MacLeod et al (95) reported that $10^{-6}M$ dopamine, a precursor of norepinephrine and epinephrine, inhibited the secretion of PRL as shown by incorporation of [³H]-leucine in purified prolactin and that it increased the stores of labelled PRL in vitro, as determined by densitometric measurements after polyacrylamide gel electrophoresis. Following the presentation of these data, MacLeod & Fontham (94) suggested that the concentration of bicarbonate ion in the in vitro medium may be more important in inhibiting or stimulating PRL secretion than the presence of catecholamines. This would imply that the inhibition of PRL observed in vitro by these several groups may be peculiar to the test system.

This supposition seems to be supported by the reports that administration of dopamine, epinephrine, or norepinephrine in vivo to adult rats did not affect plasma PRL levels (90). This might be related to the reported inability of these neurohumors to cross the blood brain barrier. Lu & Meites (92) observed that L-dopa (12 mg) treatment of adult rats decreased PRL secretion by 50% within 30 min. Since L-dopa is thought to cross the blood brain barrier, it may be that its effect is due to subsequent conversion to other forms. Similar results have been observed with humans; oral administration of L-dopa partially inhibits the rise in plasma PRL levels that is seen following administration of chlorpromazine (81). Likewise, L-dopa treatment of patients with galactorrhea (Forbes-Albright syndrome) lowered plasma PRL levels and inhibited milk secretion (150). We have observed that simultaneous administration of 50 μg L-dopa, together with 10 μg perphenazine intravenously, did not inhibit the acute rise in plasma PRL that is seen following treatment with perphenazine alone. This suggests to us that L-dopa does not directly act to inhibit PRL secretion either at the level of the brain or pituitary but must be converted into either dopamine or another catecholamine.

The data of Kamberi et al (72) would tend to support this hypothesis. They found that infusion of 1.25 μg dopamine into the third ventricle of rats caused the following decreases in plasma PRL levels; 70% preinjection level at 10 min; 47% at 20 min; 42% at 30 min; 57% at 60 min; 69% at 90 min; and 93% at 120 min. Intraventricular injection of either epinephrine or norepinephrine did not affect PRL release. They also found that infusion of dopamine, epinephrine, or norepinephrine into a hypophysial portal vein for 30 min had no effect on plasma PRL levels. Subsequently, Kamberi et al (74) found that intra-hypophysial portal infusion for 30 min at 2 μl/min of plasma taken from the hypothalamic portal vessels of another rat which had been treated with 1.25 μg dopamine via the third ventricle, caused an increase in LH and FSH secretion and a decrease in PRL secretion. Infusion of plasma taken from the femoral artery or from rats treated with saline did not significantly affect the secretion of these hormones. This suggests that dopamine causes the ultimate release of some hypothalamic compound that decreases the secretion of PRL.

SHORT FEEDBACK CONTROL OF PRL SECRETION

It has been suggested that PRL may control its secretion through a short feedback loop, since implantation of PRL into the median eminence has been claimed to reduce the duration of both pregnancy and pseudopregnancy in rats (37, 139); it was then suggested that PRL might stimulate the release of a PIF (short feedback), thereby inhibiting its own release or act directly at the level of the pituitary (ultra short feedback). Voogt & Meites (159) have observed that implantation of 250 μg of PRL into the median eminence of rats caused a marginal decrease in pituitary PRL content within 3 days. Pituitary FSH, but not LH content, was claimed to be increased in the same experiment. Concomitantly, serum LH and FSH levels were reported to increase while PRL levels remained unchanged when compared with rats receiving only implants of the control medium. No change was reportedly observed in hypothalamic PIF, LRF, or FRF content. In view of the discrepancy between the changes in plasma and pituitary levels of PRL, LH, and FSH, it may be premature to attempt to implicate PRL as a direct autoregulator of its own secretion.

T_4 AND PRL SECRETION

Chen & Meites (35) have observed that chronic treatment of rats with doses of 5 and 25 μg T_4/100 g body wt for 21 days results in an increase in the content of pituitary PRL. Chronic treatment with thiouracil for 21 days had no effect on pituitary PRL content; neither T_4 nor thiouracil treatment affected hypothalamic PIF content.

Recently, we have observed that acute treatment in vitro with T_4 ($10^{-6}M$) of either enzymatically dispersed pituitary cells or hemipituitaries, which were taken from rats treated with PTU starting before puberty, inhibits PRL secretion by 50%. This suggests that T_4 may exert an inhibitory influence on PRL secretion in vitro. Some findings by Knigge & Silverman (83) also suggest that T_4 might be involved in the regulation of PRL (and TSH) secretion. They have observed that the median eminence concentrates T_4 against a gradient. The active transport mechanism seems to be both temperature and sodium dependent and ouabain sensitive. Furthermore, they found that median eminence tissue incubated with $0.01M$ T_4 for 90 min, then transferred to fresh medium free of T_4, released 60% of the total hormone which it concentrated within 20 min. Addition of TSH to the incubation medium was found to increase T_4 concentrations and to inhibit subsequent efflux. Likewise, addition of dopamine increased T_4 uptake by 50% above controls.

In vivo data have confirmed some of the observations made in vitro; Kendall et al (79) and Knigge & Silverman (83) have shown that injection of T_4 into the lateral ventricle of rats results in an accumulation of labeled material in the median eminence. In the former study, the amount of ^{131}I–T_4 found in the anterior pituitary, cerebral cortex, posterior pituitary, and whole blood was negligible when compared to the amount that was found in the median eminence. Considering these data, the possibility exists that T_4 may be involved in the control of PRL secretion. More will be said below on possible relationships between thyroid hormones, TRF, and prolactin secretion.

Is TRF THE SUSPECTED PRF?

Nicoll et al (111) have reported that the rat hypothalamus contains PRF in addition to a PIF. This conclusion was derived from in vivo and in vitro studies using tissues taken from mammals and reptiles. Subsequently, a PRF activity was reported to be present in rat hypothalamic extracts by Valverde

& Chieffo (157); the PRF active zone appears to coincide with the TRF zone following column chromatography on G-10 Sephadex. The authors reported that intravenous injection of 100 ng of synthetic TRF into their assay (steroid pretreated) rats did not cause an elevation in plasma PRL levels; thus they concluded that TRF was not the PRF which they had detected in their fraction. Also, they found that vasopressin caused an increase in plasma PRL levels when administered to their test system. However, the PRF activity was still present after treatment of the active extract fraction with thioglycolate which would destroy vasopressin. Tashjian et al (147) have reported that chronic treatment of cloned rat pituitary tumor cells with TRF produced an increase in PRL secretion. We (155) have confirmed the original observation of Tashjian et al. Moreover, Jacobs et al (70) and Bowers et al (19) have demonstrated that injection of 10 to 800 μg of TRF into humans results in a rapid rise in plasma PRL levels. When 800 μg of TRF was given, both groups observed a tenfold increase in plasma PRL levels within 10–15 min. Concomitant elevation of plasma TSH also occurrred. There appears to be considerable species variation in the ability of TRF to induce secretion of PRL. While TRF appears to be extremely potent in stimulating the secretion of PRL in humans, monkeys,[1] and sheep,[2] large doses of TRF administered to normal rats or added in vitro to normal rat pituitary cells fail to stimulate significantly the secretion of PRL [although TRF stimulates in vitro the secretion of PRL from the pituitary of rats chronically fed PTU (151a)]. In view of the other results reported above, one may, however, speculate that the still hypothetical PRF may be closely related structurally to TRF. One might further speculate that TRF is PRF in those species in which TRF is so very active to release PRL, while PRF is a peptide different from TRF though closely related in those species in which TRF is not a powerful stimulator of PRL secretion.

STRESS AND PRL RELEASE

Raud et al (117) have shown that acute stress (noise and restraint) of adult cows for 10 min, caused a fourfold increase in plasma PRL levels as measured by specific radioimmunoassay. Neill (108, 109) also has demonstrated that plasma PRL levels in rats bled after a short exposure to ether are higher than levels found in plasma samples taken from rats following rapid decapitation. These data confirm earlier reports that stress stimulates the acute release of PRL in several species, and demonstrate that a condition other than the exogenous administration of TRF can cause a rapid release of PRL. It may be worth recalling here that acute stress, in all species studied so far, produces an acute fall in plasma TSH levels or no change at all; this would militate against TRF being the physiological mediator of the stress-induced acute release of PRL.

[1] Knobil et al. To be published.
[2] Fell, Findlay, Cumming & Goding. To be published.

Effect of Drugs on Acute Secretion of PRL

In addition to physiological data, pharmacological information suggests that PRL may be acutely released following administration of drugs such as antipsychotic tranquilizers. Ben-David et al (12) have reported that plasma PRL levels (measured by bioassay) are increased significantly within 30 min following intraperitoneal injection of perphenazine, 100 mg/kg body wt. We have observed that perphenazine in doses as low as 6.5 μg/100 g body wt given intravenously, will elevate plasma PRL levels within 10 min post-injection. This acute release is clearly not an artifact produced by ether stress; we also have evidence from in vitro studies that perphenazine does not stimulate the secretion of PRL by acting at the pituitary level. It should be noted that similar increases in plasma LH and TSH levels are seen within the same time period if LRF or TRF respectively are administered by the same route. In view of the similarity of the responses induced by the antipsychotic tranquilizers and releasing factors when related as a function of time, one might speculate that perphenazine is releasing a PRF. However, one cannot exclude the possibility that release from an inhibiting factor might follow a similar time course.

Conclusions

Our understanding of the control of PRL secretion is incomplete. At this juncture, we feel that no clear statement can be made concerning the brain control of this hormone. PRL secretion is influenced by many other hormones and it will be difficult to understand the mechanisms that control its release until we ascertain the role or roles which PRL play in the organism. The existence of the postulated hypothalamic PIF and PRF remains to be clearly proven.

CONTROL OF THE SECRETION OF THYROTROPIN

Structure of the hypothalamic TRF of ovine origin has been established as that of the tripeptide pGlu-His-Pro-NH$_2$ (26–28). TRF of porcine origin was shown to have the same structure (104). It appears that more than two mammalian TRFs may have the same structure; Bowers et al (20) have reported that TRF of human origin (based on biological activity) has, in several chromatographic systems, the same mobility as the tripeptide pGlu-His-Pro-NH$_2$. Also, there are reports (61, 100) that [^{3}H]Pro, ^{14}C-Glu, ^{14}C-His, or ^{14}C-Pro are incorporated when incubated with fragments of rat hypothalamus in vitro, into a substance which, upon chromatographic separation, has the same mobility as cold TRF or ^{125}I-labeled TRF. Furthermore, the synthetic tripeptide pGlu-His-Pro-NH$_2$ has been shown to be active in stimulating the release of TSH in all species of mammals studied so far. Although these results are inferential, they lend support to the proposal that native TRF in these various species of mammals is the tripeptide pGlu-His-Pro-NH$_2$.

This may not be the case in birds since pGlu-His-Pro-NH$_2$ is reportedly inactive in chickens (112).

Availability of unlimited quantities of synthetic TRF (11, 28, 49, 55, 156) has already led to extensive clinical studies in humans which are of considerable physiological interest; data from some of these will be presented below.

The specificity of the action of TRF exclusively to induce the secretion of TSH, as originally reported, has been considerably qualified by a series of reports demonstrating that in some species, either in vivo or in vitro, TRF is a potent stimulator of the secretion of prolactin [see above chapter on the secretion of prolactin; see also (88)]. No consistent evidence has been presented that TRF would affect secretion of growth hormone either in normal rats or in in vitro experiments dealing with tissues obtained from normal rats. The use in vitro of tumoral tissues of pituitary origin (147) and the administration in vivo of TRF to animals or patients bearing pituitary tumors may lead to entirely different results. Indeed, administration of synthetic TRF to patients with active acromegaly led to acute and striking elevations of plasma growth hormone levels (69).

Incubation in vitro of natural (ovine) or synthetic TRF (pGlu-His-Pro-NH$_2$) with rat blood, plasma, or reconstituted lyophilized serum destroyed the biological activity (120, 153). Inactivation of TRF by normal plasma took place at 0°C but at a slower rate than at 37°C. Plasma obtained from rats several weeks after hypophysectomy or after hypophysectomy and thyroidectomy inactivated TRF. TRF activity was not recovered from TRF incubated in plasma when the incubate was treated with NaCl (4 M), ethanol (80% v/v), or HCl (to pH 1). Plasma inactivation of TRF was completely prevented by pretreatment of the plasma with ethanol (80% v/v); heating of plasma at 65°C for 15 min also destroyed the ability of plasma to inactive TRF. The data reported are consistent with the hypothesis that plasma contains an enzyme or enzymes that destroy the activity of TRF. Plasma was also found to destroy the biological activity of pGlu-His-Pro-OMe and pGlu-His-Pro-OH (two synthetic tripeptides with TRF activity). The biological activity of pGlu-His-Pro-OH was destroyed in vitro at a slower rate by plasma than that of pGlu-His-Pro-NH$_2$ or natural TRF. Addition of the dipeptide analog of TRF, pGlu-His-OMe, prevented the inactivation of TRF by plasma in vitro (153).

Other studies have shown that a similar in vitro inactivation of TRF takes place in human blood (120, 121). The mechanisms involved in this enzymatic destruction of plasma in vitro have been further studied by several groups; the physiological significance of this in vitro inactivation of TRF by plasma is questionable however, in view of the observation that exogenous TRF is rapidly excreted by glomerular filtration with a large percentage of the administrated dose of TRF recovered as biologically active material in the urine (121, and Braudo et al[3]).

---

[3] Braudo, M. et al. Unpublished observations.

Porter et al (116) have demonstrated that infusion of 1 ng TRF/min into the hypophysial portal circulation caused a significant increase in peripheral TSH levels. This clearly shows that administration of a physiological dose of TRF releases TSH and supports the concept that small packets of TRF are released into the portal circulation which cause the release of pituitary hormones (TSH). Such a postulate is supported by the findings of Martin & Reichlin (96), who observed that either electrical stimulation of the medial basal hypothalamus or intravenous administration of synthetic TRF to rats induced a significant rise in plasma TSH levels within 5 min. They interpreted these findings to indicate that medial basal hypothalamus releases preformed TRF which subsequently acts on the pituitary to release TSH.

Although administration of TRF via portal vessels released TSH at nanogram doses, the administration of TRF into the cerebral spinal fluid via the lateral ventricles did not produce a more rapid release of TSH than did intravenous injection of TRF in the rat (80). This would not appear to support the proposal that TRF may be released into the CSF before it acts on the pituitary.

There is now ample evidence that synthetic TRF is highly active in stimulating secretion of TSH in humans following intravenous or oral administration as originally observed in experimental animals (151). Snyder & Utiger (137) have shown that TSH release is linear between doses of 6–400 micrograms and that while there is apparently no dependence on sex, the response to TRF in terms of elevation of plasma TSH is related to the age of the subject, older men or women showing lower responses than younger individuals of the same body weight and sex.

Hollander et al (67) have reported that administration of TRF to normal subjects causes a rapid rise in plasma TSH concentration which is accompanied and followed by a significant increase in circulating T_3 levels. In contrast to the clearcut elevation in plasma T_3, the increase in plasma T_4, though statistically significant, was apparently quite small. These interesting observations may well represent the clarification of a point that was still somewhat puzzling, namely, the reported inability of elevating plasma T_4 levels in normal individuals administered TRF. Several clinical groups have already reported considerable experience with TRF in a variety of patients (48, 58, 62). Daily testing with doses of ca 500 micrograms of TRF given intravenously appears to blunt the plasma TSH elevation response after several days of testing; however, intervals of 3 days between the intravenous administration of these doses of TRF led to normal, repeatable observations. Hyperthyroid patients with undetectable baseline TSH levels usually do not respond to TRF; patients with primary hypothyroidism with already elevated plasma TSH levels, usually show an exaggerated response to TRF. In these patients, treatment with dexamethasone appears to suppress the elevated baseline TSH levels but not the magnitude of the response to TRF. In all individuals, administration of large doses of T_4 or T_3 is able to decrease or inhibit the response to TRF. Euthyroid patients with suspected or proven pituitary tumors show a variety of possible responses to TRF ranging from normal responses to total absence of response to TRF. Of extreme interest are the reports from Grumbach's group (71, 123) that the majority of children with specific deficiencies in TSH secretion do show normal responses to TRF, leading to the conclusion that their primary defect is in the hypothalamus and not in the pituitary.

At the time of writing this review, there was already ample clinical evidence that TRF is a powerful releaser of prolactin in man [see above chapter on the secretion of prolactin; see also (58, 71)].

MECHANISM OF ACTION OF TRF

Although it seems clear that TRF is the major positive controller of TSH secretion, the mechanism by which it evokes TSH release is not fully understood. This subject has been reviewed recently (55, 141) and only a few points will be made here. It seems probable that TRF acts on the plasma membrane of the thyrotroph to bring about the release of preformed TSH. This can be inhibited by thyroid hormones as in the well-known physiological negative feedback relationships between thyroid secretion and TSH secretion. The thyroid hormones are presumed to act inside the cell to induce the synthesis of a mRNA, which in turn directs the synthesis of a regulator protein; subsequently, this protein (not characterized) inhibits the events stimulated by the binding of TRF to the plasma membrane.

The availability of [^{3}H]Pro labeled TRF has made possible the demonstration of TRF binding to the plasma membrane of the thyrotroph. Grant et al (57) have described the specific binding of labeled TRF to the membrane of mouse TSH tumor cells, dispersed cells from normal bovine, ovine, and murine pituitaries and various isolated membrane preparations. [^{3}H]TRF was found to compete with unlabeled TRF for membrane binding sites in a stoichiometric manner. LRF was reported not to compete with the labeled TRF for binding sites. Similar studies were reported by Labrie et al (89) using isolated plasma membrane from bovine anterior pituitary glands. They also reported that TRF binding was not affected by the presence of 10 μM L-T$_4$ or L-T$_3$.

Various structure-function studies described in detail by Vale et al (155) using various analogs of TRF seem to indicate that biological activity (in terms of TSH release in vivo and in vitro) is directly proportional to the affinity with which the membrane receptor or receptors bind TRF. Further, these studies demonstrate that (a) alteration of the amino acid sequence of the tripeptide TRF, (b) alteration of the N-terminal residue, or (c) alteration of the optical properties of the amino acids of TRF markedly reduces or eliminates both the binding capacity and biological activity of the molecule. Only one analog of TRF has been found to have greater specific biological activity than native TRF: the pGlu-N^{3im}Me-His-Pro-NH$_2$ derivative of TRF as described by Vale et al (156) has 8–10 times the biological potency of native TRF. This has been shown to be related to a higher binding constant (K$_a$) than that of TRF to pituitary TRF-receptor sites (155, 156).

Whether the interaction of either TRF or the thyroid hormones with the cell induces a change in the membrane electrical properties is unknown at present. York et al (175) have attempted to approach this problem by intracellular recording (in vivo) of the membrane potentials of "hypersecreting" thyrotropic cells which were induced by chronic administration of PTU to rats. They observed membrane potentials which were generally lower than those found in controls (controls being nontreated rats). This approach appears to be of doubtful significance since there is no way to identify the cell types which are penetrated by the microelectrodes, a point recognized by the investigators.

NEURAL REGULATION OF TRF RELEASE

It has been mentioned earlier that the thyroid hormones are thought to exert their major influence on TSH secretion by acting directly at the level of the pituitary. It has been suggested that these hormones might act partially at the level of the brain, possibly to modify the release of TRF. Recent studies by Knigge & Joseph (82) tend to support this contention. They reported that cats in which the basal hypothalamus had been deafferented by stereotaxic cutting exhibit a compensatory response to hemithyroidectomy similar to that of normal animals. Treatment with 2.5 μg kg^{-1} day^{-1} with T_4 for 14 days was reported to cause inhibition of thyroid function in normal cats but not in the deafferented ones, thus suggesting that T_4 acts at the level of the brain to inhibit the response. In view of this interesting observation, further studies would be worthwhile to determine the pathways involved and the nature of this possible thyroid-brain interaction. Silverman & Knigge (135) have reported in in vitro studies that the median eminence is capable of accumulating T_4 by an energy-dependent mechanism (inhibition by ouabain, iodoacetate, NaF, and KCN). Once intracellularly bound, T_4 appears to remain as unaltered hormone (T_4) in a pool readily released by addition to the in vitro system of relatively small concentrations of TSH; addition of TSH is reported also to increase uptake of T_4 by the fragment of median eminence. These results are reminiscent of the "filter theory" proposed many years back by Brown-Grant (22) in which, somehow, cellular elements of the median eminence would regulate the concentration of T_4 in the portal blood reaching the adenohypophysis. If the elegant results of Silverman & Knigge (135) are confirmed, they would have to be taken into consideration in any effort at explaining the physiological mechanisms of the negative feedback between T_4 and TRF at the level of the adenohypophysial tissues (reviews in 60, 155); they would also have to be incorporated in the recent proposal (100) that T_4 stimulates the (enzymatic) biosynthesis of TRF by cellular elements in the hypothalamus-median eminence region.

CONTROL OF THE SECRETION OF MELANOCYTE STIMULATING HORMONE

It has been proposed that the secretion of MSH is primarily inhibited by a hypothalamic MIF; the existence of a hypothalamic MRF has recently been proposed (for review, see 78).

Celis et al (32) have proposed that MIF is the tripeptide C-terminus of oxytocin, H-Pro-Leu-Gly-NH$_2$, which would be cleaved from oxytocin by a microsomal enzyme system present in the ventral hypothalamus. Nair et al (105) have isolated an MIF activity from extracts of bovine hypothalamus and have reported its structure to be H-Pro-Leu-Gly-NH$_2$; during the purification of (bovine) hypothalamic MIF, two zones of biological activity were found following thin layer chromatography as determined by a bioassay based on skin color variation of frogs previously darkened by hypothalamic lesion. The structure H-Pro-Leu-Gly-NH$_2$ corresponds to the most active zone and is considered to be native MIF by Nair et al (105).

The biological activity of H-Pro-Leu-Gly-NH$_2$ as an inhibitor of the secretion of MSH has been questioned and so has its proposed physiological role as the modulator of the secretion of MSH: Bower et al (18) could not confirm MIF-activity of synthetic H-Pro-Leu-Gly-NH$_2$ in in vitro systems using rat pituitary tissues. The same group further reported (18) that the ring structure of oxytocin, tocinoic acid (H-Cys-Tyr-Ileu-Gln-Asn-Cys-OH) is a powerful inhibitor of MSH-release in the same systems in which the tripeptide is inactive. Kastin et al (75) may have found a possible explanation for these diverging results with their report that H-Pro-Leu-Gly-NH$_2$ is apparently destroyed by plasma: injection into the dorsal lymph sac of the frog or into the aortic trunk of as much as 10 mg of the tripeptide did not produce any evidence of inhibition of the secretion of MSH, while rapid inhibition of MSH-secretion was reported following direct application of $\geqslant 1 \times 10^{-8}$g of the tripeptide to frog pituitary gland previously exposed by surgical trephination of the sphenoid bone. Incubation of H-Pro-Leu-Gly-NH$_2$ with frog serum led to disappearance of biological activity (75). Similarly, injection of the tripeptide intravenously in humans did not lead to changes in the plasma concentration of MSH (58). Nair et al (105) have reported the characterization in extracts of bovine hypothalamus of another peptide, H-Pro-His-Phe-Arg-Gly-NH$_2$ (MIF II) possessing MIF-activity, based on their assay assessing lightening of the skin of frogs previously darkened by hypothalamic lesion (75). MIF II would be a thousandth as potent as MIF I (H-Pro-Leu-Gly-NH$_2$) in inhibiting the secretion of MSH. Kastin et al (77) have reported that [^{3}H]- or ^{14}C-labeled MIF I accumulated in the pineal gland; they suggested the existence of a complex hypothalamic-pineal-pituitary axis which may involve more than one MIF-active neurohumoral substance in the physiological control of MSH secretion.

Taleisnik & Orias, who had reported (145) the existence in the hypothalamus of an MSH-releasing factor, recently isolated a pentapeptide fragment of oxytocin H-Cys-Tyr-Ile-Gln-Asn-OH from hypothalamic tissues that exhibited MSH-releasing activity (33). As in the case of the tripeptide H-Pro-Leu-Gly-NH$_2$, this pentapeptide MRF would be cleaved from oxytocin as the substrate by specific hypothalamic enzymes.

Obviously, elucidation of the physiological mechanisms involved in the regulation of the secretion of MSH is far from complete.

CONTROL OF THE SECRETION OF ADRENOCORTICOTROPIN

Despite the fact that the control of ACTH secretion by the brain was among the earliest areas studied by neuroendocrinologists, it is certainly not the one best understood at the writing of this review. Early in the 1950's posterior pituitary extracts as well as hypothalamic extracts were found to contain substances that would stimulate the release of ACTH secretion in vivo and in vitro. Subsequently, it was noted that administration of large doses of vasopressin would produce similar effects in various test systems. Although a factor could be separated from vasopressin by chromatography which would release ACTH, two schools developed, one proposing that vasopressin was the sole hypothalamic mediator of ACTH secretion, while the other maintained that the hypothalamus contained a separate corticotropin releasing factor which was the physiological controller of the secretion of ACTH (for review, see 60).

The consensus is now that vasopressin is not the physiological regulator of ACTH secretion, although the exact relationship of vasopressin to the control of corticotropin release is still unclear: Hedge & de Wied (65) have reported that atropine implants, placed in the midline just rostral to the paraventricular nuclei and caudoventral to the anterior commissure, inhibit the stress-induced release of corticotropin as determined by seconday analysis of the plasma corticosterone levels; plasma vasopressin in the same animals was unaffected by the administration of atropine. This observation indicates that the secretion of vasopressin and ACTH are regulated by separate hypothalamic mechanisms and thus further supports the concept of a separate CRF.

Although the data indicate that there exists a true CRF of hypothalamic origin, vasopressin may act together with the hypothalamic factor to regulate ACTH secretion. Yates et al (169) have reported that administration of subthreshold doses of vasopressin to rats pretreated with dexamethasone, nembutal, and morphine together with crude (ovine) hypothalamic CRF concentrate intravenously potentiated the adrenocortical response. If subthreshold doses of crude CRF were administered prior to injection of vasopressin, no potentiation was observed. They proposed that vasopressin: (*a*) may release endogenous CRF from the hypothalamus, (*b*) acts as a separate CRF, or (*c*) acts in concert with CRF to bring about the release of ACTH.

The studies of Dunn & Critchlow (44) have indicated that the hypothalamus and other forebrain structures are not necessary for vasopressin-induced ACTH release to occur in the rat. Their data suggest that the response seen with vasopressin probably occurs at the level of the pituitary.

ISOLATION OF CRF

Attempts to isolate CRF from hypothalamic tissue have had limited success. A major problem has been the unreliability of the in vivo bioassays used to assess CRF activity. It has proved difficult to block the endogenous release of ACTH, hence to evaluate the specific effect on ACTH secretion of administration of an exogenous CRF. To overcome this problem Witorsch & Brodish (166) have suggested again using rats bearing ventral medial hypothalamic lesions as a test preparation. Placement of these lesions was reported to abolish the increase in plasma corticosterone after ether stress. Unfortunately, the assay is not specific unless rigorous time parameters are observed in the testing schedule. The difficulty in suppressing spontaneous ACTH release may be noted in the data of Ondo & Kitay (113). They reported that in dexamethasone treated rats bearing isolated diencephalic islands, ACTH release could be evoked by either stress or vasopressin and histamine treatment.

As a result of the problems inherent in the direct assessment of CRF activity in vivo, various methods have been developed to measure it in vitro. Seiden & Brodish (133) have modified the Krebs-Ringer bicarbonate medium by adjusting the pH below 7.4. This modification was reported to increase the sensitivity of the assay. Further, decreasing the osmolarity of the medium seems to expand the range of the test. These investigators report a log dose response between 0.05 and 0.2 hypothalamic fragment equivalents. CRF activity was ascertained by injecting the incubation medium into hypophysectomized rats and measuring its ACTH concentration in terms of the plasma corticosterone levels (fluorometric methods) in the hypophysectomized test animals.

An elegant method for evaluating ACTH activity has been introduced by Giordano & Sayers (56). They report that isolated adrenal cells respond to ACTH with an increased steroidogenesis; when combined with Quso® (microfine silica granules) treatment, plasma ACTH levels in peripheral blood could be adequately determined. In further confirmation of the method, it was found that the isolated adrenal cells responded not only to ACTH but to cyclic AMP as well (127).

Another system which has found use in the study of CRF physiology is the monolayer pituitary cell culture described by Vale et al (154). Using this system, Rivier et al[4] have located a CRF activity in aqueous extracts of sheep hypothalamus which is not due to vasopressin or to any other known hypothalamic peptide. This observation has been confirmed in vivo using rats which were (a) acutely stressed with ether (b) bled via jugular vein (t = 0), (c) treated intravenously with crude CRF or saline and (d) decapitated 2.5 min post injection. Plasma ACTH levels were measured by highly specific radioimmunoassay and changes in plasma ACTH levels were determined following covariance analysis. At this point it is impossible to determine whether hypothalamic CRF is related to the beta and alpha CRF molecules which were isolated by Schally & Guillemin (for review, see 59) using extracts of neurohypophysial origin.

NEURAL CONTROL OF CRF RELEASE

Despite the difficulty in isolating and characterizing CRF, some progress has been made in understanding how the brain controls the secretion of the

_____

[4] Rivier, C., Vale, W., Guillemin, R. To be published.

CRF-ACTH system. The data of Weitzman et al (162) in normal human subjects suggest that the brain releases CRF in periodic bursts. They reported that plasma cortisol concentrations fluctuated throughout the 24 hr sleep-wake cycle (samples being taken every 20 min); the fluctuations were described as being characterized by sharp rises, followed by slow, smooth decline. The decay followed an exponential curve in most cases. These findings may appear to be at variance with the observations describing a circadian rhythm in plasma cortisol levels. However, the investigators indicate that if the data are averaged over 1 hr periods, the resultant curve quite closely conforms to the circadian pattern.

Scapagnini et al (128) have suggested that serotoninergic neurons may play a role in the diurnal fluctuation of pituitary-adrenal function. Their studies show that in rats, 5-hydroxytryptamine content of the hippocampus and amygdala, structures known to be involved in the trans-hypothalamic control of ACTH secretion, exhibit a diurnal rhythm; the lowest level occurred at 4 AM and the highest at 8 PM. This diurnal curve parallelled the changes in plasma corticosterone. Moreover, injection of 300 mg/kg of p-chlorophenylalanine, a drug that blocks 5-hydroxytryptamine synthesis, reversed the morning and afternoon pattern of plasma corticosterone concentration, so that there was no statistically significant fluctuation throughout the day. Serotonin contents of the hippocampus and amygdala were also reduced, though diurnal variations of 5-hydroxytryptamine content were still present in the hippocampus.

Effect of Corticosteroids on Brain-Pituitary Axis

The location at which the corticosteroids exert a modifying influence on the secretion of CRF or ACTH is not well understood, nor is the mechanism by which these agents bring out these effects. When a single injection of tritiated cortisol (F^3H) was given to an eviscerated cat, brain F^3H concentration progressively increased until after 2 hr it was equal to the levels found in the plasma. The concentration of F^3H in cerebral spinal fluid was 25% that of plasma at the same time. F^3H levels were lower in pituitary, lung, heart, and brachial muscle (160).

In an attempt to locate feedback receptors of cortisol, Bohus & Strashimirov (17) found that implantation of dexamethasone, cortisol, corticosterone, 11-dehydrocorticosterone, and 11-deoxycorticosterone in the anterior median eminence suppressed ACTH release. Implantation of dexamethasone, cortisol, and 11-deoxycorticosterone into the infundibulum also suppressed ACTH release, while dexamethasone and 11-deoxycorticosterone inhibited ACTH release when implanted bilaterally into the anterior pituitary. These data indicate that corticosteroid receptors may exist in both the hypothalamus and the pituitary.

It is obvious that considerably more work needs to be done to understand how the brain controls the secretion of ACTH. Of importance in attaining such an understanding would be learning the chemical nature of hypothalamic CRF.

LITERATURE CITED

1. Amoss, M., Blackwell, R., Guillemin, R. 1972. Stimulation of ovulation in the rabbit triggered by synthetic LRF. *J. Clin. Endocrinol.* 35:434–36

2. Amoss, M. et al 1971. Purification, amino acid composition and N-terminus of the hypothalamic luteinizing hormone releasing factor (LRF) of ovine origin. *Biochem. Biophys. Res. Commun.* 44:205–10

3. Amoss, M., Burgus, R., Ward, D. N. Fellows, R. E., Guillemin, R. 1970. Evidence for a pyroglutamic acid (PAC) N-terminus in ovine hypothalamic luteinizing hormone-releasing factor (LRF). Abstr. *Meet. Endocrine Soc., 52nd, St. Louis, Missouri,* p. 61. Philadelphia: Lippincott

4. Amoss, M., Rivier, J., Guillemin, R. 1972. Release of gonadotropins by oral administration of synthetic LRF or a tripeptide fragment of LRF. *J. Clin. Endocrinol.* 35:175–77

5. Arimura, A. 1970. Serum prolactin levels in rats with pituitary grafts. Abstr. *Meet, Endocrine Soc. 52nd, St. Louis, Missouri,* p. 127. Philadelphia: Lippincott

6. Arimura, A., Dunn, J. D., Schally, A. V. 1972. Effect of infusion of hypothalamic extracts on serum prolactin levels in rats treated with nembutal, CNS depressants, or bearing hypothalamic lesions. *Endocrinology* 90:378–83

7. Arimura, A., Matsuo, H., Baba, Y., Schally, A. V. 1971. Ovulation induced by synthetic luteinizing hormone-releasing hormone in the hamster. *Science* 174:511–12

8. Arimura, A., Saito, M., Wakabayashi, I. 1969. Effect of pig hypothalamic extracts on release of pituitary prolactin in sheep and goats. Abstr. *Meet. Endocrine Soc., 52nd, New York,* No. 31. Philadelphia: Lippincott

9. Arimura, A., Schally, A. V. 1971. Augmentation of pituitary responsiveness to LH-releasing hormone (LH-RH) by estrogen. *Proc. Soc. Exp. Biol. Med.*

136:290–93

10. Atkinson, L. E., Bhattacharya, A. N., Monroe, S. E., Dierschke, D. J., Knobil, E. 1970. Effects of gonadectomy on plasma LH concentration in the rhesus monkey. *Endocrinology* 87: 847–49

11. Baugh, C. M., Krumdieck, C. L., Hershman, J. M., Pittman, J. A., Jr. 1970. Synthesis and biological activity of thyrotropin-releasing hormone. *Endocrinology* 87:1015–21

12. Ben-David, M., Danon, A., Sulman, F. G. 1970. Acute changes in blood and pituitary prolactin after a single injection of perphenazine. *Neuroendocrinology* 6:336–42

13. Bernardis, L. L., Frohman, L. A. 1971. Plasma growth hormone responses to electrical stimulation of the hypothalamus in the rat. *Neuroendocrinology* 7: 193–201

14. Bhattacharya, A. N., Dierschke, D. J., Yamaji, T., Knobil, E. 1972. The pharmacologic blackade of the circhoral mode of LH secretion in the ovariectomized rhesus monkey. *Endocrinology* 90:778–86

15. Birge, C. A., Jacobs, L. S., Hammer, C. T., Daughaday, W. H. 1970. Catecholamine inhibition of prolactin secretion by isolated rat adenohypophyses. *Endocrinology* 86:120–30

16. Blackwell, R. et al 1972. Lack of effect of native or synthetic LRF on the secretion of prolactin *in vitro. Am. J. Physiol.* In press

17. Bohus, B., Strashimirov, D. 1970. Localization and specificity of corticosteroid "feedback receptors" at the hypothalamo-hypophysial level; comparative effects of various steroids implanted in the median eminence or the anterior pituitary of the rat. *Neuroendocrinology* 6: 197–209

18. Bower, A., Hadley, M. E., Hruby, V. J. 1971. Comparative MSH release-inhibiting activities of tocinoic acid (the ring of oxytocin) and L-Pro-L-Leu-Gly-

NH₂ (the side chain of oxyto-cin). *Biochem. Biophys. Res. Commun.* 45:1185–91
19. Bowers, C. Y., Friesen, H. G., Hwang, P., Guyda, H. J., Folkers, K. 1971. Prolactin and thyrotropin release in man by synthetic pyroglutamyl-histidyl-prolinamide. *Biochem. Biophys. Res. Commun.* 45:1033–41
20. Bowers, C. Y., Schally, A. V., Weil, A., Reynolds, G. A., Folkers, K. 1970. Chemical and biological identity of thyrotropin releasing hormones (TRH) of bovine and human origin. *Proc. Int. Thyroid Conf., 6th, Vienna, June 1970* 2:1019–40
21. Brazeau, P. et al 1972. A hypothalamic polypeptide that inhibits the secretion of pituitary growth hormone. *Science.* In press
22. Brown-Grant, K. 1956. The feedback hypothesis of the control of thyroid function. *Ciba Found. Colloq. Endocrinol.* 10:97–120
23. Brown, G. M., Schalch, D. S., Reichlin, S. 1971. Hypothalamic mediation of growth hormone and adrenal stress response in the squirrel monkey. *Endocrinology* 89:694–703
24. Burgus, R. et al 1972. Primary structure of the ovine hypothalamic luteinizing hormone-releasing factor (LRF). *Proc. Nat. Acad. Sci. USA* 69:278–82
25. Burgus, R. et al 1971. Structure moléculaire du facteur hypothalamique (LRF) d'origine ovine contrôlant la sécrétion de l'hormone gonadotrope hypophysaire de lutéinisation (LH). *Compt. Rend. Acad. Sci.* 273:1611–13
26. Burgus, R., Dunn, T. F., Desiderio, D., Guillemin, R. 1969. Structure moléculaire du facteur hypothalamique hypophysiotrope TRF d'origine ovine: évidence par spectrométrie de masse de la séquence PCA-His-Pro-NH₂. *Compt. Rend. Acad. Sci.* 269:1870–73
27. Burgus, R., Dunn, T. F., Desiderio, D., Vale, W., Guillemin, R. 1969. Dérivés polypeptidiques de synthèse doués d'activité hypophysiotrope TRF. Nouvelles observations. *Compt. Rend. Acad. Sci. Paris* 269:226–28

28. Burgus, R. et al 1970. Characterization of the hypothalamic hypophysiotropic TSH-releasing factor (TRF) of ovine origin. *Nature* 226:321–25
29. Caligaris, L., Astrada, J. J., Taleisnik, S. 1971. Biphasic effect of progesterone on the release of gonadotropin in rats. *Endocrinology* 89:331–37
30. Cargille, C. M., Ross, G. T., Rayford, P. L. 1968. Effect of oral contraceptives on plasma follicle stimulating hormone. *Gonadotropins, 1968,* ed. E. Rosemberg, 355–365. Palo Alto, Calif: Geron-X
31. Cargille, C. M., Ross, G. T., Yoshimi, T. 1969. Daily variations in plasma follicle stimulating hormone, luteinizing hormone and progesterone in the normal menstrual cycle. *J. Clin. Endocrinol.* 29:12–19
32. Celis, M. E., Taleisnik, S., Walter, R. 1971. Regulation of formation and proposed structure of the factor inhibiting the release of melanocyte stimulating hormone. *Proc. Nat. Acad. Sci. USA* 68:1428–33
33. Celis, M. E., Taleisnik, S., Walter, R. 1971. Glycoprotein metabolism: A UDP-galactose:glycoprotein galactosyltransferase of rat serum. *Biochem. Biophys. Res. Commun.* 45:56–62
34. Chen, C. L., Amenomori, Y., Lu, K. H., Voogt, J. L., Meites, J. 1970. Serum prolactin levels in rats with pituitary transplants or hypothalamic lesions. *Neuroendocrinology* 6:220–27
35. Chen, C. L., Meites, J. 1969. Effects of thyroxine and thiouracil on hypothalamic PIF and pituitary prolactin levels. *Proc. Soc. Exp. Biol. Med.* 131:576–78
36. Chen, C. L., Meites, J. 1970. Effects of estrogen and progesterone on serum and pituitary prolactin levels in ovariectomized rats. *Endocrinology* 86:503–5
37. Chen, C. L., Voogt, J. L., Meites, J. 1968. Effect of median eminence implants of FSH, LH or prolactin on luteal function in the rat. *Endocrinology* 83:1273–77
38. Corvol, M. T., Malemud, C. J., Sokoloff, L. 1972. A pituitary

growth-promoting factor for articular chondrocytes in monolayer culture. *Endocrinology* 90: 262–71

39. Dahlstrom, A. 1971. Regional distribution of brain catecholamines and serotonin. *Neurosci. Res. Program, Bull.* 9:197–205

40. Daughaday, W. H., Peake, G. T., Machlin, L. J. 1970. Assay of the growth hormone releasing factor. *Hypophysiotropic Hormones of the Hypothalamus,* ed. J. Meites, 151–170. Baltimore: Williams & Wilkins

41. Davidson, J. M., Weick, R. F., Smith, E. R., Dominguez, R. 1970. Feedback mechanisms in relation to ovulation. *Fed. Proc.* 29:1900–6

42. Dhariwal, A. P. S., Grosvenor, C. E., Antunes-Rodrigues, J., McCann, S. M. 1968. Studies on the purification of ovine prolactin-inhibiting factor. *Endocrinology* 82:1236–41

43. Dierschke, D. J., Bhattacharya, A. N., Atkinson, L. E., Knobil, E. 1970. Circhoral oscillations of plasma LH levels in the ovariectomized rhesus monkey. *Endocrinology* 87:850–53

44. Dunn, J., Critchlow, V. 1971. Vasopressin-evoked ACTH release in rats following forebrain removal. *Proc. Soc. Exp. Biol. Med.* 136:1284–88

45. Everett, J. W. 1954. Luteotrophin function of autografts of the rat hypophysis. *Endocrinology* 54: 685–90

46. Everett, J. W. 1969. Neuroendocrine aspects of mammalian reproduction. *Ann. Rev. Physiol.* 31:383–416

47. Everett, J. W., Radford, H. M. 1961. Irritative deposits from stainless steel electrodes in the preoptic rat brain causing release of pituitary gonadotropins. *Proc. Soc. Exp. Biol. Med.* 108: 604–9

48. Fleischer, N. et al 1972. Synthetic thyrotropin releasing factor as a test of pituitary thyrotropin reserve. *J. Clin. Endocrinol.* 34: 617–24

49. Flouret, G. 1970. Synthesis of pyroglutamyl-histidyl-prolinamide by classical and solid phase methods. *J. Med. Chem.* 13: 843–45

50. Freeman, M. E., Neill, J. D. 1972. The pattern of prolactin secretion during pseudopregnancy in the rat: A daily nocturnal surge. *Endocrinology* 90:1292–94

51. Freeman, M. E., Reichert, L. E., Jr., Neill, J. D. 1972. Regulation of the proestrus surge of prolactin secretion by gonadotropin and estrogens in the rat. *Endocrinology* 90:232–38

52. Frohman, L. A., Maran, J. W., Dhariwal, A. P. S. 1971. Plasma growth hormone responses to intrapituitary injections of growth hormone releasing factor (GRF) in the rat. *Endocrinology* 88:1483–88

53. Gay, V. L., Sheth, N. A., 1972. Evidence for a periodic release of LH in castrated male and female rats. *Endocrinology* 90: 158–62

54. Goebelsmann, U., Midgley, A. R., Jr., Jaffe, R. B. 1969. Regulation of human gonadotropins: VII. Daily individual urinary estrogens, pregnanediol and serum luteinizing and follicle stimulating hormones during the menstrual cycle. *J. Clin. Endocrinol.* 29:1222–30

55. Gillessen, D., Felix, A. M., Lergier, W., Studer, R. O. 1970. Synthese des "'thyrotropin-releasing" Hormons (TRF) (Schaf) und verwandter Peptide. *Helv. Chim. Acta* 53:63–72

56. Giordano, N. D., Sayers, G. 1971. Isolated adrenal cells: Assay of ACTH in rat serum. *Proc. Soc. Exp. Biol. Med.* 136:623–26

57. Grant, G., Vale, W., Guillemin, R. 1971. Interaction of thyrotropin releasing factor with membrane receptors of pituitary cells. *Biochem. Biophys. Res. Commun.* 46:28–34

58. Gual, C., Kastin, A., Schally, A. V. 1972. Clinical studies with hypothalamic hormones. *Recent. Progr. Horm. Res.* 28:173–227

59. Guillemin, R. 1964. Hypothalamic factors releasing pituitary hormones. *Recent Progr. Horm. Res.* 20:89–130

60. Guillemin, R. 1971. Hypothalamic control of the secretion of adenohypophysial hormones. *Advan. Metab. Disord.* 5:1–51

61. Guillemin, R. 1971. Biosynthesis of the hypothalamic tripeptide-amide, TRF. Abstr. Soc. Neurosci. Meet., Washington, D.C., October 1971

62. Haigler, E. D., Jr., Pittman, J. A., Jr., Hershman, J. M., Baugh, C. M. 1971. Direct evaluation of pituitary thyrotropin reserve utilizing synthetic thyrotropin releasing hormone. J. Clin. Endocrinol. 33:573–81

63. Halász, B., Schalch, D. S., Gorski, R. A. 1971. Growth hormone secretion in young rats after partial or total interruption of neural afferents to the medial basal hypothalamus. Endocrinoloy 89:198–203

64. Haun, C. K., Sawyer, C. H. 1960. Initiation of lactation in rabbits following placement of hypothalamic lesions. Endocrinology 67:270–72

65. Hedge, G. A., de Wied, D. 1971. Corticotropin and vasopressin secretion after hypothalamic implantation of atropine. Endocrinology 88:1257–59

66. Hilliard, J., Schally, A. V., Sawyer, C. H. 1971. Progesterone blockade of the ovulatory response to intrapituitary infusion of LH-RH in rabbits. Endocrinology 88:730–36

67. Hollander, C. S., Mitsuma, T., Shenkman, L., Woolf, P., Gershengorn, M. C. 1972. Thyrotropin-releasing hormone: Evidence for thyroid response to intravenous injection in man. Science 175:209–10

68. Howard, N., Martin, J. M. 1971. A stimulatory test for growth hormone release in the rat. Endocrinology 88:497–99

69. Irie, M., Tsushima, T. 1972. Increase of serum growth hormone concentrations following thyrotropin-releasing hormone injections in patients with acromegaly or gigantism. J. Clin. Endocrinol. 35:97–100

70. Jacobs, L. S., Snyder, P. J., Wilber, J. F., Utiger, R. D., Daughaday, W. H. 1971. Increased serum prolactin after administration of synthetic thyrotropin releasing hormone (TRH) in man. J. Clin. Endocrinol. 33: 996–98

71. Kaplan, S. L., Grumbach, M. M.,

Friesen, H. G., Costom, B. H. 1972. Thyrotropin releasing factor (TRF) effect on secretion of human pituitary prolactin and thyrotropin in children and in idiopathic hypopituitary dwarfism: further evidence for hypophysiotropic hormone deficiencies. J. Clin. Endocrinol. 35: In press

72. Kamberi, I. A., Mical, R. S., Porter, J. C. 1971. Effect of anterior pituitary perfusion and intraventricular injection of catecholamines on prolactin release. Endocrinology 88:1012–20

73. Kamberi, I. A., Mical, R. S., Porter, J. C. 1971. Pituitary portal vessel infusion of hypothalamic extract and release of LH, FSH, and prolactin. Endocrinology 88:1294–99

74. Kamberi, I. A., Mical, R. S., Porter, J. C. 1971. Hypophysial portal vessel infusion: In vivo demonstration of LRF, FRF and PIF in pituitary stalk plasma. Endocrinology 89: 1042–1046

75. Kastin, A. J., Schally, A. V., Viosca, S. 1971. Inhibition of MSH release in frogs by direct application of L-prolyl-L-leucyl-glycinamide to the pituitary. Proc. Soc. Exp. Biol. Med. 137: 1437–39

76. Kastin, A. J., Schally, A. V., Gual, C., Arimura, A. 1972. Release of LH and FSH after administration of synthetic LH-releasing hormone. J. Clin. Endocrinol. 34:753–56

77. Kastin, A. J., Nair, R. M. G., Viosca, S. 1972. Hypothalamic-pineal-pituitary interactions. Progr. Endocrinol., Proc. Int. Congr. Endocrinol., 4th, Washington, D.C., June 1972 Abstr. No. 574, p. 229 ICS No. 256

78. Kastin, A. J., Viosca, S., Schally, A. V. 1970. Assay of mammalian MSH release regulating factor(s). In Hypophysiotropic Hormones of the Hypothalamus, ed. J. Meites, 171–84. Baltimore: Williams & Wilkins

79. Kendall, J. W., Jacobs, J. J., Kramer, R. M. 1972. Studies on the transport of hormones from the cerebrospinal fluid to hypothalamus and pituitary. Brain-Endocrine Interaction. Median

Eminence: Structure and Function, ed. K. M. Knigge, D. E. Scott, A. Weindl, 342–349. Basel, Switzerland-Karger

80. Kendall, J. W., Rees, L. H., Kramer, R. 1971. Thyrotropin releasing hormone (TRH) stimulation of thyroidal radioiodine release in the rat: Comparison between intravenous and intraventricular administration. *Endocrinology* 88: 1503–6

81. Kleinberg, D. L., Noel, G. L., Frantz, A. G. 1971. Chlorpromazine stimulation and L-dopa suppression of plasma prolactin in man. *J. Clin. Endocrinol.* 33:873–76

82. Knigge, K. M., Joseph, S. A. 1971. Neural regulation of TSH secretion: Sites of thyroxine feedback. *Neuroendocrinology* 8:273–88

83. Knigge, K. M., Silverman, A. J. 1972. Transport capacity of the median eminence. In *Brain-Endocrine Interaction Median Eminence: Structure and Function,* ed. K. M. Knigge, D. E. Scott, A. Weindl, 350–363. Basel, Switzerland: Karger

84. Knobil, E., Meyer, V., Schally, A. V. 1968. Hypothalamic extracts and the secretion of growth hormone in the rhesus monkey. *Growth Hormone,* ed. A. Pecile, E. Muller, 226–237. Milan, Italy: Excerpta Medica Foundation. ICS No. 158

85. Koch, Y., Lu, K. H., Meites, J. 1970. Biphasic effects of catecholamines in pituitary prolactin release *in vitro. Endocrinology* 87:673–75

86. Kokka, N., Garcia, J. F., Morgan, M., George, R. 1971. Immunoassay of plasma growth hormone in cats following fasting and administration of insulin, arginine, 2-deoxyglucose and hypothalamic extract. *Endocrinology* 88:359–66

87. Krieger, D. T., Glick, S. 1971. Absent sleep peak of growth hormone release in blind subjects: Correlation with sleep EEG stages. *J. Clin. Endocrinol.* 33:847–50

88. LaBella, F. S., Vivian, S. R. 1971. Effect of synthetic TRF on hormone release from bovine anterior pituitary *in vitro. Endocrinology* 88:787–89

89. Labrie, F., Barden, N., Poirier, G., De Lean, A. 1972. Binding of thyrotropin-releasing hormone to plasma membranes of bovine anterior pituitary gland. *Proc. Nat. Acad. Sci. USA* 69: 283–87

90. Lu, K.-H., Amenomori, Y., Chen, C. L., Meites, J. 1970. Effects of central acting drugs on serum and pituitary prolactin levels in rats. *Endocrinology* 87:667–72

91. Lu, K.-H., Koch, Y., Meites, J. 1971. Direct inhibition by ergocornine of pituitary prolactin release. *Endocrinology* 89:229–33

92. Lu, K.-H., Meites, J. 1971. Inhibition by L-dopa and monoamine oxidase inhibitors of pituitary prolactin release; stimulation of methyl-dopa and *d*-amphetamine. *Proc. Soc. Exp. Biol. Med.* 137:480–83

93. MacLeod, R. M. 1969. Influence of norepinephrine and catecholamine-depleting agents on the synthesis and release of prolactin and growth hormone. *Endocrinology* 85:916–23

94. MacLeod, R. M., Fontham, E. H. 1970. Influence of ionic environment on the *in vitro* synthesis and release of pituitary hormones. *Endocrinology* 86:863–69

95. MacLeod, R. M., Fontham, E. H., Lehmeyer, J. E. 1960. Prolactin and growth hormone production as influenced by catecholamines and agents that affect brain catecholamines. *Neuroendocrinology* 6:283–94

96. Martin, J. B., Reichlin, S. 1970. Thyrotropin secretion in rats after hypothalamic electrical stimulation or injection of synthetic TSH-releasing factor. *Science* 168:1366–68

97. Matsuo, H., Arimura, A., Nair, R. M. G., Schally, A. V. 1971. Synthesis of the porcine LH- and FSH-releasing hormone by the solid-phase method. *Biochem. Biophys. Res. Commun.* 45:822–27

98. Matsuo, H., Baba, Y., Nair, R. M. G., Arimura, A., Schally, A. V. 1971. Structure of the porcine LH- and FSH-releasing hor-

mone. I. The proposed amino acid sequence. *Biochem. Biophys. Res. Commun.* 43:1334–39

99. Midgley, A. R., Jr., Jaffe, R. B. 1971. Regulation of human gonadotropins: X. Episodic fluctuation of LH during the menstrual cycle. *J. Clin. Endocrinol.* 33:962–69

100. Mitnick, M. A., Reichlin, S. 1971. Thyrotropin-releasing hormone: Biosynthesis by rat hypothalamic fragments *in vitro. Science* 172:1241–43

101. Monahan, M. et al 1971. Synthèse totale par phase solide d'un décapeptide qui stimule la sécrétion des gonadotropines hypophysaires LH et FSH. *Compt. Rend. Acad. Sci.* 273:508–10

102. Mowles, T. F., Ashkanazy, B., Mix, E., Jr., Sheppard, H. 1971. Hypothalamic and hypophyseal estradiol-binding complexes. *Endocrinology* 89:484–91

103. Muller, E. E., Schally, A. V., Cocchi, D. 1971. Increase in plasma growth hormone (GH)-like activity after administration of porcine GH-releasing hormone. *Proc. Soc. Exp. Biol. Med.* 137:489–94

104. Nair, R. M. G., Barrett, J., Bowers, C. Y., Schally, A. V. 1970. Structure of porcine thyrotropin releasing hormone. *Biochemistry* 9:1103–6

105. Nair, R. M. G., Kastin, A. J., Schally, A. V. 1971. Isolation and structure of hypothalamic MSH release-inhibiting hormone. *Biochem. Biophys. Res. Commun.* 43:1376–81

106. Nakane, P. K. 1970. Classification of anterior pituitary cell types with immunoenzyme histochemistry. *J. Histochem. Cytochem.* 18:9–20

107. Nankin, H. R., Troen, P. 1971. Repetitive luteinizing hormone elevations in serum of normal men. *J. Clin. Endocrinol.* 33:558–60

108. Neill, J. D. 1970. Effect of "stress" on serum prolactin and luteinizing hormone levels during the estrous cycle of the rat. *Endocrinology* 87:1192–97

109. Neill, J. D. 1972. Comparison of plasma prolactin levels in cannulated and decapitated rats.

Endocrinology 90:568–72

110. Neill, J. D., Freeman, M. E., Tillson, S. A. 1971. Control of the proestrus surge of prolactin and luteinizing hormone secretion by estrogens in the rat. *Endocrinology* 89:1448–53

111. Nicoll, C. S., Fiorindo, R. P., McKennee, C. T., Parsons, J. A. 1970. Assay of hypothalamic factors which regulate prolactin secretion. In *Hypophysiotropic Hormones of the Hypothalamus,* ed. J. Meites, 115–50. Baltimore: Williams & Wilkins

112. Ochi, Y., Shiomi, K., Hachiya, T., Yoshimura, M., Miyazaki, T. 1972. Failure of TRH (thyrotropin-releasing hormone) to stimulate thyroid function in the chick. *Endocrinology* 91:832–34

113. Ondo, J. G., Kitay, J. I. 1972. Pituitary-adrenal function in rats with diencephalic islands. *Neuroendocrinology* 9:72–82

114. Parsons, J. A., Nicoll, C. S. 1971. Mechanism of action of prolactin-inhibiting factor. *Neuroendocrinology* 8:213–27

115. Phifer, R., Midgley, A. R., Jr., Spicer, S. 1972. Histology of the human hypophyseal gonadotropin secreting cells. *Gonadotropins,* ed. B. B. Saxena, C. G. Beling, H. M. Gandy, 9–25. New York: Wiley-Interscience

116. Porter, J. C., Vale, W., Burgus, R., Mical, R. S., Guillemin, R. 1971. Release of TSH by TRF infused directly into a pituitary stalk portal vessel. *Endocrinology* 89:1054–56

117. Raud, H. R., Kiddy, C. A., Odell, W. D. 1971. The effect of stress upon the determination of serum prolactin by radioimmunoassay. *Proc. Soc. Exp. Biol. Med.* 136:689–93

118. Raud, H. R., Odell, W. D. 1971. Studies of the measurement of bovine and porcine prolactin by radioimmunoassay and by systemic pigeon crop-sac bioassay. *Endocrinology* 88:991–1002

119. Reeves, J. J., Arimura, A., Schally, A. V. 1970. Serum levels of prolactin and luteinizing hormone (LH) in the ewe at various stages of the estrous cycle. *Proc. Soc. Exp. Biol. Med.* 134:938–42

120. Redding, T. W., Schally, A. V. 1969. Studies on the inactivation of thyrotropin-releasing hormone (TRH). *Proc. Soc. Exp. Biol. Med.* 131:415–20

121. Redding, T. W., Schally, A. V. 1969. Studies on the thyrotropin-releasing hormone (TRF) activity in peripheral blood. *Proc. Soc. Exp. Biol. Med.* 131: 420–25

122. Rodger, N., Beck, J., Burgus, R., Guillemin, R., 1969. Variability of response in the bioassay for a hypothalamic somatotrophin releasing factor based on rat pituitary growth hormone content. *Endocrinology* 84:1373–83

123. Roth, J. C., Kelch, R. P., Kaplan, S. L., Grumbach, M. M. 1972. FSH and LH response to luteinizing hormone-releasing factor in prepubertal and pubertal children, adult males and in patients with hypogonadotropic and hypergonadotropic hypogonadism. *J. Clin. Endocr.* 35: In press

124. Rothchild, I. 1965. Interrelations between progesterone and the ovary, pituitary, and central nervous system in the control of ovulation and the regulation of progesterone secretion. *Vitam. Horm. New York* 23:209–21

125. Rubin, R. T., Kales, A., Adler, R., Fagan, T., Odell, W. 1971. Gonadotropin secretion during sleep in normal adult men. *Science*, 175:196–98

126. Saxena, B. B., Gandy, H. M., Peterson, R. E. 1968. Radioimmunoassay of FSH and LH in body fluids. In *Gonadotropins 1968*, ed. E. Rosemberg, 340–48. Palo Alto, Calif: Geron-X

127. Sayers, G., Ma, R.-M., Giordano, N. D. 1971. Isolated adrenal cells: Corticosterone production in response to cyclic AMP (adenosine-3′,5′-monophosphate). *Proc. Soc. Exp. Biol. Med.* 136: 619–22

128. Scapagnini, U., Moberg, G. P., Van Loon, G. R., De Groot, J., Ganong, W. F. 1971. Relation of brain 5-hydroxytryptamine content to the diurnal variation in plasma corticosterone in the rat. *Neuroendocrinology* 7:90–96

129. Schally, A. V. et al 1971. Isolation and properties of the FSH- and LH-releasing hormone. *Biochem. Biophys. Res. Commun.* 43:393–99

130. Schally, A. V., Arimura, A., Bowers, C. Y., Kastin, A., Sawano, S., Redding T. W. 1968. Hypothalamic neurohormones regulating anterior pituitary function. *Rec. Progr. in Horm. Res.*, 24:497–588

131. Schally, A. V. et al 1971. Gonadotropin-releasing hormone: One polypeptide regulates secretion of luteinizing and follicle-stimulating hormones. *Science* 173: 1036–38

131a. Schally, A. V., Baba, Y., Nair, R. M. G., Bennett, C. 1971. The amino acid sequence of a peptide with growth hormone-releasing activity isolated from porcine hypothalamus. *J. Biol. Chem.* 246:6647–50

132. Schally, A. V. et al 1969. Isolation of growth hormone-releasing hormone (GRH) from porcine hypothalami. *Endocrinology* 84:1493–1506

133. Seiden, G., Brodish, A. 1971. Improved parameters of pituitary incubation for the assay of corticotrophin-releasing factor. *Neuroendocrinology* 8:145–53

134. Shaar, C. J., Clemens, J. A. 1972. Inhibition of lactation and prolactin secretion in rats by ergot alkaloids. *Endocrinology* 90: 285–88

135. Silverman, A. J., Knigge, K. M. 1972. Transport capacity of median eminence thyroxine transport. *Neuroendocrinology* 10:71–82

136. Smith, G. P., Root, A. W. 1971. Dissociation of changes in growth hormone and adrenocortical hormone levels during brain stimulation of monkeys. *Neuroendocrinology* 8:235–44

137. Snyder, P. J., Utiger, R. D. 1972. Response to thyrotropin releasing hormone (TRH) in normal man. *J. Clin. Endocrinol.* 34: 380–85

138. Sorrentino, S., Jr., Reiter, R. J., Schalch, D. S. 1971. Pineal regulation of growth hormone synthesis and release in blinded and blinded-anosmic male rats. *Neuroendocrinology* 7:210–18

139. Spies, H. G., Clegg, M. T. 1971.

Pituitary as a possible site of prolactin feedback in autoregulation. *Neuroendocrinology* 8: 205–12

140. Spies, H. G., Niswender, G. D. 1971. Blockade of the surge of preovulatory serum luteinizing hormone and ovulation with exogenous progesterone in cycling rhesus (*Macaca mulatta*) monkeys. *J. Clin. Endocrinol.* 32: 309–16

141. Stevens, V. C. 1969. Comparison of FSH and LH patterns in plasma, urine and urinary extracts during the menstrual cycle. *J. Clin. Endocrinol.* 29: 904–10

142. Stumpf, W. E., Sar, M. 1971. Estradiol concentrating neurons in the amygdala. *Proc. Soc. Exp. Biol. Med.* 136:102–6

143. Swerdloff, R. S., Odell, W. D. 1969. Serum luteinizing and follicle stimulating hormone levels during sequential and nonsequential contraceptive treatment of eugonadal women. *J. Clin. Endocrinol.* 29:157–63

144. Takahashi, K., Daughaday, W. H., Kipnis, D. M. 1971. Regulation of immunoreactive growth hormone secretion in male rats. *Endocrinology* 88:909–17

145. Taleisnik, S., Orias, R. 1965. A melanocyte-stimulating hormone-releasing factor in hypothalamic extracts. *Am. J. Physiol.* 208:293–96

146. Talwalker, P. K., Ratner, A., Meites, J. 1963. *In vitro* inhibition of pituitary prolactin synthesis and release by hypothalamic extract. *Am. J. Physiol.* 205:213–18

147. Tashjian, A. H., Jr., Barowsky, N. J., Jensen, D. K. 1971. Thyrotropin releasing hormone: Direct evidence for stimulation of prolactin production by pituitary cells in culture. *Biochem. Biophys. Res. Commun.* 43: 516–23

148. Tsai, C. C., Yen, S. S. C. 1971. Acute effects of intravenous infusion of 17β-estradiol on gonadotropin release in pre- and post-menopausal women. *J. Clin. Endocrinol.* 32:766–71

149. Tsai, C. C., Yen, S. S. C. 1971. The effect of ethinyl estradiol administration during early follicular phase of the cycle on the gonadotropin levels and ovarian function. *J. Clin. Endocrinol.* 33:917–23

150. Turkington, R. W. 1972. Inhibition of prolactin secretion and successful therapy of the Forbes-Albright syndrome with L-dopa. *J. Clin. Endocrinol.* 34: 306–11

151. Vale, W., Burgus, R., Dunn, T. F., Guillemin, R. 1970. Release of TSH by oral administration of synthetic peptide derivatives with TRF activity. *J. Clin. Endocrinol.* 30:148–50

151a. Vale, W., Blackwell, R., Grant, G., Guillemin, R. 1972. TRF and thyroid hormones on prolactin secretion by rat anterior pituitary cells *in vitro*. *Endocrinology*. In press

152. Vale, W. et al 1972. Synthetic polypeptide antagonists of the hypothalamic luteinizing hormone releasing factor. *Science* 176: 933–42

153. Vale, W. W., Burgus, R., Dunn, T. F., Guillemin, R. 1971. *In vitro* plasma inactivation of thyrotropin releasing factor (TRF) and related peptides. Its inhibition by various means and by the synthetic dipeptide PCA-His-OME. *Hormones* 2:193–203

154. Vale, W., Grant, G., Amoss, M., Blackwell, R., Guillemin, R. 1972. Culture of enzymatically dispersed anterior pituitary cells: Functional validation of a method. *Endocrinology* 91: 562–72

155. Vale, W., Grant, G., Guillemin, R. 1973. Chemistry of the hypothalamic releasing factors— studies on structure-function relationships in TRF and LRF. *Frontiers in Neuroendocrinology, 1973*, ed. F. Ganong, L. Martini, New York: Oxford Univ. Press. In press

156. Vale, W., Rivier, J., Burgus, R. 1971. Synthetic TRF (thyrotropin releasing factor) analogues: II. pGlu-$N^{3 \text{im}}$Me-His-Pro-NH$_2$: A synthetic analogue with specific activity greater than that of TRF. *Endocrinology* 89:1485–88

157. Valverde, C., Chieffo, V. 1971. Prolactin releasing factor(s) in

porcine hypothalamic extracts. *Meet. Endocrin Soc. San Francisco, Calif.* No. 83. Philadelphia: Lippincott

158. Veber, D. F. et al 1971. Synthesis of a proposed growth hormone releasing factor. *Biochem. Biophys. Res. Commun.* 45:235–39

159. Voogt, J. L., Meites, J. 1971. Effects of an implant of prolactin in median eminence of pseudopregnant rats on serum and pituitary LH, FSH and prolactin. *Endocrinology* 88:286–92

160. Walker, M. D., Henkin, R. I., Harlan, A. B., Casper, A. G. T. 1971. Distribution of tritiated cortisol in blood, brain, CSF and other tissues of the cat. *Endocrinology* 88:224–32

161. Weick, R. F., Smith, E. R., Dominguez, R., Dhariwal, A. P. S., Davidson, J. M. 1971. Mechanism of stimulatory feedback effect of estradiol benzoate on the pituitary. *Endocrinology* 88:293–301

162. Weitzman, E. D. et al 1971. Twenty-four hour pattern of the episodic secretion of cortisol in normal subjects. *J. Clin. Endocrinol.* 33:14–22

163. Welsch, C. W., Squiers, M. D., Cassell, E., Chen, C. L., Meites, J. 1971. Median eminence lesions and serum prolactin: Influence of ovariectomy and ergocornine. *Am. J. Physiol.* 221:1714–17

164. White, W. F. 1970. Discussion of the Present Status of the Chemistry of PIF, FRF, and LRF. In *Hypophysiotropic Hormones of the Hypothalamus,* ed. J. Meites, 248–50. Baltimore: Williams & Wilkins

165. Wilber, J. F., Nagel, T., White, W. F. 1971. Hypothalamic growth hormone-releasing activity (GRA): Characterization by the *in vitro* rat pituitary and radioimmunoassay. *Endocrinology* 89:1419–24

166. Witorsch, R. J., Brodish, A. 1972.

Conditions for the reliable use of lesioned rats for the assay of CRF in tissue extracts. *Endocrinology* 90:552–57

167. Wuttke, W., Cassell, E., Meites, J. 1971. Effects of ergocornine on serum prolactin and LH, and on hypothalamic content of PIF and LRF. *Endocrinology* 88:737–41

168. Yamaji, T., Dierschke, D. J., Bhattacharya, A. N., Knobil, E. 1972. The negative feedback control by estradiol and progesterone of LH secretion in the ovariectomized rhesus monkey. *Endocrinology* 90:771–77

169. Yates, F. E. et al 1971. Potentiation by vasopressin of corticotropin release induced by corticotropin-releasing factor. *Endocrinology* 88:3–15

170. Yates, F. E., Russell, S. M., Maran, J. W. 1971. Brain-adenohypophysial communications in mammals. *Ann. Rev. Physiol.* 33:393–444

171. Yen, S. S. C. et al 1972. Synthetic luteinizing hormone-releasing factor: A potent stimulator of gonadotropin release in man. *J. Clin. Endocrinol.* 34:1108–11

172. Yen, S. S. C. et al 1972 Clinical studies with synthetic LRF. *Serono Conf., Acapulco, Mexico, June 1972*

173. Ying, S.-Y., Fang, V. S., Greep, R. O. 1971. Estradiol benzoate (EB)-induced changes in serum-luteinizing hormone (LH) and follicle-stimulating hormone (FSH) in immature female rats. *Fert. Steril.* 22:799–801

174. Yen, S. S. C., Tsai, C. C. 1971. The biphasic pattern in the feedback action of ethinyl estradiol on the release of pituitary FSH and LH. *J. Clin. Endocrinol.* 33:882–87

175. York, D. H., Baker, F. L., Kraicer, J. 1971. Electrical properties of cells in the adenohypophysis—an *in vivo* study. *Neuroendocrinology* 8:10–16

Ann. Rev. Physiol. 1973. 35:391–430

NEUROENDOCRINE ASPECTS OF THERMOREGULATION[1]

1101

C. C. GALE

*Regional Primate Research Center and Department of
Physiology and Biophysics
University of Washington, Seattle*

In the past five years, two excellent reviews of temperature regulation have appeared in these pages. In 1968, Hammel (44) comprehensively surveyed the control of internal body temperature, emphasing the quantitative data that led to his theoretical formulation of the hypothalamic controlling mechanism. In 1971, Chaffee & Roberts (21) thoroughly reviewed the experimental data since 1965 for acclimation to heat and cold in mammals and birds. The present survey focuses on an area of thermoregulation not emphasized previously, namely, the integration by the central nervous system of physical and chemical mechanisms of heat gain and loss. Special attention will be given to the role of the hypothalamus in synchronizing the outflow of the autonomic nervous system, particularly the sympathico-adrenomedullary system, with the conventional endocrine system comprised of the pituitary gland and its target glands, as well as the endocrine pancreas. For the reader with a more general interest in the regulation of body temperature, the published proceedings of recent international symposia provide a survey of current work: *Physiological and Behavioral Thermoregulation,* edited by Hardy, Gagge, and Stolwijk (47); *Thermorégulation Comportementale,* edited by Cabanac (16); and *Hibernation and Hypothermia,* edited by South, Hannon, Willis, Pengelley, and Alpert (102). The invited lectures at the International Symposium on Bioenergetics and Temperature Regulation, Dublin, 1971, appear in *Essays on Temperature Regulation,* edited by Bligh and Moore (12), and in *Bioenergetics,* edited by Smith, Hannon, Shields, and Horwitz (100). The short communications at the Dublin symposium have been published (109). Also the proceedings of the symposium on *Nonshivering Thermogenesis* in Prague, edited by Janský (60), have appeared, as has the symposium on *Pharmacology of Thermoregulation,* edited by Lomax and Schönbaum

[1] Preparation of this review was supported in part by NIH grants NS 06622 and RR 00166.

391

(73). Finally, Whittow has edited a three volume text with contributions from many authors on the *Comparative Physiology of Thermoregulation* (114, 115).

HISTORICAL RÉSUMÉ

In mammals the regulation of a relatively constant body temperature over a wide range of environmental conditions demands a complex interplay among all heat gain and heat loss mechanisms. Mechanisms in the defense against cold include (a) heat produced by muscular shivering, exercise, or other exothermic biochemical reactions which elevate basal metabolic rate and (b) heat conserved by cutaneous vasoconstriction or by growth of hair or fur leading to increase in peripheral insulation. Defense mechanisms against heat include (a) increase in heat loss by sweating, panting, or salivation, as well as by a rise in extracellular fluid volume and in cutaneous blood flow, with attendant increase in peripheral thermal conductance; and (b) lowering of metabolic heat production. In addition to these physiologic and metabolic adjustments, it, is now generally recognized that behavioral thermoregulation is of equal or greater importance in defense against heat and cold in most mammals, especially in man (16, 47).

Early investigators of temperature and metabolism attempted to simplify the complexities of mammalian homeothermy by sorting out and classifying thermoregulatory mechanisms. Thus, in 1902 Rubner (94a) proposed chemical thermogenesis as separable from physical thermogenesis. Physical thermogenesis was exemplified by such visible processes of heat production as muscular exercise or shivering, whereas chemical thermogenesis referred to the then little understood exothermic chemical reactions elevating the resting metabolic rate. Similarly, sweating and panting were considered physical mechanisms of heat loss, whereas reduction in metabolic rate was considered a manifestation of chemical thermosuppression. A prominent role for the endocrine system in chemical thermoregulation was suggested a priori by the action of thyroxine in modifying the metabolic rate of body tissues. The pathological hypermetabolism of Graves' disease and the hypometabolism of myxedema had been recognized by Magnus-Levy in 1895 (75a) as resulting respectively from over- and under-protection of thyroid hormone. The apparent validity of a functional dichotomy between physical and chemical thermoregulation served to advance a corollary belief that physical thermoregulation was controlled by neural outflow from the CNS (as in shivering), whereas chemical thermoregulation was controlled separately by hormones of the conventional (pituitary-target gland) endocrine system (as for thyroxine).

In 1927, Cannon reported (17a) that cats intubated with ice water released epinephrine from the adrenal medulla into the circulation; this resulted in a sustained rise in nonshivering (hence, chemical) as well as in shivering thermogenesis. Cannon's classic study served to establish chemical thermogenesis in control of body temperature but also showed that the CNS could mediate both physical and chemical thermogenesis. The sympathicoadreno-medullary (SAM) system was thus perhaps the first neuroendocrine system to be described; it is unique in that central integrative centers in the hypothalamus and brain stem regulate in common (a) a widely distributed network of noradrenergic terminals concerned with metabolic and vascular homeostasis, and (b) motor supply to the adrenal medulla for release of epinephrine into the circulation. More recently elucidated neuroendocrine systems are: hypothalamus–adenohypophysis; neurohypophysis–renal tubules; sympathicoadrenomedullary–renal juxtaglomerular apparatus; and autonomic nervous system–endocrine pancreas.

All neuroendocrine systems function importantly in thermal homeostasis, serving to mesh the great sensory and integrative capability of the CNS with endocrine motor outflow. Perhaps the first conclusive indication of the essential role of the CNS in controlling both physical and chemical thermoregulation stemmed from studies showing that laboratory rats placed chronically in the cold, 5°C ambient temperature (T_a), maintain body temperature initially by continuous shivering, but after several weeks by converting to nonshivering thermogenesis (21). Both the shivering and the nonshivering aspects of this biphasic mode of cold acclimation were shown by Leduc (71) and LeBlanc & Nadeau (69) to depend on a marked rise in catecholamine secretion, primarily of norepinephrine (NE) from adrenergic terminals but also epinephrine (E) from the adrenal medulla.

Presently, it is believed that during the shivering phase of calorigenesis the catecholamines act (a) on the cardiovascular system to increase cardiac output, to readjust organ blood flow (60a), and to mediate cutaneous vasoconstriction (83); (b) on adipose tissue to mobilize lipid substrate (54); and (c) to facilitate muscular shivering (3, 106). The conversion from shivering to nonshivering thermogenesis occurs by virtue of greatly enhanced tissue sensitivity to the calorigenic action of NE, particularly in brown adipose tissue (9, 14, 20, 21, 54, 70) and also in skeletal muscle (54, 68, 106). Cutaneous vasculature also becomes sensitized to catecholamines (70, 74, 83). Tissue sensitization to catecholamines enables acclimated rats to maintain body temperature in the cold when skeletal muscle movement is abolished by curarization but not when sympathetic nerve transmission is prevented by ganglionic blockade (19). Administration of exogenous catecholamines, especially of NE, to curarized, ganglionically-blocked, cold-acclimated rats restores thermogenesis, and body temperature is maintained in the cold (19). The marked calorigenic response to exogenously administered NE is at present the standard provocative test for acclimation to cold, including man (65, 66) and infrahuman primates (20).

At the time of these cold acclimation studies it was further recognized that thyroxine (T_4) exerted an important synergistic effect on the calorigenic action of catecholamines (19), and that adrenocorticoids were essential in the acclimation to cold (37). Collectively, the experimental evidence then available strongly suggested that hypothalamic integration of the conventional en-

docrine system with the SAM system and with the somatic system was fundamental to the thermoregulatory response to cold, and presumably the response to heat by a converse action. In the early 1960's Smith and co-workers showed that NE markedly stimulated thermogenesis in brown adipose tissue which, because of its strategic location in the interscapular, axillary, and
perirenal regions, was proposed to function as a heat generator for the spinal
cord, heart, lungs (21). Brown adipose tissue has been shown to function by
virtue of its calorigenic responsiveness to NE in (a) development and maintenance of nonshivering thermogenesis in rodents, ground squirrels, and hedgehogs (21); (b) arousal from hibernation (100, 102); and (c) nonshivering
heat production in newly born mammals, including man (21). Currently much
interest is focused on the possibility that adult, nonhibernating mammals,
particularly man (65, 66) and infrahuman primates (20, 31, 38), may regain
nonshivering thermogenesis, presumed dormant since infancy, as a form of
cold acclimation. But at present the role of brown adipose tissue in mediating
nonshivering thermogenesis in large mammals and man is little understood
(3, 14, 20, 21, 60, 66, 112).

Before proceeding with the review of current literature, it is important to
correct some misconceptions possibly remaining from Rubner's original pos-
tulation. We now recognize that all thermogenic mechanisms involve ultimately the hydrolysis of intracellular high energy phosphate bonds leading to
electron transport, oxidation of substrate, and reduction of molecular oxygen
(103). At the cellular level, then, the Rubnerian distinction between physical
and chemical thermogenesis is invalid; basically the same exothermic process
occurs in shivering muscle as in adipose tissue or liver (5, 21, 54, 103). We
recognize, however, the selective capacity for certain tissues to "loosen" or
"uncouple" oxidation from phosphorylation as an important thermogenic
mechanism in cold acclimation (5, 15, 17, 54). Similarly, the corollary concept of neural vs hormonal control of body temperature is now viewed as
inappropriate inasmuch as all endocrine systems concerned with body temperature are under central nervous control. Thus, by virtue of the powerful
sensory and integrative capability of the CNS, endocrine thermoregulatory
events are synchronized with autonomic, somatic, and behavioral activity.
One exception to this generalization may be maintenance of calcium homeostasis by cells in the parathyroid gland which secrete parathormone and in
the thyroid gland which secrete calcitonin. However, this phylogenetically
primitive endocrine system has not been implicated directly in thermoregulation.

Finally, all neurons of the central and autonomic nervous systems trans-
duce their electrical signal at the nerve terminal in the form of chemical
transmitters, which then act on specific receptors. The traditional anatomic
basis for distinguishing neural from hormonal effector systems has been the
nature of the media and the distance through which transmitters are con-
veyed in the extracellular space, e.g., over a short span in the neural synaptic
cleft, over a longer distance in the circulation. The important functional dis-

tinction between neural and hormonal effectors is the more rapid and ana-tomically discrete response to neural innervation and the slower, more general, and sustained response to hormonal innervation. Thus, our present knowledge of the physiologic role of parallel neuroendocrine systems, serving to link the great integrative capacity of the CNS to endocrine motor outflow, provides a new perspective for understanding the synchronization of hormonal, autonomic, and somatic effectors in thermoregulation.

MAMMALIAN THERMOREGULATORY SYSTEM

The temperature regulating system consists of two major functional divisions: (*a*) a quick reacting system, characterized as a neural net, with time constants of seconds or minutes, and (*b*) a slow-reacting neuroendocrine system with time constants of minutes or hours (19a). The two systems have important interactions, both centrally and peripherally, in subserving thermoregulation. In the neural net, skin receptors for warmth and "coolth" [terminology of D. Mitchell (12)] project by sensory fibers in the lateral spinal thalamic tract to synaptic relays in the reticular system of the medulla, and thence to the posterolateral ventromedial nuclei of the thalamus. Projection to cortical areas presumably mediates conscious thermal sensations. Thermal receptors exist also in the spinal cord (44, 61, 62, 97), veins (44), and the abdominal viscera (1, 44, 90). Both surface and deep body receptors are presumed to connect functionally with the preoptic anterior and posterior hypothalamus thermoregulating centers (12, 44, 47). Although specific pathways have not been identified, the ascending noradrenergic tracts connecting the brain stem with the hypothalamus, recently identified by histofluorescent techniques, may transmit the thermal sensory input (110).

In Hammel's schema (12, 44, 47, 73) the preoptic anterior hypothalamic controller possesses the unique capability of (*a*) measuring its own temperature, (*b*) generating a constant reference signal, (*c*) integrating all thermal and nonthermal inputs to adjust a virtual (optimal) set temperature, and (*d*) mobilizing physical, chemical, and behavioral thermoregulatory responses in proportion to the error signal between reference and virtual set temperature. The limitations of attributing all thermoregulatory responses to one input signal derived from a hypothetical reference temperature have been emphasized (12, 13, 101); it has been pointed out that a constant reference temperature is an abstraction, since internal temperature fluctuates in a circadian rhythm (81). The temperature controller in the hypothalamus of mammals receives many parallel negative feedback signals, e.g., thermal, chemical, and likely osmotic (101), and barostatic (22, 81), which are extremely difficult to quantitate separately by conventional open-loop techniques.

Bligh & Moore have recently edited a series of essays representing current views of leading investigators on central control of thermoregulation (12). Seven thermoregulatory effector pathways stem from the hypothalamic controller (19a). Neurons from the posterior hypothalamus convey sympathetic nervous outflow which controls (*a*) blood flow, primarily in the skin, (*b*) sweat gland activity via cholinergic innervation, (c) calorigenesis (nonshivering thermogenesis) in the cells of white and brown adipose tissue and probably in muscle, and (d) secretion of E and NE from the adrenal medulla into the circulation; somatic motor outflow from the septal area and the posterior hypothalamus controls shivering which, in turn, may be potentiated by catecholamines (3, 68, 106). The proximity of the primary motor shivering center in the posterior hypothalamus to the SAM motor outflow suggests a functional interrelationship. Recent evidence indicates that catecholamines may facilitate shivering or skeletal muscle tonus (3, 54, 106), possibly by releasing ACh at the neuromyal junction (68). In the hypothalamic-pituitary neuroendocrine systems, thermal and chemical receptors in the preoptic anterior hypothalamus (POAH) influence secretion from the anterior pituitary of thyroid stimulating hormone (TSH), ACTH, and possibly growth hormone (GH). These actions are presumably medicated via the hypothalamic releasing hormones for thyrotropin (TRH), corticotropin (CRH), and growth hormone (GRH) (Figure 1). In addition, recent evidence suggests that POAH thermoreceptors influence the secretion of the neurohypophysial hormone, ADH (50, 87).

The properties of, and interactions between, thermoreceptors in the hypothalamus (1, 3, 7, 24, 25, 32, 39–42, 47, 49, 50, 55, 61–63, 67, 81, 87, 89, 90a, 95, 113), brain stem (1, 22, 72), spinal cord (22, 61, 62, 97), and viscera (1, 3, 90) are the subject of much current study. Cooling and warming of the spinal cord evoke many of the physiological and behavioral thermoregulatory responses evoked by POAH thermal displacement, and a physiologic equivalence between the thermoregulatory capability of the thermoreceptors in the spinal cord and the POAH has been proposed (61). However, the thermoregulatory activity of the spinal cord is believed generally to depend on neural projection to the hypothalamus (12, 44, 47), and, thus, spinal cord thermoreceptive neurons may function primarily in a sensory (97) rather than integrative and motor capacity. Although dogs and rabbits subjected to high spinal cord section retain some ability to shiver when cold stressed (67a), human paraplegic patients with high spinal cord injury have impaired thermal sensation and imparied ability to shiver or to sweat (anhydrosis) which increases the propensity to develop hypothermia in a cool ambient temperature (T_a) and heat exhaustion during muscular exercise, e.g. in a wheel chair (108a).

Additional lines of evidence suggest that the spinal cord thermoreceptor mechanism lacks full functional equivalence with the hypothalamus. First, the hyperthermic response to bacterial pyrogen or to leucocytic pyrogen, which is believed to occur by a resetting upward of the regulated temperature, appears to be mediated by neurons localized to the POAH and possibly the midbrain (32) but not the spinal cord. Second, it is difficult to envisage physiologically meaningful activation of the pituitary gland, e.g. ACTH or TSH, dependent on hypothalamic neurohormones carried by the hypothalamic-pituitary portal vessels, unless the spinal cord thermoreceptors are linked by sensory input to the hypothalamus. Apparently, there are no studies of stimulation or inhibition of metabolic hormones during spinal cord thermal displacement. Third, it has been hypothesized that a rise in plasma osmolarity, or in Na^+ concentration, can elevate the regulated level of internal temperature in man at rest (101) and during exercise (43, 86, 101). The osmoreceptors, or perhaps the Na^+ receptors (4), of the hypothalamus have been postulated to contribute to regulation of heat content of the body during exercise by deriving body mass from plasma Na^+ concentration (101). Since a functional counterpart of the hypothalamic osmoreceptors has not been proposed to exist in the spinal cord, this modality of temperature control appears localized to the anterior hypothalamus. Possibly, however, changes in the gain of spinal afferent neurons, produced by local osmotic alterations, may contribute to the central response (97).

Cooling and warming in the spinal cord produce regulated changes in the cardiovascular system subserving thermoregulation in conscious, chronically prepared monkeys (22). Similar regulated changes in cardiovascular parameters and internal temperature were evoked by cooling and warming of the POAH in conscious baboons (81). The similarity of spinal cord and POAH thermal displacement in resetting the regulated levels of heart rate, blood pressure, and internal temperature suggests, but of course does not prove, that spinal thermoreceptors project to the hypothalamus. It is anticipated that high spinal cord transection would seriously impair the cardiovascular responses to spinal cord cooling and warming, inasmuch as paraplegic subjects have poor autonomic control of the cardiovascular system as well as of thermoregulation (J. A. Downey, personal communication), being particularly susceptible to orthostatic hypotension.

Cooling and warming in the medulla oblongata of conscious monkeys produced regulated changes in blood pressure, heart rate, and internal temperature, and these responses were countered by simultaneous and opposite thermal displacement in the spinal cord (22). These findings suggest the presence of thermoreceptors in the medulla which contribute to the integration of the cardiovascular system in thermal homeostasis. Local warming and cooling in the medullary-pontine region of conscious rats led to operant behavioral thermoregulation, as did thermal displacement in the POAH (72). These findings corroborate the presence of thermoreceptors in the brain stem, and suggest that they contribute to both autonomic and cortical (volitional) control of thermoregulation. In contrast, local cooling or warming in the midbrain reticular formation of the squirrel monkey (*Saimiri sciureus*) failed to evoke behavioral thermoregulatory responses, although thermal displacement in the abdomen and the posterior hypothalamus was effective, though less so than in the POAH (1).

SYMPATHICOADRENOMEDULLARY SYSTEM—COLD AND HEAT EXPOSURE

In addition to rodents (8, 9, 14, 19, 37, 54, 63, 69–71, 74, 85, 96), many medium-sized, nonhibernating mammals develop some degree of nonshivering thermogenesis in the cold, including rabbit (21, 83), cat (21), dog (21), goat (3), sheep (21, 112), rhesus monkey (*Macaca mulatta*) (20, 21), baboon (*Papio anubis*) (38), Japanese monkey (*Macaca fuscata*) (84), and man (10, 21, 57, 65, 66, 118). Yet the chemical basis for the cold-induced rise in metabolic heat production in these larger mammals has been relatively little investigated. Similarly, the adaptive changes leading to sensitization of the cardiovascular system to catecholamines and probably other hormones, e.g., renin, angiotensin, are not well understood (70, 83). Very little is known concerning physiological mechanisms leading to thicker hair or fur in the cold, although the increase in pelage has been related to photoperiodicity as well as to changes in environmental temperature (48). The possible role of neuroendocrine systems in stimulating pelage growth is suggested by the induction of cold acclimation in goats by repetitive cooling of the POAH in the summer months (3), which led to unseasonal appearance of wool. This was correlated with activation of the thyroid gland and the SAM system and, although not measured, possibly with other metabolic hormones as well, such as growth hormone and insulin. It is important to recognize that hormones function synergistically, although it is customary to study individual neuroendocrine systems separately, such as the SAM system.

The essential role of SAM catecholamines, NE and E, in mediating responses to cold exposure which lead to cold acclimation have been most completely documented in the laboratory rat (8, 9, 14, 19, 30, 37, 49, 54, 63, 69–71, 74, 85, 96, 98). Thermoregulatory responses to catecholamines are: cardiovascular adjustments leading to cutaneous vasoconstriction or selective dilatation (83), redistribution of organ blood flow (9, 60a), and increased cardiac output (9, 60a); increase in shivering thermogenesis during acute cold exposure and development of nonshivering thermogenesis in the acclimated state (19); mobilization of lipid and carbohydrate substrates, and regulation of oxidative metabolism (5, 15, 17, 54, 60, 100, 103).

Perhaps the most direct approach for evaluating activity of the SAM system in cold and heat stress is measurement of urinary excretion of free NE and E, and of their methylated metabolites, normetanephrine (*NME*) and metanephrine (*ME*). The sum of these reflects the rate of secretion of the catecholamines from sympathetic nerve terminals and adrenal medulla (98). The oxidized and methylated metabolite, 3-hydroxy-4-methoxyphenylglycol (*HMPG*) in turn reflects rate of NE synthesis in the nerve terminal (98). Because the rate of catecholamine synthesis greatly exceeds storage capacity within adrenergic granules, the intracellular oxidative enzyme, monoamine oxidase (*MAO*), continuously degrades surplus catecholamines, which then pass into the circulation where methylation occurs by catecholamine-O-methyl-transferase (*COMT*) and the end-product, HMPG, is excreted by the kidney. Thus, although only approximately 1 to 4% of free catecholamines entering the extracellular space are excreted by the kidney, urine collections of 30 min or more provide sufficient hormone to determine average SAM activity (33, 98). The measurement of urinary, tissue, and plasma catecholamines has been developed and used extensively over the past 20 years by Euler and associates (33). Ideally, simultaneous measurement of methylated and deaminated metabolites as well as of free catecholamines assures that alterations in rates of hormone degradation have not influenced the excretion rates of NE and E. However, it is currently accepted that excretion rate of free NE and E provides a valid estimate of average SAM activity (2, 3, 7, 31, 33, 38, 39, 56, 64, 69, 71, 75, 89, 98, 112).

A tabulation of urine concentrations of NE and E compiled from the literature on thermoregulation studies is presented in Table 1, including values for rat (64, 69, 71, 98), rhesus monkey (31), baboon (38, 39, 42), pig (7), goat (3), man (56, 75), sheep (112), and cow (2). The species are listed in order of ascending body weight. The low ratio of mass to body surface in very small mammals necessitates a much higher rate of oxidative metabolism for maintenance of thermal equilibrium in the cold than is required of larger mammals. In view of the known calorigenic actions of catecholamines, it might be anticipated that secretion of catecholamines per kilogram body weight would fall progressively with increase in size of mammals exposed to environmental cold. This relationship holds as an approximation. However, it is evident that age, weight, and strain are factors determining the SAM response to cold even within one species, e.g., rat. Generally, the larger and older rats secreted proportionately greater amounts of catecholamines, particularly of NE, per kilogram of body weight. This relationship between weight, age, and SAM activity in cold acclimation was also related in rats to the ratio of brown adipose tissue to body weight (21). It was reported (71) that when rats weighing 180 g were placed in $3°C$ T_a, urinary NE rose from control level of 2.78 ng kg^{-1} min^{-1} to 13.89 within 24 hr and remained elevated for approximately four weeks, but then fell slowly to plateau at 5.56 at eight weeks. Urinary E showed a smaller response which roughly paralleled NE. On the other hand, it was found (69) that 400-g rats, which at $22°C$ T_a excreted 3.19 ng kg^{-1} min^{-1} of NE, when placed in $10°C$ T_a increased their urinary NE to 16.68 after 210 days. The sustained elevation is presumed due to relative insensitivity of older and larger rats to the calorigenic action of NE (21), and hence the need to secrete more catecholamines to maintain body temperature.

Recently the effects were studied of acute and chronic cold exposure, as well as of heat exposure, on urinary NE, E, and their metabolites NME and ME (98). Urinary free catecholamines and methylated metabolites were summed to assess the secretion (release) rate of free catecholamines, since methylation occurs primarily after the catecholamine enters the extracellular synaptic cleft. In addition, the synthesis rate was calculated by urinary excretion of HPMG, the principal metabolite of NE degraded by intraneuronal oxidation when synthesis exceeds storage capacity in granules. In contrast to the previous studies, groups of four rats were caged together, and the lower control excretion of NE at $22°C$ T_a of 1.0 ng kg^{-1} min^{-1}, and the moderate rise to 3.52 ng kg^{-1} min^{-1} acutely upon exposure to $4°C$ T_a reflect the protec-

TABLE 1. Urinary Catecholamines (ng kg^{-1} min^{-1})[a]

Ref	Species	Wt(kg)	Neutral T_a NE	E	°C	Acute cold NE	E	°C	Chronic cold NE	E	°C	Warm NE	E	°C
71	Rat	.180	2.78	0.69	22°	13.89 (6 days)	4.17	3°	5.56 (60 days)	1.04	3°			
98	Rat	.260	1.00	0.27	30°	3.52 (24 hr)	1.38	4°	2.53 (30 days, 4 rats/cage)	0.43	4°	1.18	0.31	36°
64	Rat	.350	0.63	0.19	27°				4.16 (12 weeks)	0.68	4°			
64	Hypothyroid rat (methimazole)		0.59	0.17	27°				8.67 (3 weeks)	1.39	4°			
69	Rat	.400	3.19	0.23	25°				16.68 (210 days)	1.11	10°			
31	Rhesus	5.7	0.58	0.44	25°				up to 8 fold rise		5°			
39	Baboon	12	0.33	0.38	25°	1.00 (6 days)	0.58	6°	1.23 (60 days)	0.46	6°			
42	Thyrx[b]	12	0.92	1.85	25°									
7	Pig[b]	26 (estimated)	0.17	0.06	25°	0.41	0.14	10°				0.12	0.06	35°
3	Goat[b]	40	0.25	0.08	22°	0.88	0.14	−3°						
3	Thyrx[b]	40	0.67	0.26	22°	1.13	1.03	−3°						
75	Man[c]	70	2.85	0.76	25°	5.2	0.76	5°	2.5	0.76	5°			
56	Man[b]	70	0.44	0.10								0.67 (25–40 min)	0.14	75°
112	Sheep	80	0.76	0.28	25°				1.53	0.56	5°			
									3.12	0.76	− 3°			
									3.12	1.10	−10°			
									4.93	3.61	−25°			
2	Cow	591	0.069	0.028	18°	0.083 (48 hr)	0.034	2°				0.084 (48 hr)	0.031	37°

[a] Based on 24 hr urine collection unless otherwise noted.
[b] Urine collected for 3 hr during the day.
[c] Urine collected for 8 hr during the day.

tive effects of huddling. Although the excreted levels of NE and its principal metabolite NME increased in parallel in urine during acute cold, the level of HMPG rose nearly twice as steeply. This suggests that the measurement of NE alone provides a reasonable estimate of hormone secretion and that cold stimulated synthesis of NE proceeded at twice the rate of secretion upon acute cold exposure. However, after 24 hours the rate of synthesis fell and stabilized at a level approximating secretion rate for four weeks. When rats were transferred from T_a 22° to 36°C (heat stress), excretion of NE and NME rose significantly but the excretion of HMGP fell (98). These results were interpreted as showing differential effects of ambient temperature on the synthesis vs the secretion of catecholamines. Further evidence for dissociation of catecholamine synthesis from secretion was obtained during ganglionic blockade, which reduced the cold-induced rise in NE (secretion) but not the cold-induced rise in HMPG (synthesis) (99).

In studies of cold acclimation in infrahuman primates, exposure of baboons (*Papio anubis*) to 6°C for ten weeks led promptly to a sustained, threefold rise in urinary NE, and to a lesser rise in urinary E (38). Failure of NE secretion to decline in baboons after four weeks in the cold may be related to the fact that this infrahuman primate shivers very little if at all at 6°C T_a. Seemingly the prompt increase in thermoregulatory nonshivering thermogenesis upon cold exposure was not mediated via NE-induced hypertrophy of brown adipose tissue, as occurs in rats. Maintenance of nonshivering thermogenesis would therefore presumably require continued secretion of NE at the initial high levels. The sustained rise of SAM activity and of adrenocortical glucocorticoid secretion in the cold, shown by 50% rise in urinary 17-ketogenic steroids (38), was associated with a 20 to 30% rise in resting metabolic rate (measured at 6°C T_a), a doubling of food intake, and persistent cutaneous vasoconstriction. Acceleration by 15% in fractional disappearance of T_4^{I-125} from plasma during cold exposure, which suggested increased thyroid hormone secretion, appeared to be related to a rise in enterohepatic clearance of unmetabolized hormone secondary to elevated food intake rather than to peripheral tissue utilization (38). These findings suggest that the rise in SAM and adrenocortical activity in chronically cold exposed baboons contributes importantly to cold acclimation by increasing the capacity for nonshivering thermogenesis, by improving substrate mobilization and synthesis (gluconeogenesis), and by sensitizing the peripheral vasculature to cold. The neuroendocrine response of rhesus monkeys (*Macaca mulatta*) to six weeks of chronic cold exposure (5°C) is similar to that of baboons. In a preliminary report (31) urinary catecholamines and 17-ketogenic steroids were increased several fold in conjunction with a doubling of food intake. The monkeys shivered very little if at all (J. W. Mason, personal communication). When cold-acclimated baboons were returned to neutral T_a (25°C), urinary catecholamines and 17-ketogenic steroids fell below the pre-cold exposure level (38). This rebound effect may be related to sensitization (increased gain) of the hypothalamic thermoregulatory mechanism mediating chemical thermosuppresion. A similar decline in SAM and adrenocortical activity occurs when the POAH of baboons is acutely warmed in neutral T_a (89).

The rhesus monkey remains in good condition for months or years when individually caged in constant ambient temperature ranging from 5° to 38°C, and becomes respectively cold-acclimated or warm-acclimated at these temperature extremes (20). Acclimation was evaluated by changes in resting metabolic rate measured in thermal neutral zone (between 10° and 31°C), and by the metabolic response to intramuscular injection of NE. The mean resting metabolic rate was 672 ml O_2 kg$^{-0.7}$ hr^{-1} for warm-acclimated monkeys, 936 for monkeys acclimated to 25°C T_a, and 1380 for cold-acclimated animals. Thus, the difference between resting metabolic rate in cold-acclimated and warm-acclimated monkeys is much greater, 100%, than between Korean women divers in winter and summer, 17% (66). When these monkeys were administered NE intramuscularly, resting metabolic rate rose 33%

in cold-acclimated animals but failed to increase in warm-acclimated animals (20). The metabolic response was intermediate in monkeys acclimated to 25°C T_a, suggesting that this temperature, usually regarded as thermoneutral, may constitute some degree of cold stress. Monkeys which were acclimated to 5 and 25°C had brown adipose tissue in the axillary region, whereas warm-acclimated monkeys had none (20). This suggests that brown adipose tissue may fulfill some thermoregulatory role in infrahuman primates, and may provide an explanation for the greater metabolic response to NE in cold-acclimated rhesus monkeys, 33%, than in cold-acclimated men, 15% (65), and cold-acclimated women, 7% (66).

Since heat-acclimated rhesus monkeys survived acute heat exposure, 40°C T_a, whereas cold-acclimated monkeys suffered heat stroke, and, conversely, since warm-acclimated monkeys were unable to maintain body temperature in acute severe cold, $-6°C$, whereas cold-acclimated animals maintained homeothermy, this infrahuman primate is capable of acclimating to temperature extremes by increasing nonshivering thermogenesis in the cold and by metabolic thermosuppression in the heat (20). The metabolic response of the Japanese monkey (*Macaca fuscata*) to 5°C T_a is greater than that of the rhesus monkey (84). This species inhabits colder regions than the rhesus and grows a considerably thicker coat in the winter (84), and thus acclimates by both increased metabolic heat production and more efficient peripheral insulation. In contrast to the rhesus and Japanese monkey, the pigtail monkey (*Macaca nemestrina*) has apparently much less resistance to cold. The native habitat of this species is limited to tropical zones in Asia. Of several species of infrahuman primates living in outdoor compounds in the state of Washington, only pigtail monkeys were observed to die of exposure in the cooler autumn and early winter nights (personal communication, W. R. Morton). Rhesus monkeys and baboons survived the cooler weather in good condition. The apparent poor cold resistance of the pigtail monkey may partially account for the deterioration of space monkey Bonny in orbit in June, 1969 (46). The mean internal temperature of this adult male pigtail was 34.8°C for days 1 to 5 and 33.2°C for days 5 to 9 in space orbit. The continuous movement of 20°C air within the space capsule may have constituted an appreciable cold stress which, combined with the state of weightlessness, central redistribution of blood volume, and dehydration, contributed to the animal's progressive deterioration (46). This seems plausible in light of recent findings that 25°C may represent a mild cold stress for the more cold-resistant rhesus monkey (20), and that the pigtail monkey will perform an operant task to obtain infrared heat reward up to 32°C T_a (18). The squirrel monkey (*Saimiri sciureus*), a New World primate with a thermal habitat comparable to that of the pigtail, will also work to maintain ambient temperature at approximately 32°C (1).

When goats (3) and pigs (7) are subjected to three hours of cold exposure, urinary NE rises approximately threefold and E twofold. Although goats show clear evidence of acclimation to chronic cold by developing nonshivering thermogenesis and growing wool (3), the pig apparently does not develop nonshivering thermogenesis but rather increases its capacity for shivering thermogenesis (14). Pigs placed in hot (35°C) T_a for three hours suppress urinary NE below control (25°C T_a) level; this reduction suggests hypothalamically mediated chemical thermosuppression. The important influence of cutaneous thermoreception in determining the level of SAM activity in pigs was demonstrated by measuring urinary catecholamines during POAH cooling or warming in cold (10°C), neutral (25°C), and hot (35°C) ambient temperatures (7). An interrelationship between the regulation of the SAM system and the thyroid gland has been shown by surgical thyroidectomy in goats (3) and baboons (42), and by drug-induced hypothyroidism in rats (37, 64, 74). The condition of hypothyroidism leads to compensatory increase in SAM activity, as reflected by increased urinary catecholamines, especially of E, in neutral T_a (3, 42), in cold T_a (3, 37, 42), and during POAH cooling (3, 42). Administration of exogenous T_4 to induce a hyperthyroid condition suppressed urinary catecholamines below control levels in neutral T_a (3, 42), cold T_a (3), and during POAH cooling (3).

Exposure of lightly clad men to 5°C for 8 hr/day for five weeks resulted initially in a twofold rise in urinary NE excretion but none in E. After six days of such intermittent cold stress, urinary NE returned to control levels (75). This apparently is the only study of urinary catecholamines in men subjected to cold under controlled laboratory conditions. Even taking into account that SAM activity is greater during the waking hours (33), the control excretion rate of catecholamines was considerably higher than in other studies in man based on 24-hr mean values (33). The relative increase in NE during acute cold exposure, however, represents a real rise in SAM activity (M. Mager, personal communication). Exposure of adult men to 14°C T_a for two weeks resulted in acclimation to cold, as shown by a 15% rise in nonshivering thermogenesis (O_2 consumption) in response to iv infusion of NE (65). Urinary catecholamines were not measured during cold acclimation or during NE infusion.

The high incidence of cardiac arrhythmia during NE infusion perhaps illustrates the dissimilarity of NE iv infusion from NE released endogenously at adrenergic nerve terminals (65). Since cold acclimation in all probability sensitized cardiac beta receptors to catecholamines, it might be expected that NE infused directly into the venous return to the heart might provoke cardiac arrhythmia. The relatively small increase in metabolic rate, therefore, might be partly due to discomfort and anxiety. Obviously it would be helpful to measure plasma levels of endogenously released catecholamines during cold exposure, but the technical difficulties of measuring trace levels in plasma (33) are complicated further by a circulatory half life of only 2-3 min (33). The relatively large volumes of blood that would have to be drawn frequently would thus create the risk of SAM activation by hypovolemia. Recent studies indicate, however, that during maximal exercise plasma NE may reach 10 ng /ml (45), higher than the calculated concentration in plasma in the NE infusion test for cold acclimation (65), and suggest that NE in the blood stream may mediate physiological as opposed to pharmacological effects.

When men were exposed to dry heat, 75°C (Finnish sauna) for 25 to 40 min, urinary catecholamines rose significantly; this rise presumably reflected SAM mediation of increased cutaneous blood flow (56). Similarly, in non-acclimated men exercising in 50°C for 90 min significantly elevated urinary NE in association with a rise in rectal temperature (76). The SAM activation is related to demands on the cardiovascular system to increase blood flow both to working muscle and to skin for heat loss. After heat acclimation, exercise no longer increased urinary NE in the heat and internal temperature rose significantly less (76).

Sheep respond to exposure to 5°C by elevating urinary catecholamines, with a further marked rise during exposure at −3° to −25°C (112). Although sheep become cold-acclimated, they show no calorigenic response to exogenous NE, possibly because they lack brown adipose tissue (112). Oxen exposed to heat, or subjected to local heating of the POAH, increase SAM activity as shown by rises in blood pressure and heart rate (113), presumably to effect greater cutaneous blood flow. Cows excrete increased amounts of catecholamines during cold as well as during heat exposure (2), illustrating the dual capacity of the SAM system in this species to mediate both cold and heat defense mechanisms. Plasma catecholamines were continuously elevated in cows during 24 days of exposure to 35°C; plasma glucocorticoids were only transiently increased, whereas internal temperature remained significantly elevated (M. B. Alvarez and H. D. Johnson, personal communication).

SAM RESPONSE TO POAH COOLING AND WARMING

Another experimental approach used to investigate the thermoregulatory role of the SAM system is local cooling and warming (so-called "thermal clamping") of the POAH region (3, 7, 24, 25, 39, 44, 49, 50, 55, 63, 67, 87, 89, 90a, 113). The procedure is performed in conscious animals following stereotaxic implantation in the hypothalamus of water-perfused thermodes, or of guide sleeves for acute insertion of thermodes. The POAH region of the diencephalon is the site of specialized neurons which monitor local brain temperature over a range of approximately 32 to 42°C (12, 32, 44). Most of these thermodetector neurons show a steep linear increase in firing rate as local brain temperature rises, i.e., they are primary "warmth receptors" (12, 32, 44, 47). "Cold receptors" i.e., neurons that show a linear increase in firing rate as brain temperature falls over a range of 42 to 32°C, have also been reported in the POAH, although in fewer numbers than warmth receptors. However, the existence of primary cold receptors in the POAH has been questioned by Eisenman (32) who has suggested that in light of the greater sensitivity of these receptors to the depressant action of barbiturates (compared to warmth receptors), they may be interneurons linking the POAH warmth receptors with the SAM and shivering motor centers in the posterior hypothalamus.

At normal brain temperature, the POAH warmth receptors may be viewed as maintaining a tonic inhibition on the interneurons (Figure 1). Suppression of the tonic inhibition by local POAH cooling would lead to an increase in interneuron firing rate and to mobilization of cold defense mechanisms. Conversely, local POAH warming would augment the tonic inhibition of the interneurons leading to heat loss responses. In a thermally neutral ambient temperature, i.e., one in which cutaneous thermoreceptors project little or no thermal information to the CNS, the POAH thermodetector neurons are functionally deafferented. Since brain temperature is determined primarily by the temperature of the blood perfusing it, the metabolic heat production of the CNS being quite constant (50a), the responses evoked by thermal displacement in the POAH in neutral T_a reflect the capability of the central warmth receptors to measure local temperature displacement and to mobilize neural and hormonal mechanisms for thermal homeostasis. When ambient temperature is above or below thermal neutrality, or when the level of nonthermal inputs to the hypothalamus is altered, as in states of alertness or drowsiness, the sensitivity of the POAH to local temperature displacement is altered accordingly. For example, the POAH must be cooled more deeply in a warm ambient temperature, or in a drowsy animal, to elicit the same intensity of shivering as in a cool ambient temperature, or in an alerted animal (3, 44, 55). This alteration in POAH thermosensitivity has been ascribed to resetting to an optimal level of the set (threshold) temperature for individual thermoregulatory responses, e.g., shivering, vasoconstriction, sweating, panting, etc. (12, 44).

In this schema, thermal input from internal thermodetector neurons, principally in the POAH but also in the spinal cord (22, 61, 62, 97), midbrain (1, 22), and viscera (90), is integrated in the hypothalamus with various nonthermal as well as peripheral thermal sensory inputs. The integrated signal then continuously modulates SAM outflow to maintain cardiovascular and metabolic homeostasis (21, 53) and probably to influence neuromuscular tonus (3, 68) as well.

In goats (3), pigs (7), and baboons (39) local POAH cooling provoked a rise in SAM activity, as determined by increased urinary catecholamine excretion, in association with shivering, cutaneous vasoconstriction, rise in metabolic rate, and elevation in core temperature of 1–2°C. Local warming of the POAH in these species produced the reverse thermoregulatory effects and suppressed urinary catecholamine excretion (3, 7, 89). An apparent exception is the ox, which responded to POAH warming with augmented SAM activity, manifested as a rise in blood pressure and heart rate (113) which mediate greater cutaneous blood flow. Compared to the SAM reactivity to environmental cold, characterized by a predominent rise in urinary NE, local cooling for 2–3 hr of the POAH in goats evoked a relatively greater increase in E (117%) than in NE (48%), associated with activation of the thyroid gland but not of the adrenal cortex (3). In contrast, the baboon, which also excretes proportionately more NE in environmental cold stress (38), responded to POAH cooling with a proportionately greater rise in NE (100%) than in E (68%) (39). This was always associated with stimulation of adrenogluco-corticoid secretion but inconsistent thyroidal activation. Under the conditions of chronic restraint in a primate chair in neutral T_a, the baboon excretes much more E relative to NE than the goat (3), pig (7), rat (69, 71), cow (2), sheep (112), or man (56, 75). In this respect, the baboon resembles the rhesus monkey adapted to primate chair restraint (31). The higher E to NE ratio in these infrahuman primates possibly reflects the stress of chair confinement, although the plasma levels of 17-hydroxycorticosteroids existing prior to central cooling were not particularly elevated (39).

It has been proposed that elevations in urinary E in man are associated with mental states of anxiety or fear, whereas rises in urinary NE are related to aggression and anger (33). The greater secretion of NE than of E during physical exercise, however, is mainly related to cardiovascular and metabolic activities (33, 45). Mason (78) has cautioned that in evaluating the physiological activities of stress hormones, e.g. ACTH, catecholamines, GH, and TSH, it is more difficult to control or eliminate psychological influences in physiological studies than vice versa. This is particularly relevant, of course, to studies in primates.

The pig responded to environmental cooling (10°C) with a 176% rise in NE and a 121% rise in E, and to local POAH cooling with a 93% rise in NE and a lesser 45% rise in E (7). Observations on the influence of cold (10°C), neutral (25°C), and warm (35°C) ambient temperatures led to the conclusion that input from cutaneous thermal receptors can modify SAM activation by POAH cooling (7). Thus local POAH cooling for 3 hr conducted in a cold (10°C) or neutral (25°C) ambient temperature elevated urinary NE 100%, but POAH cooling in a warm T_a (25°C) had no effect. These changes were associated with a 1°C rise in core temperature at each ambient temperature, which is a smaller hyperthermic response than in the goat (2°C) (3) or baboon (1–1.5°C) (39, 81) in neutral T_a. Local warming of the POAH for 3 hr in the pig led to a fall in urinary NE (7) at 35°C, but not at 10°C T_a. These results show that a strong thermal stimulus at skin thermoreceptors can counter an opposite thermal displacement in the POAH. In contrast, however, POAH warming in the goat (3) inhibited the rise in urinary catecholamines customarily evoked by ruminal cooling with ice water. Similarly, warming the POAH of goats in 5°C T_a inhibited catecholamine excretion and cold defense mechanisms, and led to progressive fall in internal temperature to 31°C within several hours. Cessation of POAH warming in this situation was followed by maximal shivering thermogenesis and marked rise in urinary catecholamines. Epinephrine was excreted in proportionally greater amounts when internal temperature was very low (31°C), whereas NE was preferentially increased with moderate hypothermia (35°C), (3). This accords with the view (71) that NE is the principal catechol released in cold exposure, with E serving as a secondary defense against extreme cold stress.

In the baboon, POAH warming in neutral T_a for several hours lowered both urinary NE and E in association with a 2°C fall in internal temperature, 35% decline in oxygen consumption, cutaneous vasodilatation, and lassitude (89). Plasma 17-hydroxycorticosteroids, glucose, free fatty acids (FFA), and insulin also fell significantly during POAH warming, suggesting that hypothalamic thermoreceptors serve to adjust substrate mobilization to metabolic requirements. These findings demonstrate hypothalamic integration of both physical and chemical thermosuppression. POAH warming not only inhibited shivering and vasoconstriction, thus causing a fall in internal temperature, but lowered the resting metabolic rate and suppressed lipolysis and glycogenolysis.

The observation that during 1–2 hr of POAH warming in baboons internal temperature stabilized at a lower level and cutaneous vasoconstriction returned, indicates that thermodetectors elsewhere in the body core, presumably in the brainstem (1, 22, 72), spinal cord (21, 61, 62, 97), and viscera (1, 90), respond to the core hypothermia and, by sensory input to the hypothalamus, serve to counteract POAH warming. However, the complete inhibition of shivering at an internal temperature of 35°C demonstrates the thermoregulatory predominance of locally warmed POAH thermoreceptors. Warmth receptors in the spinal cord show a similar thermoregulatory predominance. Intensive spinal cord warming in oxen in 12°C T_a led to continuous fall in internal temperature to 33°C; core thermoreceptors elsewhere were apparently incapable of countering the progressive hypothermia (62). Cessation of POAH warming in baboon (81, 89) and of spinal cord warming in oxen (62) resulted in prompt shivering thermogenesis, and internal temperature rose steeply. In baboon, urinary catecholamines, plasma glucose, FFA, insulin, 17-hydroxycorticosteroids, and growth hormone rose significantly as O_2 consumption increased threefold above the nadir (89). A related study showed that behavioral thermoregulatory responses are elicited in baboon by POAH cooling and warming (40), as indicated by operant bar pressing to receive infrared heat reward. Furthermore, POAH cooling and warming led to regulated changes in blood pressure and heart rate which paralleled and correlated significantly with alterations in internal temperature (81). Thus, POAH thermal displacement in baboon evoked synchronized responses involving cortical (volitional), autonomic, and neuroendocrine thermoregulatory motor systems.

Ganglionic blockade.—Recent experiments designed to elucidate more definitively the fundamental role of the SAM system in the adaptive changes in cold stress have involved chemical blockade of the sympathetic ganglia or of adrenergic receptors in tissues (3, 41). In the goat, iv injection of Ecolid (chlorisondamine), a long acting ganglionic blocker, led to cutaneous vasodilatation and a slight fall in rectal temperature (3). The customary 2°C rise in rectal temperature during several hours of POAH cooling in goats was inhibited, and instead rectal temperature fell 1.2°C. Despite the combination of general hypothermia and the normally powerful thermogenic stimulus of POAH cooling, shivering was sporadic and weak, and internal temperature did not rise. Inhibition by ganglionic blockade of the expected thermogenic response was associated with a marked decline in urinary catecholamines, reflecting SAM suppression. When NE was administered iv during ganglionic blockade and POAH cooling, strong shivering thermogenesis was restored and rectal temperature rose 1.2°C in one hour.

A similar experimental protocol has been more recently applied to the baboon and has yielded comparable results (41). In the baboon adapted to primate chair restraint, iv administration for one hour of Arfonad (trimethaphan comphorsulfonate), a ganglionic blocker which acts rapidly but becomes ineffective quickly at stop of infusion, caused peripheral vasodilatation, marked fall in blood pressure, and a 1.7°C fall in internal temperature (41). There also occurred a decline in plasma FFA and glucose, little change in oxygen consumption, and decline in turnover (utilization) rate of FFA measured by iv infusion of ^{14}C palmitate tracer. Suppression of SAM activity during Arfonad was shown by the decline in urinary catecholamines, primarily in NE. Despite the fall in internal temperature during ganglionic blockade, shivering was only weak and sporadic. When the POAH was cooled for one hour during ganglionic blockade, none of the parameters was altered appreciably (41). However, if at this point, ganglionic blockade were stopped, or, alternatively, exogenous catecholamines were given iv during blockade, strong shivering thermogenesis was promptly restored and internal temperature rose 1.5 to 2°C, within one hour. This was associated with a 50 to 100% rise in metabolic rate, cutaneous vasoconstriction, elevation of blood pressure to the mildly hypertensive levels customary for POAH cooling, mobilization of plasma FFA and glucose, and a 100–150% increase in FFA turnover rate (41).

These studies in goat (3) and baboon (41) and earlier studies in the rat (19) demonstrate that catecholamines must be released and react at receptor sites for the normal thermogenic response to cold. The marked impairment by ganglionic blocking agents of shivering in cold stress and the restoration of strong shivering by administration of catecholamines during ganglionic blockade (3, 41) or after high cervical cord section (106) suggest that catecholamines importantly facilitate the shivering mechanism. Although a central facilitatory action of systemic catecholamines on shivering has been postulated (3), the low permeability of the blood brain barrier to catecholamines would tend to reduce the likelihood of this possibility. Alternatively, the catecholamines may act centrally indirectly via baroreceptor reflexes, or by direct action on the neuromyal junction of skeletal muscle to enhance ACh release (68, 106).

Blockade of adrenergic receptors.—Although ganglionic blockade abolished the normal thermoregulatory responses to cold stress in goat (3), rat (19, 71), and baboon (41), attempts to produce a similar degree of intervention with adrenergic receptor blocking agents have been unsuccessful. In goats, administration of phenoxybenzamine, an alpha-adrenergic blocker, caused cutaneous vasodilatation and marked increase in excretion of catecholamines, but did not impair the thermogenic response to POAH cooling (3). Indeed, shivering was potentiated. In baboons, iv infusion of an alpha-adrenergic blocker, phentolamine, caused cutaneous vasodilatation, a 0.5 to 1.0°C fall in internal temperature, and a decline in plasma glucose (41). However, the metabolic response to POAH cooling was not prevented, but rather was greater than in the absence of alpha blockade, O_2 consumption rising 100% and FFA turnover increasing 30%. During alpha blockade there was a selective rise in urinary NE. Thus, the principal effect of alpha blockade was cutaneous vasodilatation which, by increasing heat loss, attenuated the hyperthermia normally evoked by POAH cooling, but as a consequence elevated metabolic heat production. Blockade of beta-adrenergic receptors by iv infusion of propranolol also failed to inhibit the thermogenic response to POAH cooling. Mobilization of FFA and glycerol was, however, impaired, and the rise in internal temperature and increase in metabolic rate (50%) apparently occurred at the expense of circulating pools or muscle stores of substrate. Urinary E rose 75% during beta-adrenergic blockade and POAH cooling, thus reflecting a strong SAM response.

Sheep may respond uniquely to cold exposure (112). Although urinary catecholamines rose to high levels in sheep exposed to cold (Table 1), iv infusion of NE or E failed to increase metabolic rate in either cold- or warm-acclimated sheep. Propranolol reduced cold thermogenesis in warm- and cold-acclimated sheep by 8% and 12%, respectively. Phenoxybenzamine nearly abolished cold thermogenesis in warm-acclimated sheep, but cold-acclimated sheep so treated maintained homeothermy during severe cold stress. It was concluded that sheep can develop nonshivering thermogenesis, i.e. become cold-acclimated, but that the direct thermogenic action of catecholamines observed in rodents (9, 14, 19, 21, 54) and hibernating mammals (102), mediated by brown adipose tissue, does not occur in sheep and may not occur in other large mammals lacking brown adipose tissue. An exception may be the calorigenic response of cold-acclimated rhesus monkeys to im NE (20) and cold-acclimated man to iv NE (65, 66).

In contrast to the uncertainty of the role of alpha- and beta-adrenergic receptors in mediating thermogenesis in large mammals, considerable evidence points to beta-adrenergic mediation of nonshivering thermogenesis in cold-acclimated rodents, including neonates. Administration of pronethalol, a beta-adrenergic blocker, to cold-acclimated or newborn guinea pigs caused a rise in electrical activity of skeletal muscle as metabolic rate and internal temperature fell (14). This was interpreted as a switching to shivering thermogenesis as nonshivering thermogenesis declined. Similarly, in anesthetized cold-acclimated rats blockade of beta-adrenergic receptors with propranolol led to a fall in rectal temperature and a marked rise in shivering monitored electromyographically (96). Propranolol did not inhibit shivering in anesthetized warm-acclimated (23°C) rats placed in the cold (96). The interactions of brown adipose tissue, catecholamines, and nonshivering thermogenesis in smaller mammals and neonates have been extensively reviewed recently (21, 54).

THYROID AND ADRENOCORTICAL INTERACTIONS WITH SAM

Thyroid.—Recognizing that the thyroid gland sets an optimal level of metabolism for most tissues, earlier investigators conjectured that the rise in metabolic rate in acute or chronic cold exposure might be mediated by increased production and utilization of thyroid hormones (37, 60). Recent study of thyroid function in cold stressed laboratory rats, however, suggests that there is little or no rise in peripheral tissue utilization of T_4 (21). Although normal levels of thyroid hormones are essential for cold defense, e.g., hypothyroid rats do not maintain body temperature in the cold (21, 37, 64, 74), such evidence for thyroid hyperfunction as glandular hypertrophy, rise in plasma TSH, increase in thyroid uptake of iodide, and rise in hormone secretion may be related to augmented enterohepatic clearance of unmetabolized hormone (21). Rats in the cold increase food uptake, and hence excrete more thyroid hormone in the greater fecal bulk (21). Additionally, however, it has very recently been suggested that cold acclimated rats preferentially increase secretion of triiodothyronine (T_3) (30, 85). Thus, plasma T_3 and TSH are significantly elevated in cold acclimated rats (30, 85), as is hypothalamic activity of thyrotropin releasing hormone (*TRH*) synthetase (91), but plasma T_4 is unchanged or decreased (30, 85). Therefore, the increased enterohepatic clearance of T_4 in rats in the cold may be balanced by augmented secretion of T_3 (S. Reichlin, personal communication). Whether this augmentation leads to a net increase in peripheral utilization of thyroid hormone is uncertain. Similarly it is unknown whether the greater calorigenic potency of T_3 relative to T_4 may lead to a net increase in metabolic stimulation. In contrast to these findings, however, a recent study (8) of cold acclimation in rats indicated no increase in plasma TSH, and it was concluded that increase in thyroid activity is not required for acclimation. Recent evidence in rats that cold exposure (*a*) elevates plasma free fatty acids which in turn increase plasma free T_4 by reducing binding to plasma globulins (37), and (*b*) stimulates catecholamine secretion leading to more rapid hepatic deiodination of T_4 (37), suggests that the augmented turnover rate of thyroid hormones may be directly related to metabolic stimulation.

Currently, the evidence is compelling that acclimation to cold involves a synergistic action between thyroid hormones and SAM catecholamines on adrenergic mechanisms in various tissues (3, 9, 21, 37, 42, 54, 60, 64, 70, 74, 106). For the laboratory rat acclimating to cold, this synergism occurs most importantly in brown adipose tissue, which in response undergoes hypertrophy and, by mobilizing and oxidizing lipid stores, serves as a heat generator for special organs, e.g., heart, spinal cord, lungs (9, 14, 21, 54, 60, 70). Furthermore, brown adipose tissue in rats is postulated to confer the property of nonshivering thermogenesis on skeletal muscle, presumably by a humoral factor (54, 70). At present it is unwarranted to extrapolate this mechanism of cold acclimation to larger mammals for which there is inconclusive evidence for hypertrophy or even the presence of brown adipose tissue in chronic cold exposure.

The interaction between catecholamines and thyroid hormones on the vasculature and heart may require a higher tissue concentration of catecholamines (saturation) as well as increased receptor sensitivity (70, 74). A current question of interest is whether cold-acclimated infrahuman primates and man secrete and utilize increased amounts of thyroid hormones to maintain thermal homeostasis, or whether the synergistic action of catecholamines so sensitizes receptors that no increase in T_4 or T_3 is required. There is little experimental evidence to elucidate this question.

Rhesus monkeys exposed for six weeks to 5°C increased urinary catecholamines and 17-ketogenic steroids markedly (31), but the evidence for increased thyroidal activity is less clear. There were small but consistent increments in total and free T_4 in plasma, and in one monkey plasma TSH rose progressively on three consecutive cold exposures. Since food intake also rose, these indications of thyroidal activation may be secondary to fecal loss of hormone. In these animals plasma growth hormone and insulin were unchanged, but urinary excretion of testosterone was suppressed. When adolescent male baboons adapted to primate chair restraint were exposed to 6°C for ten weeks, urinary catecholamines, particularly NE, were consistently elevated as were 17-ketogenic steroids (38). The evidence for thyroidal activation was less clear. When $T_4{}^{I-125}$ was given iv on three occasions during cold exposure, the fractional disappearance rate from plasma was 15% higher than in the pre- and post-cooling periods (38). Because plasma T_4 level was unaltered in the cold, the more rapid disappearance of T_4 from plasma indicates a corresponding rise in secretion into plasma. The rise in fractional disappearance of $T_4{}^{I-125}$ was largely accounted for by enterohepatic clearance of intact hormone, as in rats (21), since the rise in fecal radioactivity correlated with the greater fecal bulk (38). Although plasma TSH was not significantly elevated in cold-exposed baboons, the homeostasic regulation of thyroid hormone secretion may function so precisely that augmented hormone secretion occurred without measureable change in plasma TSH. Whether cold acclimated primates preferentially increase secretion of T_3, as reported in rats (30, 85), is unknown but deserves study.

Man may adapt[2] to cold by increasing surface insulation secondary to intense cutaneous vasoconstriction, as in the Australian aborigine (19), or by marked elevation in resting metabolic rate, as in the Alacaluf Indian (19), or by a combination of these mechanisms, as in the Eskimo (19), Caucasian (19), or Ama (66). Little is known of the neuroendocrine mechanisms by which man acclimates to cold. Intermittent exposure to 5°C led to a twofold

[2] "Adaptation" refers to long-term, genetically mediated adjustments in a population, as opposed to physiological changes in an individual occurring over weeks or months in "acclimation."

rise in urinary NE, which then fell to control level after a week (75). Continuous exposure of lightly clad men to 13°C for 48 hr caused alterations in the diurnal rhythm of plasma cortisol but did not change its urinary excretion (35). Thyroid function was studied in men undergoing five weeks of physical conditioning and cold acclimation (118). Measurement of plasma TSH, long acting thyroid stimulator (*LATS*), PBI, PBI[131], and thyroid uptake and urinary excretion of ^{131}I failed to show indications of increased thyroidal activity. Although resting metabolic rate rose 20%, this was attributed to physical conditioning rather than cold exposure per se.

Perhaps the most thorough study of human thyroid function in chronically cold stressed human subjects was conducted some years ago (10, 57). Lightly clad men were exposed for two weeks to 14 or 15°C, under carefully controlled conditions which excluded the opportunity to exercise and thus avoided the complications of physical conditioning. Cold-induced stimulation of thyroid activity was indicated by a rise in fractional disappearance rate of T_4^{I-131} following iv injection, a fall in plasma PBI, increased thyroidal and renal clearance of inorganic iodide, and increased uptake of radioiodide in the thyroid (57). Resting metabolic rate rose approximately 20 to 25% in the cold (10). These results were interpreted as indicating greater peripheral degradation of thyroid hormone with compensatory rise of secretion into plasma (57). However, at the time of this study it was not recognized that increased fecal bulk resulting from greater food intake leads to a rise in enterohepatic clearance of thyroxine (21, 38). Thus, the possibility remains that the augmented secretion represented compensation for fecal loss rather than greater tissue utilization. Clearly additional experimentation is needed to elucidate the contribution of T_3 and T_4 to cold acclimation in man and infrahuman primate.

It is unlikely that the hypermetabolism secondary to excessive thyroid secretion in man (thyrotoxicosis) simulates nonshivering thermogenesis of cold acclimation. Whereas an increase in SAM activity is a universal response to cold exposure in mammals (2, 3, 7, 31, 37, 38, 64, 69, 71, 74, 98), experimental production of hyperthyroidism by T_4 or T_3 administration is associated with suppression of urinary catecholamine excretion (3, 42), and the marked rise in plasma T_4 in thyrotoxicosis contrasts with unchanged or slightly lowered levels of T_4 in cold-acclimated man (57, 118). Most likely the rise in resting metabolic rate in cold-acclimated man (57, 118), baboon (38), and rhesus monkey (20) is determined by the synergism between fluctuating levels of catecholamines and constant levels of thyroid hormones on tissues of high metabolic activity.

Evidence has recently been presented that the increased calorigenesis of experimental hyperthyroidism in rats given T_3 or T_4 (58, 59) is quantitatively related to activation of Na^+-K^+ ATPase in the plasma membrane of liver, skeletal muscle, and kidney cells. Thyroid hormone activates the Na^+ pump in these tissues and elevates oxidative metabolism by increasing (*a*) Na^+-transport-dependent respiration, and (*b*) the transmembrane electrochemical gradient for Na+. The lower basal metabolic rate of hypothyroid rats appears to be related to less activity of the Na+ pump (58). The hyperthermia characteristic of dehydrated exercising men, e.g. marathon runners, may be in part related to stimulation of Na+ pump activity by plasma hyperosmolarity, but also to sensitivity of the hypothalamic thermal controller to elevated plasma Na+ (43, 86, 101).

As an alternative to exposure to environmental cold or heat, local cooling and warming of the POAH has been used to elucidate interactions between central thermoreceptor neurons and autonomic and neuroendocrine motor systems. Earlier studies in smaller laboratory animals such as rat, guinea pig, and hamster demonstrated that acute cold exposure led to prompt activation of the thyroid gland. Presumably a combination of peripheral cold stimuli and fall in central temperature served to activate the hypothalamic-pituitary axis. The anatomical proximity of the thermoregulatory center in the POAH to the neurons in the anterior hypothalamus regulating TSH (presumably by secretion of TRH) has suggested to many workers (3, 39, 90a) a functional interrelationship between temperature control and thyroid activity. A recent study in euthyroid and hypothyroid rats failed to support the hypothesis that hypothalamic thermal sensitivity stimulates TSH secretion during cold acclimation or inhibits it upon rewarming or exposure to heat (8). An earlier report that POAH cooling in rats led to thyroidal activation, as determined by release of ^{131}I from the thyroid (90a), was not confirmed when plasma TSH and T_4 were measured in centrally cooled rats (63). However, placement of the thermode in the POAH and the degree of brain cooling are critical factors, as emphasized in experiments in goats (3), rhesus monkeys (50), and baboons (39, 67, 81).

In chronically prepared conscious goats, local POAH cooling promptly activated the thyroid gland, as determined by increases in plasma PBI[131] and PBI as well as by concomitant fall in thyroid gland radioactivity (3). The thyroid response was always accompanied by increased SAM activity, as measured by urinary catecholamine excretion, but not by stimulation of adrenal glucocorticoid secretion. Because plasma TSH was not measured in these studies, an alternative explanation for thyroidal activation should be considered, namely, that sympathetic innervation or circulating catecholamines may directly release hormone stored in colloid. In support of this possibility administration of sympathetic biogenic amines (79), and electrical stimulation of the cervical sympathetic supply to the thyroid (80), have been reported in cat and mouse to evoke droplet formation in colloid and to increase secretion of thyroid hormone into the circulation. These responses are prevented by administration of the alpha-adrenergic blocking agent, phentolamine (80). The physiological significance of direct adrenergic stimulation of the thyroid which bypasses hypothalamic-pituitary control deserves further study. Of related interest, induction of ganglionic blockade in rats at neutral T_a led to a 1°C fall in body temperature and a rise in plasma TSH (77). However, ganglionic blockade in rats at 6°C T_a resulted in deeper hypothermia and no rise in plasma TSH, presumably because of inhibitory effects of the greater stress.

Local warming of the POAH in goats led to a synchronous suppression of thyroid and SAM activity in conjunction with panting, cutaneous vasodilatation, and decline in rectal temperature (3). Thus, hypothalamic thermoreceptors in this species can mediate chemical thermogenesis when cooled and chemical thermosuppression when warmed. Peripheral interaction between thyroid hormones and catecholamines is believed to contribute to the sustained elevation in rectal temperature during seven days of POAH cooling in goats and perhaps to the growth of wool in response to repetitive POAH cooling; cold acclimation is thus suggested (3). In a recent study, cooling of the POAH for seven days in rats led to sensitization to the calorigenic action of administered NE characteristic of cold acclimation in this species (49), but the neuroendocrine mechanisms conferring sensitivity were not elucidated.

That hypothalamic thermoreceptors may regulate thyroid function in infrahuman primates was suggested recently by the febrile response to exogenous pyrogen (119). During the acute phase of fever following the administration of *Diplococcus pneumoniae* to rhesus monkeys, the accelerated clearance of labeled T_4 and T_3 from peripheral pools without alteration in plasma levels suggested increased secretion of thyroid hormones. Because bacterial pyrogens release leucocytic pyrogen which then acts primarily on the POAH controller to reset the regulated level of internal temperature (32, 44), the febrile response to pyrogen resembles that to POAH cooling (44). Theoretically, POAH cooling should lead to TSH secretion. However, POAH cooling in conscious baboons (39) led to activation of the thyroid gland, measured by increment in plasma PBI[131], in only 50% of cases. It was concluded that thyroidal stimulation per se is not essential to the acute cold defense response.

The observation that plasma TSH is elevated in human neonates (34) and in children subjected to deep hypothermia for cardiac surgery (116) suggests that thermal stress can stimulate the hypothalamic-pituitary axis, presumably by activation of TRH synthetase (91). However, adults exposed acutely to peripheral cold (34) or to general hypothermia via ingestion of ice (91) do not have elevated plasma TSH. It has been long known that stress-induced release of glucocorticoids may inhibit release of pituitary TSH, and recently evidence of such action has been documented in humans (117). Thus, the interrelation between the hypothalamic thermal controller and metabolic hormones, remains complex. There appear to be important species differences. For example, although cold exposure stimulates growth hormone release in rats, there is no consistent growth hormone release in baboons subjected to POAH cooling (39), nor in deeply hypothermic human infants (11), nor in human adults rendered mildly hypothermic by ingesting ice (91).

The reciprocal regulation of the thyroid and SAM system and the synergistic action between thyroid hormones and catecholamines at tissue receptor sites was studied in thyroidectomized goats (3). Surgical thyroidectomy followed by treatment with ^{131}I to destroy ectopic thyroid tissue led to increased secretion of catecholamines, particularly of E, in neutral T_a, and to a further marked increase in cold T_a ($-3°C$), or during POAH cooling. The increased catecholamine secretion presumably compensated for the absence of thyroid hormones, and thus enabled the animals to maintain internal temperature during acute cold exposure and to respond to POAH cooling with customary hyperthermia. Administration of exogenous T_4 to induce a hyperthyroid condition resulted in suppression of catecholamine secretion below presurgical levels and inhibited the response to POAH cooling.

A similar reciprocal regulation between the thyroid gland and the SAM system has since been demonstrated in rats rendered hypothyroid with antithyroid drugs (37, 64, 74) and in baboons surgically thyroidectomized (42). Inhibition of synthesis of thyroid hormones by administration of methimazole to rats acclimated to 4°C T_a led to a twofold rise in urinary NE and E (64). After the third week of treatment in the cold, body temperature and metabolic rate of rats fell significantly. These results suggest that cold-acclimated rats rendered hypothyroid increase secretion of catecholamines and thereby compensate for a time for thyroid hormone deficiency (64). In a comparable study, rats acclimated to 25°C T_a were given propylthiouracil to inhibit thyroid hormone synthesis, and were then restrained acutely in 5°C T_a to determine the rate of body cooling (37). Although urinary E rose 3.2 and NE 1.2 times relative to control rats similarly stressed, the hypothyroid rats cooled significantly faster. This was interpreted as reflecting a loss of sensitivity by cutaneous vasculature to the constrictor action of catecholamines and, hence, loss of peripheral insulation rather than failure of metabolic heat production.

Surgical removal of the thyroid in baboons led to a twofold rise in urinary NE and E (42). Although resting metabolic rate fell, thyroidectomized baboons living in primate chairs in 25°C T_a maintained normal body temperature and responded to POAH cooling with augmented excretion of catecholamines and rise in internal temperature. Conversely, POAH warming lowered urinary catecholamines in conjuction with a fall in internal temperature. These findings suggest that hypothyroid baboons regulate SAM activity at a higher level to compensate thyroid hormone deficiency. In mild chronic cold, 19°C T_a, internal temperature fell 2 to 3°C in hypothyroid baboons, indicating that the compensatory action of heightened SAM activity in thermoregulation is limited. Replacement with T_4 to restore euthyroidism caused catecholamines to fall to presurgical control levels, whereas production of hyperthyroidism by excess T_4 replacement suppressed urinary catecholamines below the normal level. Thus, in the goat (3), rat (37, 64, 74), and baboon (42), the SAM system and thyroid gland appear to be regulated reciprocally in maintenance of thermal homeostasis. The synergistic action of catecholamines and thyroid hormones on peripheral receptors to mediate cardiovascular, metabolic, and substrate mobilizing activity, in turn feed back to modulate central control. These studies point to the importance of interactions between catecholamines and thyroid hormones in peripheral tissues.

The details of these interactions are as yet little understood but the effect of hypothyroidism in impairing sympathetically mediated lipolysis in adipose tissue has been clarified by recent in vitro studies on human cells (92, 93) and in vivo observations on dogs (88). During fasting lipolysis in man it has been proposed (92, 93) that beta-adrenergic receptors on adipocytes are stimulated by NE and thyroid hormones acting synergistically. The resulting activation of membrane adenyl cyclase and increase in intracellular cyclic AMP stimulates hormone sensitive lipase and, hence, causes hydrolysis of triglycerides. The results of observations on adipocytes from hypothyroid humans suggested that the absence of thyroid hormone selectively increases the sensitivity of alpha-adrenergic receptors to NE (92, 93). The resulting predominance of alpha-adrenergic stimulation in adipocytes in turn leads to inhibition of membrane adenyl cyclase and to a decrement in intracellular cyclic AMP. Hence, lipolysis is inhibited. Addition of either phentolamine, an alpha-adrenergic blocking agent, or prostaglandin E_1, inhibited alpha-adrenergic stimulation of hypothyroid adipocytes by catecholamines. In this circumstance, the action of NE in stimulating beta-adrenergic receptors became predominant again, and the normal lipolytic response was restored (92, 93).

The suggested role of thyroid hormones in maintaining beta-adrenergic stimulation of fat cells may explain the recent findings of deficient lipolysis in hypothyroid dogs (88). When compared with normal dogs in neutral T_a, surgically thyroidectomized dogs displayed a 26% lower resting metabolic rate. Although able to maintain a normal plasma level of FFA, thyroidectomized dogs had a 35% lower FFA turnover rate (plasma disappearance rate) as measured by palmitate ^{14}C infusion. In both groups of animals lipid oxidation accounted for the same proportion of total caloric expenditure. These data indicate that FFA mobilization is defective in the absence of thyroid hormones, in agreement with in vitro studies in man (92, 93), but that tissue oxidation of FFA is not impaired, in agreement with in vivo studies in hypothyroid rats (37, 74). When thyroidectomized dogs were placed in 5°C T_a, their metabolic rate rose 100%, as compared with a 50% rise in normals, but the total caloric expenditures in the two groups were similar because of the lower resting metabolic rate in hypothyroid dogs (88). Although plasma FFA rose equally in both groups, FFA turnover rate was 33% lower in the thyroidectomized dogs, reflecting impaired FFA mobilization. The thyroidectomized animals, however, achieved the same caloric expenditure from FFA as did normals because they oxidized a much greater percentage of mobilized FFA (88). These results indicate that thyroid hormones participate in the regulation of FFA mobilization but apparently not directly in regulation of tissue oxidation of FFA. An excess of thyroid hormones, however, would be expected to increase FFA oxidation in connection with activation of membrane Na^+-K^+ ATPase and the Na^+ pump (58, 59).

Recent studies have also shown that thyroid hormones may interact with catecholamines to maintain tissue levels of cyclic AMP and thereby subserve thermoregulation in rats (74). Rats acclimated to neutral T_a were rendered hypothyroid by treatment with aminotriazole and then restrained in 7°C T_a

to determine cooling rate. Hypothyroid rats cooled five times more rapidly than controls, despite a marked rise in urinary catecholamines. The rise in catecholamine secretion was interpreted as a functional response to hypothermia inasmuch as administration of T_4 to hypothyroid rats prevented hypothermia in the cold and suppressed the rise in urinary catecholamines. When hypothyroid rats were treated with aminophylline to retard the enzymatic degradation by phosphodiesterase of intracellular cyclic AMP, their internal temperature did not fall in the cold. These data suggest that the thyroid hormones and catecholamines interact synergistically on a common mechanism, possibly on a common receptor, to increase cyclic AMP. Because adenyl cyclase is commonly believed to be activated by beta-adrenergic stimulation, and in view of recent evidence that thyroid hormone deficiency leads to a preferential stimulation of alpha-adrenergic receptors by NE (92, 93), the normal balance of thyroid hormones and catecholamines at adrenergic receptors may modulate cyclic AMP formation. As a ubiquitous intracellular second messenger, cyclic AMP in turn mediates a variety of processes subserving thermal homeostasis, such as mobilization of lipid and carbohydrate substrates, level of metabolism, and cardiovascular responses.

Recently Christensen (120) reported that plasma NE is threefold higher in hypothyroid human patients than in normal controls in both supine and standing positions. Treatment of these patients with thyroxine restored plasma NE to normal. In hyperthyroid patients, plasma NE was lower than in controls.

In summary, the evidence is compelling for peripheral synergism between thyroid hormones and catecholamines, and for central reciprocal control of the two neuroendocrine motor systems. Finally, the role of other metabolic hormones in thermoregulation is largely unknown. Of particular interest are the functions of growth hormone, cortisol, insulin, and glucagon for thermal homeostasis.

Adrenal cortex.—Maintenance of thermal homeostasis in cold and heat exposure requires intact, normally functioning adrenal cortices (37). Glucocorticoids regulate fasting gluconeogenesis via protein catabolism, act permissively on lipolysis, and maintain the reactivity of the cardiovascular system to catecholamines. Exposure to cold led to hypertrophy of the adrenal cortex and increased secretion of glucocorticoids (37). Adrenalectomized rats maintained on 1% salt could not maintain or restore body temperature in the cold. Rhesus monkeys (31) and baboons (38) placed in 5 and 6°C for six and ten weeks, respectively, showed a persistent increase in urinary 17-ketogenic steroid excretion, reflecting greater glucocorticoid secretion. This may be related to stimulation of gluconeogenesis in support of the 20 to 30% rise in resting metabolic rate. The doubling of food intake in the cold would increase protein substrate for mandatory catabolism. In this connection, when lightly clad men were exposed to 13°C for 48 hrs, rectal temperature fell significantly and plasma cortisol levels were altered (35). The associated fall in plasma tryptophan and tyrosine, and rise in urinary metabolites of tryptophan, suggest that hepatic enzymes catabolic to protein had been activated. In general, cold exposure stimulates secretion of glucocorticoids (27), whereas heat exposure suppresses secretion (27), at least until internal temperature rises to a critical threshold of hyperthermia (26). In men unacclimated to heat, acute heat exposure led to progressive hyperthermia, and when internal temperature exceeded 38.3°C, plasma cortisol rose significantly (26). In contrast, heat-acclimated men exposed to the same conditions did not become hyperthermic and plasma cortisol did not rise (26). Thermal displacement of the POAH alters plasma cortisol via the hypothalamic-pituitary axis. Local POAH cooling led to elevated plasma cortisol in baboons (39), dogs (25), and cats (95), but not goats (3). Local POAH warming led to a fall in plasma cortisol in baboons (89), caused little change in cats (95), and produced a transient elevation in dogs (24).

HORMONAL, OSMOTIC, AND BARORECEPTOR INFLUENCES ON THERMOREGULATION

Nonthermal as well as thermal modalities converge on the hypothalamic controller to modify temperature regulation. For example, the activity of the reticular activating system in adjusting the level of alertness of the cerebral cortex, as in sleep vs wakefulness, alters the sensitivity of the hypothalamus to peripheral thermal input (3, 44, 55). Most recently it has been suggested that sensory inputs related to other hypothalamically regulated vegetative functions also interact importantly in thermoregulation. Thus, plasma levels of certain steroids (progesterone, estradiol, cortisol) (28, 36, 94, 111), plasma osmolarity or Na^+ concentration (43, 86, 101), and level of blood pressure (22, 81) are modalities continuously monitored in the diencephalon which interact with thermal sensory input in regulation of body temperature.

Steroids and prostaglandins.—It has been recognized of over 100 years that early morning (basal) temperature of ovulating women is about 0.75°C higher during the luteal phase of the menstrual cycle, i.e. when progesterone is secreted from the corpus luteum. Although there is no direct evidence for progesterone's site of action in elevating basal temperature (36, 94), it has been proposed that the steroid acts on the hypothalamus to raise the thermal set point (28). It is unlikely that a peripheral action to increase heat production would per se elevate basal temperature, since heat dissipation mechanisms would prevent a rise in core temperature. Progesterone might act analogously to leucocytic pyrogen, i.e. to elevate regulated temperature by directly facilitating interneurons of the thermoregulatory effector system (32). More likely, however, since progesterone has important feedback effects on hypothalamic regulation of pituitary gonadotrophins (111), the central effects are mediated by specific protein receptors in the cytoplasm of specialized chemoreceptor neurons. Therefore, a simplified explanation is that progesterone-sensitive neurons in the anterior hypothalamus facilitate the activity of interneurons linking primary thermoreceptors in the POAH with heat gain and conservation motor centers in the posterior hypothalamus (Figure 1). Estradiol may act in a reverse manner to lower the regulated level of internal temperature, inasmuch as this steroid lowers basal temperature about 1°C in rats (111). Because estradiol acts on neurons in the POAH and basal hypothalamus to modulate gonadotrophin secretion, it is plausible that neurons specifically receptive to estradiol also mediate the changes in food intake, energy expenditure, and body temperature which are correlated with the surge of estrogen secretion during the rat estrous cycle, shown by Brobeck, Wheatland & Strominger in 1948 (111). Thus, estradiol might lower basal temperature by inhibiting the interneurons linking the POAH thermoreceptors with heat gain and conservation effectors.

Cortisol also influences internal temperature by inhibiting the febrile response to bacterial pyrogen (23), as shown by microinjection of the steroid into the POAH. Inasmuch as cortisol is believed to exert negative feedback on the anterior hypothalamus to block pituitary ACTH by inhibiting CRH release, it is plausible to envisage mediation of its thermoregulatory action by a specific chemoreceptor. The temperature effect of cortisol might be similar to that of estradiol, i.e. inhibition of interneurons mediating heat gain and conservation. In addition, cortisol may prevent the febrile response by stabilizing the membranes of interneurons against leucocytic pyrogen. Etiocholanolone, a metabolite of androgens, causes fever apparently by stimulating formation of leucocytic pyrogen, which then acts on the POAH (6).

Finally, prostaglandins (PG) injected in very small amounts (ng) into the POAH of rabbits (104) produce very rapid thermogenic responses, e.g., shivering and vasoconstriction, leading to prompt rise in internal temperature. Unlike steroids, these fatty acid derivatives are present in all cells, and appear to mediate inhibitory actions. Thus, it is possible that PG E_1 may interdict the inhibitory neurotransmitter function of NE, presumably released by primary warmth receptors at the interneuron (52, 108). In this schema, disinhibition (by PG E_1) of the interneuron from POAH suppression would lead to a rise in internal temperature.

Plasma osmolarity or Na+ concentration.—Conventionally, two thermal inputs, mean skin temperature and mean core temperature (including POAH temperature), converge on the hypothalamic controller to determine thermoregulatory effector output (44). However, when man exercises in warm T_a, the rate of sweating does not correlate with either mean skin or core temperature (43, 86, 101). Apparently, the rise in plasma osmolarity secondary to dehydration incurred before (43) or during exercise (101), or by ingesting saline (86), leads to an elevation in regulated internal temperature. Conversely, hyperhydration and resultant lowering of plasma osmolarity is associated with a fall in regulated internal temperature during rest or exercise (43, 86, 101). Snellen has hypothesized that during exercise in man, heat content of the body rather than body temperature per se may be regulated (101). He has proposed that plasma osmolarity, or perhaps more accurately, plasma Na+

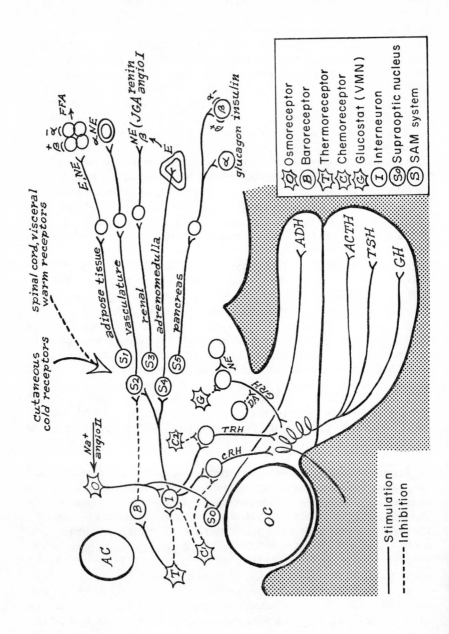

concentration, may be "read" by central osmoreceptors as a derivative of body mass. Integration by the hypothalamic controller of derived body mass with mean body temperature yields instantaneous heat content. Thus, continuous monitoring of plasma osmolarity (or Na^+ concentration) by hypothalamic osmoreceptors is suggested as a sensory modality which, upon integration with thermal, chemical, and psychological inputs, determines thermoregulatory effector output. Recently neurons specifically sensitive to hypertonic NcCl have been identified in the POAH of conscious monkeys (51).

Hyperosmolarity of plasma is believed to stimulate hypothalamic osmoreceptors to reflexly release antidiuretic hormone (ADH) from the neurohypophysis and also to elicit thirst (4). In addition, activation of hypothalamic Na^+ receptors by plasma hyperosmolarity may facilitate the elevation by the interneuron of regulated level of body temperature. The associated increase in

---

←◀◀◀

FIGURE 1. The schema depicts hypothetical interactions between thermal and nonthermal modalities regulating body temperature in the hypothalamus. Primary warmth receptor T tonically inhibits interneuron I, which in turn drives SAM effector cells in the posterior hypothalamus. The SAM neuron pool subserves five general functions: (a) lipolysis, (b) cardiovascular homeostasis, (c) renin release from the juxtaglomerular apparatus (JGA) in the kidney, (d) epinephrine release from the adrenal medulla, (e) modulation of insulin and glucagon secretion from the endocrine pancreas. The SAM effector pool, or interneuron I, or both, are facilitated by cutaneous cold receptors and inhibited by cutaneous, spinal cord, and visceral warmth receptors. The osmoreceptor O mediates reflex release of ADH from the neurohypophysis in response to plasma hyperosmolarity (or rise in Na^+), and also may elevate the regulated level of internal temperature by facilitating interneuron I. Increased SAM output to the renal JGA releases renin causing formation of angiotensin I and II. Angiotensin II acts on the osmoreceptor to facilitate entrance of Na^+ and thus increases the sensitivity (gain) of the system. Primary warmth receptor T facilitates the baroreceptor reflexogenic neuron in the POAH, and thereby modulates baroreceptor sensory input. Thus, during POAH warming, hypotension and bradycardia occur in parallel with fall in the body temperature, whereas during POAH cooling hypertension and tachycardia parallel the rise in body temperature. Progesterone, estradiol, and cortisol bind to receptors in cytoplasm of chemoreceptors C which in turn may facilitate or inhibit interneuron I to alter internal temperature. Leucocytic pyrogen acts directly on I to produce fever. Cortisol and thyroid hormones may exert feedback actions via similar chemoreceptors on neurons synthesizing releasing hormones (CRH, TRH) to regulate pituitary secretion. Elevation in plasma glucose, monitored by glucostat G, inhibits noradrenergic stimulation of GRH, which is also inhibited by dopaminergic axo-axonal nerve linkage. Although not shown, chemoreception of estradiol and progesterone regulates pituitary secretion of gonadotropins. Primary warmth receptors influence ACTH and TSH secretion by altering the level of activity of interneuron I. In adipose tissue and the beta cell of the pancreatic islets, beta-adrenergic receptors stimulate lipolysis and insulin release, respectively, whereas alpha-adrenergic receptors are inhibitory. Adrenergic regulation of alpha cells of the pancreatic islets remains to be elucidated.

SAM outflow to the renal juxtaglomerular apparatus would stimulate beta-adrenergic receptors, directly by sympathetic nerves or indirectly by circulating E, to release renin. The resulting formation of angiotensin I and II in the circulation would act homeostatically by (*a*) stimulating release of aldosterone to conserve Na^+ and thus restore contracted extracellular space, (*b*) facilitating the entrance of Na^+ into the hypothalamic osmoreceptor, thereby increasing central sensitivity or gain, and (*c*) stimulating thirst by central dipsogenic action of angiotensin II (4). It is also possible that contracted blood volume secondary to dehydration would stimulate atrial volume receptors to reflexly increase SAM outflow.

The suggestion has been made that the ratio of Na^+ to Ca^{2+} in the posterior hypothalamus determines the thermal set point (82), since microinjections of Na^+ lowered internal temperature, and Ca^{2+} elevated internal temperature in conscious monkeys. In view of the very high concentrations of electrolytes injected, however, these thermal responses may reflect nonspecific stimulation by Na^+ and inhibition by Ca^{2+} of heat gain-heat conservation neural pathways. The hypothesis that osmo- or Na^+ receptors continuously monitor a derivative of body mass, which upon integration with mean body temperature yields the regulated parameter of heat content, is supported by experimental documentation of Na^+ sensitive receptors in the POAH (51) and by the fact that alterations in regulated internal temperature resulted from physiological changes in plasma osmolarity, e.g. by dehydration during exercise.

Baroreceptor influence on temperature.—Recent evidence indicates that the reflex regulation of blood pressure and heart rate by the autonomic nervous system is intimately related to homeostatic control of internal temperature. Local cooling of the POAH of conscious baboons and rhesus monkeys leads to regulated rises in blood pressure (50, 81), heart rate (81), and internal temperature (50, 81), while warming of the POAH of conscious baboons lowers blood pressure, heart rate, and internal temperature (81). The changes in blood pressure of 15 to 20 mm Hg evoked by POAH cooling and warming are of sufficient magnitude to elicit baroreceptor reflex alteration in heart rate. However, the finding that heart rate rose during the hypertension of POAH cooling and fell during the hypotension of POAH warming suggests that POAH thermoreceptors can override the effect of sensory input from the carotid sinus and aortic arch on central reflexogenic neurons. Recent evidence (53) indicates the existence of neurons in the POAH which mediate baroreceptor reflex control of blood pressure and heart rate, and has led to the suggestion that the neural network integrating reflex regulation of blood pressure and heart rate extends from the medulla oblongata through the basal brain stem to the POAH. Thus, primary thermoreceptors in the POAH may modify or reverse baroreceptor sensory input by facilitating reflexogenic cells in the POAH during central warming, or by inhibiting them during central cooling. It is likely that thermally initiated inhibition or facilitation of the baroreceptor reflex is also mediated via reflexogenic neurons in the medulla, since local cooling and warming in the medulla of conscious monkeys produced similar cardiovascular changes (22).

That spinal cord cooling and warming evoked parallel changes in blood pressure, heart rate, and internal temperature comparable to those during POAH (81) and medullary thermal displacement (22), suggests that thermoreceptors in the spinal cord project sensory pathways to the medulla and POAH. The observed synchronous changes in cardiovascular and thermal parameters probably can not occur without participation of the hypothalamic controller. Although the comparatively large changes in POAH temperature, about 1 to 1.5°C, required to alter blood pressure, heart rate, and internal temperature in conscious primates (50, 81) suggest a relative thermal insensitivity, more moderate temperature displacement in the POAH selectively altered blood flow in the descending abdominal aorta without altering blood pressure or heart rate (67). This response is presumably due to the extreme sensitivity of cutaneous vasomotor tone to POAH temperature change. Thus, the rise in abdominal aortic flow may be viewed as a compensatory response to cutaneous vasodilatation and increased skin blood flow (67).

Hypothalamic integration of thermoregulation with cardiovascular regulation has been shown by another experimental method, namely, central infusion of biogenic amines. Infusion of NE into the POAH of conscious baboons led to a 1.2°C fall in internal temperature which correlated temporally with cutaneous vasodilatation, fall in blood pressure and heart rate, and decline in plasma glycerol (measured as an index of lipolysis) (108). The SAM suppression indicated by these synchronous responses and the evocation of such responses by POAH warming in baboons (89) further suggest a role for NE as a hypothalamic heat loss neurotransmitter (52). Approximately one hour after central NE infusion, hypothermic baboons restored their internal temperature in association with cutaneous vasoconstriction, shivering, rise in blood pressure and heart rate, increase in plasma glucose and glycerol (reflecting mobilization of both carbohydrate and lipid substrates, and a rise in urinary catecholamines (108). Thus, restoration of temperature was associated with a generalized increase in SAM activity.

The action of hypothalamically infused NE in supressing SAM activity and lowering blood pressure suggests that this central neurotransmitter may normally exert a direct negative feedback action on the SAM system. Thus, NE released endogenously from adrenergic terminals in the brain may act to prevent systemic hypertension. Indeed, it has been suggested that the antihypertensive drug, catapressin, mimics the central action of NE, i.e. it stimulates alpha-adrenergic receptors (108). The hypothermic, hypotensive response of baboons to hypothalamically infused NE appears to be specific for the POAH. When NE was microinjected into or near the ventromedial nucleus in the basal hypothalamus in conscious baboons, internal temperature, blood pressure, and heart rate were not altered, but growth hormone was consistently released from the anterior pituitary (107). In contrast, infusion of dopamine into the third brain ventricle of conscious baboons led to a selective inhibition of growth hormone secretion (108).

Two examples of chemical messengers contributing to metabolic regulation in a hibernating mammal and a poikilothermic vertebrate have been cited which suggest at least the possibility of analogous functions in higher mammals: Ground squirrels can be induced to enter hibernation in the summer if infused iv with plasma from spontaneously hibernating ground squirrels, thus demonstrating a blood borne hibernating trigger (29); and metabolism is suppressed by an antimetabolite extracted from the brains of estivating lungfish (105). Elucidating the significance of these mechanisms to higher mammals remains a challenge for future research.

LITERATURE CITED

1. Adair, E. R. 1971. Evaluation of some controller inputs to behavioral temperature regulation. *Int. J. Biometeorol.* 15:121-25
2. Alvarez, M. B., Johnson, H. D. 1970. Urinary excretion of adrenaline and noradrenaline in cattle during heat and cold exposure. *J. Dairy Sci.* 53:928-30
3. Andersson, B. 1970. Central nervous and hormonal interaction in temperature regulation of the goat. *Physiological and Behavioral Temperature Regulation,* ed. J. D. Hardy, A. P. Gagge, J. A. J. Stolwijk, 634-47. Springfield: Thomas
4. Andersson, B., Eriksson, L. 1971. Conjoint action of sodium and angiotensin on brain mechanisms controlling water and salt balance. *Acta Physiol. Scand.* 81:18-29
5. Andersen, H. T., Christiansen, E. N., Gray, H. J., Pedersen, J. I. 1971. Mitochondrial regulation of thermogenesis in brown adipose tissue. *J. Physiol. Paris* 63: 194-97
6. Atkins, E., Bodel, P. 1972. Fever. *N. Engl. J. Med.* 286:27-34
7. Baldwin, B. A., Ingram, D. L., LeBlanc, J. A. 1969. The effects of environmental temperature and hypothalamic temperature on excretion of catecholamines in the urine of the pig. *Brain Res.* 16:511-15
8. Bakke, J. L., Lawrence, N. L. 1971. Effects of cold adaptation, rewarming and heat exposure on thyrotropin (TSH) secretion in rats. *Endocrinology* 89:204-12
9. Bartůňková, R., Janský, L., Mejsnar, J. 1971. Nonshivering thermogenesis and cold adaptation. *Nonshivering Thermogenesis,* ed. L. Janský, 39-56. Prague: Academia
10. Bass, D. E. 1958. Metabolic and energy balance of men in a cold environment. *Transactions of 6th Conference on Cold Injury,* ed. S. M. Horvath, 317-38. New York: J. Macy, Jr. Foundation. 375 pp.
11. Baum, D., Gale, C. C., Dillard, D. H. 1968. Plasma growth hormone in the infant undergoing deep hypothermic cardiovascu-

lar surgery. *Proc. Soc. Exp. Biol. Med.* 138:70-75
12. Bligh, J., Moore, R. E., Ed. 1972. *Essays on Temperature Regulation.* Amsterdam: North-Holland. 186 pp.
13. Brown, A. C., Brengelman, G. L. 1970. The interaction of peripheral and central inputs in the temperature regulation system. *Physiological and Behavioral Temperature Regulation,* ed. J. D. Hardy, A. P. Gagge, J. A. J. Stolwijk, 684-702. Springfield: Thomas
14. Brück, K., Wunnerberg, W., Zeisberger, E. 1969. Comparison of cold-adaptive metabolic modifications in different species, with special reference to the miniature pig. *Fed. Proc.* 28:1035-41
15. Bulychev, A., Kramar, R., Drahota, Z., Lindberg, O. 1972. Role of specific endogenous fatty acid fraction in the coupling-uncoupling mechanism of oxidative phosphorylation of brown adipose tissue. *Exp. Cell Res.* 72:169-87
16. Cabanac, M., Ed. 1971. Symposium International de Thermorégulation Comportementale, Lyon. *J. Physiol. Paris* 63:187-472
17. Cannon, B. 1971. Control of fatty-acid oxidation in brown-adipose-tissue mitochondria. *Eur. J. Biochem.* 23:125-35
17a. Cannon, W. B., Querido, A., Britton, S. W., Bright, E. M. 1926. The role of adrenal secretion in the chemical control of body temperature. *Am. J. Physiol.* 79: 466-507
18. Carlisle, H. J. 1971. Behavioral temperature regulation in cynomolgus and pig-tailed macaques (I). *J. Physiol Paris* 63: 226-28
19. Carlson, L. D. 1969. Temperature regulation and acclimation. Brody Memorial Lecture IX, 1-27. *Special Report, Univ. Missouri, Columbia*
19a. Carlson, L. D. 1973. Central and peripheral mechanisms in temperature regulation. *The Pharmacology of Thermoregulation,* ed. P. Lomax, E. Schönbaum, 7-21. Basel, Switzerland: Karger

20. Chaffee, R. R. J., Allen, J. R. 1972. Studies on resting metabolic rate (RMR), nonshivering thermogenesis (NST), thermoneutral zone (TNZ) and survival to temperature extremes in cold and heat acclimated *Macaca mulatta*. *Comp. Biochem. Physiol.* 40B. In press

21. Chaffee, R. R. J., Roberts, J. C. 1971. Temperature acclimation in birds and mammals. *Ann. Rev. Physiol.* 33:155–202

22. Chai, C. Y., Lin, M. T. 1972. Effects of heating and cooling the spinal cord and medulla oblongata on thermoregulation in monkeys. *J. Physiol. London.* 225:297–308

23. Chowers, I., Conforti, N., Feldman, S. 1968. Local effect of cortisol in the preoptic area on temperature regulation. *Am. J. Physiol.* 214:538–42

24. Chowers, I., Hammel, H. T., Eisenman, J., Abrams, R. M., McCann, S. M. 1966. Comparison of effect of environmental and preoptic heating and pyrogen on plasma cortisol. *Am. J. Physiol.* 210:606–10

25. Chowers, I., Hammel, H. T., Stromme, S. B., McCann, S. M. 1964. Comparison of effect of environmental and preoptic cooling on plasma cortisol levels. *Am. J. Physiol.* 207:577–82

26. Collins, K. J., Few, J. D., Forward, T. J., Giec, L. A. 1969. Stimulation of adrenal corticoid secretion in man by raising the body temperature. *J. Physiol. London* 202:645–60

27. Collins, K. J., Weiner, J. S. 1968. Endocrinological aspects of exposure to high environmental temperatures. *Physiol. Rev.* 48:785–839

28. Cunningham, D. J., Cabanac, M. 1971. Evidence from behavioral thermoregulatory responses of a shift in setpoint temperature related to the menstrual cycle. *J. Physiol. Paris* 63:236–38

29. Dawe, A. R. 1973. Autopharmacology of hibernation. *The Pharmacology of Temperature Regulation*, ed. P. Lomax, E. Schönbaum, 359–63. Basel, Switzerland: Karger.

30. Dulac, S., Jobin, M. 1972. Comparison of plasma disappear-ance of triiodothyronine and thyroxine in rats. *Proc. Can. Fed. Biol. Sec. 15* Abstr. 127

31. Ehle, A. L., Mougey, E. H., Wherry, F. E., Mason, J. W. 1971. Multiple endocrine responses to cold exposure in the monkey. *Physiologist* 14:138

32. Eisenman, J. 1972. Unit activity studies of thermo-responsive neurons. *Essays on Temperature Regulation*, ed. J. Bligh, R. E. Moore, 55–69. Amsterdam: North-Holland. 186 pp.

33. von Euler, U. S. 1964. Quantitation of stress by catecholamine analysis. *Clin. Pharmacol. Ther.* 5:398–404

34. Fisher, D. A., Odell, W. D. 1971. Effect of cold on TSH secretion in man. *J. Clin. Endocrinol. Metab.* 33:859–62

35. Francesconi, R. P., Boyd, A. E., Mager, M. 1972. Human tryptophan and tyrosine metabolism: effects of acute exposure to cold stress. *J. Appl. Physiol.* 33:165–169

36. Freeman, M. E., Crissman, J. K., Jr., Louw, G. N., Butcher, R. L., Inskeep, E. K. 1970. Thermogenic action of progestrone in the rat. *Endocrinology* 86:717–20

37. Fregly, M. J. 1973. Hormonal interactions in thermoregulation. *The Limbic System*, ed. G. J. Mogenson, F. R. Calaresu. Toronto: Univ. Toronto Press. In press

38. Gale, C. C. et al 1972. Endocrine responses to chronic cold exposure in baboon. *Physiologist* 15:141

39. Gale, C. C., Jobin, M., Proppe, D. W., Notter, D., Fox, H. 1970. Endocrine thermoregulatory responses to local hypothalamic cooling in unanesthetized baboons. *Am. J. Physiol.* 219:193–201

40. Gale, C. C., Mathews, M., Young, J. 1970. Behavioral thermoregulatory responses to hypothalamic cooling and warming in baboons. *Physiol. Behav.* 5:1–6

41. Gale, C. C., Muramoto, K., Toivola, P. T. K., Stiner, D. 1971. Sympathetic control of substrates and thermogenesis during central cooling. *Int. J.*

Biometeorol. 15:162–67

42. Gale, C. C., Williams, R., Toivola, P. 1971. Thyroid-sympathetic nervous system interactions in thermoregulation. *Acta Endocrinol. Suppl.* 155:34

43. Greenleaf, J. E. 1973. Blood electrolytes and exercise in relation to temperature regulation in man. *The Pharmacology of Temperature Regulation*, ed. P. Lomax, E. Schönbaum, 72–89. Basel, Switzerland: Karger.

44. Hammel, H. T. 1968. Regulation of internal body temperature. *Ann. Rev. Physiol.* 30:641–710

45. Häggendal, J., Hartley, L. H., Saltin, B. 1970. Arterial noradrenaline concentration during exercise in relation to the relative work levels. *Scand. J. Clin. Lab. Invest.* 26:337–42

46. Hahn, P. M., Hoshizaki, T., Adey, W. R. 1971. Circadian rhythms of the *Macaca nemestrina* monkey in Biosatellite III. *Aerosp. Med.* 42:295–304

47. Hardy, J. D., Gagge, A. P., Stolwijk, J. A. J., Eds. 1970. *Physiology and Behavioral Thermoregulation.* Springfield: Thomas. 944 pp.

48. Hart, J. S. 1964. Geography and season: mammals and birds. Adaptation to the environment. *Handbook of Physiology*, ed. D. B. Dill, E. F. Adolph, C. G. Wilber, 295–321. Washington, DC: Am. Physiol. Soc.

49. Hartner, W. C., South, F. E. 1972. Effect of chronically lowered preoptic area temperature on metabolism in rat. *Fed. Proc.* 31:889

50. Hayward, J. N., Baker, M. A. 1968. Diuretic and thermoregulatory response to preoptic cooling in the monkey. *Am. J. Physiol.* 214:843–50

50a. Hayward, J. N., Baker, M. A. 1968. Role of cerebral arterial blood in the regulation of brain temperature in the monkey. *Am. J. Physiol.* 215:389–403

51. Hayward, J. N., Vincent, J. D. 1970. Osmosensitive single neurons in the hypothalamus of unanesthetized monkeys. *J. Physiol. London* 210:947–72

52. Hellon, R., 1972. Central transmitters and thermoregulation. *Essays on Temperature Regula-*

tion, ed. J. Bligh, R. E. Moore, 71–85. Amsterdam: North-Holland. 186 pp.

53. Hilton, S. M., Spyer, K. M. 1971. Participation of the anterior hypothalamus in the baroreceptor reflex. *J. Physiol. London* 218:271–93

54. Himms-Hagen, J. 1972. Lipid metabolism during cold exposure and during cold-acclimation. *Lipids* 7:310–23

55. Hunter, W. S., Adams, T. 1971. Interactions of skin and hypothalamic temperatures as inputs to thermoregulation in the unanesthetized cat. *Physiologist* 14:166

56. Huikko, M., Jouppila, P., Kärki, N. T. 1966. Effect of Finnish bath (sauna) on the urinary excretion of noradrenaline, adrenaline, and 3-methoxy-4-hydroxy-mandelic acid. *Acta Physiol. Scand.* 66:316–21

57. Ingbar, S. H., Bass, D. E. 1957. Effects of prolonged exposure to cold on production and degradation of thyroid hormone in man. *J. Endocrinol.* 15:ii–iii

58. Ismail-Beigi, F., Edelman, I. S. 1970. Mechanism of thyroid calorigenesis: role of active sodium transport. *Proc. Nat. Acad. Sci. USA* 61:1071–78

59. Ismail-Beigi, F., Edelman, I. S. 1971. The mechanism of the calorigenic action of thyroid hormone. *J. Gen. Physiol.* 57:710–22

60. Janský, L., Ed. 1971. *Nonshivering Thermogenesis.* Prague: Academia. 310 pp.

60a. Janský, L., Hart, J. S. 1968. Cardiac output and organ blood flow in warm- and cold-acclimated rats exposed to cold. *Can. J. Physiol. Pharmacol.* 46:653–59

61. Jessen, C., Mayer, E. T. 1971. Spinal cord and hypothalamus as core sensors of temperature in the conscious dog. I. Equivalence of responses. *Pfluegers Arch.* 324:189–204

62. Jessen, C., McLean, J. A., Calvert, D. T., Findlay, J. D. 1972. Balanced and unbalanced temperature signals generated in spinal cord of the ox. *Am. J. Physiol.* 222:1343–47

63. Jobin, M., Endröczi, E., Hon-

tela, S., Fortier, C. 1971. Effect of hypothalamic cooling on the behaviour and the pituitary-thyroid activity of the rat. *J. Physiol. Paris* 63:309–11

64. Johnson, G. E., Flattery, K. V., Schönbaum. E. 1967. The influence of methimazole on the catecholamine excretion of cold-stressed rats. *Can. J. Physiol. Pharmacol.* 45:415–21

65. Joy, R. T. J. 1963. Responses of cold acclimatized men to infused norepinephrine. *J. Appl. Physiol.* 18:1209–12

66. Kang, B. S. et al 1970. Calorigenic action of norepinephrine in the Korean women divers. *J. Appl. Physiol.* 29:6–9

67. Kastella K. G., Brown, A. C. 1970. Effect of hypothalamic temperature waveforms on peripheral blood flow in the baboon. *Am. J. Physiol.* 29:499–507

67a. Klussman, F. W., Pierau, Fr.-K. 1972. Extra-hypothalamic deep body thermosensitivity. *Essays on Temperature Regulation*, ed. J. Bligh, R. E. Moore, 87–104. Amsterdam: North-Holland. 186 pp.

68. Kuba, K., Tomita, T. 1971. Noradrenaline action on nerve terminal in rat diaphragm. *J. Physiol. London* 217:19–31

69. LeBlanc, J. A., Nadeau, G. 1961. Urinary excretion of adrenaline and noradrenaline in normal and cold-adapted animals. *Can. J. Biochem. Physiol.* 39:215–17

70. LeBlanc, J., Villemaire, A. 1970. Thyroxine and noradrenaline on noradrenaline sensitivity, cold resistance, and brown fat. *Am. J. Physiol.* 218:1742–45

71. Leduc, J. 1961. Catecholamine production and release in exposure and acclimation to cold. *Acta Physiol. Scand.* 53:Suppl. 183, 1–101

72. Lipton, J. M. 1971. Behavioral temperature regulation in the rat: Effects of thermal stimulation of the medulla. *J. Physiol. Paris* 63:325–28

73. Lomax. P., Schönbaum, E., Eds. 1973. *The Pharmacology of Thermoregulation.* Basel, Switzerland: Karger. In press

74. Lutherer, L. O., Fregly, M. J., Anton, A. H. 1969. An interrela-tionship between theophylline and catecholamines in the hypothyroid rat acutely exposed to cold. *Fed. Proc.* 28:1238–42

75. Mager, M., Robinson, S. M. 1969. Substrate mobilization and utilization in fasting men during cold exposure. *Bull. NJ Acad. Sci.*, Special Symposium Issue, 26–30

75a. Magnus-Levy, A. 1895. Über den respiratorischen Gaswechsel unter dem Einfluss der Thyreoidia sowie unter verschiedenen pathologischen Zuständen. *Berlin Klin. Wschr.* 32:650

76. Maher, J. T., Bass, D. E., Heistad, D. D., Angelakos, E. T., Hartley, L. H. 1972. Effect of posture on heat acclimatization in man. *J. Appl. Physiol.* In press

77. Martin, J. B., Reichlin, S. 1971. Neural regulation of the pituitary-thyroid axis. *Proc. 6th Midwest Thyroid Meeting,* 1–24. Columbia, Mo.: Univ. Missouri Press

78. Mason, J. W. 1971. A re-evaluation of the concept of 'non-specificity" in stress theory. *J. Psychiat. Res.* 8:323–33

79. Melander, A. 1970. Amines and mouse thyroid activity. *Acta Endocrinol.* 65:371–384

80. Melander, A., Nilsson, E., Sundler, F. 1972. Thyroid hormone secretion induced by sympathetic stimulation. *Acta Physiol. Scand.* 84:43A

81. Morishima, M. S., Gale, C. C. 1972. Relationship of blood pressure and heart rate to body temperature in baboons. *Am. J. Physiol.* 223:387–95

82. Myers, R. D., Yaksh, T. L. 1971. Thermoregulation around a new "set-point" established in the monkey by altering the ratio of sodium to calcium ions within the hypothalamus. *J. Physiol. London* 218:509–33

83. Nagasaka, T., Carlson, L. D. 1971. Effects of blood temperature and perfused norepinephrine on vascular reponses of rabbit ear. *Am. J. Physiol.* 220:289–92

84. Nakayama, T., Hori, T., Nagasaka, T., Tokura, H., Takadi, E. 1971. Thermal and metabolic responses in the Japanese monkey at temperatures of 5–38°C. *J.*

Appl. Physiol. 31:332–37
85. Nejad, I. F., Bollinger, J. A., Mitnick, M. A., Reichlin, S. 1972. Importance of T₂ (triiodothyronine) secretion in altered states of thyroid function in the rat: cold exposure, subtotal thyroidectomy, and hypophysectomy. *Trans. Assoc. Am. Physicians.* In press
86. Nielsen, B., Hansen, G., Jorgensen, S. O., Nielsen, E. 1971. Thermoregulation in exercising man during dehydration and hyperhydration with water and saline. *Int. J. Biometeorol.* 15: 195–200
87. Olsson, K. 1969. Studies on central regulation of secretion of antidiuretic hormone (ADH) in the goat. *Acta Physiol. Scand.* 77:465–74
88. Paul, P., Holmes, W. L. 1972. Free fatty acid metabolism in thyroidectomized and normal dogs during rest and acute cold exposure—shivering. *J. Appl. Physiol.* In press
89. Proppe, D. W., Gale, C. C. 1970. Endocrine thermoregulatory responses to local hypothalamic warming in unanesthetized baboons. *Am. J. Physiol.* 219: 202–7
90. Rawson, R. O., Quick, K. P. 1972. Localization of intra-abdominal thermoreceptors in the ewe. *J. Physiol. London.* 222:665–77
90a. Reichlin, S. 1964. Function of the hypothalamus in regulation of pituitary-thyroid activity. *Brain-Thyroid Relationships. Ciba Foundation Study Group No. 18,* ed. M. P. Cameron, M. O'Connor, 17–34. Boston: Little, Brown
91. Reichlin, S. et al 1972. The hypothalamus in pituitary-thyroid regulation. *Recent Progr. Horm. Res.* 28:229–77
92. Rosenqvist, U. 1972. Adrenergic receptor response in hypothyroidism: an in vitro study on human adipose tissue and rabbit aorta. *Acta Med. Scand., Suppl.* 532:1–28
93. Rosenqvist, U., Efendíc, S., Jereb, B. Östman, J. 1971. Influence of the hypothyroid state on lipolysis in human adipose tissue in vitro. *Acta Med. Scand.* 189: 381–84

94. Rothchild, I. 1969. The physiological basis for the temperature raising effect of progesterone. *Metabolic Effects of Gonadal Hormones and Contraceptive Steroids,* ed. H. A. Salhanick, D. M. Kipnis, R. L. Vande Wiele, 668–675. New York, Plenum, 762 pp.
94a. Rubner, M. 1902. *Die Gesetze des Energieverbrauch bei der Ernährung.* Leipzig und Wien: Franz Denticke. 426 pp.
95. Ruch, W. et al 1972. CNS-endocrine interactions in thermoregulation. *Fed. Proc.* 31: 139
96. Schönbaum, E., Johnson, G. E., Sellers, E. A., Gill, M. J. 1966. Adrenergic β-receptors and nonshivering thermogenesis. *Nature* 210:426
97. Simon, E. Iriki, M. 1971. Sensory transmission of spinal heat and cold sensitivity in ascending spinal neurons. *Pfluegers Arch.* 328:103–20
98. Shum, A., Johnson, G. E., Flattery, K. V. 1969. Influence of ambient temperature on excretion of catecholamines and metabolites. *Am. J. Physiol.* 216: 1164–69
99. Shum, A., Johnson, G. E., Flattery, K. L. 1970. Influence of ganglionic blockade on catecholamine and metabolite excretion. *Am. J. Physiol.* 219: 58–61
100. Smith, R. E., Hannon, J. P., Shields, J. C., Horwitz, B. A., Eds. 1972. *Bioenergetics. Proceedings of the International Symposium on Environmental Physiology, Dublin.* Washington: Federation of American Societies for Experimental Biology. 195 pp.
101. Snellen, J. W. 1972. Set point and exercise. *Essays on Temperature Regulation,* ed. J. Bligh, R. E. Moore, 139–48. Amsterdam: North-Holland. 186 pp.
102. South, F. E., Hannon, J. P., Willis, J. S., Pengelley, E., Alpert, N. R., Eds. 1972. *Hibernation and Hypothermia, Perspectives and Challenges,* Amsterdam: Elsevier. 1743 pp.
103. Steiner, G. 1973. Biochemical basis and regulation of thermogenesis. *The Pharmacology of*

Thermoregulation, ed. P. Lomax, E. Schönbaum, 42–56. Basel, Switzerland: Karger

104. Stitt, J. T., Hardy, J. D. 1972. Effect of prostaglandin E_1 injected into the brainstem on the body temperature of rabbits. *Fed. Proc.* 31:831

105. Swan, H., Jenkins, D. Knox, K. 1968. Antimetabolic extract from the brain of *Protoperus aethiopicus*. *Nature* 217:671

106. Tanche, M., Therminarias, A. 1969. Thyroxine and catecholamines during cold exposure in dogs. *Fed. Proc.* 28:1257–61

107. Toivola, P. T. K., Gale, C. C. 1972. Stimulation of growth hormone release by microinjection of norepinephrine into hypothalamus of baboons. *Endocrinology* 90:895–902

108. Toivola, P., Gale, C. C. 1970. Effect on temperature of biogenic amine infusion into hypothalamus of baboons. *Neuroendocrinology* 6:210–19

108a. Totel, G. L., Johnson, R. E., Fay, F. A., Goldstein, J. A., Schick, J. 1971. Experimental hyperthermia in traumatic quadriplegia. *Int. J. Biometeor.* 15:346–55

109. Tromp, W. H., Weihe, W. H., Eds. 1972. Proceedings of the Symposium on Temperature Regulation, Dublin. *Int. J. Biometeorol.* 15:101–361

110. Ungerstedt, U. 1971. Stereotaxic mapping of the monoamine pathways in the rat brain. *Acta Physiol. Scand. Suppl.* 367:1–48

111. Wade, G. N. 1972. Gonadal hormones and behavioral regulation of body weight. *Physiol. Behav.* 8:523–34

112. Webster, A. J. F., Heitman, J. H., Hays, F. L., Olynyk, G. P. 1969. Catecholamines and cold thermogenesis. *Can. J. Physiol. Pharmacol.* 47:719–24

113. Whittow, G. C. 1968. Cardiovascular response to localized heating of the anterior hypothalamus. *J. Physiol. London.* 198:541–48

114. Whittow, G. C., Ed. 1970. *Comparative Physiology of Thermoregulation.* Vol. I: *Invertebrates and Nonmammalian Vertebrates.* New York: Academic. 333 pp.

115. Whittow, G. C., Ed. 1971. *Comparative Physiology of Thermoregulation.* Vol. II: *Mammals.* New York: Academic. 420 pp.

116. Wilber, J. F., Baum, D. 1970. Elevation of plasma TSH during surgical hypothermia. *J. Clin. Endocrinol.* 31:372–75

117. Wilber, J. F., Utiger, R. D. 1969. The effect of glucocorticoids on thyrotropin secretion. *J. Clin. Invest.* 48:2096–103

118. Wilson, O. 1966. Metabolic rate and thyroid function. Part VIII, A field study of physiological adjustment to increased muscular activity with and without cold exposure, ed. K. L. Andersen, O. Wilson, 1–43. *Acta Univ. Lund*, Lund, Gleerup.

119. Woeber, K. A., Harrison, W. A. 1971. Alterations in thyroid hormone economy during acute infection with *Diplococcus pneumoniae* in the rhesus monkey. *J. Clin. Invest.* 50:378–87

120. Christensen, N. J. 1972. Increased levels of plasma noradrenalin in hypothyroidism. *J. Clin. Endocrinol. Metab.* 35:359–63

Ann. Rev. Physiol. 1973. 35:431–452

SECRETION OF GASTROINTESTINAL HORMONES 1102

SVEN ANDERSSON

Department of Pharmacology, Karolinska Institutet, Stockholm, Sweden

Compared with development in other fields of hormone research, one must describe advances in the knowledge of gastrointestinal hormones as stumbling. The first evidence suggesting the existence of hormones in the mucosa of the gastrointestinal tract was provided by Bayliss & Starling—for secretin in 1902 (13), and by Edkins—for gastrin in 1905 (25). Apart from occasional important discoveries, gastrointestinal hormone research was then more or less dormant for almost 50 years. During this time there was much controversy as to whether the postulated hormones really existed; in fact, this debate continued until the hormones had been chemically identified and their specific biological actions subsequently demonstrated.

As a result of the participation of research workers from several different branches of medical science, a considerable amount of new information on gastrointestinal hormones has accumulated during the last ten years, and this has acted as a strong stimulus to further research in this area. Morphologists have provided evidence on particular cells in the mucosa of the gastrointestinal tract that might harbor various hormonal substances. Biochemists have succeeded in identifying, determining the structures of, and synthesizing the three "old" hormones, gastrin, secretin, and cholecystokinin-pancreozymin. Access to pure hormonal substances has made it possible for immunologists to work out sensitive and specific radioimmunoassays whereby the hormones can be detected and measured in tissues and body fluids.

WHAT ARE THE CRITERIA FOR A GASTROINTESTINAL HORMONE?

In recent years the number of possible candidates for new hormones has increased considerably. Evidence for a new gastrointestinal hormone has been based either on purely physiological observations or on the chemical isolation of a new agent from the gastrointestinal tract. It is therefore particularly important for the following discussion to decide criteria that must be fulfilled before an agent can be classified as a gastrointestinal hormone. By definition, a hormone is a discrete chemical substance secreted by a specific tissue and transported to a distant site where it exerts its effect upon other specific tissues. Thus, in order to prove the existence of a gastrointestinal hormone by physiological means one must show that the application of a physio-

431

logical stimulus to some part of the gastrointestinal tract causes a response in some other part of the tract or in some other organ, and that this effect persists when all neural connections between the two sites have been eliminated. It must also be shown that a stimulatory substance absorbed and transported by the body fluids is not itself the stimulus for the effector organ. To prove that a chemically isolated and identified substance is a hormone one must show that this substance is present in the stimulated organ, that it is released into the body fluids upon stimulation and that it has biological actions similar to those of the endogenous hormone. From Table 1 it is evident that only a limited number of postulated gastrointestinal hormones fulfil the criteria of a true hormone. In the group of "old" hormones four substances can be considered as established gastrointestinal hormones, namely cholecystokinin-pancreozymin (*CCK-PZ*), enterogastrone, gastrin, and secretin. The name enterocrinin was given to a principle extractable from the small intestine which had a stimulatory action on the secretion of fluid and enzymes by the small intestine (79). However, the physiological evidence that enterocrinin might be a gastrointestinal hormone is still incomplete. The recent findings (11) that several of the chemically identified gut polypeptides (e.g. gastric inhibitory polypeptide and vasoactive intestinal polypeptide) stimulate small intestinal secretions indicate that enterocrinin-like activity of intestinal extracts could be due to the presence of one or several such polypeptides.

Urogastrone has been isolated from the urine and is a well-known inhibitor of gastric acid secretion. Its inclusion in Table 1 may be questioned, since it is not known if it is derived from the gastrointestinal canal. On the other hand, it is in fact a highly active gastric inhibitory polypeptide (41) which is believed to constitute an excretory product of some endogenous inhibitory hormone. Hopefully, future work will show whether or not this assumption is correct.

The group of "new" hormones contains several substances which may be considered as presumptive gastrointestinal hormones. The evidence for a hormonal function of these agents is based on data that are either purely physiological or more or less purely biochemical. The existence of a specific inhibitory agent named bulbogastrone in the upper duodenum has been extensively documented in a series of physiological studies. This agent is released by a specific and physiological stimulus, it has specific actions on a target organ other than its site of origin, and its effect persists after removal of all nervous connections between the target organ and site of release. Bulbogastrone will therefore be discussed in the following review as a strong candidate for inclusion in the list of gastrointestinal hormones. Its definite place in the group of well-established hormones must await its chemical isolation and identification.

The presence of a glucagon-like substance within the wall of the small intestine is fairly well established. Its release is stimulated during intestinal absorption of for example glucose, and intestinal extracts have been shown to possess glucagon-like actions. The gut glucagon cross-reacts immunologically with pancreatic glucagon. Further investigation is needed to establish its status as a hormone, as well as its physiological function.

Three other chemically well-defined polypeptides have been isolated from the small intestine, namely, gastric inhibitory polypeptide (*GIP*), motilin, and vasoactive intestinal polypeptide (*VIP*). GIP is a 43 amino acid residue polypeptide with a calculated molecular weight of 5105 (19). It has a strong chemical homology with secretin and glucagon. It was originally isolated from impure preparations of cholecystokinin-pancreozymin, and it inhibits gastric secretion and motility. The spectrum of biological actions of GIP has been said to be identical with that produced by the instillation of fat and fatty acids in the intestine. Therefore, it has been claimed that GIP is identical with the "old" enterogastrone. Whether this is true is open to question. The main difficulty in accepting GIP as a possible gastrointestinal hormone is that the physiological stimulus for its release is at present unknown. However, since GIP has been chemically identified, this important difficulty may be resolved if its presence in blood and possible variations in its plasma levels can be demonstrated by radioimmunoassay.

Motilin is a polypeptide isolated from the mucosa of the small intestine of hog (20). It contains 22 amino acid residues and has a calculated molecular weight of 2700. The peptide has been isolated as a by-product in the purification of secretin but it has no chemical similarities with any of the identified gastrointestinal polypeptides. Motilin stimulates gastric motor activity in both fundic and antral gastric pouches. In a previous study (17) it was demonstrated that alkalinization of the duodenum in dogs caused stimulation of motor activity in transplanted fundic pouches. The possibility was raised that this humoral stimulation of motility was due to release of motilin by duodenal alkalinization. It is debatable whether such alkalinization of the duodenum—instillation of buffer of pH 9.0—occurs under physiological conditions. In addition, there is no evidence that the agent released by such alkalinization is identical with motilin. It is known that other gastrointestinal polypeptides (e.g. gastrin) also influence gastric motor activity.

The VIP isolated from porcine upper intestinal wall by Said & Mutt (93) is composed by 28 amino acid residues. By relaxation of smooth muscle in peripheral and splanchnic blood vessels, VIP produces an increase in both splanchnic and peripheral blood flow. In this respect the polypeptide resembles secretin and CCK-PZ since both can produce splanchnic vasodilation. Structurally VIP resembles both secretin and glucagon and it has recently been shown that VIP has secretin-like effects on the cat pancreas (93). On a molar basis, its activity is 5–10% of that of secretin. VIP has also been shown to have glucagon-like activity. The status of VIP as a gastrointestinal hormone is today unclear, and its physiological role during normal digestion has still to be elucidated.

Thus, it is in many respects too early to classify many of the agents shown in Table 1 as gastrointestinal hormones, despite the fact that they evidently occur in the intestinal wall and in many cases there is rather good

TABLE 1. GASTROINTESTINAL HORMONES

A gastrointestinal hormone should fulfill all A or all B criteria.
A. Physiological criteria:
  i. Is released from a specific site of origin by physiological stimuli.
  ii. Has specific actions on specific structures or organs, other than its site of origin.
  iii. Its effect persists after eliminating all nervous connections between site of origin and site of action (or, effect can be shown in vitro)
B. Biochemical criteria:
  i. Chemically identified in extracts from the stimulated tissue or organ.
  ii. Chemically or immunologically identified in blood (or lymph).
  iii. Administration of physiological amounts of exogenous agent produces actions similar to those of the endogenous one (criterion closely related to A: i and ii).

Substances and references	A. Physiological criteria			B. Biochemical criteria		
	i	ii	iii	i	ii	iii
"Old" hormones						
Cholecystokinin-pancreozymin (44, 50, 76, 78, 105)	+	+	+	+	(+)	(+)[a]
Enterocrinin (47, 79)	(+)	−	(+)	−	−	(+)[a]
Enterogastrone (30, 31, 63)	+	+	+	−	−	(+)[a,b]
Gastrin (25, 38, 40, 42, 55, 102)	+	+	+	+	+	+
Secretin (13, 77, 105)	+	+	+	+	(+)	+[a]
Urogastrone (37, 41)	−	+?	−	−	−	−
"New" hormones						
Bulbogastrone (2, 103)	+	+	+	−	−	(+)
Entero-glucagon (46, 68)	+	+	−	−	(+)	(+)[a,b]
Gastric inhibitory polypeptide (GIP) (18, 19)	−	+	−	+	−	−
Motilin (17, 20)	(+)	+	+	+	−	−
Vasoactive intestinal polypeptide (VIP) (93)	−	+	−	+	−	−

[a] Physiological plasma levels not known.
[b] Crude extracts have shown a certain degree of specificity.

+ Has been demonstrated
(+) Evidence doubtful
− Has not been demonstrated
? Criterion partly fulfilled

evidence that the agent has a physiological role. For most of these substances a major criterion has not yet been fulfilled, namely the demonstration of a physiological stimulus for their release. Since the aim of this review is to discuss mechanisms related to the release of gastrointestinal hormones, only established hormones with defined physiological stimuli for release can be considered. The hormones will be described in the order in which they appear as one proceeds down the gastrointestinal canal.

Species differences, especially in the biological actions of the various hormones, have been found. In some instances, possible species differences have also been demonstrated for the release mechanisms of the hormones. Furthermore, species variations are both quantitative and qualitative. The scope of this review does not permit a detailed description of such differences, but some major points will be considered.

CONTROL OF GASTRIN SECRETION

The hormone gastrin is a straight-chain polypeptide composed of 17 amino acid residues. It occurs in two forms, gastrin I and gastrin II (40). Recently an immunoreactive gastrin of larger size was demonstrated in radioimmunological studies on gastrin in plasma (109). The physiological significance of the presence of different sized gastrins in tissues and blood is not clear.

The major source of gastrin in all the species so far studied is the mucosa of the pyloric gland area (antrum) of the stomach. Small amounts of immunoreactive gastrin have been demonstrated in the duodenum of various species. Interestingly enough, the human has the highest concentration of all species studied, and the whole duodenum contains totally almost as much gastrin as the human antrum (82).

The location of gastrin within the mucosa was first determined by bioassay in the early sixties (26). The full paper first appeared in 1968 (16) about the time that the first reports on the location of gastrin by immunofluorescence technique appeared (69). Irrespective of the technique used, gastrin has been found mainly in the deeper portion of the pyloric glands. Today the gastrin cell can be identified with certainty by histochemical and electron microscopical methods (21, 96), as well as by immunological techniques (21, 70). The cells are specialized endocrine cells—G-cells—and contain gastrin stored in granules.

The physiological release of gastrin from the pyloric antrum mucosa is controlled by two main stimulatory mechanisms. The intake of food gives rise to cephalic stimulation which causes release of gastrin by means of vagal reflexes. Gastrin is also released by chemical and mechanical stimulation of the antrum mucosa by food and its digestion products. Gastrin release is subject to an autoregulatory control: high acidity within the antrum inhibits the mechanisms of gastrin release. The stimulatory mechanisms involved in gastrin release could not be studied quantitatively until this pH-dependency had been recognized (83).

The first evidence that the release of gastrin was under vagal control was presented by Uvnäs in 1942 (102). Since then the importance of vagal release of gastrin in the regulation of the secretion of hydrochloric acid in the stomach has been established by various means. For example, exclusion of the antrum from contact with acid gastric contents resulted in a several-fold increase in gastric acid output in response to cephalic stimulation by insulin hypoglycemia and sham feeding (1, 84). These observations suggest that following the removal of the inhibitory influence of acid on the gastrin release mechanism, the vagal release of gastrin is considerably increased. From a physiological point of view, it should be emphasized that the vagal phase of gastrin release in connection with meals operates when the pH of the antral content is close to neutrality, due to the buffering action of food. On the other hand, removal of the antrum more or less completely eliminated the gastric acid response to vagal stimulation by sham feeding in dogs (85). The crucial physiological evidence for vagal release of gastrin came when it was shown that sham feeding induced acid responses from vagally-denervated gastric pouches (87). The success of those particular experiments depended on the use of dogs with vagally-innervated antral pouches wherein vagal release of gastrin could occur without any inhibitory interference by acid.

The results obtained by these purely physiological means have been confirmed using radioimmunoassay methods. Jaffe, McGuigan & Newton (51) studied the effect of insulin hypoglycemia on gastric secretion and portal vein gastrin levels in dogs with gastrostomies and portal vein cannulae. They found that insulin hypoglycemia was accompanied by an increased rate of gastric secretion and a significant rise in gastrin levels in portal blood. In dogs with a gastric fistula and a vagally-innervated fundic pouch, sham feeding caused increases in serum gastrin concentration, accompanied by acid responses from the fundic pouch (81). With the gastric fistula closed, and thereby allowing full acidification of the antral mucosa, the rise in serum gastrin level was of relatively short duration. In experiments with the gastric fistula open, sham feeding caused a prolonged rise in serum gastrin levels. These findings verify two important concepts concerning gastrin release, namely that vagal stimulation by physiological means releases gastrin and that acidification of the antrum due to the secretory activity in the stomach during stimulation is an important inhibitor of vagal release of gastrin.

Transmission of vagal impulses to the gastrin cells had long been thought to involve cholinergic mechanisms. The studies concerning this question are few and there is indeed very sparse direct evidence for this concept. The only support for a cholinergic mechanism of release of gastrin is the well-known fact that bathing the antral mucosa with acetylcholine causes acid secretory responses from fundic pouches.

The availability of radioimmunoassay techniques for measuring gastrin in plasma has greatly facilitated studies on the release mechanisms. Walsh, Yalow & Berson (104) studied the plasma levels following an ordinary meal in eight human subjects with and without atropinization. In contrast to what was expected, they found that the rise in plasma levels after eating was greater during atropinization than without atropine in the majority of subjects. The interpretation of these results is difficult, since the conditions under which these experiments were performed were rather complex. A test meal gives rise to gastric secretory stimulation by cephalic, intragastric, and intestinal mechanisms. According to the authors the most probable explanation is that after atropinization the oxyntic glands secrete less acid, so that the normal acid feedback on gastrin release is eliminated. This would then lead to higher gastrin release rates. However, in several of their atropinized subjects the increase in plasma gastrin, compared with that of the non-atropinized subjects, was greater almost immediately after the meal. Due to the buffering action of the food, the gastric pH would at that time be similar, regardless of atropinization. However, although the reduced acid response to a meal after atropinization may partly explain their results, other factors must be considered. The human duodenum contains as much immunoreactive gastrin as the human antrum, release mechanisms for duodenal gastrin are unknown, and, finally, radioimmunoassay is not yet able to distinguish between plasma gastrin derived from antral and duodenal sources. Such factors could influence the results of such studies. Another possible explanation for the atropine resistant gastrin release will be discussed below.

Two recent studies have taken up the question of cholinergic and noncholinergic release of gastrin. Nilsson et al (81) studied gastric acid secretion and plasma gastrin concentrations following feeding and sham feeding in dogs with Pavlov pouches and gastric fistulae. Gastric acid and plasma gastrin responses were determined with or without prior atropinization. It was found that atropinization virtually abolished the plasma gastrin response to sham feeding, whereas no major change was observed in plasma gastrin responses to feeding after atropinization. Atropine completely suppressed acid gastric responses to both sham feeding and feeding. In a similar experimental study in dogs with Pavlov pouches and innervated antral pouches, Csendes, Walsh & Grossman (23) studied the influence of atropine on plasma gastrin responses to insulin hypoglycemia. In essence, their results were similar— atropine eliminated insulin-stimulated plasma gastrin responses, as well as gastric acid responses. However, they had to use a higher dose of atropine in two of the four dogs in order to eliminate the plasma response. They also studied the effect of atropine on gastrin responses to feeding in two other dogs with Pavlov pouches. Again, the results agreed with previous findings that atropine had no significant effect on the rise in plasma gastrin following feeding, whereas the acid response from the Pavlov pouch was completely eliminated.

Thus, it is evident from these studies that gastrin release in response to cephalic stimulation involves a cholinergic release mechanism and that gastrin release in connection with meals includes also a noncholinergic release mechanism. In dogs, interference of duodenal gastrin is unlikely, since, compared to man, this species has insignificant amounts of immunoreactive gastrin in the duodenum (82). In view of these findings, what kind of a atropine-resistant gastrin releasing mechanism could be envisaged?

The intake of food releases gastrin by the chemical and mechanical stimulation of the antrum mucosa (38, 42). In studies in which the extractable amounts of gastrin in the antrum mucosa in cats were assayed biologically, Fyrö (35) found a significant reduction in the content of gastrin after feeding. More recently, Forssman & Orci (33) using electron microscopy studied intracellular changes in the gastrin-producing cells in the antral mucous membrane of the cat. In fasting cats the gastrin cells contained electron dense secretory granules, whereas after feeding these cells were degranulated, showing clear secretory granules. This finding indicates an intracellular storage site for gastrin and cyclic variation in the granules during the digestion process.

It is still not known which food products constitute the physiological stimuli for gastrin release. It has long been believed that the natural stimuli for gastrin release are proteins or large molecular-weight polypeptides. Experimental studies on gastrin release from isolated antral pouches by chemical means have shown that the most active gastrin releasing agents are small molecules such as amino acids, lower aliphatic alcohols, and choline. By comparing the stimulatory efficacy of a number of amino acids, Elwin (26) has found a clear structure-activity relationship among the various acids. For example, glycine and β-alanine are potent gastrin releasers, whereas α-alanine is almost ineffective. The same is true for the alcohols—n-propanol is a potent gastrin releaser but isopropanol is not (27). Thus, the gastrin releasing potency of these agents seems to be associated with a relatively simple molecular structure, which supports the concept of a common receptor mechanism for gastrin release by chemical stimulants. The recent observation by Elwin (29) that among various fractions of a protein hydrolysate only the small molecular fractions are effective gastrin releasers also supports the concept of a receptor for small molecular agents in food.

The stimulatory action of chemical agents is thought to be transmitted from mucosal surface receptors to the gastrin cells through a local cholinergic reflex mechanism. The experimental evidence for this hypothesis is the finding that topical application of local anesthetics abolishes the stimulatory action of chemical stimulation of the antrum mucosa. Also, the inhibition of gastrin release in response to chemical stimuli produced by local atropinization supports the concept of such a cholinergic reflex mechanism (94). The studies upon which this hypothesis is based are in fact few and are not as extensive as those we demand today for proving the existence of a physiological mechanism by pharmacological means. In addition, no nerve endings or other neural structures have ever been observed close to the lumen or any possible specialized chemoreceptor. Recent ultrastructural studies have shown that the gastrin cells are in direct contact with the lumen of the pyloric glands and that the cells extend into the glandular lumen a "bouquet" of microvilli (95). In their paper, Solcia, Vassallo & Sampietro (95) suggested that "the microvilli apparatus extending into the glandular lumen seems in keeping with the hypothesis that some luminal content, perhaps acting as a chemical stimulus for hormone secretion, may be absorbed by the cell." This very attractive hypothesis may explain the recent findings (23, 81, 104) that the gastrin releasing action of food in the stomach is atropine resistant. The hypothesis is supported by the observation (8) that one potent stimulus for gastrin release, namely choline, is in fact readily absorbed through the antral mucosa, and the better the absorption the higher is the acid response from an indicator fundic pouch. However, choline has other actions in addition to releasing gastrin (28). Therefore, interpretation of these results is difficult and other experimental designs are needed to prove the existence of a noncholinergic mechanism for release of gastrin.

A potent feedback mechanism for all modes of gastrin release is related to the degree of acidity within the antrum. The final proof that high acidity within the antrum inhibits release of gastrin is the observation that acidification of the antrum greatly reduced the plasma levels of gastrin (23, 81). Physiologically, the antral pH varies between 1 and 7, and the effectiveness with which gastrin is released is therefore greatly dependent on the actual acidity of the antral content. The optimal pH for gastrin release is pH 5–7. Below pH 5 the release mechanism is gradually inhibited, the degree of inhibition depending on the stimulant. In comparing the efficacy of various gastrin-releasing agents applied to the antral mucosa at various pH levels, it was found that the stimulatory effect of ethanol was not blocked until the antral pH had been depressed to below pH 2 (7). The same was true for vagal release of gastrin in response to sham feeding (3). On the other hand, gastrin release induced by glycine and choline was more sensitive to acidity (7): in both instances inhibition began when the pH was reduced to pH 5 and became progressively greater as the pH was reduced further. Above pH 1–2 the inhibitory effect of acid could be overcome by increasing the concentration of the stimulant applied to the antrum mucosa.

The mechanism by which acid interferes with gastrin release is unknown. Evidence against a reflex mechanism can be found in the observation that local anesthesia of the antral mucosa does not abolish the inhibitory effect of acid on gastrin release in response to bathing the antrum mucosa with acetylcholine (90). In addition, the same objection can be raised to the hypothesis of luminal reflex inhibition as was raised to the hypothesis of luminal reflex stimulation of gastrin release, namely, the absence of any nervous elements in or close to the mucosal surface. The observations cited above (3, 7, 28) suggest a dual mechanism of action of acid. For agents like glycine, it was proposed that low pH might produce changes of a physico-chemical nature such that the compounds lose their gastrin releasing properties, i.e. that their ability to reach or react with a specific receptor mechanism is decreased. It is reasonable to assume that another mechanism of acid inhibition is operating when release of gastrin is induced by ethanol and vagal stimulation. Possibly high antral acidity might strengthen the intracellular binding of gastrin (54).

Other possible modulators of gastrin release have been postulated recently. Intravenous administration of secretin has been found to lower the plasma gastrin levels both in humans and in dogs (43, 101). The mechanism behind the plasma gastrin lowering effect of secretin is unknown. Apart from interference with antral gastrin release, it was speculated that secretin might affect the metabolism or the excretion of gastrin. Whether this effect of secretin constitutes a physiological inhibition of gastrin release is uncertain. An argument against secretin being a physiological regulator of gastrin release is that in both cited studies relatively high doses of secretin had to be used

(92). Further analysis of the mechanism of action of secretin upon plasma gastrin levels is needed before a physiological role of secretin in the regulation of gastrin release can be accepted.

Intravenous infusion of calcium increases plasma gastrin (91) and this increase is particularly great in patients with very high plasma levels of gastrin, for example in the Zollinger-Ellison syndrome (98). It is well known that calcium ions are of considerable importance for the processes involved in the release of many biological agents. However, the above-mentioned observations on the influence of calcium on plasma gastrin do not allow any conclusion about the possible interrelationship between physiological variations of serum calcium and the release of gastrin.

RELEASE OF BULBOGASTRONE

During digestion, when gastric chyme starts to enter the duodenum, various mechanisms having inhibitory effects upon gastric functions are brought into action. This view is based on old observations that constituents of gastric content, such as hydrochloric acid and fats, inhibit gastric secretion and motility when introduced into the duodenum. There has been much controversy as to whether the mechanism of acid inhibition is humoral or nervous in nature, and even the physiological role of duodenal acid inhibition has been questioned. Today, the existence of a pH-sensitive duodenal mechanism inhibiting gastric acid secretion by humoral pathways is well established (103).

The observation (2) that acidification of isolated pouches of the duodenal bulb could produce the same degree of inhibition as that produced by acidification of the whole duodenum indicated that the pH-sensitive mechanism is mainly located in the duodenal bulb. This concept is further supported by the fact that acidification of a considerably longer segment of the distal duodenum had no inhibitory effect (5). Furthermore, the demonstration of a pH-gradient in the duodenum in both humans (4) and dogs (15), with a more acid pH in the duodenal bulb than in the postbulbar duodenum, strongly indicates a physiologically important mechanism in controlling the secretion of hydrochloric acid in the stomach.

The inhibitory agent released by acid from the mucosa of the duodenal bulb has been called bulbogastrone. Its release is pH-dependent and stimulated by an acid pH within the duodenal bulb. In contrast to the situation during the release of secretin, no correlation has been found between the release of bulbogastrone and the absorption of hydrogen ions (6). The stimulus is specific insofar as the mechanism cannot be activated by bathing the bulbar mucosa with digested fat (9). The pH-threshold for release of bulbogastrone is well within the limits of the physiological pH-variations in this part of the duodenum. Postprandial and interprandial pH in the duodenal bulb can go down to pH 1–2 both in man and in dog (4, 15). With a physiological stimulus, such as sham feeding, inhibition of gastric acid secretion can be detected at a bulbar pH of around 4 (80). A lower pH is required to inhibit the maximal response of the stomach to, for example, pentagastrin (6). Since the mucosa of the duodenal bulb can be expected to contain secretin and since acid is also a stimulus for secretin release, it was of great importance to learn whether bulbogastrone is identical with secretin. This question was answered by experiments in which the effect of bulbar acidification was studied in dogs provided with gastric and pancreatic fistulae (103); acid perfusion of the bulb produced pronounced gastric secretory inhibition without any detectable change in the volume and bicarbonate concentration of pancreatic secretion. In addition, bulbar acidification did not cause any change in the output and concentration of pancreatic amylase. Therefore, the humoral agent released from the duodenal bulb following acidification is neither secretin nor CCK-PZ. Recent investigations from two other laboratories (59, 106) support the concept of a specific inhibitory hormone in the duodenal bulb mucosa. It has also been possible to prepare extracts from the duodenal bulb mucosa which are active in the microgram range in inhibiting gastric acid secretion in response to gastrin (103). No details of the extraction procedure or the chemical nature of bulbogastrone have yet been published.

CONTROL OF SECRETIN RELEASE

The complete amino acid sequence of porcine secretin was determined by Mutt, Jorpes & Magnusson in 1970 (77). Secretin contains 27 amino acid residues and shows a high degree of sequence homology with porcine glucagon.

The distribution of secretin along the gastrointestinal tract is well established (34). The highest concentration is found in the duodenum. In the dog the concentration decreases with the distance from the pyloric sphincter, and in the distal ileum there is hardly any detectable secretin activity. In recent studies, Konturek and co-workers (57, 58) have confirmed older work (107) on the distribution of secretin by instilling acid at various levels in the small intestine and measuring the volume and bicarbonate response from pancreatic fistulae. In both dogs (58) and cats (57) acid infusion into the duodenum produced the greatest pancreatic response. Acidification of the jejunum gave smaller responses and no responses were obtained upon acidification of the ileum.

The first attempts to demonstrate the location of the secretin-producing cells in the intestinal mucosa were made by Krawitt, Zimmerman & Clifton (64). They sectioned the duodenal mucosa of dogs horizontally so that the villous layer was separated from the crypts of Lieberkühn. Preparation of crude secretin extracts from the tissues showed that secretin activity was almost exclusively restricted to the villous layer. It was concluded that the source of secretin was either the cells located in the stroma of the villi or those in the villous epithelium. Two groups of workers (88, 97) have shown that it is the latter type of cell which contains the hormone. By the use of an immunofluorescence technique with secretin antibodies, numerous cells with green fluorescence were found scattered in the epithelium lining both the crypts and the villi of the pig duodenum and the upper jejunum. In the dog, these cells were mainly located in the so-called transitional zone of the duodenal mucosa. When the ultrastructural appearance of the fluorescent cells is compared with the various nonenterochromaffin endocrine cell types studied previously, the fluorescent cells are most likely to be identified as the so-called S-cells. Furthermore, distribution of the S-cells along the intestinal tract compares favorably with the previous findings on secretin distribution. The S-cells are numerous in the duodenum and in the upper jejunum. S-cells could not be detected in the terminal ileum or in the stomach. Previous assertions that the pyloric antrum mucosa contains secretin can now be explained by the fact that gastrin possesses secretin-like activity.

When the stomach begins to empty an ingested meal into the duodenum the pancreas starts to secrete. Pancreatic stimulation in response to the passage of food through the duodenum is believed to be due mainly to the release of secretin and CCK-PZ. However, we do not yet know definitely what kind of digestive products are the most important stimuli for the release of secretin and hence, as with gastrin, there are uncertainties regarding the physiological stimuli for release. By tradition, acid is regarded as the most potent stimulus for secretin release. This concept is based on the assumption that the gastric content passing into the duodenum during gastric emptying is sufficiently acid to be an adequate stimulus for the release of secretin. In addition, Wang & Grossman (105) found that, in comparison with other secretin releasing agents, hydrochloric acid was the most efficient agent for stimulating the flow of pancreatic juice from a transplanted pancreas. Fatty acids and amino acids produced only half of the response of that to hydrochloric acid. To assess the importance of hydrochloric acid for secretin release during normal digestion it is necessary to know the pH-threshold for secretin release and also the intraduodenal pH-levels occurring physiologically. The pH-threshold for secretin release has been shown to be 4.5 (74). The pH of the duodenal content during digestion not only fluctuates with time but also varies with the distance from the pylorus. As mentioned previously, under normal conditions, the duodenal bulb has a much more acid pH than the rest of the duodenum. On the other hand, the release of secretin from the limited duodenal bulb area is probably of minor importance quantitatively for the overall control of pancreatic secretion. Acidification of the duodenal bulb did not cause any detectable pancreatic response (103). Therefore, the most important site for secretin release is the rest of the duodenum and possibly also the upper jejunum. Measurements of the acidity in the postbulbar duodenum of dogs in connection with a meal have shown pH as low as 3 which suffices to induce secretin release (15, 100).

For several reasons it is difficult to assess the role of duodenal acidity in physiological secretin release. Measurements of the normal pancreatic response to a meal are hampered by the fact that the removal of alkaline pancreatic juice from the duodenum may disturb physiological events. Annis & Hallenbeck (10) demonstrated that the removal of pancreatic juice during digestion altered the pattern of the pancreatic response. They found that if collected pancreatic juice was returned to the duodenum, the total pancreatic secretion was much less than when the juice was not returned. From this study it is evident that the release of secretin in response to acid is subject to an autoregulatory inhibitory influence by the secretion of alkaline juices from the pancreas, which is in close analogy to the acid inhibition of gastrin release from the antrum mucosa. Another reason why it is so difficult to determine the relative importance of acidity for normal secretin release is related to the significance of peptides, amino acids, and fatty acids for secretin release. As pointed out by Wang & Grossman (105), such agents, when introduced into the duodenum, increase the volume of pancreatic secretion and the amount of bicarbonate in it. The problem became even more complicated when it was shown by Henriksen & Worning (48) that exogenously administered secretin and CCK-PZ had a potentiating effect on the pancreatic secretion of bicarbonate. Subsequently it was shown that endogenously released CCK-PZ could also potentiate the pancreatic bicarbonate response to exogenous secretin (73). Since both amino acids and fatty acids are known to release CCK-PZ, it seemed difficult to decide whether these agents are true secretin releasers or stimulate pancreatic bicarbonate secretion by their release of CCK-PZ. However, the problem was solved when it was shown by Meyer, Spingola & Grossman (73) that duodenal infusion of L-phenylalanine —a potent CCK-PZ releaser—did not augment bicarbonate secretion in response to a high background stimulation with exogenous CCK-PZ, whereas a dose of secretin that was subthreshold when given alone caused a marked increase. From these studies it was concluded (74) that L-phenylalanine does not release secretin and that all its effects on both protein and bicarbonate secretion can be fully accounted for by release of CCK. The authors assumed that this applies to all amino acids but noted that this assumption remained to be tested. Whether the same statement applies to fatty acids is still not known. In conclusion, these authors (74) stated that hydrogen ions are the only potent releasers of scretin. The final proof for this concept must await radioimmunological determinations of secretin in plasma following the introduction into the duodenum of the various agents discussed above.

Since we can accept acid as a major stimulant for secretin release, what closer relations exist between the intraduodenal pH and the degree of secretin release? This question has recently been carefully investigated by Meyer, Way & Grossman (71, 72). They found that there was a close correlation between pH and rate of secretin release within the range from the threshold pH 4.5 down to pH 3. At and below pH 3 the secretin release was maximal. However, below pH 3 the release mechanism seemed to be sensitive to variations in the total amount of acid introduced into the duodenum, i.e. altering the volume inflow rate and holding the acid concentration constant resulted in different bicarbonate responses of the pancreas. In addition, they showed that there was a direct linear relation between the acid load and the length of intestine acidified, so that the larger the amount of acid introduced into the duodenum the longer was the segment of the gut that was acidified. Furthermore, a direct correlation was found between the length of gut acidified and the amount of secretin released, and the secretin releasing capacity per unit length of intestine did not decrease in the first 90 cm from the pyloric sphincter. They therefore concluded that the acid load introduced into the duodenum is important not only as a determinant of the length of gut acidified, but also as a determinant of the amount of secretin released by a segment already acidified in the optimal pH range, namely below pH 3. It is easy to reconcile the pH-dependent secretin release with the physiological pH conditions in the duodenum during digestion. For the same reason, it is difficult to accept the control of secretin release below pH 3 by the acid load as a mechanism operating under physiological conditions, unless this mechanism can also be expected to function within the pH-range between pH 3 and 4.5.

An important question, which is closely related to the physiological regulation of secretin release, is how much secretin can be released maximally during normal digestion. The question is of considerable importance for investigations in which the spectrum of biological actions of secretin is studied since, for example, the plasma levels obtained by doses of exogenous secretin necessary for maximal stimulation of pancreatic secretion will perhaps never occur physiologically. Direct methods for measuring the release rates of secretin are not yet available, but reasonably valid calculations have been made. Thus, Rune & Worning (92) calculated the maximal amount of secretin released from the normal human duodenum to be about 0.5 clinical units per kg and hour. A similar figure was suggested by Lagerlöf (65).

There is no conclusive evidence on the intimate mechanism of secretin release by acid—whether acid releases secretin by direct action on the secretin cells or through a mechanism involving neuronal elements. Harper (45) has recently analyzed in great detail previous studies on the possible participation of local reflexes in secretin release. The role of the vagi in the release of secretin is uncertain. There is no conclusive evidence for vagal release of secretin (89). However, recent studies suggest that vagal innervation might facilitate the release of secretin by acid (49, 61).

So far, no specific mechanisms inhibiting secretin release have been found apart from the above-mentioned autoregulatory inhibition by the pancreatic juice itself.

REGULATION OF SECRETION OF CCK-PZ

The hormone that we today call cholecystokinin-pancreozymin can be said to have been discovered twice. The gall-bladder contracting activity in intestinal extracts was demonstrated by Ivy & Oldberg (50) in 1928 and, logically, they named the active principle cholecystokinin. Harper & Raper (44) showed in 1943 that, besides secretin, there exists in extracts of the small intestinal mucosa a second substance having an action on the exocrine pancreas. Since it mainly stimulated the pancreatic secretion of enzymes, it was called pancreozymin. Not until the final stages of the purification of intestinal extracts containing cholecystokinin- and pancreozymin-like activities had been reached in the middle of the sixties, did it become evident that one single polypeptide possessed the actions of both cholecystokinin and pancreozymin. In a recent communication (78) Mutt & Jorpes reported the complete amino acid sequence of CCK-PZ. It is a polypeptide composed of 33 amino acid residues. The C-terminal pentapeptide sequence of CCK-PZ is identical with that of the gastrins.

The distribution of CCK-PZ has been less extensively studied than that of secretin. It is believed that the distribution of CCK-PZ corresponds closely to that of secretin. Recently, Konturek, Tasler & Obtulowicz (60) measured the pancreatic protein output following perfusion of isolated intestinal segments with a solution containing L-leucine and L-tryptophan. They found that the maximal protein output from the pancreas was obtained during perfusion of a duodeno-jejunal loop; perfusion of a distal jejunal loop caused only slight increase in enzyme output and there was no response during irrigation of a distal ileal loop.

The cells containing CCK-PZ have not yet been identified. However, the solution of this problem is almost certainly only a matter of time, and Solcia et al (97) have in fact recently proposed that CCK-PZ originates in the so-called I-cells.

According to Wang & Grossman (105), the most potent stimulus for CCK-PZ release is peptone: amino acids and fatty acids were less effective. Hydrochloric acid produced about 50% of the response obtained with peptone. However, the relative importance of various food constituents for the release of CCK-PZ is still not known. In view of the above-mentioned observations one should expect to find the physiological releasers of CCK-PZ among peptides, amino acids and fatty acids. Taking pancreatic enzyme secretion as a measure of CCK-PZ release, the ability of several individual amino acids to release CCK-PZ has been studied recently in man (36) and in dog (74). In the dog, only neutral amino acids were effective and among the various amino acids phenylalanine and tryptophan were the most active. In the case of phenylalanine, only the L-isomer was active (74). A similar structure-activity relationship seems to exist among the fatty acids, so that only fatty acids with carbon chains longer than eight carbons are effective CCK-PZ releasers (74). The studies in man (36) have shown that only essential amino acids are effective in stimulating pancreatic enzyme secretion. When the essential amino acids were examined individually, stimulation of enzyme output was found only with phenylalanine, methionine, and valine. The responses to these amino acids individually were less than those obtained with a mixture of essential amino acids. All the effective amino acids are believed to be transported by the same system and it is conceivable that the absorption process is closely related to the mechanism of release of CCK-PZ. In any case, these investigations suggest that there is a specific receptor mechanism for essential amino acids which have certain physico-chemical characteristics in common.

Barbezat & Grossman (12) have shown unequivocally that hydrochloric acid can stimulate release of CCK-PZ. The pancreas was stimulated by a supramaximal dose of secretin and when a plateau of secretion had been attained hydrochloric acid was infused into the duodenum, resulting in a definite rise in protein output by the pancreas. However, the physiological role of hydrochloric acid in the release of CCK-PZ cannot be settled by these experiments because quite large amounts of the acid were introduced into the duodenum.

Another approach to the study of the release of CCK-PZ has been made by Berry & Flower (14). They used isolated strips of rabbit gall-bladder to assay CCK-PZ in blood. Various test agents were perfused through the duodenum of anesthetized dogs and cats and blood samples were collected from the portal vein and assayed on the isolated gall-bladder strip. In contrast to the results of others, hydrochloric acid was found to be the most potent stimulus for CCK-PZ release in this assay system. Release of CCK-PZ could also be demonstrated following duodenal perfusion with fatty acids and peptone. Because of rather large individual variations, no quantitative comparisons between the various stimuli could be made. The results of this study are in many respects surprising and differ from those of others. It is therefore necessary to carry out further studies and analyze the release of CCK-PZ in this particular assay system in order to explain the discrepancies.

It seems unlikely that vagal stimulation releases CCK-PZ (61, 75). However, as with secretin, vagal innervation is assumed to facilitate release of CCK-PZ in response to chemical agents. Other physiological stimuli for CCK-PZ release have to be considered. Two recent studies have given strong support for the view that bile may be a physiological releaser of CCK-PZ. Forell (32) and Wormsley (108) have both shown a clearcut stimulation of pancreatic enzyme output upon introduction of bile salts into the human duodenum. However, the exact mechanism whereby bile salts stimulate the pancreas has not yet been defined.

In anesthetized dogs with pancreatic cannulae and stimulated with a constant background of secretin, distention of the jejunum caused increased protein output from the pancreas (22). If the experiments were repeated with an extracorporeal circulation for the jejunum and ileum, no stimulation of enzyme output was observed. It was concluded that the results provided evidence for the release of a blood-borne agent by jejunal distention and, since it stimulated particularly the enzyme secretion from the pancreas, it was assumed that the agent was identical with CCK-PZ. Further investigations are needed to assess the role of intestinal mechanical stimuli in physiological CCK-PZ release.

RELEASE OF ENTEROGASTRONE

No other gastrointestinal hormone has for so long defied identification as enterogastrone. The name enterogastrone was created in 1930 (63) for a humoral principle that was released from the small intestine by neutral fat and its digestion products. Since several recent comprehensive reviews (39, 53) of the story of enterogastrone are available, the present review will only summarize the present status of the hormone and discuss in more detail only the most recent work.

Introduction of fat or fatty acids into the duodenum inhibits both gastric motility and secretion. The inhibitory action of fat in the intestine has been demonstrated in fully denervated gastric pouches. It has been shown that fat must be present in an absorbable form to produce inhibition. Recent studies (56, 66) have demonstrated that the degree of inhibition in connection with the presence of fat in the intestine is closely associated with the rate of absorption of fat. Konturek & Grossman (56) demonstrated inhibition from all levels of the small intestine but inhibition was most effective from the jeunum where the rate of fat absorption was also fastest.

The inhibitory pattern produced by fat in the small intestine has been discussed. One of the major questions has been whether or not the inhibitory action of enterogastrone shows any selectivity against various types of gastric secretion. In older studies on the hormone, histamine-stimulated secretion was more or less resistant against the inhibition produced by fat. Later, several investigators claimed that histamine-induced gastric secretion could also be inhibited by the presence of fat in the intestine. It is difficult to analyze the various experimental conditions under which these divergent results have been obtained and to try to explain the discrepancies. It is therefore still an open question whether or not any selectivity is associated with the inhibitory action of enterogastrone. One recent study (24) gives strong support for the concept that fat in the intestine exclusively inhibits secretory responses to both endogenous and exogenous gastrin but not responses to histamine.

The most recent discussion has centered on the question as to whether enterogastrone is identical with any of the identified gastrointestinal hormones. The most probable candidate has been CCK-PZ, which is also released by fatty acids. This is still debated but there are in fact more arguments against such an assumption than for it (52).

Great efforts have been made to isolate enterogastrone but the purification of the active principle has evidently involved major difficulties, and the results obtained so far have been disappointingly inconclusive. In a recent paper, Lucien, Itoh & Schally (67) reported that purification of an active inhibitor of gastric secretion extracted from pig intestinal mucosa. The inhibitor, which they called enterogastrone, did not possess any secretin- or CCK-PZ-like activities and, upon intravenous infusion in doses of 0.5–2.0 mg, it produced inhibition of histamine-stimulated secretion. A more potent inhibitor of gastric acid secretion is the GIP of Brown (19). In a recent study, Pederson & Brown (86) have shown that GIP in a dose as low as 0.25 microgram per kg and hour significantly inhibited gastric secretory responses to both pentagastrin and histamine. It is tempting to believe that the GIP is in fact the "old" enterogastrone, but we have to await further investigations in order to establish a definite connection between GIP and enterogastrone.

LITERATURE CITED

1. Andersson, S., Elwin, C. E., Uvnäs, B. 1958. The effect of exclusion of the antrum and duodenum and subsequent resection of the antrum, on the acid secretion in Pavlov pouch dogs. *Gastroenterology* 34:636–57
2. Andersson, S., Uvnäs, B. 1961. Inhibition of postprandial gastric secretion in Pavlov pouches by instillation of hydrochloric acid into the duodenal bulb. *Gastroenterology* 41:486–90
3. Andersson, S., Olbe, L. 1964. Inhibition of gastric acid response to feeding in Pavlov pouch dogs by acidification of antrum. *Acta Physiol. Scand.* 61:1–10
4. Andersson, S., Grossman, M. I. 1965. Profile of pH, pressure and potential difference at gastroduodenal junction in man. *Gastroenterology* 49:364–71
5. Andersson, S., Nilsson, G., Uvnäs, B. 1967. Effect of acid in proximal and distal duodenal pouches on gastric secretory responses to gastrin and histamine. *Acta Physiol. Scand.* 71: 368–78
6. Andersson, S., Nilsson, G. 1969. pH-dependence of the mechanism in the duodenal bulb inhibiting gastric acid responses to exogenous gastrin. *Acta Physiol. Scand.* 76:182–90
7. Andersson, S., Elwin, C. E. 1971. Relationship between antral acidity and gastrin releasing potency of chemical stimulants. *Acta Physiol. Scand.* 83:437–45
8. Andersson, S., Elwin, C. E. 1972. Release of gastrin in relation to antral acidity and absorption of chemical stimulants. *Gastrointestinal Hormones*, ed. L. Demling, 1–6. Stuttgart, Germany: Georg Thieme
9. Andersson, S. Unpublished data.
10. Annis, D., Hallenbeck, G. A. 1951. Effect of excluding pancreatic juice from duodenum on secretory response of pancreas to a meal. *Proc. Soc. Exp. Biol. Med.* 77:383–85
11. Barbezat, G. O., Grossman, M. I. 1971. Intestinal secretion:

Stimulation by peptides. *Science* 174:422–24
12. Barbezat, G. O., Grossman, M. I. 1971. Cholecystokinin released by duodenal acidification. *Gastroenterology* 60:761
13. Bayliss, W. M., Starling, E. H. 1902. The mechanism of pancreatic secretion. *J. Physiol. London* 28:325–53
14. Berry, H., Flower, R. J. 1971. The assay of endogenous cholecystokinin and factors influencing its release in the dog and cat. *Gastroenterology* 60:409–20
15. Brooks, A. M., Grossman, M. I. 1970. Postprandial pH and neutralizing capacity of the proximal duodenum in dogs. *Gastroenterology* 59:85–89
16. Broomé, A., Fyrö, B., Olbe, L. 1968. Localization of gastrin activity in the gastric antrum. *Acta Physiol. Scand.* 74:331–39
17. Brown, J. C., Johnson, L. P., Magee, D. F. 1966. Effect of duodenal alkalinization on gastric motility. *Gastroenterology* 50:333–39
18. Brown, J. C., Pederson, R. A., Jorpes, J. E., Mutt, V. 1969. Preparation of highly active enterogastrone. *Can. J. Physiol. Pharmacol.* 47:113–14
19. Brown, J. C., Dryburgh, J. R. 1971. A gastric inhibitory polypeptide. II. The complete amino acid sequence. *Can. J. Biochem.* 49:867–72
20. Brown, J. C., Cook, M. A., Dryburgh, J. R. 1972. Motilin, a gastric motor activity-stimulating polypeptide: final purification, amino acid composition, and C-terminal residues. *Gastroenterology* 62:401–4
21. Bussolati, G., Canese, M. G. 1972. Electron microscopic identification of the immunofluorescent gastrin cells in the cat pyloric mucosa. *Histochemie* 20:198–206
22. Chung, R. S. K., Fromm, D., Trencis, L., Silen, W. 1970. Gastric and pancreatic responses to jejunal distension. *Gastroenterology* 59:387–95

23. Csendes, A., Walsh, J. H., Grossman, M. I. 1972. Effects of atropine and of antral acidification on gastrin release and acid secretion in response to insulin and feeding in dogs. *Gastroenterology* 63:257–63

24. Debas, H. T., Bedi, B. S., Gillespie, G., Gillespie, I. E. 1969. Mechanism by which fat in the upper small intestine inhibits gastric acid. *Gastroenterology* 56:483–87

25. Edkins, J. S. 1905. On the chemical mechanism of gastric secretion. *Proc. Roy. Soc. B.* 76:376

26. Elwin, C. E., Uvnäs, B. 1966. Distribution and local release of gastrin. *Gastrin*, ed. M. I. Grossman p. 69–82. Los Angeles: Univ. Calif. Press

27. Elwin, C. E. 1969. Stimulation of gastric acid secretion by irrigation of the antrum with some aliphatic alcohols. *Acta Physiol. Scand.* 75:1–11

28. Elwin, C. E., Andersson, S. 1972. Relation between stimulatory effect on gastric acid secretion and antral absorption of chemical compounds. *Scand. J. Gastroenterol.* 7:247–55

29. Elwin, C. E. Release mechanism of gastrin. *Nobel Symposium XVI, Frontiers in Gastrointestinal Hormone Research*, ed. S. Andersson. Uppsala, Sweden: Almquist & Wiksell. In press

30. Farrell, J. I., Ivy, A. C. 1926. Studies on the motility of the transplanted gastric pouch. *Am. J. Physiol.* 76:227–28

31. Feng, T. P., Hou, H. C., Lim, R. K. S. 1929. On the mechanism of the inhibition of gastric secretion by fat. *Chin. J. Physiol.* 3:371–78

32. Forell, M. M. Bile salts as stimulants of pancreatic secretion. *Nobel Symposium XVI, Frontiers in Gastrointestinal Hormone Research*, ed. S. Andersson. Uppsala, Sweden: Almquist & Wiksell. In press

33. Forssman, W. G., Orci, L. 1969. Ultrastructure and secretory cycle of the gastrin-producing cell. *Z. Zellforsch. Mikrosk. Anat.* 101:419–32

34. Friedman, M. H. F., Thomas, J. E.

1950. The assay and distribution of secretin. *J. Lab. Clin. Med.* 35:366–72

35. Fyrö, B. 1968. Effect of feeding on antral and duodenal gastrin activity. *Acta Physiol. Scand.* 74:166–72

36. Go, V. L. W., Hofman, A. F., Summerskill, W. H. J. 1970. Pancreozymin bioassay in man based on pancreatic enzyme secretion: Potency of specific amino acids and other digestive products. *J. Clin. Invest.* 49:1558–64

37. Gray, J. S., Culmer, C. U., Wieczorowski, E., Adkison, J. L. 1940. Preparation of pyrogen-free urogastrone. *Proc. Soc. Exp. Biol. Med.* 43:225–28

38. Gregory, R. A., Ivy, A. C. 1941. The humoral stimulation of gastric secretion. *Quart. J. Exp. Physiol.* 31:111–28

39. Gregory, R. A. 1962. *Secretory Mechanisms of the Gastro-intestinal Tract*, 117–28. London: Edward Arnold

40. Gregory, R. A., Tracy, H. J. 1964. The constitution and properties of two gastrins extracted from hog antral mucosa. *Gut* 5:103–17

41. Gregory, H. 1970. Some polypeptides influencing gastric acid secretion. *Am. J. Dig. Dis.* 15:141–48

42. Grossman, M. I., Robertson, C. R., Ivy, A. C. 1948. The proof of a hormonal mechanism for gastric secretion—the humoral transmission of the distension stimulus. *Am. J. Physiol.* 153:1–9

43. Hansky, J., Soveny, C., Korman, M. G. 1971. Effect of secretion on serum gastrin as measured by immunoassay. *Gastroenterology* 61:62–68

44. Harper, A. A., Raper, H. S. 1943. Pancreozymin, a stimulant of the secretion of pancreatic enzymes in extracts of the small intestine. *J. Physiol. London* 102:115–25

45. Harper, A. A. 1967. Hormonal control of pancreatic secretion. *Handbook of Physiology. Section 6: Alimentary Canal. Vol. II: Secretion*, ed. C. F. Code,

969-95. Washington, DC: Am. Physiol. Soc.

46. Heding, L. G. 1971. Radioimmunological determination of pancreatic and gut glucagon in plasma. *Diabetologia* 7:10-19

47. Heggeness, F. W., Nasset, E. S. 1951. Purification of enterocrinin. *Am. J. Physiol.* 167:159-65

48. Henriksen, F. W., Worning, H. 1967. The interaction of secretin and pancreozymin on the external pancreatic secretion in dogs. *Acta Physiol. Scand.* 70:241-49

49. Henriksen, F. W., Rune, S. J. 1969. Cholinergic effect on the canine pancreatic response to acidification of the duodenum. *Scand. J. Gastroenterol.* 4:203-8

50. Ivy, A. C., Oldberg, E. A. 1928. A hormone mechanism for gallbladder contraction and evacuation. *Am. J. Physiol.* 86:599-613

51. Jaffe, B. M., McGuigan, J. E., Newton, W. T. 1970. Immunochemical measurement of the vagal release of gastrin. *Surgery* 68:196-201

52. Johnson, L. R., Grossman, M. I. 1969. Effect of fat, secretin and cholecystokinin on histamine-stimulated gastric secretion. *Am. J. Physiol.* 216:1176-79

53. Johnson, L. R., Grossman, M. I. 1971. Intestinal hormones as inhibitors of gastric secretion. *Gastroenterology* 60:120-44

54. Jorpes, J. E. The ionic mechanisms for accumulation and release of peptide hormones. *Nobel Symposium XVI, Frontiers in Gastrointestinal Hormone Research,* ed. S. Andersson. Uppsala, Sweden: Almquist & Wiksell. In press

55. Komarov, S. A. 1942. Studies on gastrin. I. Methods of isolation of a specific gastric secretagogue from the pyloric mucous membrane and its chemical properties. *Rev. Can. Biol.* 1:191-205

56. Konturek, S., Grossman, M. I. 1965. Effect of perfusion of intestinal loops with acid, fat or dextrose on gastric secretion. *Gastroenterology* 49:481-89

57. Konturek, S. J., Dubiel, J., Gabrys, B. 1969. Effect of acid infusion into various levels of the intestine on gastric and pancreatic secretion in the cat. *Gut* 10:749-53

58. Konturek, S. J., Tasler, J., Obtulowicz, W. 1971. Localization of secretin release by acid in small intestine of the dog. *Am. J. Physiol.* 220:124-27

59. Konturek, S. J., Tasler, J., Obtulowicz, W. 1971. Duodenal mechanisms for inhibition of gastric acid secretion in the dog. *Am. J. Physiol.* 220:918-21

60. Konturek, S. J., Tasler, J., Obtulowicz, W. 1972. Localization of cholecystokinin release in intestine of the dog. *Am. J. Physiol.* 222:16-20

61. Konturek, S. J., Radecki, T., Biernat, J., Thor, P. 1972. Effect of vagotomy on pancreatic secretion evoked by endogenous and exogenous cholecystokinin and caerulein. *Gastroenterology* 63:273-78

63. Kosaka, T., Lim, R. K. S. 1930. Demonstration of the humoral agent in fat inhibition of gastric secretion. *Proc. Soc. Exp. Biol. Med.* 27:890-91

64. Krawitt, E. L., Zimmerman, G. R., Clifton, J. A. 1966. Location of secretin in hog duodenal mucosa. *Am. J. Physiol.* 211:935-38

65. Lagerlöf, H. Estimation of endogenous release of secretin and cholecystokinin. *Nobel Symposium XVI, Frontiers in Gastrointestinal Hormone Research,* ed. S. Andersson. Uppsala, Sweden: Almquist & Wiksell. In press

66. Long, J. F., Brooks, F. P. 1965. Relation between inhibition of gastric secretion and absorption of fatty acids. *Am. J. Physiol.* 209:447-51

67. Lucien, H. W., Itoh, Z., Schally, A. V. 1970. Inhibitory effects of a purified entero-gastrone, secretin and cholecystokinin on histamine stimulated gastric acid secretion. *Gastroenterology* 59:707-11

68. Makman, M. H., Sutherland, E. W. 1964. Use of liver adenyl cyclase for assay of glucagon in

human gastrointestinal tract and pancreas. *Endocrinology* 75: 127–34

69. McGuigan, J. E. 1968 Gastric mucosal intracellular localization of gastrin by immunofluorescence. *Gastroenterology* 33: 315–27

70. McGuigan, J. E., Greider, M. H., Grawe, L. 1972. Staining characteristics of the gastrin cell. *Gastroenterology* 62:959–69

71. Meyer, J. H., Way, L. W., Grossman, M. I. 1970. Pancreatic bicarbonate response to various acids in the duodenum. *Am. J. Physiol.* 219:964–70

72. Meyer, J. H., Way, L. W., Grossman, M. I. 1970. Pancreatic response to acidification of various lengths of proximal intestine in the dog. *Am. J. Physiol.* 219:971–77

73. Meyer, J. H., Spingola, L. J., Grossman, M. I. 1971. Potentiation of pancreatic response to exogenous secretin by endogenous cholecystokinin in dog. *Am. J. Physiol.* 221:742–47

74. Meyer, J. H., Grossman, M. I. 1972. Release of secretin and cholecystokinin. *Gastrointestinal Hormones*, ed. L. Demling, 43–55. Stuttgart, Germany: Georg Thieme

75. Moreland, H. J., Johnson, L. R. 1971. Effect of vagotomy on pancreatic secretion stimulated by endogenous and exogeneous secretin. *Gastrtroenterology* 60: 425–31

76. Mutt, V., Jorpes, J. E. 1968. Structure of porcine cholecystokinin-pancreozymin. I. Cleavage with thrombin and with trypsin. *Eur. J. Biochem.* 6:156–62

77. Mutt, V., Jorpes, J. E., Magnusson, S. 1970. Structure of porcine secretin. The amino acid sequence. *Eur. J. Biochem.* 15: 513–19

78. Mutt, V., Jorpes, J. E. 1971. Hormonal polypeptides of the upper intestine. *Biochem. J.* 125:57–58 P

79. Nasset, E. S., Pierce, H. B., Murlin, J. R. 1935. Proof of a humoral control of intestinal secretion. *Am. J. Physiol.* 111: 145–58

80. Nilsson, G. 1969. Effect of acid in

the duodenal bulb on gastric secretory responses to sham feeding. *Acta Physiol. Scand.* 77: 308–15

81. Nilsson, G., Simon, J., Yalow, R. S., Berson, S. A. 1972. Plasma gastrin and gastric acid responses to sham feeding and feeding in dogs. *Gastroenterology* 63:51–59

82. Nilsson, G., Yalow, R. S., Berson, S. A. Distribution of gastrin in the gastrointestinal tract of human, dog, cat and hog. *Nobel Symposium XVI, Frontiers in Gastrointestinal Hormone Research*, ed. S. Andersson. Uppsala, Sweden: Almquist & Wiksell. In press

83. Oberhelman, H. A., Jr., Woodward, E. R., Zubiran, J. M., Dragstedt, L. R. 1952. Physiology of the gastric antrum. *Am. J. Physiol.* 169:738–48

84. Olbe, L. 1963. Significance of vagal release of gastrin during the nervous phase of gastric secretion. *Gastroenterology* 44: 463–68

85. Olbe, L. 1964. Effect of resection of gastrin releasing regions on acid response to sham feeding and insulin hypoglycemia in Pavlov pouch dogs. *Acta Physiol. Scand.* 62:169–75

86. Pederson, R. A., Brown, J. C. 1972. Inhibition of histamine-, pentagastrin-, and insulin-stimulated canine gastric secretion by pure "gastric inhibitory polypeptide." *Gastroenterology* 62:393–400

87. Pe Thein, M., Schofield, B. 1959. Release of gastrin from the pyloric antrum following vagal stimulation by sham feeding in dogs. *J. Physiol. London* 148: 291–305

88. Polak, J. M., Bloom, S., Coulling, J., Pearse, A. G. E. 1971. Immunofluorescent localization of secretin in the canine duodenum. *Gut* 12:605–10

89. Preshaw, R. M. 1967. Integration of nervous and hormonal mechanisms for external pancreatic secretion. *Handbook of Physiology. Section 6: Alimentary Canal. Vol. II: Secretion*, ed. C. F. Code, 997–1005. Wash-

ington, DC: Am. Physiol. Soc.
90. Redford, M., Schofield, B. 1965. The effect of local anesthesia of the pyloric antral mucosa on acid inhibition of gastrin-mediated acid secretion. *J. Physiol. London* 180:304–20
91. Reeder, D. D. et al 1970. Influence of hypercalcemia on gastric secretion and serum gastrin concentrations in man. *Ann. Surg.* 172:540–46
92. Rune, S. J., Worning, H. 1970. The pancreatic response to instillation of acid into the duodenum and to exogenous secretin in man. *Scand. J. Gastroenterol.* 6:291–296
93. Said, S. I., Mutt, V. 1972. Isolation from porcine-intestinal wall of a vasoactive octacosapeptide related to secretin and to glucagon. *Eur. J. Biochem.* 28:199–204
94. Schofield, B., Redford, M., Grabham, A. H., Nuaimi, K. 1965. Neural factors in the control of gastrin release. *Gastric Secretion: Mechanisms and Control*, ed. T. K. Shnitka, J. A. L. Gilbert, R. C. Harrison, 91–104. New York: Pergamon
95. Solcia, E., Vassallo, G., Sampietro, R. 1967. Endocrine cells in the antro-pyloric mucosa of the stomach. *Z. Zellforsch. Mikrosk. Anat.* 81:474–86
96. Solcia, E., Vassallo, G., Capella, C. 1969. Studies on the G-cells of the pyloric mucosa, the probable site of gastrin secretion. *Gut* 10:379–88
97. Solcia, E., Capella, C., Vezzadini, P., Barbara, L., Bussolati, G. 1972. Immunohistochemical and ultrastructural detection of the secretin cell in the pig intestinal mucosa. *Experientia* 28:549–50
98. Trudeau, W. L., McGuigan, J. E. 1969. Effects of calcium on serum gastrin levels in Zollinger-Ellison syndrome. *N. Engl. J. Med.* 281:862–66
100. Thomas, J. E. 1940. The maximal

acidity of the intestinal contents during digestion. *Am. J. Dig. Dis.* 7:195–97
101. Thompson, J. C., Bunchman, H. M., II, Reeder, D. D. 1972. Inhibition of gastrin release by secretin in man and in dogs. *Gastrointestinal Hormones.* ed. L. Demling, 86–90. Stuttgart, Germany: Georg Thieme
102. Uvnäs, B. 1942. The part played by the pyloric region in the cephalic phase of gastric secretion. *Acta Physiol. Scand.* 4: Suppl. 13
103. Uvnäs, B., Nilsson, G., Andersson, S., Sjödin, L. Mechanism of duodenal inhibition of gastric acid secretion. *Nobel Symposium XVI, Frontiers in Gastrointestinal Hormone Research*, ed. S. Andersson. Uppsala, Sweden: Almquist & Wiksell. In press
104. Walsh, J. H., Yalow, R. S., Berson, S. A. 1971. The effect of atropine on plasma gastrin response to feeding. *Gastroenterology* 60:16–21
105. Wang, C. C., Grossman, M. I. 1951. Physiological determination of release of secretin and pancreozymin from intestine of dogs with transplanted pancreas. *Am. J. Physiol.* 164:527–45
106. Way, L. W., Grossman, M. I. 1970. Gastric and pancreatic response to acid in the duodenum after partial duodenectomy. *Am. J. Physiol.* 219:449–54
107. Weaver, M. M. 1927. Distribution of pancreatic secretin in the gastrointestinal tract. *Am. J. Physiol.* 82:106–12
108. Wormsley, K. G. 1970. Stimulation of pancreatic secretion by intraduodenal infusion of bile salts. *Lancet* 2:586–88
109. Yalow, R. S., Berson, S. A. 1970. Size and charge distinctions between endogenous human plasma gastrin in peripheral blood and heptadecapeptide gastrins. *Gastroenterology* 58:609–15

SOME RELATED ARTICLES APPEARING
IN OTHER *ANNUAL REVIEWS*

From the *Annual Review of Biochemistry*, Volume 42 (1973)
   Surface Membranes of Animal Cells, *M. M. Burger, A. R. Oseroff, P. Robbins*
From the *Annual Review of Biophysics and Bioengineering*, Volume 2 (1973)
   Frequency Dynamics of Peripheral Vascular Blood Flow, *E. O. Attinger*
   Biophysics of Flagellar Motility, *J. J. Blum, J. Lubliner*
   Interpretation of Some Microelectrode Measurements of Electrical Properties of Cells, *A. Peskoff, R. S. Eisenberg*
   Electric and Magnetic Field of the Heart, *D. Geselowitz*
   Optimization of the Mammalian Respiratory Gas Transport System, *F. S. Grodins, S. M. Yamashiro*
From the *Annual Review of Entomology*, Volume 18 (1973)
   The Fine Structure of Membranes and Intercellular Communication in Insects, *P. Satir, N. B. Gilula*
   Neuro-Hormonal Control of Sexual Behavior, *R. H. Barth, L. J. Lester*
From the *Annual Review of Medicine*, Volume 24 (1973)
   Insulin Receptors, *B. Desbuquois, P. Cuatrecasus*
   Secretion and Action of Thyrotropin-Releasing Factor, *J. F. Wilber*
   Glucagon and Homeostasis of Metabolic Fuels, *R. H. Unger*
   Extraction of Insulin by the Liver, *J. B. Field*
   Nature and Biological Activities of Degradation Products of Fibrinogen and Fibrin, *H. C. Kwaan, G. H. Barlow*
   Renal Metabolism in Relation to Renal Function, *R. H. Kessler, N. W. Levin, A. P. Quintanilla*
From the *Annual Review of Pharmacology*, Volume 13 (1973)
   Sympathetic Mechanisms in Blood Vessels: Nerve and Muscle Relationships, *J. A. Bevan, C. Su*
   Serotonin and Central Nervous System Function, *T. N. Chase, D. L. Murphy*
Micropharmacology of Vertebrate Neuromuscular Transmission, *J. I. Hubbard, D. Quastel*
From the *Annual Review of Psychology*, Volume 24 (1973)
   Visual Sensitivity, *J. L. Brown*
   The Sense of Smell, *T. Engen*
   Physiological Psychology: Sleep, *H. L. Williams, F. A. Holloway, W. J. Griffiths*

REPRINTS

The conspicuous number aligned in the margin with the title of each review in this volume is a key for use in the ordering of reprints.

Available reprints are priced at the uniform rate of $1 each postpaid. Payment must accompany orders less than $10. The following discounts will be given for large orders: $5–9, 10%; $10–$24, 20%; $25 and over, 30%. Current discounts on reprint orders will expire June 30, 1973, after which a single discount of 20% will be given on orders of $20 or more. All remittances are to be made payable to Annual Reviews, Inc. in US dollars. California orders are subject to sales tax. One-day service is given on items in stock.

For orders of 100 or more, any *Annual Reviews* article will be specially printed and shipped within 6 weeks. Reprints that are out of stock may also be purchased from the Institute for Scientific Information, 325 Chestnut Street, Philadelphia, Pa. 19106. Direct inquiries to the Annual Reviews Inc. reprint department.

The sale of reprints of articles published in the *Reviews* has been expanded in the belief that reprints as individual copies, as sets covering stated topics, and in quantity for classroom use will have a special appeal to students and teachers.

AUTHOR INDEX

SUBJECT INDEX

A

Acetylcholine
brain synthesis of, 279
coronary vessels and, 154
kidney circulation and,
156
spreading vasodilation from,
132
stomach secretion and, 436,
439
subcellular localization of,
279, 280
sweating control and, 212,
213
transmitter role of, 277-80,
288, 289
Acidosis
bronchial effects of, 183
Acromegaly
lung volume and function in,
172
ACTH
adrenal effects of, 380
assay of, 380
secretion of
atropine and, 379
cold defense and, 396
control of, 379-81
corticosteroids and, 381
hypothalamus and, 380
stress and, 380
vasopressin and, 379

Adenohypophysis
cells of
FSH and LH in, 362
extracts of
chondrocyte mitosis and,
363
prolactin secretion by, 365-
75
secretion by
hypothalamic control of,
357-81
somatotropin secretion by,
358-65
thyrotropins in
TSH secretion and, 376
see also Gonadotropins,
pituitary
Adenosine
coronary blood flow and,
152
kidney circulation and, 155
splenic blood flow and,
160
Adenosine monophosphate,
cyclic
brain synthesis of, 292
effects of
cardiac calcium uptake
and, 71
catecholamines and, 70,
71
neurotransmitter action and,
292

thermoregulatory role of,
416, 417
Adenylcyclase
brain actions of, 292
kidney function and, 44
Adipose tissue
circulation in
control of, 160
lipolysis in
control of, 416
Adipose tissue, brown
cold acclimation and
hormonal role in, 410
temperature regulation and,
393, 394, 396, 402
Adrenal cortex
ACTH action on, 380
temperature regulation and,
417, 418
Adrenal cortical hormones
ACTH secretion and, 381
cold acclimation and, 393
glucocorticoids
cold defense and, 401,
417
preoptic area cooling and,
406, 407
secretion of
social behavior and, 232
Adrenergic mechanisms
adrenergic neuron destruction
6-hydroxydopamine and,
283

Adrenergic neurons
catecholamine synthesis in, 285
Adrenergic receptors
adipose tissue lipolysis and, 416
beta
cold sensitization of, 403
nonshivering thermogenesis and, 409
blocking of
temperature regulation and, 408-10
Afferent mechanisms, 243-65
cellular level studies, 243, 244
dorsal column role in, 261
cortical function and, 261, 262
functional relations of, 243-65
sensations and, 243
telencephalic mechanisms for, 261-64
see also Olfaction, Vision, etc
Aggressive behavior
see Behavior, aggressive
Aldosterone
secretion of
heat stress and, 194-96
sodium reabsorption and
collecting duct role in, 42
mechanism of, 46
Amines, aromatic
brain synthesis of, 282, 283
degradation of, 290
half-time turnovers of, 284
release from synaptosomes, 288
transmitter roles of, 282-84
Amino acids
brain regional distribution of, 281
brain transport of, 281, 282, 289
CCK-PZ secretion and, 445
gastrin release and, 438, 439
kidney transport of, 26-32
sugar inhibition of, 18, 19
neurotransmitter role of, 275, 276, 278
L-phenylalanine
pancreatic secretion and, 443, 445
synthesis of, 284, 285
tissue uptake of

synaptosomes and, 275
transmitter role of, 280-82, 289
AMP, cyclic
see Adenosine monophosphate, cyclic
Amygdala
aggressive behavior and, 335-39, 346
5-HT content of
diurnal rhythm of, 381
interactions with hypothalamus, 338, 339
lesions of
social behavior and, 223, 234
neural connections of, 335, 338, 339
Angiotensin
pulmonary circulation and, 158
Antidiuretic hormone (ADH)
kidney actions of
see Kidney, ADH effects on
secretion of
hypothalamic thermoreceptors and, 396
urea excretion and, 42
Aortic valve
closure of
vortices and, 96
stenosis of
jet flow into arteries from, 96
Arfonad
temperature regulation and, 408
Arterial pulse
transmission into venules, 129, 130
Arteries
atherosclerosis in
factors favoring, 99, 100
plaque distortion of flow from, 100
blood flow in
measurement of, 93-95
text on, 87
branching tubes in
dynamics of, 95
cholesterol transfer in
wall shear and, 100
elasticity of, 96-101
factors changing, 99
large deformations and, 97
reviews on, 96
variation among arteries in, 98
vascular smooth muscles and, 98, 99
viscoelastic properties and, 97, 98
Young's modules of, 97-99

hemodynamics of, 92-104
reviews on, 87
impedance of, 103, 104
cardiac work minimization and, 103
cardiovascular abnormalities and, 103
particular vascular beds and, 104
reflection and, 103
jet flow into, 96
nonlaminar flow in, 95, 96
pathological changes in walls of, 99, 100
poststenotic dilatation of, 99
pressure-flow relations in, 92-96
oscillatory, 95, 96
pressure in
measurement of, 92
pressure injury of, 99
Reynold's numbers in, 96
"tethering" of, 99
velocity profiles in, 95
vibration effects on, 99
wave transmission in, 101-3
reflection and, 102, 103
wave equation, 101-3
wave velocity in, 102, 103
yield stress of, 99
Artery, pulmonary
elastic properties of, 100
ATPase
activity of
calcium and, 69
kidney function and, 44-47
sodium and, 45, 46
Atrium, left
pressure in
airway resistance and, 185
Atropine
ACTH secretion and, 379
bronchial elasticity and, 174-76
Attention
amygdaloid stimulation and, 336
Audition
neural mechanisms for, 252-54
cellular unit activity and, 253
olivocochlear bundle and, 254
sound localization and, 253
see also Cochlea
Autonomic nervous system

C

Caffeine
calcium movements and,
72, 73
cyclic AMP degradation and,
73
heart effects of, 71-73
Calcium
heart contraction and, 60-
70
calcium fluxes and, 70,
71
mitochondrial role in, 68
quantitative relations between, 76
species differences in, 64,
66
kidney sugar transport and,
20
mitochondrial uptake of,
68
movements of, 72, 73
caffeine and, 72, 73
control of, 74-80
digitalis and, 73
myocardial compartments
and, 65
myocardial localization of,
55-65
myocardial release of
excitation and, 61-63, 65,
66
myocardial transport of, 58-
64
membrane potential and,
60
secretion release and,
44
skeletal muscle function
and, 66, 67
thermoregulation and
proptic area and, 422
two compounds of
myocardial contraction and,
62-64
Capacitance vessels
see Venous circulation
Capillaries
blow flow in
techniques for, 118
capillary bed design, 118-21
dimesions of, 119
module of, 118, 119
neurogenic control of, 120,
121
preferential channels in,
119, 120
shunting in, 121
sphincters in, 120
compliance of, 130
exchange across, 132-36
mathematical models of,
139, 140
pathways for, 133, 134
pinocytosis and, 134
single vessels and, 132,

133
fluid movement across
capillary filtration coefficients, 133
Starling concept of, 132,
133, 138
hydrodynamic coefficient of,
132
oxygen tensions around,
135
permeability of
basement membrane and,
123, 124
blood flow rate and, 134,
135
fenestrae and, 123, 128
polysaccharide endothelial
layer, 122, 123
protein concentration and,
133
regional differences in,
132, 133
reviews on, 117
symposium on, 140
techniques for, 118
pressures in
pressure waves in, 129,
130
regulation of, 128, 129
techniques for, 128
surface properties of, 123
theoretical models of, 138-
40
see also Microcirculation
Carbon dioxide
brain circulation and,
157
bronchial effects of, 183,
184
laryngeal resistance and,
185
pulmonary circulation and,
158
Cardiac output
exercise in heat and, 198,
199
methods for, 106, 107
temperature regulation and,
204, 205
Carotid sinus
elastic properties of, 100,
101
microanatomy of, 101
Catapressin
central actions of, 423
Catecholamines
brain synthesis of, 292,
284
cold acclimation and, 399,
400
cold defense role of, 393,
396, 398
cyclic AMP and, 70
heart effects of
excitation-contraction
bondings, 70, 71
relaxation and, 71

high-affinity transport of,
283
metabolic derivatives of,
398
"post-denervation supersensitivity", 291
prolactin secretion and,
369, 370
secretion of
cold exposure and, 403-11,
415, 417
temperature regulation and,
393, 396, 399-403
subcellular localization of,
282-84
synthesis vs release of,
400
urinary excretion of, 398-
401
Cerebellum
Purkinje cells of
neurotransmitters of, 290-
92
Cholecystokinin-pancreozymin
chemistry of, 445
digestive role of, 444
hormonal nature of, 434,
444
location of, 445
pancreatic secretion and,
443
secretion of
acid and, 446
bile and, 446
food constituents and,
445
jejunal distention and,
446
regulation of, 444-46
vagus nerve and, 446
Choline acetyltransferase
acetylcholine-synthesis by,
279, 280
Chlorisondamine
ganglionic blockade by
temperature regulation
and, 407
**Circulation, pulmonary, 158-
60**
angiotensin effects on,
159
capacitance vessels of, 158
capillary volume in, 159
carbon dioxide effects on,
158, 183
fetal
autoregulation in, 158
segmental resistance in,
159
hyperosmolar effects on,
158
hypoxia effects on, 158, 159
impedance of, 124
right ventricular work and,
104
indicator dilution methods
for, 105

CUMULATIVE INDEXES

VOLUMES 31-35

INDEX OF CONTRIBUTING AUTHORS

INDEX OF CHAPTER TITLES

VOLUMES 31-35